Complications of Laparoscopic and Robotic Urologic Surgery

Reza Ghavamian

Complications of Laparoscopic and Robotic Urologic Surgery

Springer

Editor
Reza Ghavamian
Albert Einstein College
of Medicine
Montefiore Medical Center
Department of Urology
Bainbridge Avenue 3400
10461 Bronx, New York
USA
rghavami@montefiore.org

ISBN 978-1-4899-8124-0 ISBN 978-1-60761-676-4 (eBook)
DOI 10.1007/978-1-60761-676-4
Springer New York Dordrecht Heidelberg London

Softcover re-print of the Hardcover 1st edition 2010

Printed on acid-free paper

Springer is part of Springer Science+Business Media (www.springer.com)

This book is dedicated to

All my mentors who taught me medicine and surgery
To my patients from whom I have learned abundantly
To my loving wife Ann and my dearest daughter Roya who give me ever-present support, joy, and raison d'etre

Preface

There has been an explosion in minimally invasive surgery (MIS) in urology. As surgical subspecialists, urologists were slow to embrace minimally invasive surgery at its inception. However, in the last decade, the interest in MIS has grown exponentially in urology. Laparoscopic renal procedures are commonplace, and more and more complex oncologic and reconstructive procedures are performed laparoscopically. Much of this exponential growth has been due to the rapid dissemination of robotic technology, specifically for prostatectomy. Soon afterward, robotic technology was applied to other complex lower tract oncologic and reconstructive procedures. Robotic assistance has also been applied to upper tract urologic procedures such as pyeloplasty but its application for partial nephrectomy is more recent. It has become apparent that robotic technology can serve as an interface between open and laparoscopic surgery for the laparoscopically naïve surgeon. It has certainly been shown to be so for prostatectomy, and whether the same pans out for partial nephrectomy is yet to be seen.

As more experience is gained in MIS, more and more complex procedures are performed laparoscopically and robotically. Contrary to logical expectation, the incidence of complications has indeed increased with increasing experience in MIS. This is purely a reflection of the complexity of the procedures performed rather than surgical ineptitude. Increased surgical experience and surgeon volume with a certain procedure can decrease perioperative morbidity. As in open surgery, complications will be ever present in the laparoscopic management of our patients and cannot be eradicated in all instances. They can, however, be avoided and measures can be taken to decrease their incidence. Much of this knowledge is gained purely from surgical experience. Certain clinical scenarios and comorbidities predispose the patient to complications. Specific to surgical technique, certain maneuvers increase the likelihood of intra-operative and perioperative complications and increase the likelihood of adverse outcomes. On the contrary, certain precautions and maneuvers can serve to prevent complications.

This textbook is intended to familiarize the modern urologist with the common and the more eccentric complications of laparoscopic and robotic urologic surgery. Recognized urologic experts in MIS have contributed to making this the first comprehensive textbook specifically dedicated to complications in minimally invasive urologic surgery. The book is divided into three specific parts. In the first part, medical and general considerations are discussed. In the second part, generalized discussion of common surgical complications is presented. Complications specific to robotic surgery in general are emphasized in a separate unique chapter. The third part is dedicated to procedure-specific complications. Complications of upper tract and lower tract laparoscopic and robotic procedures are discussed in different subsections. In most chapters, a brief description of the procedure is provided as well as an in-depth discussion of the diagnosis and management of complications associated with that particular procedure. In each chapter, a discussion of preventive measures is emphasized. The last segment in this section deals with special topics such as single port surgery, ablative procedures, and pediatric laparoscopy. Finally, a comprehensive chapter on medico-legal implications of laparoscopic and robotic technology is presented.

Certain complications are common in a variety of procedures and thus are emphasized and repeated in more than one chapter. Although an attempt is made to decrease repetition, the organization of this book is designed to lend itself to being a user-friendly and quick reference textbook. It also at times presents unique perspectives of different experts within the field who address the same issues in different fashions. The organization of each chapter is left to the discretion of the authors and ample illustrations and images are presented when appropriate. As more urologists embrace laparoscopy and robotics and more fellows and residents are trained in this subspecialty, the use of this technology is sure to increasingly expand in our field. Prior knowledge of potential complications is a valuable adjunct in their diagnosis and management. It is my hope that this textbook serves as a useful reference for management of complications in urologic MIS. I also believe that it can serve to educate surgeons in certain new procedures before they actually embark on performing them. I wish to thank all authors who have contributed to this textbook. It is my sincere hope that the reader finds this textbook user-friendly and that it can serve as a valuable resource for urologists who wish to incorporate MIS in their surgical armamentarium.

New York, NY — Reza Ghavamian

Contents

Contributors

Bobby S. Alexander, MD New York Medical College, Westchester Medical Center, Valhalla, NY, USA

Mohamed A. Atalla, MD Smith Institute for Urology, Hofstra University School of Medicine, North Shore – LIJ Health System, New Hyde Park, NY, USA, atalla@att.net

Akshay Bhandari, MD Chief Resident, Vattikutti Urology Institute, Henry Ford Health System, Detroit, MI, USA, abhanda1@hfhs.org

Jay T. Bishoff, MD, FACS Director, Intermountain Urological Institute, Intermountain Health Care, Associate Clinical Professor of Surgery and Urology, University of Utah College of Medicine, Salt Lake City, UT, USA

Ugur Boylu, MD Endourology Fellow, Department of Urology, Center for Minimally Invasive & Robotic Surgery, Tulane University School of Medicine, New Orleans, LA, USA

Christopher Bryan-Brown, MD Professor and Interim Chairman, Department of Anesthesiology, Montefiore Medical Center/Albert Einstein college of Medicine, Bronx, NY, USA

Jeffrey A. Cadeddu, MD Professor of Urology and Radiology, University of Texas Southwestern Medical Center, Dallas, TX, USA, jeffrey.cadeddu@utsouthwestern.edu

Sean T. Corbett, MD Assistant Professor, Division of Pediatric Urology, University of Virginia, Charlottesville, VA, USA, stc2u@virginia.edu

Philip J. Dorsey Jr, MD, MPH Research Associate, James Buchanan Brady Foundation Department of Urology, Lefrak Institute of Robotic Surgery, Weill Medical College of Cornell University, New York Presbyterian Hospital, USA

Reza Ghavamian, MD Professor of Urology, Director of Urologic Oncology and Robotics, Montefiore Medical Center, Albert Einstein College of Medicine, Bronx, NY, USA, rghavami@montefiore.org

Ahmed Ghazi, MD Department of Urology, Elisabethinen Hospital Linz, Austria

Raj K. Goel, MD Fellow, Section of Laparoscopic and Robotic Urology, Glickman Urological and Kidney Institute, Cleveland Clinic, Cleveland, OH, USA

Erin C. Grantham, MD New York medical College, Westechester Medical Center, Valhalla, NY, USA

Michael Grasso, III MD Chairman of Urology, Saint Vincent Medical Center, Vice Chairman of Urology, New York Medical College, New York, NY, USA, mgrasso3@earthlink.net

David A. Green, MD Resident in Urology, Westchester Medical Center, Valhalla, NY, USA

Khurshid A. Guru, MD Assistant Professor of Oncology, Attending Surgeon Department of Urologic Oncology, Director of Robotic Surgery, Roswell Park Cancer Institute, Buffalo, NY, USA, khurshid.guru@roswellpark.org

Abraham Ari Hakimi, MD Resident in Urology, Montefiore Medical Center/Albert Einstein College of Medicine, Bronx, NY, USA

David M. Hoenig, MD Associate Professor of Urology, Director of Endourology, Montefiore Medical Center/Albert Einstein College of Medicine, Bronx, NY, USA, dhoenig@montefiore.org

Michael H. Hsieh, MD, PhD Assistant Professor, Department of Urology, University Tenure Line, Stanford University School of Medicine, Stanford, CA, USA

Elias Hyams, MD Resident in Urology, New York University Langone Medical Center, New York, NY, USA

Gunter Janetschek, MD Department of Urology, Elisabethinen Hospital Linz, Austria, guenter.janetschek@elizabethinen.or.at

Jihad H. Kaouk, MD Director, Section of Laparoscopic and Robotic Urology, Glickman Urological and Kidney Institute, Cleveland Clinic, Cleveland, OH, USA, kaoukj@ccf.org

Louis R. Kavoussi, MD Smith Institute for Urology, Hofstra University School of Medicine, North Shore – LIJ Health System, New Hyde Park, NY, USA

Kathleen C. Kobashi, MD Head, Section of Urology and Renal Transplantation, Virginia Mason, Medical Center, Associate Clinical Professor, University of Washington, Seattle, WA, USA, urokck@vmmc.org

Jaime Landman, MD Associate Professor of Urology, Director of Minimally Invasive Urology, Columbia University Medical Center, New York, NY, USA, landman.jaime@gmail.com

Philip Lebowitz, MD Professor of Anesthesiology, Montefiore Medical Center/Albert Einstein college of Medicine, Bronx, NY, USA, plebowit@montefiore.org

Alvaro Lucioni, MD Clinical Fellow, Section of Urology and Renal Transplantation, Virginia Mason Medical Center, Seattle, WA, USA, alvaro.lucioni@vmmc.org

Ahmed M. Mansour, MD, MRCS (ENG) Department of Urologic Oncology, Roswell Park Cancer Institute, Buffalo, NY, USA

Pedro Maria, DO Fellow in Endourology and laparoscopy, Montefiore Medical Center/Albert Einstein College of Medicine, Bronx, NY, USA

Maxwell V. Meng, MD, FACS Associate Professor in Residence, Urologic Oncology Fellowship Director, Department of Urology, University of California, San Francisco, CA, USA, mmeng@urology.ucsf.edu

Mani Menon, MD Rajendra and Padma Vattikuti Distinguished Chair in Oncology, Director, Vattikuti Urology Institute, Henry Ford Health System, Detroit, MI, USA; Clinical Professor of Urology, Case School of Medicine, University of Toledo, and New York University, NY, USA, mmenon1@hfhs.org

Ravi Munver, MD Vice Chairman & Associate Professor of Urology, Chief, Minimally Invasive & Robotic Urologic Surgery, Hackensack University Medical Center, Touro University College of Medicine, Hackensack, NJ, USA, rmunver@humed.com

Ricardo A. Natalin, MD Fellow in Minimally Invasive Urology, Columbia University Medical Center, New York, NY, USA

Michael A. Palese, MD Associate Professor of Urology, Director of Minimally Invasive Urology, Mount Sinai Medical Center, New York, NY, USA, michael.palese@mountsinai.org

James O. Peabody, MD, FACS Senior Staff Surgeon, Vattikutti Urology Institute, Detroit, MI, USA

John L. Phillips, MD Associate Professor of Urology, Director of Urologic Oncology and Robotics, New York Medical College, Westechester Medical Center, Valhalla, NY, USA, john_phillips@nymc.edu

S. Scott Putman, MD Associate Clinical Professor of Surgery and Urology, Intermountain Urological Institute, Intermountain Health Care, University of Utah College of Medicine, Salt Lake City, UT, USA, scott.putman@imail.org

Mahesan Richards, MD Assistant Professor, Department of Anesthesiology, Montefiore Medical Center/Albert Einstein college of Medicine, Bronx, NY, USA

Matthew Sand, MD Resident in Urology, New York University Medical Center, New York, NY, USA

Michael Stifelman, MD Associate Professor of Urology, Director of Robotics and Minimally Invasive Urology, New York University Langone Medical Center, New York, NY, USA, michael.stifelman@nyumc.org

Gerald Y. Tan, MB, ChB (Edin) Fellow in Robotic Surgery, James Buchanan Brady Foundation Department of Urology, Lefrak Institute of Robotic Surgery, Weill Medical College of Cornell University, New York, NY, USA, gyt2001@med.cornell.edu

Daniel Tare, MD Resident in Urology, Montefiore Medical Center/Albert Einstein College of Medicine, Bronx, NY, USA

Ashutosh K. Tewari, MD, MCh Director, LeFrak Institute of Robotic Surgery, Director, Prostate Cancer Institute, Ronald P. Lynch Professor of Urologic Oncology, James Brady Foundation Department of Urology, Weill Medical College of Cornell University, New York Presbyterian Hospital, 525 East 68th Street, Starr 900, New York, NY 10065, USA, ashtewarimd@gmail.com

Raju Thomas, MD, FACS, MHA Chairman, Professor of Urology, Department of Urology, Center for Minimally Invasive & Robotic Surgery, Tulane University School of Medicine, New Orleans, LA, USA, rthomas@tulane.edu

Chad R. Tracy, MD Fellow in Minimally Invasive Surgery and Endourology, University of Texas Southwestern Medical Center, Dallas, TX, USA

Jayant Uberoi, MD Fellow in Endourology, Laparoscopy and Robotic Surgery, Hackensack University Medical Center, Hackensack, NJ, USA

Steve W. Waxman, MD Fellow, Minimally Invasive Urologic Surgery, University of Iowa, Iowa City, IA, USA

Alexei Wedmid, MD Department of Urology, Mount Sinai Medical Center, New York, NY, USA

Wesley M. White, MD Fellow, Section of Laparoscopic and Robotic Urology, Glickman Urological and Kidney Institute, Cleveland Clinic, Cleveland, OH, USA

Steve K. Williams, MD Resident in Urology, Montefiore Medical Center/Albert Einstein College of Medicine, Bronx, NY, USA

Howard N. Winfield, MD Urology Associates of West Alabama, 701 University Blvd., E., Tuscaloosa, AL, USA, hnwinfield@mchsi.com

Eboni J. Woodard Smith Institute for Urology, Hofstra University School of Medicine, North Shore – LIJ Health System, New Hyde Park, NY , USA

Reinhold Zimmermann, MD Department of Urology, Elisabethinen Hospital Linz, Austria

Part I
General and Medical Considerations

Physiology of Laparoscopy and Pneumoperitoneum

Steve W. Waxman and Howard N. Winfield

Keywords Laparoscopy · Physiology · Pneumoperitoneum

Introduction

Laparoscopy requires the creation and maintenance of pneumoperitoneum or retroperitoneum in order to visualize the operative field within the abdominal and pelvic cavities. Pneumoperitoneum is a complex and dynamic environment with significant potential alterations on a patient's mechanical, physiologic, and immunologic state [1]. The various effects of pneumoperitoneum have been studied extensively by researchers in many fields. We are continuing to learn new information on the various immunologic responses of the human body to pneumoperitoneum [2]. This chapter will explore the basic physiologic responses to pneumoperitoneum that all urologists performing laparoscopy should appreciate.

Background

Laparoscopy has been in general use in gynecologic and general surgery for over a quarter century. Investigators in these fields as well as anesthesiology have elucidated the mechanical and physiologic effects of pneumoperitoneum on the human body. In the past 15 years due to the rapid increase in laparoscopic surgical procedures, urologic researchers have significantly added to the knowledge of the human responses to pneumoperitoneum. We will limit our discussion of pneumoperitoneum to the abdominal insufflation of carbon dioxide (CO_2) gas, as it is most commonly used.

Pulmonary, Cardiovascular, and Hemodynamic Effects

When CO_2 is insufflated into the peritoneal cavity of a patient at a pressure of 15 mmHg, it can have significant effects owing to both the mechanical pressure on organ systems and its absorption into the blood and tissues [3]. The hemodynamic effects of laparoscopy are primarily due to hypercarbia and increased intra-abdominal pressure [4]. The tissues are highly permeable to CO_2 resulting in a rapid diffusion of CO_2 into the bloodstream. The hypercarbia can usually be compensated for by hyperventilation of the lungs by anesthesia [5]. The increase in intra-abdominal pressure limits diaphragmatic motion [6].

Functional reserve capacity decreases while peak airway pressure increases to maintain tidal volume in the face of increased intra-abdominal pressure [3]. Vital capacity and compliance are both decreased. Most healthy patients tolerate the increase in CO_2 pressure and decrease in pH well as they increase their elimination of CO_2 from the lungs, while endogenous buffering systems within the body accommodate the increased acid load. Patients with decreased pulmonary

H.N. Winfield (✉)
Urology Associates of West Alabama, 701 University Blvd., E., DCH Medical Towers, Suite 908, Tuscaloosa, AL 35401, USA
e-mail: hnwinfield@mchsi.com

R. Ghavamian (ed.), *Complications of Laparoscopic and Robotic Urologic Surgery*,
DOI 10.1007/978-1-60761-676-4_1, © Springer Science+Business Media, LLC 2010

reserves such as those with chronic obstructive pulmonary disease (COPD) and restrictive lung disease will have more difficulty breathing off the excess CO_2 [2].

The effects on hemodynamic function by the increase in intra-abdominal pressure are dependent on the patients' intravascular volume, level of intra-abdominal pressure, and the position [7]. Many studies have shown an increase in systemic vascular resistance (SVR), mean arterial pressure (MAP), and myocardial filling pressures, along with a fall in cardiac index (CI), and little change in heart rate [8]. Although studies show significant changes in respiratory and hemodynamic function after insufflation of the abdomen, these findings rarely have a clinically significant negative impact on most patients [9]. Patients with significant cardiac disease, including low ejection fraction, may not tolerate the cardiovascular and hemodynamic affects associated with the increased abdominal pressure of pneumoperitoneum. A summary of the physiologic changes of pneumoperitoneum is listed in Table 1.

Arrhythmias during laparoscopy can occur due to the associated hypercarbia; however, they can also be a result of pneumothorax, hypoxia, or gas embolism [3, 6]. Hypercarbia stimulates the sympathetic nervous system, increasing serum catecholamines which produce vasoconstriction, and increase heart rate, blood pressure, and the chances of arrhythmias [2]. Bradycardia from vagal stimulation is also possible due to peritoneal irritation from insufflated CO_2.

Table 1 Pressure effects of 10 and 20 mmHg pneumoperitoneum

Effects	10 mmHg	20 mmHg
Heart rate	I	I
Mean arterial pressure	I	I
Systemic vascular resistance	I	I
Venous return	I or D	I or D
Cardiac output	U or I	U or D
Glomerular filtration rate	D	Larger D
Urine output	D	Larger D
End-tidal CO_2	U or I	U or I
PCO_2	I	I
Arterial pH	U or D	D

I increase, *D* decrease, *U* unchanged
Adapted from Eichel et al. [6]

CO_2 insufflation may stimulate the renin–angiotensin–aldosterone and the sympatho-adrenal systems resulting in further cardiovascular effects. Central venous pressure may rise or fall as a result of pneumoperitoneum and is therefore an unreliable indicator of intravascular volume [6]. Depending on the hydration status of the patient, low levels of insufflation pressure early on may increase venous return to the heart, while higher sustained pressures will decrease venous return through the vena cava, resulting in a lowered stroke volume.

Extraperitoneal or retroperitoneal insufflation of CO_2 results in increased absorption into the tissues and bloodstream. The insufflated gas is more apt to dissect into the mediastinal and pleural spaces. Increased insufflation pressures and subcutaneous emphysema also result in more CO_2 gas absorption.

Pediatrics

Children have a decreased pulmonary reserve, which results from a relatively low functional reserve capacity and lower oxygen reserve [10]. Therefore, children do not tolerate decreases in oxygen saturation as well as adults. Neonates are even more prone to oxygen desaturation because of their lower functional pulmonary reserve and their higher oxygen consumption [10].

Cerebral Blood Flow

Insufflation with CO_2 causes a rise in intracranial pressure (ICP). The causes are multifactorial. Hypercarbia causes cerebral vasodilation causing an increase in ICP. Trendelenburg position exacerbates the increase in ICP during pneumoperitoneum [8].

Patient Position

The Trendelenburg (head-down tilt) position during pelvic laparoscopy results in increased cardiac output, increased arterial pressure, and decreased vascular resistance [3]. The reverse Trendelenburg (head-up) position results in an increase in the heart rate and systemic vascular resistance while decreasing the cardiac output. Lateral decubitus positioning such as with renal laparoscopic surgery decreases vascular resistance and creates a ventilation–perfusion mismatch. Careful control of ventilation will usually manage the pulmonary consequences of positioning [3]. Patients undergoing laparoscopic procedures can develop hypothermia if the insufflated gas is not warmed or if external warming devices are not placed on the patient. Use of energy devices such as the argon beam coagulator laparoscopically must take into account rapid increases in intra-abdominal pressure generated by the device. Venting a laparoscopic port or actively suctioning during use of the argon beam will lessen the chance of over-pressurization of the abdomen.

CO_2 Embolus

CO_2 embolus is a rare but potentially lethal complication of pneumoperitoneum. It usually occurs during placement of the Verres needle or first trocar. As CO_2 is much more soluble in blood than air or nitrogen, it has a greater margin of safety should embolization occur [3]. The gas embolus causes either an "air lock" in the atrium, blocking right-sided cardiac output, or blockage at the level of the pulmonary arterial tree, directly blocking the pulmonary microcirculation. Gas embolism is suspected with hypotension, cyanosis, and arrhythmia. A precordial stethoscope may or may not detect the classic "mill wheel" murmur. As the embolized gas is CO_2, the end-tidal CO_2 usually drops suddenly. Patients should be emergently ventilated with 100% oxygen, placed in a head-down, left lateral position (right side elevated), and the embolus aspirated from the right heart via a central line catheter [3]. Obviously, the pneumoperitoneum needs to be immediately desufflated.

Metabolic Changes and Procedure Duration

During prolonged laparoscopic and robotic procedures, only minor changes are noted in hemodynamic and acid–base parameters. Minute ventilation is adjusted by anesthesia according to blood gas analyses to maintain pH, $PaCO_2$, bicarbonate, and base excess within physiologic norms [11]. Morbidly obese patients are affected by pneumoperitoneum in the same fashion as the nonobese; however, increased abdominal pressure can reduce femoral blood flow, leading to increased venous stasis. The use of sequential compression devices can minimize venous stasis so as to decrease the chance for deep venous thrombosis [12]. CO_2 is also stored in the viscera, bones, and muscles. During longer laparoscopic cases, more CO_2 builds up in these reservoirs. Postoperatively, the CO_2 is released from these sites and expired from the lungs. It is important to monitor patients closely in the postoperative period for hypercarbia, especially following long procedures and in those with underlying pulmonary disease such as COPD [6]. Absorption of CO_2 is greater during extraperitoneal insufflation; therefore, patients with underlying pulmonary disease must be monitored closely as they may not be able to adequately exhale the CO_2 during a retroperitoneoscopic approach [13].

Effects on Urine Output

The increased intra-abdominal pressure of pneumoperitoneum appears to decrease both renal blood flow and renal function during the procedure. The degree of suppression of the renal parameters is correlated with the state of hydration, insufflation pressure, patient position, and duration of the pneumoperitoneum [14]. Therefore, the reduction in renal function results in intraoperative oliguria. Despite this oliguria, prolonged laparoscopic procedures do not appear to adversely affect postoperative renal function [15]. Anesthesia should provide adequate maintenance fluids during laparoscopy, with the realization that urine output will be decreased and is thus unreliable as a measure of hydration during the procedure. One exception is during laparoscopic donor nephrectomy, where it is crucial to aggressively hydrate the patient and promote a brisk diuresis with diuretics prior to transecting the vasculature.

Physiological Changes with Immune Function

Both open and laparoscopic operations affect the immune status of the patient. Animal experiments and clinical trials looking at cytokine- and cell-mediated immune responses have shown less effect on the systemic stress response in laparoscopic procedures as compared to their open counterparts [2, 16, 17].

Insufflation of CO_2 into the abdomen causes a metabolic acidosis and hypercarbia. CO_2 acidification of the peritoneal surface may mediate suppression of macrophage function at that level [18]. Although port site metastasis has been reported, the etiology is not completely understood and felt to be multifactorial. Suggested contributing factors include tumor seeding from poor technique, aggressive tumor biology, local effects of CO_2, and immunosuppression [2].

Conclusions

Laparoscopy requires creation of a pneumoperitoneum which is commonly performed by insufflating CO_2 intra-abdominally. Urologists must be cognizant that insufflated CO_2 is physiologically active and dynamic in patients, having a host of effects on the patient's pulmonary, cardiovascular, metabolic, renal, and immune systems. Although most patients tolerate CO_2 pneumoperitoneum well, some patients will not and others will be at higher risk for morbidity should they undergo a laparoscopic procedure. The surgeon must not only recognize signs of laparoscopic complications but also anticipate the physiologic changes their patients will undergo in response to CO_2 pneumoperitoneum.

References

1. Safran DB, Orlando R. Physiologic effects of pneumoperitoneum. Am J Surg. 1994;167:281–6.
2. Ost MC, Tan BJ, Lee BR. Urological laparoscopy: basic physiological considerations and immunological consequences. J Urol. 2005;174:1183–8.
3. Stoller ML, Wolf JS. Physiologic considerations in laparoscopy. In: Crawford ED, Das S, editors. Urologic laparoscopy. Philadelphia: Saunders; 1994.
4. Sharma KC, Brandstetter RD, Brensilver JM, Jung LD. Cardiopulmonary physiology and pathophysiology as a consequence of laparoscopic surgery. Chest. 1996; 110:810–5.
5. Tan PL, Lee TL, Tweed WA. Carbon dioxide absorption and gas exchange during pelvic laparoscopy. Can J Anaesth. 1992;39:677–81.
6. Eichel L, McDougall EM, Clayman RV. Basics of laparoscopic urologic surgery. In: Wein AJ, Kavoussi LR, Novick AC, Partin AW, Peters CS, editors. Campbell-Walsh urology. 9th ed. Philadelphia: Saunders; 2007.
7. Grabowski JE, Talamini MA. Physiological effects of pneumoperitoneum. J Gastrointest Surg. 2009;13(5):1009–16.
8. O'Malley C, Cunningham AJ. Physiologic changes during anesthesia. Anesthesiol Clin North Am. 2001;19:1–19.
9. Hardacre JM, Talamini MA. Pulmonary and hemodynamic changes during laparoscopy – are they important? Surgery. 2000;127:241–4.
10. Docimo SG, Peters CA. Pediatric endourology and laparoscopy. In: Wein AJ, Kavoussi LR, Novick AC, Partin AW, Peters CS, editors. Campbell-Walsh urology. 9th ed. Philadelphia: Saunders; 2007.
11. Nguyen NT, Wolfe BM. The physiologic effects of pneumoperitoneum in the morbidly obese. Ann Surg. 2005;241:219–26.
12. Meininger D, Byhahn C, Bueck M, Binder J, Kramer W, Kessler, Westphal K. Effects of prolonged pneumoperitoneum on hemodynamics and acid-base balance during totally endoscopic robot-assisted radical prostatectomies. World J Surg. 2002;26:1423–7.
13. Glascock JM, Winfield HN, Lund GO, Donovan JF, Ping ST, Griffiths DL. Carbon dioxide homeostasis during transperitoneal or extraperitoneal laparoscopic pelvic lymphadenectomy: a real-time intraoperative comparison. J Endourol. 1996;10:319–23.
14. Demyttenaere S, Feldman LS, Fried GM. Effect of pneumoperitoneum on renal perfusion and function: a systematic review. Surg Endosc. 2007;21:152–60.
15. Nguyen NT, Perez RV, Fleming N, Rivers R, Wolfe BM. Effect of prolonged pneumoperitoneum on intraoperative urine output during laparoscopic gastric bypass. J Am Coll Surg. 2002;195:476–83.
16. Corrigan M, Cahill RA, Redmond HP. The immunomodulatory effects of laparoscopic surgery. Surg Laparosc Endosc Percutan Tech. 2007;17:256–61.
17. Buunen M, Gholghesaei M, Veldkamp R, Meijer DW, Bonjer HJ, Bouvy ND. Stress response to laparoscopic surgery. Surg Endosc. 2004;18:1022–8.
18. Neuhaus SJ, Watson DI. Pneumoperitoneum and peritoneal surface changes. Surg Endosc. 2004;18:1316–22.

Anesthesia and Management of Anesthetic Complications of Laparoscopic Urological Surgery

Philip Lebowitz, Mahesan Richards, and Christopher Bryan-Brown

Keywords Anesthetic · Complications · Urological Laparoscopy

Patients undergoing laparoscopic urological surgery are subjected by definition to non-physiological trespass that threatens to destabilize their homeostasis. Consequently, the anesthesiologist needs to take an active role in the process from the outset and must work closely with the surgical team in order to bring the patient through the operation without adverse outcome. This coordinated effort involves preoperative patient evaluation, optimization of the patient's composite organ function or dysfunction, provision of an appropriate anesthetic with appropriate physiological monitoring, careful patient positioning, preservation of cardiovascular stability, maintenance of oxygenation and ventilation, protection of renal function, and smooth emergence from the anesthetized state to the recovering state. This chapter will consider this process in three parts: preoperative evaluation and preparation; maintenance of cardiovascular, including renal, function during the procedure; and management of oxygenation and ventilation in the context of laparoscopy and non-supine positioning.

Preoperative Evaluation and Preparation

No rational surgeon would choose to operate on a patient whose medical conditions and physiological instability would lead (if one could predict it with certainty) to postoperative organ dysfunction and a complicated, protracted recovery, perhaps with permanent morbidity or even death. Medical outcomes exist in the realm of probabilities, and time is limited by operating room schedules. As a result, we are forced to make decisions with imperfect knowledge and under the pressure of timed performance. However, in the interest of uncomplicated postoperative lives for our patients and for ourselves, we must consider what we do know and what we think we know about the factors (other than the surgery itself) that promote successful surgical outcomes.

The most basic stratification of preoperative patient health is the American Society of Anesthesiologists' (ASA) Physical Status classification system [1] that dates back to 1941. Although relatively uncomplicated, it offers a time-honored method of categorizing the level of concern that an anesthesiologist should apply in considering a given patient's anesthetic.

ASA Physical Status Classification

- I A normal healthy patient
- II A patient with mild systemic disease
- III A patient with severe systemic disease
- IV A patient with severe systemic disease that is a constant threat to life
- V A moribund patient who is not expected to survive without the operation

P. Lebowitz (✉)
Department of Anesthesiology, Montefiore Medical Center, Albert Einstein College of Medicine, 111 E. 210 St., Bronx, NY 10467, USA
e-mail: plebowit@montefiore.org

R. Ghavamian (ed.), *Complications of Laparoscopic and Robotic Urologic Surgery*,
DOI 10.1007/978-1-60761-676-4_2, © Springer Science+Business Media, LLC 2010

VI A declared brain-dead patient whose organs are being removed for donor purposes

E Emergency operation [appended to the foregoing, e.g., III E]

Although anesthesiologists have debated for decades precisely which patients fall into which categories, the ASA has declared that "there is no additional information that will help you further define these categories." Just the same, the Cleveland Clinic has publicized on its web site the following examples (http://my.clevelandclinic.org/services/Anesthesia/hic_ASA_Physical_Classification_System.aspx):

I – No organic, physiologic, or psychiatric disturbance; excludes the very young (<2 years) and very old (>70 years); healthy with good exercise tolerance

II – No functional limitations; has a well-controlled disease of one body system; controlled hypertension or diabetes without systemic effects, cigarette smoking without chronic obstructive pulmonary disease (COPD); mild obesity, pregnancy

III – Some functional limitation; has a controlled disease of more than one body system or one major system; no immediate danger of death; controlled congestive heart failure (CHF), stable angina, old heart attack, poorly controlled hypertension, morbid obesity, chronic renal failure; bronchospastic disease with intermittent symptoms

IV – Has at least one severe disease that is poorly controlled or at end stage; possible risk of death; unstable angina, symptomatic COPD, symptomatic CHF, hepatorenal failure

V – Not expected to survive >24 h without surgery; imminent risk of death; multiorgan failure, sepsis syndrome with hemodynamic instability, hypothermia, poorly controlled coagulopathy

This system was not conceived as a means of stratifying risk, but rather a means of getting anesthesiologists to think about their patients' preoperative condition with an eye toward modifying the anesthetic that they would be administering. Just the same, the ASA Physical Status Classification appears to be as good a prognosticator of postoperative complications as more recent and complex methodologies such as the well-known Cardiac Risk Index published by Goldman et al. in 1977 [2].

In order to classify a patient's preoperative physical state, it is necessary to obtain a detailed history, perform a physical examination, and consider relevant laboratory test results. The presence of volunteered symptoms or the finding of an abnormal lab result does not necessarily mean that a patient has organic disease. As Roizen describes, for tests reported over a continuous range of results, the distribution in a population is Gaussian, i.e., a normal distribution. Arbitrarily, 2.5% of lab test results for healthy patients will fall above the "normal" range and another 2.5% of the same test results for healthy patients will fall below the "normal" range. Furthermore, ordering multiple tests increases the probability of an "abnormal" finding in a healthy patient [3].

There is no established standard among anesthesiologists as to what testing needs to be done preoperatively. Rather, it is more logical to obtain laboratory information on the basis of the patient's underlying conditions and medications. For example, a patient receiving diuretics may become hypokalemic and alkalotic; knowing that patient's recent electrolytes, BUN, and creatinine is highly relevant to the subsequent conduct of an anesthetic. While healthy patients undergoing minor, non-invasive procedures need not have any laboratory testing whatsoever, a patient with multi-system disease undergoing major surgery needs extensive testing. Essentially, a thorough history and physical examination in the context of the intended surgery should dictate preoperative laboratory testing. The best uses of preoperative testing are to confirm clinical diagnoses and optimize the patient's readiness for surgery.

Even so, many surgeons have had the unfortunate experience of having evaluated (or having had evaluated for them by an internist or an anesthesiologist) a patient some days prior to surgery, only to have a different anesthesiologist on the day of surgery hold up the surgery by requiring additional testing. It goes without saying that it is insufficient simply to have had an internist "clear" the patient without that person's understanding the implications of that patient's medical condition on the conduct of the anesthetic and surgery. In effect, only the anesthesiologist on the day of surgery can "clear" the patient. Good anesthesiologists, however, do look to a good internist's or a colleague's evaluation of a patient's physical status, particularly from the beneficial viewpoint of a relevant longitudinal history, as an important means of assessing that patient's optimization for surgery.

The best way to avoid having a patient's surgery delayed (or worse, having the patient unsafely undergo the procedure) is to apply consistently an appreciation of the interactions of a patient's medical condition with anesthesia and surgery. A group of anesthesiologists should ideally gravitate to a consistent approach over time, particularly with regard to required laboratory testing. Having already stated that there is no standard among anesthesiologists in this regard, we might suggest the following schema (modified from Roizen [3]) for adult patients undergoing invasive laparoscopic urological surgery:

- CBC, including platelet count
- Electrolytes (Na^+, Cl^-, K^+, HCO_3^-), BUN, creatinine, glucose
- INR, PTT
- Liver function tests
- ECG for age > 50 or symptomatic
- Chest x-ray only for patients with worsening pulmonary symptoms

This list is not exhaustive nor does it preclude other testing as indicated by the patient's history or physical examination. Likewise, it includes testing where the yield is likely to be low. Its purported value is its sharing a common ground for most anesthesiologists in order to minimize delays or cancellations on the day of surgery. This discussion may be moot if hospital policies have been elaborated that dictate the extent and timing of the preoperative evaluation and laboratory testing.

To that last point, there is no standard among anesthesiologists regarding how recently the history, physical examination, and laboratory testing need to have been done in order to be considered useful. We would again suggest that the rule of reason be applied. In the absence of new symptoms and to the degree that a given patient is known to have been stable in terms of medical conditions and medications, the less the urgency in repeating testing. Conversely, new or interval change in symptoms, medical instability, and/or changed medication regimens all heighten the need for testing close to the day of surgery.

The preceding general discussion of preoperative evaluation and preparation can be more definitively refined for adult patients with cardiac disease undergoing non-cardiac surgery. The American College of Cardiology (ACC) and the American Heart Association (AHA) jointly published their most recently revised set of practice guidelines for this subgroup of patients in 2007 [4]. This algorithm, based on active clinical conditions, known cardiovascular disease, or cardiac risk factors for patients 50 years of age or greater, provides a stepwise description of the types of further cardiac investigation that are recommended for patients with cardiac disease relative to the type of surgery planned. A summary of the algorithm follows:

- Emergency non-cardiac surgery requires no further workup. The procedure needs to be performed, so perioperative surveillance and treatment are implemented both in the operating room and during recovery.
- Non-emergency surgery allows greater discretion on the part of the caregivers to assess the patient's cardiac status and, if needed, define the extent of disease and treat it accordingly.
- Active cardiac disease encompasses unstable or severe angina, recent MI, decompensated heart failure (i.e., New York Heart Association Class IV patients who should be at complete rest, confined to bed or chair; any physical activity brings on discomfort and symptoms occur at rest), significant arrhythmias, and severe valvular disease.
- Low-risk surgery (risk of cardiac death and non-fatal myocardial infarction <1%) includes endoscopic and superficial procedures, while intermediate-risk surgery (cardiac risk 1–5%) includes prostate surgery and intra-peritoneal surgery. High-risk surgery (cardiac risk >5%) relates to vascular surgery.
- A person with an exercise tolerance of four metabolic equivalents (METs) can climb a flight of stairs or walk up a hill, walk on level ground at 4 mph (6.4 km/h), run a short distance, do heavy work around the house like scrubbing floors or lifting or moving heavy furniture, participate in moderate recreational activities like golf, bowling, dancing, doubles tennis, or throwing a baseball or football.
- A patient without active cardiac disease having low-risk surgery or exhibiting functional capacity equivalent of greater than or equal to four METs without symptoms can proceed to surgery without further workup.
- A patient with active cardiac disease undergoing low-risk surgery can proceed directly to surgery.

- A patient with active cardiac disease with a functional capacity equal to or greater than four METs without symptoms undergoing intermediate- or high-risk surgery can proceed to surgery if non-invasive testing will not alter treatment.
- A patient with active cardiac disease undergoing intermediate- or high-risk surgery with less than four METs exercise tolerance needs an evaluation of his/her clinical risk factors. These include ischemic heart disease, compensated or prior heart failure, diabetes mellitus, renal insufficiency, and cerebrovascular disease.
- If the person does not have any of these clinical risk factors, the planned surgery should proceed. Otherwise, it is recommended to proceed with surgery in patients with one to three clinical risk factors unless non-invasive testing will change management.
- Patients with three or more clinical risk factors requiring vascular surgery need further testing if it will change anesthetic management.
- Assessment for coronary artery disease risk and functional capacity includes a 12-lead electrocardiogram, exercise stress testing, and pharmacological stress testing.
- Supplemental preoperative cardiac evaluation consists of left ventricular function by radionuclide angiography, echocardiography, and contrast ventriculography.

While the foregoing algorithm is complicated, its application, in brief, is that patients undergoing laparoscopic urological surgery (intermediate risk) who do not have functional capacity greater than four METs or who do have cardiac symptoms need to be evaluated by a cardiologist or internist. If that patient is appraised as having no clinical risk factors (listed above), one may proceed with the planned surgery. Patients with one, two, or three clinical risk factors may proceed to surgery, particularly with heart rate control, if management will not likely be affected. Alternatively, these patients should undergo non-invasive testing if it will likely change the patient's perioperative management. The nebulous nature of these last two statements suggests that the surgeon, anesthesiologist, and cardiologist or internist confer prior to the day of surgery in order to arrive at a common ground.

A patient's integrated cardiopulmonary performance can be limited by lung disease in the absence of heart problems. Identifying pulmonary disease by history, according to Roizen [3], can be done by asking the following questions:

- Have you ever had pneumonia?
- Have you ever undergone lung surgery?
- Do you have shortness of breath, wheezing, chest pain, bronchitis, asthma, or emphysema?
- Do you cough regularly or frequently?
- Do you cough up mucus?
- In the last 4 weeks have you had a fever, chills, cold, or flu?
- Do you smoke or have you ever smoked?
- Do you ever spit or chew tobacco?

Auscultation of the lungs with a stethoscope can quickly determine the presence or absence of rhonchi, wheezes, or rales. A chest x-ray, in the absence of history or physical examination findings suggestive of cardiopulmonary disease, is unlikely to add any useful information and is an unnecessary screening test. In the presence of positive historical or physical evidence, however, a chest x-ray can serve as a valuable basis for postoperative comparison.

Pulmonary function testing (PFT) is an objective means by which to quantify a patient's respiratory dysfunction beyond that achieved after obtaining a medical history and performing a physical examination. PFTs are done to predict how well a patient with lung disease will deal with the stressors of surgery and anesthesia so as to avoid perioperative pulmonary complications (PPCs), such as atelectasis, pneumonia, respiratory failure, and exacerbation of long-standing lung disease.

Useful PFTs include arterial blood gas measurement and spirometry. The latter includes forced expiratory volume in the first second (FEV_1), forced vital capacity (FVC), the FEV_1/FVC ratio, peak flow, and forced expiratory flow between 25 and 75% of lung volume ($FEF_{25-75\%}$) – before and after bronchodilator treatment. Examination of the flow-volume loop configuration, in addition to providing the aforementioned data, can be informative about the location of fixed or variable airway obstruction. Essentially, PFTs, including arterial blood gas analysis, offer information about whether a patient's pulmonary disease is obstructive vs. restrictive, whether the patient has a propensity to retain carbon dioxide, and whether the patient's pulmonary disease has a reversible component.

Asthmatic patients will tell you specifically what makes them better and what makes them worse. Continuing their established treatment or prevention regimen through the day of surgery and prophylactically by administering an inhalable bronchodilator before induction of anesthesia will, along with a smoothly conducted anesthetic, serve to minimize perioperative bronchospasm.

In 2006 the American College of Physicians elaborated a set of guidelines for risk assessment and reduction of PPCs [5]. They stated that significant preoperative risk factors for PPCs are chronic obstructive pulmonary disease, age > 60 years, ASA Physical Status Class II or higher, serum albumin levels <3.5 g/dL, functional dependence, and recumbent congestive heart failure. They also determined that surgery >3 h duration, abdominal surgery, and general anesthesia were significant risk factors for PPCs in these patient populations. The guidelines concluded that these patients at risk should receive preoperative PFTs and postoperative incentive spirometry.

Preoperative measures to improve lung function include smoking cessation, mobilization of secretions, bronchodilator treatment, and improved stamina. Although smoking-induced destruction of lung architecture cannot be reversed, smoking cessation results in decreased airway secretions, decreased airway reactivity, and improved mucociliary transport. Just the same, these benefits may not be realized for 2–4 weeks. Smoking cessation on the day prior to surgery will only improve the picture by decreasing the carbon monoxide carried by blood. Reducing the percentage of circulating carboxyhemoglobin will, however, improve the amount of oxygen carriage by the blood.

A related and, given the current obesity epidemic, an increasingly important issue is that of obstructive sleep apnea (OSA). OSA is characterized by periodic, partial, or complete obstruction of the upper airway during sleep. Clinical signs and symptoms that suggest the presence of OSA include BMI > 35 kg/m^2, neck circumference 17 in. in men or 16 in. in women, craniofacial abnormalities affecting the airway, tonsils nearly touching or actually touching in the midline, and anatomical nasal obstruction. OSA is characterized by daytime somnolence, difficulty concentrating, headaches, and memory impairment. During sleep, symptoms include apnea, hypopneas, and snoring.

Potential physiological consequences of these symptoms are hypoxemia, hypercarbia, pulmonary hypertension, systemic vasoconstriction, and secondary polycythemia. The obesity hypoventilation syndrome, eponymically termed the Pickwickian Syndrome, is a manifestation of severe OSA that culminates in right ventricular failure from chronic hypoxic pulmonary vasoconstriction.

A sleep study – polysomnography – can confirm the diagnosis of OSA and quantify it, though physical findings and observed apnea during sleep lead to a presumptive diagnosis. The reason why OSA has interested anesthesiologists and for which the ASA has issued a set of guidelines [6] is that OSA patients risk airway obstruction during induction of anesthesia and upon emergence from anesthesia. Coupled with their increased sensitivity to anesthetics, manifested as respiratory depression, OSA patients in the supine position tend more than other patients to have their tongue, tonsils, and soft palate come to rest against their hypopharynx, thus obstructing airflow above the level of the larynx. The insertion of an endotracheal tube effectively stents the upper airway, allowing free passage of air or anesthetic gases to the lungs. Even if tracheal intubation has been performed successfully (though not necessarily easily), removal of the endotracheal tube at the end of surgery can result in life-threatening airway obstruction.

Consequently, the ASA guideline urges that extubation be performed in the semi-upright, upright, or non-supine position after full neuromuscular recovery has been verified and the patient has fully awakened. Problems arise in these patients when the patient struggles against the presence of the endotracheal tube but has not sufficiently regained consciousness so as to maintain airway patency. Deep extubation is clearly contraindicated. The principle of avoiding extubation while the patient is excitedly emerging from anesthesia but has not yet achieved sufficient recovery so as to protect the airway needs to be followed in these patients scrupulously.

In performing a preoperative evaluation, the anesthesiologist should always examine the patient's airway anatomy to determine whether ventilation of the patient's lungs by anesthesia face mask or direct laryngoscopy and intubation of the patient's trachea might prove to be difficult. The airway examination consists of assessing the patient's cervical range of motion (particularly active neck extension), maxillary–mandibular alignment (otherwise referred to as the thyromental distance), mouth opening, state of dentition, and the patient's Mallampati airway classification [7].

Although the Mallampati airway classification does not by itself provide an infallible correlation between class score and ease of laryngoscopy, its simplicity has earned it widespread application. The examiner directs the patient to sit up straight, open the mouth, stick out the tongue, but not phonate. Class 1: visualization of soft palate, fauces, uvular, and tonsillar pillars; Class 2: visualization of soft palate, fauces, and uvula; Class 3: visualization of soft palate and uvular base; Class 4: visualization of the hard palate only.

The guiding principle holds that alignment of the oral, pharyngeal, and laryngeal axes for direct visualization of the larynx is most easily accomplished in patients with full neck extension at the atlanto-occipital joint, matched maxillary–mandibular alignment, BMI < 25 kg/m^2, neck circumference <40 cm, normal mouth opening, and Mallampati 1 classification, aided by the absence of maxillary dentition. Conversely, limited neck extension, retrognathia, BMI > 30 kg/m^2, neck circumference >40 cm, limited mouth opening, and Mallampati 4 classification made more difficult by full maxillary dentition, separately or in combination can lead to poor alignment of the oral, pharyngeal, and laryngeal axes and an inability to visualize the larynx directly. Other airway features such as a large or immobile tongue, radiation fibrosis of airway structures, or tumors of the head and neck can likewise complicate the ease of lung ventilation by anesthesia face mask and/or tracheal intubation.

The anesthesiologist, in planning for a general endotracheal anesthetic, must decide whether, given the constellation of physical findings, he or she believes that ventilation of the patient's lungs by anesthesia face mask and direct laryngoscopic visualization of the patient's larynx can be accomplished without inordinate difficulty and without subjecting the patient to undue risk, once anesthesia induction has commenced. When difficult ventilation and/or difficult tracheal intubation is contemplated, the anesthesiologist must make provision for these potential difficulties by arranging for the availability and usability of auxiliary airway management devices and, if possible, the assistance of a second anesthesiologist. The anesthesiologist, furthermore, has to decide whether these auxiliary devices can be safely employed after the patient has been anesthetized or, if not, whether the airway needs to be secured prior to the patient having received an anesthetic. The commonest approach in such patients is awake/sedated fiber-optic laryngoscopy and tracheal intubation. Although all patients would prefer to be asleep before having an endotracheal tube placed through their mouth or nose, most patients can be persuaded to cooperate in the interest of their safety. On the other hand, in the interest of patient happiness, the anesthesiologist should not proceed to awake fiber-optic laryngoscopy without good reason.

Even so, despite careful evaluation and sound clinical judgment, the anesthesiologist will occasionally encounter a patient whom he or she believed to be safely intubatable but whose larynx eludes visualization and whose trachea eludes intubation. In such situations the anesthesiologist should apply the principles of the ASA Difficult Airway Algorithm [8], a stepwise sequence of branched decision-making, the goal of which is an unharmed patient.

If, for example, initial intubation attempts have proved unsuccessful, the anesthesiologist must ventilate the patient's lungs by anesthesia face mask. If ventilation is adequate, a non-emergency pathway can be followed where alternative approaches to intubation can be tried, including allowing the patient to awaken. If, however, face mask ventilation is not adequate, a laryngeal mask airway (LMA) should be inserted, if feasible. If LMA ventilation proves adequate, the anesthesiologist can return to the non-emergency pathway. If LMA ventilation is not adequate, the anesthesiologist must follow the emergency pathway which leads either to the patient's awakening or to the insertion of an emergency invasive airway access device, i.e., a tracheostomy or a cricothyroidotomy.

Another issue that unites (but sometimes divides) surgeon and anesthesiologist is NPO (Latin: *nil per os* = nothing by mouth) status. No one would choose to have a patient regurgitate or vomit gastrointestinal contents while under the influence of an anesthetic, which suppresses the reflexes that protect the trachea and lungs from intrusion by anything other than airway gases. Except for the extreme elderly and brain-injured individuals, the presence of solids or liquids in the pharynx leads to "trap-door" closure of the epiglottis over the larynx as well as vocal cord approximation so that food and drink follow their intended course from the mouth to the esophagus. Malfunction of these protective mechanisms can result in the trachea being confronted with solids or liquids, whether they are on their way to the stomach or on the way back out.

The consequence of aspiration of solids or liquids into the trachea can range from obstruction of the airway to soilage of the pulmonary parenchyma and, potentially, pneumonitis and even death. Pulmonary aspiration of acidic gastric contents is particularly problematic: Pulmonary morbidity from aspiration is proportional to the volume of aspirate and inversely proportional to the pH of the aspirated material. Risk factors for pulmonary aspiration include a "full stomach," pregnancy, obesity, gastroesophageal dysfunction (including prior esophageal surgery, symptomatic hiatal hernia, and dysphagia), functional or mechanical obstruction to digestion, and vocal cord malfunction. Gastroparesis, idiopathic or associated with diabetes mellitus, compounds the problem. Alkalinizing the gastric contents with proton pump inhibitors, histamine-2 antagonists, and/or a non-particulate antacid like sodium citrate by mouth can ameliorate the potential injury to the lungs by eliminating the acid component of the aspirate.

Because these conditions occur not uncommonly in routine practice, the anesthesiologist needs to deal with the added risk of pulmonary aspiration by adjusting the anesthetic induction method. In these situations, the anesthesiologist modifies routine practice by performing a rapid sequence induction, doing an awake fiber-optic intubation, or entirely avoiding general anesthesia, where possible. A rapid sequence induction involves preoxygenation, the administration of a rapidly acting induction drug, and the near-simultaneous administration of a rapidly acting muscle relaxant, usually while an assistant applies cricoid pressure to compress the esophagus between the cricoid cartilage and the vertebral column. Although the utility of cricoid pressure has lately been criticized as ineffectual and, what is worse, distorting to the intubator's laryngoscopic view, the cardinal principle is that the trachea be protected by a cuffed endotracheal tube in as short a time period as possible after loss of consciousness (with the attendant loss of protective airway reflexes).

The downside of performing a rapid sequence induction is that the anesthesiologist has "burned his (or her) bridges," i.e., the anesthesiologist has paralyzed the patient before assuring that either ventilation or tracheal intubation is doable. Clearly, the anesthesiologist must appraise the situation before embarking on this path and feel confident that the airway is controllable. The unexpected inability to control the airway requires the anesthesiologist to follow the difficult airway algorithm that was previously discussed – and accept the risks inherent in the process.

The best way to avoid such risks is to keep the patient's stomach empty. Hence, the traditional NPO dictum that elective patients have nothing to eat or drink after midnight. But what should we do if a patient sneaks in a cup of coffee at 6 A.M. before coming into the hospital, or has a few bites of a bagel before remembering that he was told not to eat or drink, or is given a full breakfast by a well-meaning nurses' aide?

The ASA, having examined the literature on this subject, helpfully offers us some guidelines to consider in making go/no-go decisions [9]. In summary, a patient may consume clear liquids (liquids through which one can see, e.g., water, non-pulp fruit juice, carbonated beverages, clear tea, black coffee) up to 2 h prior to anesthetic induction. There is some evidence that ingestion of clear liquids actually aids gastric emptying. The guidelines state that breast milk requires 4 h for gastric emptying. More directly applicable to adults, the guidelines suggest 6 h for a modest amount of non-human milk, infant formula, or a light meal, such as toast and clear liquids. The guidelines get less prescriptive after that: "Meals that include fried or fatty foods or meat may prolong gastric emptying time. Both the amount and type of foods ingested must be considered when determining an appropriate fasting period" [9].

Consequently, most anesthesiologists are willing to accept the ASA guidelines as far as 6 h for clear liquids, breast milk, non-human milk, or formula, but some anesthesiologists are uncomfortable with what patients may consider a "light meal." Furthermore, if NPO after midnight means that a patient can consume a pizza and beer by 11:59 the evening before a 7:30 A.M. surgery, is it logical to conclude that 7.5 h is a sufficient period of time to allow 2 P.M. surgery after a full breakfast at 6:30 A.M. that day?

No one knows the answer. Every experienced practitioner can remember a patient who had been NPO for 15 h, yet had retained partially digested food in the stomach. Alternatively, practitioners can point to countless examples of rapid sequence inductions because of the need to perform surgery on an emergency basis, where patients were safely anesthetized despite having "full stomachs." Until these questions can be answered definitively, our version of today's best practice requires patients to be NPO after midnight, discouraged from having that pizza and beer at 11:59, allowed – even encouraged – to have clear liquids up to 2 h preoperatively, and considered to have a "full stomach" the entire calendar day after ingesting a full meal. Establishing an agreement on principles among a hospital's surgeons and anesthesiologists can prevent confusion and conflict when patients fail to do what they are asked to do.

Maintenance of Cardiovascular Function

Hemodynamic changes and complications associated with robotic-assisted laparoscopic genitourinary surgery may be divided into four categories:

- Induction
- Intra-peritoneal insufflation
- Positioning
- End of surgery and postanesthesia

Induction

The incidence of hemodynamic changes and complications during induction for robotic laparoscopic urological surgery is no different from that encountered during non-robotic surgery. Blood pressure may vary from hypotension to hypertension, and heart rate may vary from bradycardia to tachycardia.

Patients with a history of high blood pressure and who are not well controlled may be subject to very labile blood pressure at induction. These patients are volume depleted and may require volume expansion, i.e., administration of IV fluids, which by itself may not be sufficient, therefore requiring the use of vasopressors. If acute changes of blood pressure in either direction are not corrected, they may lead to myocardial ischemia, renal ischemia, and cerebral ischemia. It is of paramount importance to maintain the mean arterial pressure above 50–60 mmHg to avoid these complications.

Most patients presenting for robotic urological surgery are older and are more likely to have coexisting myocardial ischemia. Tachycardia should be prevented at all costs in these patients, either by administration of intravenous fluid if hypovolemia is the cause, with medications to reduce the heart rate, or by deepening the level of the anesthetic to counter the stress influences of surgery. Dealing with these hemodynamic perturbations at the time of anesthetic induction must be continued throughout the surgical procedure.

The insensible fluid losses and third spacing are minimal during laparoscopic procedure as compared with open body cavity surgery; hence the intravenous fluid requirements are modest but must be sufficient to maintain renal perfusion. Failure to limit intraoperative fluid administration may result in postoperative congestive heart failure.

Intra-peritoneal Insufflation

Carbon dioxide is the gas of choice for intra-peritoneal insufflation because it has a high diffusion coefficient, is highly soluble in plasma, is physiologic, and can be ventilated out of the body. Although gas (CO_2) embolization is very rare, its occurrence can lead rapidly to cardiovascular collapse and death. The greatest risk for its occurrence is at the beginning of the procedure with direct intravenous or intra-arterial injection via the Veress needle. Signs of CO_2 embolization include a mill wheel cardiac murmur, decreased end-tidal CO_2, and cyanosis with a precipitous fall in O_2 saturation. Treatment includes rapid decompression of the pneumoperitoneum, hyperventilation with 100% O_2, placement of the patient in the left lateral decubitus and Trendelenburg position, and aspiration via a central venous catheter, if one is already in place.

Intra-peritoneal insufflation reduces the patient's functional residual capacity. The consequent decrease in pulmonary compliance results in ventilation–perfusion mismatching, leading to hypoxemia, hypercarbia, respiratory acidosis, and, potentially, metabolic acidosis. The increased abdominal pressure also causes compression of the inferior vena cava with the result that less blood is delivered to the right atrium. In addition, the increased pressure on the aortic runoff can cause a rise in cardiac afterload with either systemic hypertension or a reduction in cardiac output. High intra-abdominal pressure can also compress the iliac veins, further reducing venous return to the heart as well as increasing the potential for deep vein thrombosis and pulmonary thromboembolization. The incidence of deep vein thrombosis can be reduced by application of elastic stockings, intermittent calf compression, and preoperative subcutaneous injection of heparin.

Cardiac arrhythmias, especially sinus bradycardia to the point of sinus arrest, occur in up to 27% of laparoscopic procedures due to increased vagal tone as a result of the relatively rapid build-up of intra-abdominal pressure from insufflation [10]. Treatment includes immediate reduction of insufflation pressure below 15 mmHg and IV atropine – an anti-cholinergic to counteract the muscarinic cholinergic vagal stimulus. Prolonged massive increased intra-abdominal pressure can also cause a reduction in renal blood flow, decreased glomerular filtration, and consequent oliguria.

Positioning

Patient positioning varies from mild to extreme Trendelenburg (30–40° head-down) for robotic-assisted laparoscopic prostatectomy and to lateral decubitus with an elevated kidney rest for laparoscopic nephrectomy. The combination of flexion in the lateral position and elevation of the kidney bar can result in compression of the inferior vena cava and subsequent reduction in venous return to the heart leading to hypotension. Prolonged lateral decubitus positioning with a raised kidney rest can result in rhabdomyolysis, manifested by a metabolic acidosis and dark discoloration of the urine. This complication in severe cases can be fatal.

The anesthesiologist, in addition to sharing with the surgeon the responsibility of assuring that the patient's trunk, arms, and legs have been positioned without undue stretching or pressure, must also assure that intravenous lines, the arterial monitoring catheter (if used), the blood pressure cuff tubing, and the breathing circuit are arranged properly since, as a practical matter, access to them is limited during the procedure.

End of Surgery and Postanesthesia

Trendelenburg positioning, worse with extreme Trendelenburg positioning, for any extended period of time causes swelling of the soft tissues of the head and neck. The conjunctivae become chemotic, notably. This gravitationally induced edema, though cosmetically unappealing, resolves gradually with reversal of the gravitational gradient, namely nursing the patient postoperatively in a head-up position. Of concern, however, is the edema that occurs at the level of the larynx. A patient with a narrowed laryngeal aperture secondary to pre-existing vocal cord palsy, laryngeal disease, or traumatic tracheal intubation can develop critical narrowing so as to impair air movement through the larynx, once tracheal extubation has been performed. Recognition of this problem is vital at the time of or soon after extubation. Depending on the degree of impaired gas exchange, re-intubation may be required. In less critical situations, nursing in the head-up position, limitation of IV fluids, and, possibly, treatment with nebulized racemic epinephrine solution may obviate the need for re-intubation. After extubation patients may become distressed because they feel it is difficult to breathe as a result of laryngeal and hypopharyngeal swelling, as well as a completely blocked nasal passages. The authors have found that a nasal airway and head-up positioning will usually relieve the patient's symptoms.

In addition, patients with congestive heart failure are at risk for developing postoperative pulmonary edema, particularly when IV fluids have been given to excess. Patients with good cardiac function, in contrast, can maintain alveolar–pulmonary capillary integrity and stay clear of pulmonary edema, despite the head-down positioning, copious IV fluids, and evidence of soft tissue swelling.

Management of Oxygenation and Ventilation

During laparoscopic surgery, a major challenge for the anesthesiologist is to maintain the anesthetized patient's oxygenation and ventilation within acceptable parameters when the patient is in a steep head-down position. The physiological alterations that are encountered are the same irrespective of the actual procedure, so relevant interchangeable data are derived from patients having gynecological, urological, and bariatric operations.

Pulmonary function is optimal in the standing subject. The resting lung volume at the end of expiration (functional residual capacity, FRC) is maximal, about 3.0 L in the normal man. This is reduced by 30% in the supine position, and a little more with a 30° head-down tilt [11]. By the age of 44 years the closing capacity (CC) (the lung volume at which there develops measurable reduction of alveolar ventilation due to the diminution of lung volume and small airway collapse) begins to exceed the FRC in the supine subject [12]. The effect is more lung units have a low ventilation/perfusion (V/Q) ratio, develop a venoarterial shunt, and become atelectatic. FRC is further diminished by the induction of anesthesia, mechanical ventilation, and possibly paralysis [13]. The use of muscle relaxants may not have a significant effect on FRC [14], but their use is indicated for most major laparoscopic surgeries. The application of a pneumoperitoneum causes further cephalad movement of the diaphragm, reducing FRC even more.

There is very little oxygen stored in the body. In a normal man there is less than a liter, and most of that is in the blood. By the time half is used, the oxygen tension has fallen to a state of severe hypoxia. The FRC provides the largest reservoir, but in the supine air-breathing patient (FRC about 2.0 L) the alveolar oxygen fraction (F_AO_2) is around 0.13. This provides an additional 250 mL of oxygen. Again, when half is used, hypoxic levels are reached. This results in less than 2 min of apnea before severe hypoxia is evident. Before induction, preoxygenation (denitrogenation) has become a standard of care. During apnea there is seven times more oxygen available stored in the lungs, and the patient may take over 5 min to start desaturating. Anything that reduces the FRC during the induction of anesthesia will therefore reduce the safety margin for apnea and diminish the time needed for securing the airway. Obesity markedly reduces FRC, and, if a supine overweight patient is put in the 25° head-up position during induction, oxygenation is better maintained. In one study [15] on morbidly obese patients (BMI about 45 kg/m^2) the time from the onset of apnea to an arterial saturation (pulse oximeter) reduced to 92% was 201 s for the head-up and 155 s for the supine patients. The head-up patients also achieved an initial arterial oxygen tension (PaO_2) 23% higher than the supine patients. Extrapolating from Nunn's data [11] the head-up group could have expanded their FRCs by 20%.

When the patient is anesthetized and paralyzed in the steep head-down position, the anesthesiologist is faced with the problem of providing carbon dioxide elimination and oxygenation when compliance is restricted and FRC reduced by the weight of the abdominal contents and a pneumoperitoneum pushing a paralyzed diaphragm cephalad. In one study [16], head-down positioning decreased the compliance by 20% and the pneumoperitoneum by a further 30%. Restraints stabilizing the patient on the operating table compress the chest wall. From a practical point of view, the pressure of the pneumoperitoneum should be kept as low as possible, preferably no higher than 15 mmHg. When the patient is anchored to the table, strapping should be as high on the chest wall as possible to allow free movement of the lower rib cage. To avoid high peak inflation pressures, potentially a cause of lung damage, low tidal volumes should be used. The best tidal volume and plateau pressure (pressure at the end of inspiration when flow has ceased) are hard to define in the anesthetized patient. Certainly, when the plateau pressure is above 30 cm H_2O, lung units may not be over-distended when compliance is elevated by obesity, head-down position, and pneumoperitoneum. Current thinking would suggest that tidal volumes should not be more than 10 mL/kg in people with healthy lungs under anesthesia for routine surgical procedures and 6 mL/kg in patients with compromised pulmonary function or considered at risk [17]. Increasing respiratory rate appears less efficient at removing CO_2 than increased tidal volume, because of an increase in the dead space [16]. It is unclear how important it is to keep the $PaCO_2$ within the normal range. Elevated CO_2 tensions increase cerebral blood flow and potentially increase the possibility of cerebral edema, particularly in the steep head-down position. Unfortunately there is a paucity of studies as to the safety of permissive hypercapnia in this situation.

When pressure-controlled and volume-controlled ventilations are compared, the better mode for patients with a reduced compliance has been shown to be pressure controlled [18, 19]. It provides an instantaneous higher peak flow, with a probably greater rate of recruitment of alveoli, while limiting the inflation pressure to a preset value. Its major disadvantage is that tidal volumes will vary with variations in compliance due to changes in the patient's position or intra-abdominal pressure, so the ventilation pressure may have to be reset frequently.

The optimal inspired oxygen fraction (F_IO_2) is not easily defined. When there is likely to be a high incidence of wound infection, a high concentration is indicated [20]. In a study on patients receiving 30 and 80% oxygen in the perioperative period (up to 8 h), there were only minor differences and no discernable difference in pulmonary function after 24 h [21]. High alveolar oxygen tensions initiate atelectasis within minutes, converting lung units with low V/Q ratios to full shunt [22]. Atelectasis is much greater with general anesthesia when the F_IO_2 is 1.0 compared to 0.8 (5.6 and 1.3%, respectively, in one study [23]), but this is easily countered by elevating the positive end-expiratory pressure (PEEP) [23–25] which is used by most anesthesiologists in any case to maintain lung volume when it is reduced by external forces.

References

1. Saklad M. Grading of patients for surgical procedures. Anesthesiology. 1941;2:281–4.
2. Goldman L, Caldera DL, Nussbaum SR, et al. Multifactorial index of cardiac risk in noncardiac surgical procedures. N Engl J Med. 1977;297:845.
3. Roizen MF. Preoperative evaluation. In: Miller RD, editors. Miller's anesthesia. 6th ed. Philadelphia: Elsevier Churchill Livingstone; 2005. pp. 927–98.
4. Fleisher LA, Beckman JA, Brown KA, et al. ACC/AHA 2007 Guidelines on perioperative cardiovascular evaluation and care for noncardiac surgery. J Am Coll Cardiol. 2007; 50:159–242. doi:10.1016/j.jacc.2007.09.003. Published online 27 Sept 2007.
5. Qaseem A, Snow V, Fitterman N, et al. Risk assessment for and strategies to reduce perioperative pulmonary complications for patients undergoing noncardiothoracic surgery: a guideline from the American college of physicians. Ann Int Med. 2006;144:575–80, 581–95, 596–608.
6. Practice guidelines for the perioperative management of patients with obstructive sleep apnea. A report by the American Society of Anesthesiologists Task Force on Perioperative Management of Patients with obstructive sleep apnea. Anesthesiology. 2006;104:1081–93.
7. Mallampati S, Gatt S, Gugino L, et al. A clinical sign to predict difficult tracheal intubation: a prospective study. Can Anaesth Soc J. 1985;32:429–34.
8. Practice guidelines for management of the difficult airway – An updated report by the American Society of Anesthesiologists Task Force on Management of the difficult airway. Anesthesiology. 2003;98:1269–77.
9. Practice guidelines for preoperative fasting and the use of pharmacologic agents to reduce the risk of pulmonary aspiration: application to healthy patient undergoing elective procedures – a report by the American Society of Anesthesiologists Task Force on preoperative fasting. Anesthesiology. 1999;90:896–905.
10. Van Appledorn S, Costello A. Complications of robotic surgery and how to prevent them. In: Patel VR, editor. Robotic Urologic Surgery. New York: Springer; 2007, pp. 169–172.
11. Nunn J. Nunn's applied respiratory physiology. 4th ed. Oxford: Butterworth-Heinemann; 1993.
12. Leblanc P, Ruff F, Milic-Emili J. Effects of age and body position on "airway closure" in man. J Appl Physiol. 1970;28:448–541.
13. Hedenstierna G, Strandberg A, Brismar B, Lundquist H, Svensson L, Tokics L. Functional residual capacity: thoracoabdominal dimensions, and central blood volume during general anesthesia with muscle paralysis and mechanical ventilation. Anesthesiology. 1985;62:247–54.
14. Bergman N. Reduction of resting end-expiratory position of the respiratory system with induction of anesthesia and neuromuscular paralysis. Anesthesiology. 1982; 57:14–17.
15. Dixon BJ, Dixon JB, Carden JR, Burn AJ, Schachter LM, Playfair JM, Laurie CP, O'Brien PE. Preoxygenation is more effective in the 25° head-up position than in the supine position in severely obese patients. Anesthesiology. 2005;102:1110–5.
16. Hirvonen EA, Nuutinen LS, Kauko M. Ventilatory effects, blood gas changes, and oxygen consumption during laparoscopic hysterectomy. Anesth Analg. 1995;80:961–5.
17. Schultz MJ, Haitsma JJ, Slutsky AS, Gajic O. What tidal volumes should be used in patients without acute lung injury? Anesthesiology. 2007;106:1226–31.
18. Cadi P, Guenoun T, Journois D, Chevallier J-M, Diehl J-L, Safran D. Pressure-controlled ventilation improves oxygenation during laparoscopic obesity surgery compared with volume-controlled ventilation. Br J Anaesth. 2008;100:709–15.
19. Hans GA, Sottiaux TM, Lamy ML, Joris JL. Ventilatory management during routine general anaesthesia. Eur J Anaesthesiol. 2009;26:1–8.
20. Greif R, Akça O, Horn EP, Kurz A, Sessler DI. Supplemental perioperative oxygen to reduce the incidence of surgical-wound infection. N Engl J Med 2000; 342:161–7.
21. Akça O, Podolsky A, Eisenhuber E, Panzer O, Hetz H, Lampl K, Lackner FX, Wittmann K, Grabenwoeger F, Kurz A, Schultz A-M, Negishi C, Sessler DI. Comparable postoperative pulmonary atelectasis in patients given 30 or 80% oxygen during and 2 hours after colon resection. Anesthesiology. 1999;91:991–8.
22. Dantzker DR, Wagner PD, West JB. Instability of lung units with low V_A/Q ratios during O_2breathing. J Appl Physiol. 1975;38:886–95.
23. Rothen HU, Sporre B, Engberg G, Wegenius G, Hogman M, Hedenstierna G. Influence of gas composition on recurrence of atelectasis after a re-expansion maneuver during general anesthesia. Anesthesiology. 1995;832–42.
24. Meininger D, Byhahn C, Mierdi S, Westphal K, Zwissler B. Positive end-expiratory pressure improves arterial oxygenation during prolonged pneumoperitoneum. Acta Anesthesiol Scand. 2005;49:778–83.
25. Neumann P, Rothen HU, Berglund JE, Valtysson J, Magnusson A, Hedenstierna G. Positive end-expiratory pressure prevents atelectasis during general anaesthesia even in the presence of a high inspired oxygen concentration. Acta Anesthesiol Scand. 1999;43:295–301.

Metabolic and Renal Complications and Immunologic Implications of Laparoscopic Urologic Surgery

Steve K. Williams and David M. Hoenig

Keywords Complications · Laparoscopy · Immunology

Introduction

Laparoscopic surgery has had a revolutionary impact on the field of urology. The benefits of decreased postoperative pain, reduced hospital stay, and faster return to work have all been well documented. The number of laparoscopic procedures performed in the United States has increased rapidly over the past few decades with increasingly more complex procedures performed in older patients with more preexisting comorbid conditions [1]. The laparoscopic surgeon must be aware of the complex physiologic consequences of laparoscopic surgery as well as the potential metabolic risks of renal surgery. A thorough understanding of the impact of laparoscopic surgery on the various body systems is necessary to effectively assess risk that a prospective laparoscopic patient may face. In this chapter our aim is to review the main metabolic and immunologic effects of laparoscopy and pneumo peritoneum.

D.M. Hoenig (✉)
Department of Urology, Montefiore Medical Center, Albert Einstein College of Medicine, Bronx, NY, USA
e-mail: dhoenig@montefiore.org

Laparoscopic Gas Insufflation Physiology

Following the creation of a pneumoperitoneum, there are two immediate effects. The first effect is due to the increased pressure within the peritoneum from the instillation of a gas under pressure. The second effect is the result of the gaseous diffusion allowing the gas to reach equilibrium with the peritoneum and the bloodstream and as a result produce systemic effects. The summated force of gaseous molecules colliding at a surface divided over the surface area is the pressure that a gas exerts, and this pressure is directly proportional to the concentration of the gas and its temperature. The concentration of a gas in solution is determined by its pressure and its solubility coefficient. The higher the solubility for a gas, the more of that gas is dissolved at any given pressure [2]. The principal determinant of movement of gases in tissues is the rate at which gases diffuse across tissue water which is in turn determined by the solubility of the gas in the fluid, the cross-sectional area, the molecular weight of the gas, the temperature of the fluid, and the distance through which the gas must diffuse.

The ideal laparoscopic insufflation gas should be readily available, relatively inexpensive, colorless, highly soluble in plasma, and suitable to use for most patients and procedures. It also should be chemically stable, physiologically inert, and non-explosive. Various gasses have been used for abdominal insufflation during laparoscopy. In the early days of laparoscopy, room air was used for the creation of a pneumoperitoneum. Air is colorless and odorless, but supports combustion and has a potential for venous embolism because of its poor solubility in blood [3].

R. Ghavamian (ed.), *Complications of Laparoscopic and Robotic Urologic Surgery*,
DOI 10.1007/978-1-60761-676-4_3,

Nitrous oxide (N_2O) is a colorless and odorless nonirritating gas with low solubility in blood and has been used in the past as an insufflant [3]. Colton was the first to administer N_2O in 1844, and in 1879 Bert demonstrated its ability to induce general anesthesia when administered under hyperbaric conditions [3]. Nitrous oxide is not absorbed as rapidly as CO_2 from the peritoneal surface but its absorption is rapid enough that prolonged postoperative distension does not occur. Robinson et al. first drew attention in 1975 to the possibility of an explosion hazard if N_2O were used as the insufflating gas, theorizing that hydrogen and methane could diffuse from the bowel into the peritoneal cavity creating a potentially explosive gaseous mixture [4]. The subsequent report by El-Kady et al. of an intraperitoneal explosion resulting in the death of a patient undergoing laparoscopic surgery in which N_2O was used, as well as other reports of less severe episodes of intraperitoneal combustion, has led to the abandonment of nitrous oxide as an insufflant [5].

Carbon dioxide (CO_2) has become the primary gas used in laparoscopy due to its ability to suppress combustion and its high solubility in water. It was first discovered at the end of the 18th century by Priestly with its role in respiration described later by Lavoisier [3].

Carbon Dioxide Gas Physiology

The changes in acid–base balance and hemodynamics during a CO_2 pneumoperitoneum have been well described in the literature [6–10]. An appreciation of the basic physiology of CO_2 is essential to the understanding of the effects of the CO_2 pneumoperitoneum. A full discourse on this topic is beyond the scope of this chapter, but we will review some basic principles here.

Carbon dioxide gas is one of the main end-products of metabolism and is transported in the blood in three forms: in the form of bicarbonate (90%), in a dissolved form in plasma (5–10%), and the remainder complexed to hemoglobin. Dissolved CO_2 reacts with water to form carbonic acid which dissociates into hydrogen and bicarbonate ions. The hydrogen ions so created are buffered by hemoglobin and this pathway is essential in the regulation of acid–base balance. Carbon dioxide is transported in the blood to the lungs where it readily diffuses from the bloodstream across the alveolar membrane.

Under normal resting conditions approximately 4 ml of CO_2 is transported from the tissues to the lungs for each 100 ml of blood. During physiological or pathological states where CO_2 production exceeds its elimination of acid–base, respiratory homeostasis is altered. As described previously, an increase in CO_2 concentration also increases hydrogen ion production and therefore creates an acidemic state. This acidosis affects alveolar ventilation by stimulation of respiratory chemoreceptors in the medulla. The resulting effect is an increase in ventilation with the elimination of CO_2 from the blood and maintenance of homeostasis. During a CO_2 pneumoperitoneum, a large amount of CO_2 gas is absorbed through the peritoneum. Ho et al. showed that, on the average, 200 ml/kg of CO_2 is absorbed every hour of insufflation [9]. An average 70 kg patient would therefore absorb 14 L of CO_2 gas every hour. The total storage capacity of the body is approximately 120 L with bone being the largest potential reservoir [11]. Absorbed CO_2 entering the body initially equilibrates with peripheral tissue stores before diffusing out of the tissue cells in a gaseous form to enter the bloodstream.

Cardiovascular Consequences of Laparoscopic Surgery

Cardiac output is determined by cardiac function and by venous return. Cardiac function depends on the afterload as well as the chronotropic and inotropic properties of the myocardium which may be affected by intrinsic or extrinsic factors [2]. Both the mechanical (i.e., pressure related) and the CO_2 absorption-related effects of CO_2 pneumoperitoneum affect the cardiovascular system. Venous return during raised intra-abdominal pressure is dependent on the venous resistance as well as the mean systemic pressure. The mean systemic pressure is primarily determined by the pressure within the capacitance vessels of the systemic vasculature, i.e., the small veins and venules, and is determined by vascular tone, blood volume, and the pressure in the tissues surrounding the capacitance vessels. Increased intra-abdominal pressure increases both the mean systemic pressure and the venous resistance.

The hemodynamic changes observed during laparoscopy are primarily a result of the combined effects of the raised intra-abdominal pressure and hypercapnia from the absorbed CO_2. The degree to which cardiac output is affected, however, depends on a number of variables including a patient's intravascular volume, patient position, insufflating gas and intra-abdominal pressure, duration of the procedure, and the patient's age and comorbidities [12–14]. Although, in general, laparoscopic surgery is tolerated well by most patients, cardiovascular changes could have adverse effects in those patients with limited cardiac reserve [15].

Mechanical Effects of Pneumoperitoneum on the Cardiovascular System

Increased intra-abdominal pressure causes compression of the abdominal venous and arterial vasculature. Aortic compression results in an increase in cardiac afterload and systemic vascular resistance, which leads to a decrease in cardiac output. In addition, compression of the venous system results in a decline in preload, further decreasing cardiac output [16]. Kashtan et al. [17] studied the hemodynamic effects of increased intra-abdominal pressure in anesthetized 20–30 kg male dogs. The authors increased intra-abdominal pressure to 40 mmHg by infusing fluid into the abdomen in normovolemic, hypovolemic, and hypervolemic dogs. Cardiac output decreased by 53% in hypovolemic dogs and by 17% in normovolemic dogs, but increased by 50% in hypervolemic dogs. The physiologic basis for these findings was demonstrated to be due to reduced inferior vena cava (IVC) flow. When the pressure in the IVC is high as in the hypervolemic dogs in this study, the compression of the cava is minimized and venous resistance rises little. In hypovolemic conditions, however, the caval pressure is low and the cava is easily compressed, resulting in a high venous resistance.

Raised intra-abdominal pressure (IAP) increases both mean systemic pressure and venous resistance. In dogs, venous resistance is insignificant below 5–7 mmHg intra-abdominal pressure, and at such a low pressure there is an increase in venous flow. Above this pressure, venous resistance becomes dominant and caval flow decreases. Contrast studies of the IVC during insufflations have demonstrated that in humans the anatomic site of maximum resistance is just below the diaphragm at which point the IVC collapses with raised intra-abdominal pressure [18]. Although venous return decreases and ventricular volumes are not increased, there is an increase in the measured central venous pressure and pulmonary artery wedge pressure. These changes are due to the cephalad shift of the diaphragm with transmission of increased pressure from the abdomen to the mediastinum and chest.

Cardiovascular changes are proportional to the IAP attained. The safe upper limit of intra-abdominal pressure was investigated by Dexter and colleagues [19]. The author reported on 20 patients who were randomized to either high-pressure (15 mmHg) or low-pressure (7 mmHg) pneumoperitoneum. Arterial blood pressure was measured invasively while heart rate, stroke volume, and cardiac output were measured by trans-esophageal Doppler. In the high-pressure group, heart rate and mean arterial blood pressure increased during insufflations, while stroke volume and cardiac output were depressed by a maximum of 26 and 28%. In the low-pressure group, insufflations produced a rise in arterial pressure and a peak rise in both stroke volume and cardiac output of 10 and 28%, respectively. The authors concluded that low-pressure pneumoperitoneum is feasible and minimizes the adverse effects of peritoneal insufflation. Similarly, Motew et al. demonstrated elevated arterial and central venous pressures with minimal change in cardiac output, tachycardia, and acidosis with CO_2 insufflation to a pressure of 20 mmHg in healthy women [20]. When the authors increased the IAP to 30 mmHg, they noted a decrease in central venous return, arterial pressures, and cardiac output. It is a recommendation that the lowest IAP allowing adequate exposure of the operative field be used for laparoscopic procedures [21]. An IAP of lower than 14 is generally considered safe in a healthy patient. In ASA I and II patients, low-pressure pneumoperitoneum appears to minimize adverse effects without compromising laparoscopic feasibility [22]. In older and compromised patients (ASA III and IV), an elevated IAP of 12–15 mmHg showed considerable cardiac alterations in some studies [23, 24]. In these patients, invasive monitoring and adequate volume loading may be necessary to keep cardiac function stable.

In summary, the pressure-related effect of a pneumoperitoneum is a decrease in preload which results in a slight decrease in cardiac output. Pressures of 40 mmHg as used in the above studies are rarely used clinically in establishing a pneumoperitoneum, but it is important for the laparoscopic surgeon to be aware of the pressure-related physiologic changes which occur on the cardiovascular system. The European Association for Endoscopic Surgery practice guidelines have suggested that for intra-abdominal pressures up to 15 mmHg, the decrease in venous return and cardiac output is minimal in healthy patients [21]. At this pressure, adequate volume resuscitation reduces the cardiovascular effects of pneumoperitoneum, which are most pronounced at induction of anesthesia [25].

Effect of CO_2 Absorption and Hypercarbia on the Cardiovascular System

Absorption of CO_2 during pneumoperitoneum causes minimal hypercarbia which leads to a mixed response impact in cardiac function [26]. The direct effect of associated academia on the myocardium and the indirect effect via CO_2 stimulation of the autonomic nervous system have an overall depressant effect on myocardial contractility [9]. Severe hypercarbia stimulates the sympathetic nervous system, with a two- to threefold elevation in plasma catecholamines resulting in a rise in the heart rate and blood pressure, systemic vasoconstriction, and possible cardiac dysrhythmia [27]. Excessive hypercarbia is also detrimental as cardiac work is increased and myocardial oxygen requirement outpaces supply, resulting in potential endocardial ischemia [27]. It is therefore important that end-tidal CO_2 is controlled by adjustment of the minute volume during ventilation.

Effects of Laparoscopy on Renal Perfusion and Function

Urine output is markedly decreased during the insufflation of the abdominal cavity during laparoscopy. Decreased renal vein blood flow and direct renal parenchymal compression mimicking a Page kidney have been shown to be the likely reasons for the oliguric state [28–30]. Changes in antidiuretic hormone (ADH) levels have also been suggested to play a role in the oliguria seen in patients during increased intra-abdominal pressure. Other proposed mechanisms such as ureteral compression, decreased cardiac output, and renal ischemia have not been shown to have a causal role in laparoscopy-associated oliguria [25, 28, 31].

Razvi et al. inflated a pressure cuff to 15 mmHg around the renal parenchyma of six canine kidneys which resulted in a decreased urine output of 63% as well as a decreased GFR and effective renal blood flow. Dunn and McDougall conducted a non-systematic review and concluded that the cause of oliguria was vascular and parenchymal compression, as well as systematic hormonal effects [25, 31]. The decrease in renal blood flow during pneumoperitoneum appears to be pressure dependent. Chiu et al. studied the effects of intra-abdominal pressure on renal tissue perfusion in six pigs comparing a laser Doppler probe placed in the renal parenchyma with a flow probe around the renal artery [29]. The authors reported an almost exponential decrease in renal blood flow with increasing intra-abdominal pressure. With an intra-abdominal pressure of 15 mmHg, the renal blood flow decreased to 25% of baseline.

Bradley et al. studied the effect of raised intra-abdominal pressure on renal plasma flow, glomerular function, and tubular function in 17 normal human subjects [32]. The authors measured renal plasma flow by the diodrast or *p*-aminohippurate (PAH) clearances while GFR was measured by mannitol or insulin clearances. The maximal rate of tubular glucose reabsorption was determined to estimate tubular function and to assess the distribution of filtrate and perfusate to tubular tissue. The pressure within the abdomen was increased by inflating a rubber bladder with air to an intra-abdominal pressure which averaged 20 mmHg. The authors noted that effective renal plasma flow and glomerular filtration rate were always reduced by the effects of increased intra-abdominal pressure by 24 and 27%, respectively. There was no change in the filtration fraction or the percentage of the plasma filtered at the glomerulus and it was noted that the increase in renal venous pressure was sufficient to account for the reduction in plasma flow. Maximum tubular diodrast excretion was reduced significantly in all patients.

Data from trials evaluating the effect of pneumoperitoneum on renal function in randomized clinical trials are also available. Nguyen et al. in a randomized control trial comparing open and laparoscopic gastric bypass reviewed the effects of pneumoperitoneum on renal function [33]. They reported that urine output was decreased in the laparoscopic group, but there were no significant differences in postoperative creatinine levels. The authors concluded that pneumoperitoneum significantly reduced intraoperative urine output, but did not adversely affect postoperative renal function. Similarly, Miki et al. reported a decrease in urine output and effective renal plasma flow in patients undergoing laparoscopic cholecystectomy, but not when an abdominal wall lift device was used instead of pneumoperitoneum [34].

The data suggest that renal blood flow decreases during pneumoperitoneum and that this decrease is pressure dependent. Renal blood flow is worsened in certain positions (head elevated), is improved with hydration, and is not dependent on the gas used. The clinical significance of these findings is not immediately clear as it appears that renal function returns to normal after the pneumoperitoneum is released.

Laparoscopic Surgery and the Systemic Immune Response

The body's acute-phase response to surgical trauma represents a complex interplay between neuroendocrine, metabolic, and immune systems. The inflammatory response to surgical trauma is proportional to the degree of the initial insult and is directed toward host defense [35]. This response is composed of an initial proinflammatory phase characterized by activation of cellular processes designed to restore tissue function and eradicate invading microorganisms, followed by a compensatory anti-inflammatory phase important for preventing excessive proinflammatory activities [36]. The amplitude of this proinflammatory–immunosuppressive cycle also is proportional to the degree of the initial insult. Surgical trauma-induced immune dysfunction results from a disruption of homeostatic mechanisms with effects proportional to the magnitude of the injury. Local injuries of limited duration are usually followed by functional restoration with minimal intervention, while major insults may be associated with an overwhelming inflammatory response which may adversely impact patient survival.

A number of investigators have questioned the effect of laparoscopic techniques on overall markers of immune function [37, 38]. In general, these studies have shown that the systemic immune function is better preserved after laparoscopic surgery when compared with laparotomy. In this section, we will review these studies, outlining the systemic, metabolic, and immune responses to laparoscopic surgery in context of surgery and injury in general. Related issues of injury induced activation of the coagulation cascade; the role of innate immune system and sympathetic nervous system is beyond the scope of this review and will not be discussed here. It is important to understand, however, that these issues are all interrelated and are relevant to a full understanding of the pathophysiology of the response to injury.

Cytokine and Acute-Phase Proteins Response to Injury

Cytokines are soluble mediators of host defense responses that act through paracrine, autocrine, and hemocrine mechanisms to regulate T and B lymphocytes. They comprise a diverse collection of proteins that, by activation of specific cell-surface receptors, regulate many cellular processes, including the immune and inflammatory systems, and differentiation processes such as hematopoiesis and leukopoiesis. This family includes the interleukins (IL), the tumor necrosis factors (TNF-α and -β), the interferons (IFN-α, -β, and -γ), the macrophage and granulocyte colony-stimulating factors (M-CSF/CSF-1, G-CSF, and GM-CSF), and several other molecules. Monocytes, macrophages, and T-helper cells are the most important sources of cytokines, but they are also produced by many other cells, including mast cells, glial cells, fibroblasts, keratinocytes, bone marrow stromal cells, eosinophils, endothelial cells, mesangial cells, and endocrine glands.

Surgical injury to the abdominal viscera has been shown to have a profound influence on the generation of inflammatory mediators and homeostatic responses such as acute-phase protein production. Following acute injury or during infections, TNF-α is among the earliest and most potent mediators of subsequent host responses. Tumor necrosis factor induces marked metabolic and hemodynamic changes and activates mediators distally in the cytokine cascade such as IL-1. Interleukin-1 is primarily released by activated macrophages and endothelial cells. Interleukin-1 induces the classic inflammatory febrile response to injury by stimulating local prostaglandin activity in the anterior hypothalamus.

TNF-α and IL-1 are potent inducers of IL-6 production from virtually all cells and tissues. After injury, IL-6 levels in the circulation are detectable by 60 min, peak between 4 and 6 h, and can persist for as long as 10 days. Circulating IL-6 levels appear to be proportional to the extent of tissue injury during an operation, more so than the duration of the surgical procedure itself. Interleukin-6 regulates the hepatic component of the acute-phase response resulting in the production of acute-phase proteins [39–41]. IL-6 also induces neutrophil activation during injury and inflammation and may delay the disposal of such neutrophils, thereby prolonging the injurious effects mediated by these cells. IL-6 also possesses anti-inflammatory properties during injury by attenuating TNF-α and IL-1 activity while promoting the release of soluble tumor necrosis factor receptors (sTNFR) and IL-1 receptor antagonists. Serum IL-6 levels are early and sensitive markers of tissue damage and rise in proportion to the surgical trauma and associated injury [41]. Alterations in IL-6 levels have also been directly correlated with procedure duration and the amount of blood loss during surgery [42].

The acute-phase proteins are nonspecific biochemical markers produced by hepatocytes in response to tissue injury, infection, or inflammation. C-reactive protein has a physiologic role in the innate immune response to infection and may participate in the clearance of necrotic and apoptotic cells. C-reactive protein is the most widely studied acute-phase protein after surgery. The C-reactive proteins rise approximately 4–12 h after surgery and peak at 24–72 h. Subsequently, C-reactive proteins remain elevated for approximately 2 weeks [42].

Effects of Pneumoperitoneum on Acute-Phase Response and Cytokines

Several investigators have examined how laparoscopic surgery affects the acute-phase response by measuring C-reactive proteins. Squirrell et al. in a prospective randomized trial of laparoscopic versus small incision open cholecystectomy demonstrated significantly lower C-reactive protein levels following laparoscopic cholecystectomy [43]. The C-reactive protein remained significantly elevated at 24 and 48 h in patients with open cholecystectomy compared with those undergoing a laparoscopic procedure. The degree of alteration of C-reactive proteins was noted to be 20-fold after open cholecystectomy but only a 5-fold increase after laparoscopic cholecystectomy. Other studies have shown that although both open and laparoscopic colorectal surgery are associated with elevated plasma CRP levels, there is a more rapid return to baseline preoperative levels following the latter [44]. Many of these studies, however, have shown these differences in the level of inflammatory cytokines to be short lived and most pronounced 1–6 h postoperatively and no longer detectable on postoperative day 2 [45, 46]. These variable results have been attributed to the small size and nonrandomized nature of these studies, the timing of blood collection, and heterogenous population groups.

The acute-phase response after laparoscopic surgery has been studied in several clinical trials measuring IL-6 levels after laparoscopic surgery [47–49]. The outcomes of some clinical and experimental studies tend to show a less impaired systemic immune response after laparoscopic surgery. Schwenk and colleagues in a randomized controlled trial of laparoscopic versus conventional colonic resection demonstrated a postoperative rise of IL-6 in both groups, with a more marked response after open surgery. Duchene reviewed differences in the systemic and cell-specific immune response to open and laparoscopic nephrectomy in the porcine model [50]. The CRP concentration increased more in the open than the laparoscopic groups in the first 48 h ($P = 0.01$). Production of IL-10 decreased in the laparoscopic nephrectomy animals, while increasing after open nephrectomy. The authors concluded that in a porcine model, open nephrectomy caused greater immune suppression than laparoscopic nephrectomy.

Other authors, however, have reported contradictory findings. In a randomized prospective study of primary inguinal hernia repair, no significant differences in postoperative IL-6 levels were detected between laparoscopic and open herniorrhaphy groups. (The authors suggested that this may be due to the fact that overall tissue damage for the open procedure is significantly less than during a formal laparotomy.) Similarly, McMahon showed no significant difference between laparoscopic cholecystectomy and mini-laparotomy cholecystectomy groups [51]. This study found that IL-6 levels in both laparoscopic and mini-cholecystectomy groups were similar to historical reports of standard cholecystectomy levels. Further, Fukushima et al. also reported that IL-6 levels were more elevated after laparoscopic colectomy when compared to open colectomy [52]. The authors suggested that this rise in IL-6 levels may be due to the longer operation time in the laparoscopic group as well as the greater intestinal manipulation inherent to the procedure.

Regarding urologic surgical procedures, Landman et al. prospectively compared the systemic immune and stress response of patients who underwent laparoscopic total nephrectomy and open nephrectomy for renal cell carcinoma [53]. Peripheral venous blood was collected preoperatively and intraoperatively and 24 h, 2 weeks, 4 weeks, and 3 months postoperatively. Blood was analyzed for stress markers (adrenalin, noradrenalin, and cortisol), inflammatory response markers (C-reactive protein, white blood count, and leukocyte count), lymphocytic response markers (CD3, CD4, and CD8), cytokines (interleukin-2 and -4, interferon-alpha, and tumor necrosis factor α), HLA-DR expression and the proliferative response to mitogen stimulation using concanavalin A, phytohemagglutinin 10, and pokeweed mitogen. The authors reported that the inflammatory and stress response markers were statistically similar in both groups at all time points postoperatively. They concluded that the immunological and stress responses after LRN and ON for renal cell carcinoma were without significant difference.

In summary, with some exceptions, the majority of studies suggest that the systemic immune response is less intense following minimally invasive surgery when compared to open surgery. Inherent difficulties exist in assessing the data from available clinical studies due to the unavailability of well-constructed randomized prospective studies.

Cell-Mediated Immunity and the Response to Surgical Trauma

Cell-mediated immunity is central in host defense against intracellular pathogens such as viruses and in combating tumor cells and is also a central part of the immunological response to surgery. The constituents of the cell-mediated immune system include macrophages, which present the antigen to T cells; helper T cells, which participate in antigen recognition and in regulation (helper and suppressor) functions; natural killer (NK) cells, which can inactivate pathogens; and cytotoxic T cells, which can kill virus-infected cells with or without antibody [36].

Surgical trauma is associated with acute impairment of cell-mediated immunity and macrophage function. Impaired postoperative cell-mediated immune functions including decreased delayed-type hypersensitivity responses, downregulation of T-helper type cytokine response as well as decreased lymphocyte proliferation have all been described after open surgery [38, 54, 55]. Major open surgery may further significantly suppress natural killer cell function, cytokine elaboration, neutrophils and lymphocyte chemotaxis, and monocyte human leukocyte antigen (HLA)-DR expression [38, 56, 57]. Surgery also results in defects in immunoregulatory T lymphocytes and natural killer cells and causes a shift in the immunoregulatory helper to suppressor ratio. Dysfunction of the neutrophils and monocytes cell population after surgery-induced immunosuppression may lead to an increased risk of postoperative infection [58].

Effect of Laparoscopy on the Cell-Mediated Inflammatory Response

Several investigators have reviewed the changes in cellular immunity after laparoscopic surgery. Evidence from these studies seems to show that a laparoscopic approach may attenuate the cellular immunosuppression after surgery. Wu et al. reported that postoperative leukocyte counts normalized earlier in patients with colonic carcinoma after laparoscopic colectomy than after open surgery [56].

Neutrophil function has been evaluated by measuring their production of hypochlorous acid. Hypochlorus acid is a product of superoxide anion production involved in the activation of elastase and collagenase and is a central enzyme in microbial killing. Carey et al. showed that hypochlorous acid production fell significantly greater after laparotomy when compared with patients after laparoscopy [58]. The changes in hypochlorous acid production returned to preoperative levels in both groups by the sixth day of surgery. These findings suggest preserved enzymatic activity of neutrophils in laparoscopic patients. Redmond et al. reported an increased monocyte and neutrophil production of superoxide anion in open versus laparoscopic cholecystectomy and showed a correlation between these findings and septic complications in the open group [59]. Similarly, polymorphonuclear elastase has been assayed as an index of neutrophils function after surgery. Neutrophils contain high concentrations of this serine proteinase, which is stored in intracellular vacuoles. The primary role of elastase is to digest any pathogens that the neutrophil has phagocytosed, and it is upregulated with neutrophil activation [40]. Gal et al. [60] found that although elastase levels were similar on the first postoperative day, levels returned to normal by the third day in those who had undergone laparoscopy but remained elevated in those patients who had undergone laparotomy.

Postoperative changes in T-cell function have been studied using the delayed-type hypersensitivity induced by phytohemagglutinin (PHA). Whelan et al. confirmed a better cell-mediated immunity as measured by delayed-type hypersensitivity challenges after laparoscopic colectomy [54]. Kloosterman et al. similarly found that PHA skin testing showed relative anergy after an open but a normal reaction after laparoscopic cholecystectomy [61].

Expression of class II major histocompatibility (MHC-II) molecule, human leukocyte antigen DR (HLA-DR) is essential for mediating specific immune responses in humans [62]. HLA-DR expression shows little variation with age, sex, or race, and as a result, it provides a reliable measure for the relative immunologic capacity of the host. Kloosterman et al. found that HLA-DR expression on monocytes was unimpaired in patients who underwent laparoscopic cholecystectomy [61]. They reported a significant reduction in HLA-DR expression 1 day after conventional surgery, but not after laparoscopy. This would seem to suggest that patients would remain immunocompetent during the early postoperative period, which may be critical in minimizing postoperative infections.

In summary, comparative studies of cellular immunity after laparoscopic and conventional surgery have produced objective evidence of an immunologic advantage conferred by laparoscopy.

Peritoneal Immunity and the Immune Response to Surgery

The normal peritoneal cavity contains less than 100 ml of serous fluid, which is essentially an ultrafiltrate of plasma. It contains fewer than 300 cells/mm^3, mostly macrophages, but with some desquamated mesothelial cells and lymphocytes as well [63]. Peritoneal macrophages are scavengers that play a central role in the local immune response of the peritoneal cavity [64]. The peritoneal cavity is protected by a mechanical system of clearance (diaphragmatic stomas, abscess formation, natural killer cells, polymorphonuclear neutrophils, and macrophages) and a specific immune system mediated by both T- and B-cell lymphocytes.

The cellular response to intraperitoneal inflammation occurs in two phases, an early phase characterized by activation of local macrophages, mast cells, and lymphocytes, followed by a second phase consisting of a rapid influx of neutrophils. Degranulation of peritoneal mast cells releases vasoactive substances (increasing vascular permeability), complement (components of which are chemotactic for macrophages), and opsins. In addition, cytokines secreted by polymorphs upregulate macrophage phagocytic functions. Two proinflammatory cytokines, tumor necrosis factor α (TNF-*a*) and interleukin-1 (IL-1), exhibit increased expression in peritoneal macrophages within hours of peritonitis in an animal model [65]. A similar cytokine response has been documented in humans with the measurement of elevated peritoneal levels of TNF and IL-6 in patients with scheduled repeat laparotomy for peritonitis [66].

Local macrophages are central to the regulation of this acute-phase response and the release of these cytokines within the peritoneum. The number of peritoneal macrophages as well as their capacity for cytokine production is hence important in determining the host's ability to control intraperitoneal infection in the postoperative period. The surgical stress of intra-abdominal surgery can manifest itself in impaired phagocytosis, increased activation of peritoneal macrophages, and increased cytokine production.

Effect of Laparoscopic Surgery on Peritoneal Immunity

Laparotomy has been reported to cause a temporary but significant impairment in both local and systemic macrophage functions [67]. There is mounting evidence, however, that CO_2 laparoscopy may cause less impairment of peritoneal immunity when compared to open surgery. Collet et al. investigated the effect of laparoscopy and laparotomy on peritoneal host defenses in 16 pigs [68]. The authors reported that peritoneal and systemic monocyte class 2 antigen expression and serum TNF activity was greater after laparotomy and that peritoneal bacterial clearance was more efficient in the laparoscopic groups. The authors concluded that there may be a potential immune benefit of laparoscopic surgery, at least in terms of the ability to clear bacterial contamination. Mathew et al. found that peritoneal macrophages harvested from rats that had undergone laparoscopy with CO_2 24 h earlier produced significantly less TNF alpha in vivo than macrophages from rats that had undergone laparoscopy or laparotomy [69]. This response was still present when macrophages were collected 3 days after operation [70]. More recently, Lee et al. evaluated the functions of rat peritoneal macrophages after open and laparoscopically assisted cecum resections [71]. They reported higher levels of TNF-a secreted by stimulated peritoneal macrophages explanted from an open group than from either a laparoscopically assisted group or an anesthesia control group. This increase in macrophage cytokine production after laparotomy demonstrates a significantly stronger inflammatory activation of peritoneal host defenses than that observed after laparoscopy.

The mechanism by which the laparoscopic approach confers a better preservation of peritoneal immunity remains unclear. Studies seem to suggest that a major component of the anti-inflammatory effects of laparoscopic surgery is related to the insufflation of carbon dioxide during the procedure [72]. Carbon dioxide diffuses rapidly into cells and produces intracellular acidification and impaired cellular function and immunomodulation. Swallow et al. showed that intracellular acidification resulted in a pH-dependent inhibition of H+ ATPase activity as well as superoxide production in peritoneal macrophages [73]. West et al. suspended peritoneal macrophages in medium and bubbled air, CO_2, or helium (as an anoxic control) for 1 h [74]. Cells were then resuspended in fresh medium and stimulated with endotoxin. CO_2 exposure caused near-complete inhibition of TNF compared to room air, and helium, which had little effect. Human macrophages also have been shown to produce less TNF-a when placed in a hypercapnic environment [75]. In this study, Kopernik and colleagues showed that CO_2 blocked the superoxide release from activated polymorphonuclear leukocytes and significantly reduced the secretion of IL-1 from human peritoneal macrophages [75].

While these effects on macrophages may be beneficial in elective surgery, concern has arisen on this effect on macrophages in the setting of infection [76]. In a study by Chekan et al., the immune competence of mice, based on their ability to clear intraperitoneally administered *Listeria monocytogenes* following CO_2 vs. helium (He) insufflation, was tested. Eighty-five mice were divided between the following four treatment groups: CO_2 insufflation, helium insufflation, abdominal laparotomy, and control (anesthesia only). Immediately postoperatively, each group was inoculated percutaneously and intraperitoneally with a sublethal dose of virulent *L. monocytogenes*. Half of the animals were killed on postoperative day 3 and half on day 5. Spleens and livers (sites of bacterial predilection) were harvested, homogenized, and plated on TSB agar. The laparoscopic group (3.44×10^6 LM/spleen and liver) had significantly more bacteria than the controls. There were no significant differences between any of the groups on day 5. The clinical significance of this finding remains unknown. In studies where laparoscopy was compared to open surgery for peritoneal infection such as appendicitis, there was no clear increase of infectious complications associated with the use of CO_2 pneumoperitoneum [77].

In summary, studies seem to suggest that laparoscopic surgery better preserves peritoneal macrophage number and viability, improves bacterial clearance, and stimulates cytokine production in a manner less so than patients at laparotomy. As a result, the laparoscopic approach appears to be advantageous to peritoneal host defenses, as compared with open surgery.

Laparoscopy and Tumor Immunity

Primary tumor growth rates have been shown to be influenced by the degree of operative trauma [78]. Laparoscopy may cause less suppression of immune function and therefore be less likely to facilitate tumor growth [68]. The application of laparoscopy for cancer surgery, however, remains controversial, with concerns remaining about the potential for laparoscopic approaches to compromise longer term outcomes [79]. Port-site metastases, a phenomenon of tumor implantation at the port of entry of the laparoscopic trocar, has been one such area of concern.

Studies have shown immunosuppression after laparotomy tends to be more severe and prolonged in patients with cancer [80]. Wu et al. found that postoperative leukocyte counts and leukocyte subpopulations normalized earlier in patients with colonic carcinoma after laparoscopic colectomy than after open surgery [56]. In addition, on postoperative day 4, monocyte HLA-DR expression was more suppressed in the open colectomy group than in the laparoscopic group. This reduced monocyte HLA-DR expression causes suppressed antigen presentation capacity which, in turn, may increase patient susceptibility to infection and impair tumor immunosurveillance. It appears that decreasing perioperative stress and reducing immune system activation may affect tumor dissemination and growth. As a result, the laparoscopic approach may be particularly beneficial for oncologic patients.

A number of experimental studies have investigated the role of laparoscopy on tumor growth. Southall et al. injected B16 melanoma cell lines into the dorsal skin of a mouse model. The mice were subsequently subjected to pneumoperitoneum, laparotomy, or no procedure [81]. Larger and more readily established tumors were found in animals that had undergone laparotomy rather than laparoscopic or sham procedures. In a similar study, Da Costa et al. subjected mice to laparotomy or laparoscopy after a flank injection of B16 melanoma cells [82]. Significant increases in flank tumor growth were seen in the laparotomy group during the second 48 h after surgery.

Reservations have been raised as to the applicability of laparoscopy for cancer patients. Concerns exist for potential inadequate exploration of the abdominal cavity and reduced accessibility of the tumor mass, and the potential for violations of surgical oncologic principles has been cited [47]. In addition, earlier reports suggested an increased incidence of port-site recurrences and tumor dissemination as well as reduced survival and higher recurrence rates [62].

At present, there are no randomized studies available in the urologic literature comparing laparoscopic and open oncologic procedures. A comparative study of open and laparoscopic radical nephrectomy for renal cell carcinoma of similar grade and stage showed equal cancer control for both groups (mean follow-up period was 35 months for the laparoscopic group and 44 months for the open group) [83]. Makhoul et al. published similar findings for T1 renal cell carcinoma [84]. McNeill et al. reviewed the oncological effectiveness and outcome of laparoscopic nephroureterectomy [85], which determined that there was no increase in positive surgical margins, or extravesical or port-site recurrence, compared with open surgery, and that long-term survival was equivalent. These results and others confirm the oncologic safety of laparoscopic resection of urological cancer.

Port-Site Metastases

Tumor seeding after open and laparoscopic surgery is a potential risk and has been reported in general surgery literature. The incidence of port-site metastases in general laparoscopic surgery is reported to be between 0.8 and 21% [86]. The first report of urological tumor seeding occurred after a laparoscopic lymphadenectomy for bladder cancer [87]. Subsequently, Bangma et al. noted a 0.1% rate of port-site metastases in laparoscopic pelvic lymph node dissection, while an incidence of 0–6.25% has been reported after laparoscopic radical nephrectomy [88, 89]. Metastases typically present as hard, painful nodules at the previous site of one or more of the laparoscopic cannulas [90]. Kruitwagen et al. assessed the effect of port-site metastasis on patient survival and confirmed that the presence of a metastasis at the site of a trocar or paracentesis access wound correlated adversely with survival [91]. By comparison, the incidence of incisional scar metastases after open radical nephrectomy for renal cell carcinoma is 0.4% [92].

Experimental and clinical studies of tumor seeding indicate multiple potential etiologies including aerosolization of tumor cells, instrument contamination or tumor spillage during dissection/extraction, and preexisting peritoneal tumor cells [93]. Violation of the primary tumor boundaries or damage of tumor-bearing lymph nodes may promote tumor cells dissemination.

Local factors at the sites of port placement may also contribute to the localization of tumor metastases. It has been shown that tumor preferentially spreads to recently traumatized tissues and that malignant cells tend to grow easily in areas of high cellular proliferation [78]. While the intact peritoneum is resistant to tumor cell implantation the port site provides a localized peritoneal breach and an area of high cellular proliferation associated with the healing wound. Pneumoperitoneum-related factors may also contribute. Nduka et al. have suggested that the pneumoperitoneum acts as a closed system through which airborne particulate matter must circulate, whereas during open surgery this particulate matter tends to be drawn away by the theatre ventilation system [90]. The rate of seeding has been shown to vary with the tumor type, with a higher incidence of seeding related to highly aggressive tumors [94].

There have been few reports of port-site metastases in the urological literature. Castilho et al. reported two cases of abdominal wall metastases after laparoscopic radical nephrectomy for a clinical stage T1N0M0 renal cell carcinoma and low Fuhrman grade [95]. The specimen was retrieved by mechanical morcellation in a plastic bag and not a bag specifically designed for morcellation. In the other case reported in this series, there was the presence of ascites at surgery, which may have already contained malignant tumor cells. Barrett et al. reported a port-site recurrence after laparoscopic nephrectomy in a patient with T3N0M0 grade IV renal cell carcinoma (and an 862 g pathological specimen) at 25-month follow-up [96]. The specimen had been entrapped in the Cook Lap Sac and fragmented with the Cook electrical mechanical morcellation (Cook Urological, Inc., Spencer, Indiana). This specimen was large and weighed 862 g and had an aggressive Fuhrman grade IV/IV with sarcomatoid elements which may have contributed to risk.

In summary, it is likely that the mechanism of wound metastasis is multifactorial. Laparoscopy can result in the mechanical redistribution of tumor cells directly by spread from contaminated instruments and indirectly due to the mechanical effect of the insufflation gas. Metabolic and immunological factors specific to carbon dioxide insufflation, acting locally at the port site, may also be important. The use of a plastic bag for specimen retrieval is an important method of avoiding contact between malignant tissue and peritoneum or subcutaneous tissue, and morcellation should be performed only in an organ entrapment sac designed for this purpose.

Renal Function Complications Following Laparoscopic Renal Surgery

Long-term renal function is clearly a dramatically important parameter when embarking upon renal surgery. Both total and partial nephrectomies will decrease the overall number of nephrons, but there is additional concern regarding the potential implications when temporary ischemia is used for hemostatic control during partial nephrectomy.

Uzzo and Novick reported on a review of the literature comparing cancer control for partial vs. total nephrectomy and concluded that, stage for stage, equivalent cancer control was possible in each approach [97]. Zincke et al. confirmed equivalent cancer cure, but described a significant difference between partial and total nephrectomies as far as future renal function was concerned: There was progression of renal insufficiency (defined as serum creatinine > 2.0) in 11% of patients who underwent partial nephrectomy vs. 22% of patients undergoing radical nephrectomy [98]. Using the more precise measurement of glomerular filtration rate (GFR), Hwang et al. reported that the 3-year probability of freedom from decline of GFR below 60 was 80% after partial nephrectomy, but only 35% after radical nephrectomy [99].

Laparoscopic partial nephrectomy is a viable technique for localized tumor management developed with, among concerns regarding oncologic cure, also a concern regarding the preservation of maximal function. Godoy et al. suggest, based on a review of 101 patients undergoing laparoscopic partial nephrectomy, that the greatest significant changes occur after warm ischemia time (WIT) of greater than 40 min [100]. Techniques to reduce WIT have been described and continue to be explored [101, 102].

Lifshitz et al. have recently reported on predictors for prolonged warm ischemia time (WIT) during laparoscopic partial nephrectomy. Their study suggests that central tumor location, tumor size greater than 4 cm, and Body Mass Index (BMI) greater than 30 kg/m^2 are independent predictors of WIT greater than 30 min and created a nomogram with 75.4% accuracy [103].

Overall, however, the impact of WIT on renal function appears to be primarily in the acute postoperative period, with no significant GFR changes noted at approximately 1 year postoperative, except in patients with underlying medical renal disease [104].

Therefore, partial nephrectomy, when feasible, offers greater security from progression of renal failure, particularly in the setting of such comorbidities as smoking, hypertension, diabetes mellitus, obesity, hypercholesterolemia, and vascular disease. However, prolonged warm ischemia time during laparoscopic partial nephrectomy can negatively impact on postoperative renal function and should clearly be minimized as much as possible.

Conclusion

Minimally invasive surgery has several short-term benefits including early mobilization, shorter hospital stay, and less pain. Various gases have been used for maintenance of a pneumoperitoneum with CO_2 used most often due to its predictable effects and overall safety. It is important that the operating surgeon be familiar with the physiologic consequences of laparoscopy and is aware of strategies to prevent complications. The physiologic effects of laparoscopy are related to the intra-abdominal pressure, the type of gas insufflated as well as the position of the patient. Minimizing intra-abdominal pressure during insufflation decreases the risk of perioperative myocardial and renal events or organ dysfunction. At the cellular level, laparoscopy may be associated with preservation of the systemic immune response with attenuation of peritoneal immunity at the level of macrophages.

References

1. Wolfe BM, Gardiner B, Frey CF. Laparoscopic cholecystectomy. A remarkable development. JAMA. 1991 Mar 27;265(12):1573–4.
2. Barrett KE, Barman SM, Boitano S, Brooks H. Chapter 36: Gas transport & pH in the lung. In: Barrett KE, Barman SM, Boitano S, Brooks H, editors. Ganong's review of medical physiology, 23rd ed., McGraw-Hill Companies.
3. Barrett KE, Barman SM, Boitano S, Brooks H. Goodman and gilman's the pharmacological basis of therapeutics. In: Barrett KE, Barman SM, Boitano S, Brooks H, editors. Ganong's review of medical physiology. 23rd ed.
4. Robinson JS, Thompson JM, Wood AW. Letter: laparoscopy explosion hazards with nitrous oxide. Br Med J. 1975 Sep 27;3(5986):764–5.
5. El-Kady AA, Abd-El-Razek M. Intraperitoneal explosion during female sterilization by laparoscopic electrocoagulation. A case report. Int J Gynaecol Obstet. 1976;14(6):487–8.
6. Johannsen G, Andersen M, Juhl B. The effect of general anaesthesia on the haemodynamic events during laparoscopy with CO_2-insufflation. Acta Anaesthesiol Scand. 1989 Feb;33(2):132–6.
7. Wittgen CM, Andrus CH, Fitzgerald SD, Baudendistel LJ, Dahms TE, Kaminski DL. Analysis of the hemodynamic and ventilatory effects of laparoscopic cholecystectomy. Arch Surg. 1991 Aug;126(8):997–1000; discussion 1000–1.
8. Liu SY, Leighton T, Davis I, Klein S, Lippmann M, Bongard F. Prospective analysis of cardiopulmonary responses to laparoscopic cholecystectomy. J Laparoendosc Surg. 1991 Oct;1(5):241–6.
9. Ho HS, Saunders CJ, Gunther RA, Wolfe BM. Effector of hemodynamics during laparoscopy: CO_2 absorption or intra-abdominal pressure? J Surg Res. 1995 Oct;59(4):497–503.
10. Leighton T, Pianim N, Liu SY, Kono M, Klein S, Bongard F. Effectors of hypercarbia during experimental pneumoperitoneum. Am Surg. 1992 Dec;58(12):717–21.
11. Callery MP, Soper NJ. Physiology of the pneumoperitoneum. Baillieres Clin Gastroenterol. 1993 Dec;7(4):757–77.
12. Ciofolo MJ, Clergue F, Seebacher J, Lefebvre G, Viars P. Ventilatory effects of laparoscopy under epidural anesthesia. Anesth Analg. 1990 Apr;70(4):357–61.
13. Ivankovich AD, Albrecht RF, Zahed B, Bonnet RF. Cardiovascular collapse during gynecological laparoscopy. IMJ Ill Med J. 1974 Jan;145(1):58, 61 passim.
14. Williams MD, Sulentich SM, Murr PC. Laparoscopic cholecystectomy produces less postoperative restriction of pulmonary function than open cholecystectomy. Surg Endosc. 1993 Nov–Dec;7(6):489–92; discussion 493.
15. Cunningham AJ. Myocardial ischemia – association with perioperative cardiac morbidity. Yale J Biol Med. 1993 Sep–Oct;66(5):339–48.
16. Ortega AE, Richman MF, Hernandez M, Peters JH, Anthone GJ, Azen S, et al. Inferior vena caval blood

flow and cardiac hemodynamics during carbon dioxide pneumoperitoneum. Surg Endosc. 1996 Sep;10(9):920–4.
17. Kashtan J, Green JF, Parsons EQ, Holcroft JW. Hemodynamic effect of increased abdominal pressure. J Surg Res. 1981 Mar;30(3):249–55.
18. Rubinson RM, Vasko JS, Doppman JL, Morrow AG. Inferior vena caval obstruction from increased intra-abdominal pressure. Experimental hemodynamic and angiographic observations. Arch Surg. 1967 Jun;94(6):766–70.
19. Dexter SP, Vucevic M, Gibson J, McMahon MJ. Hemodynamic consequences of high- and low-pressure capnoperitoneum during laparoscopic cholecystectomy. Surg Endosc. 1999 Apr;13(4):376–81.
20. Motew M, Ivankovich AD, Bieniarz J, Albrecht RF, Zahed B, Scommegna A. Cardiovascular effects and acid-base and blood gas changes during laparoscopy. Am J Obstet Gynecol. 1973 Apr 1;115(7):1002–12.
21. Neudecker J, Sauerland S, Neugebauer E, Bergamaschi R, Bonjer HJ, Cuschieri A, et al. The European association for endoscopic surgery clinical practice guideline on the pneumoperitoneum for laparoscopic surgery. Surg Endosc. 2002 Jul;16(7):1121–43.
22. Popesco D, Le Miere E, Maitre B, Darchy B, Domart Y. Coronary gas embolism after laparoscopic surgery. Ann Fr Anesth Reanim. 1997;16(4):381–5.
23. Dhoste K, Lacoste L, Karayan J, Lehuede MS, Thomas D, Fusciardi J. Haemodynamic and ventilatory changes during laparoscopic cholecystectomy in elderly ASA III patients. Can J Anaesth. 1996 Aug;43(8): 783–8.
24. Frank SM, Fleisher LA, Breslow MJ, Higgins MS, Olson KF, Kelly S, et al. Perioperative maintenance of normothermia reduces the incidence of morbid cardiac events. A randomized clinical trial. JAMA. 1997 Apr 9;277(14):1127–34.
25. Harman PK, Kron IL, McLachlan HD, Freedlender AE, Nolan SP. Elevated intra-abdominal pressure and renal function. Ann Surg. 1982 Nov;196(5):594–7.
26. Safran DB, Orlando R 3rd. Physiologic effects of pneumoperitoneum. Am J Surg. 1994 Feb;167(2): 281–6.
27. Rasmussen JP, Dauchot PJ, DePalma RG, Sorensen B, Regula G, Anton AH, et al. Cardiac function and hypercarbia. Arch Surg. 1978 Oct;113(10):1196–200.
28. McDougall EM, Monk TG, Wolf JS Jr, Hicks M, Clayman RV, Gardner S, et al. The effect of prolonged pneumoperitoneum on renal function in an animal model. J Am Coll Surg. 1996 Apr;182(4):317–28.
29. Chiu AW, Azadzoi KM, Hatzichristou DG, Siroky MB, Krane RJ, Babayan RK. Effects of intra-abdominal pressure on renal tissue perfusion during laparoscopy. J Endourol. 1994 Apr;8(2):99–103.
30. Razvi HA, Fields D, Vargas JC, Vaughan ED Jr, Vukasin A, Sosa RE. Oliguria during laparoscopic surgery: evidence for direct renal parenchymal compression as an etiologic factor. J Endourol. 1996 Feb;10(1):1–4.
31. Kirsch AJ, Hensle TW, Chang DT, Kayton ML, Olsson CA, Sawczuk IS. Renal effects of CO_2 insufflation: Oliguria and acute renal dysfunction in a rat pneumoperitoneum model. Urology. 1994 Apr;43(4):453–9.
32. Bradley SE, Bradley GP. The effect of increased intra-abdominal pressure on renal function in man. J Clin Invest. 1947 Sep;26(5):1010–22.
33. Nguyen NT, Perez RV, Fleming N, Rivers R, Wolfe BM. Effect of prolonged pneumoperitoneum on intraoperative urine output during laparoscopic gastric bypass. J Am Coll Surg. 2002 Oct;195(4):476–83.
34. Miki Y, Iwase K, Kamiike W, Taniguchi E, Sakaguchi K, Sumimura J, et al. Laparoscopic cholecystectomy and time-course changes in renal function. The effect of the retraction method on renal function. Surg Endosc. 1997 Aug;11(8):838–41.
35. Davies MG, Hagen PO. Systemic inflammatory response syndrome. Br J Surg. 1997 Jul;84(7):920–35.
36. Ni Choileain N, Redmond HP. Cell response to surgery. Arch Surg. 2006 Nov;141(11):1132–40.
37. Daphan CE, Agalar F, Hascelik G, Onat D, Sayek I. Effects of laparotomy, and carbon dioxide and air pneumoperitoneum, on cellular immunity and peritoneal host defences in rats. Eur J Surg. 1999 Mar;165(3): 253–8.
38. Vittimberga FJ Jr, Foley DP, Meyers WC, Callery MP. Laparoscopic surgery and the systemic immune response. Ann Surg. 1998 Mar;227(3):326–34.
39. Perlmutter DH, Dinarello CA, Punsal PI, Colten HR. Cachectin/tumor necrosis factor regulates hepatic acute-phase gene expression. J Clin Invest. 1986 Nov;78(5):1349–54.
40. Pullicino EA, Carli F, Poole S, Rafferty B, Malik ST, Elia M. The relationship between the circulating concentrations of interleukin 6 (IL-6), tumor necrosis factor (TNF) and the acute phase response to elective surgery and accidental injury. Lymphokine Res. 1990 Summer;9(2): 231–8.
41. Cruickshank AM, Fraser WD, Burns HJ, Van Damme J, Shenkin A. Response of serum interleukin-6 in patients undergoing elective surgery of varying severity. Clin Sci (Lond). 1990 Aug;79(2):161–5.
42. Ohzato H, Yoshizaki K, Nishimoto N, Ogata A, Tagoh H, Monden M, et al. Interleukin-6 as a new indicator of inflammatory status: detection of serum levels of interleukin-6 and C-reactive protein after surgery. Surgery. 1992 Feb;111(2):201–9.
43. Squirrell DM, Majeed AW, Troy G, Peacock JE, Nicholl JP, Johnson AG. A randomized, prospective, blinded comparison of postoperative pain, metabolic response, and perceived health after laparoscopic and small incision cholecystectomy. Surgery. 1998 May;123(5):485–95.
44. Braga M, Vignali A, Zuliani W, Radaelli G, Gianotti L, Martani C, et al. Metabolic and functional results after laparoscopic colorectal surgery: a randomized, controlled trial. Dis Colon Rectum. 2002 Aug;45(8):1070–7.
45. Schietroma M, Carlei F, Franchi L, Mazzotta C, Sozio A, Lygidakis NJ, et al. A comparison of serum interleukin-6 concentrations in patients treated by cholecystectomy via laparotomy or laparoscopy. Hepatogastroenterology. 2004 Nov–Dec;51(60):1595–9.
46. Ordemann J, Jacobi CA, Schwenk W, Stosslein R, Muller JM. Cellular and humoral inflammatory response after laparoscopic and conventional colorectal resections. Surg Endosc. 2001 Jun;15(6):600–8.

47. Schwenk W, Jacobi C, Mansmann U, Bohm B, Muller JM. Inflammatory response after laparoscopic and conventional colorectal resections – results of a prospective randomized trial. Langenbecks Arch Surg. 2000 Jan;385(1):2–9.
48. Glaser F, Sannwald GA, Buhr HJ, Kuntz C, Mayer H, Klee F, et al. General stress response to conventional and laparoscopic cholecystectomy. Ann Surg. 1995 Apr;221(4):372–80.
49. Joris J, Cigarini I, Legrand M, Jacquet N, De Groote D, Franchimont P, et al. Metabolic and respiratory changes after cholecystectomy performed via laparotomy or laparoscopy. Br J Anaesth. 1992 Oct;69(4): 341–5.
50. Duchene DA, Gallagher BL, Ratliff TL, Winfield HN. Systemic and cell-specific immune response to laparoscopic and open nephrectomy in porcine model. J Endourol. 2008 Jan;22(1):113–20.
51. McMahon AJ, O'Dwyer PJ, Cruikshank AM, McMillan DC, O'Reilly DS, Lowe GD, et al. Comparison of metabolic responses to laparoscopic and minilaparotomy cholecystectomy. Br J Surg. 1993 Oct;80(10):1255–8.
52. Fukushima R, Kawamura YJ, Saito H, Saito Y, Hashiguchi Y, Sawada T, et al. Interleukin-6 and stress hormone responses after uncomplicated gasless laparoscopic-assisted and open sigmoid colectomy. Dis Colon Rectum. 1996 Oct;39 Suppl 10:S29–34.
53. Landman J, Olweny E, Sundaram CP, Chen C, Rehman J, Lee DI, et al. Prospective comparison of the immunological and stress response following laparoscopic and open surgery for localized renal cell carcinoma. J Urol. 2004 Apr;171(4):1456–60.
54. Whelan RL, Franklin M, Holubar SD, Donahue J, Fowler R, Munger C, et al. Postoperative cell mediated immune response is better preserved after laparoscopic vs. open colorectal resection in humans. Surg Endosc. 2003 Jun;17(6):972–8.
55. Brune IB, Wilke W, Hensler T, Holzmann B, Siewert JR. Downregulation of T helper type 1 immune response and altered pro-inflammatory and anti-inflammatory T cell cytokine balance following conventional but not laparoscopic surgery. Am J Surg. 1999 Jan;177(1):55–60.
56. Wu FP, Sietses C, von Blomberg BM, van Leeuwen PA, Meijer S, Cuesta MA. Systemic and peritoneal inflammatory response after laparoscopic or conventional colon resection in cancer patients: a prospective, randomized trial. Dis Colon Rectum. 2003 Feb;46(2):147–55.
57. Hewitt PM, Ip SM, Kwok SP, Somers SS, Li K, Leung KL, et al. Laparoscopic-assisted vs. open surgery for colorectal cancer: comparative study of immune effects. Dis Colon Rectum. 1998 Jul;41(7):901–9.
58. Carey PD, Wakefield CH, Thayeb A, Monson JR, Darzi A, Guillou PJ. Effects of minimally invasive surgery on hypochlorous acid production by neutrophils. Br J Surg. 1994 Apr;81(4):557–60.
59. Redmond HP, Watson RW, Houghton T, Condron C, Watson RG, Bouchier-Hayes D. Immune function in patients undergoing open vs. laparoscopic cholecystectomy. Arch Surg. 1994 Dec;129(12):1240–6.
60. Gal I, Roth E, Lantos J, Varga G, Jaberansari MT. Inflammatory mediators and surgical trauma regarding laparoscopic access: free radical mediated reactions. Acta Chir Hung. 1997;36(1–4):97–9.
61. Kloosterman T, von Blomberg BM, Borgstein P, Cuesta MA, Scheper RJ, Meijer S. Unimpaired immune functions after laparoscopic cholecystectomy. Surgery. 1994 Apr;115(4):424–8.
62. Novitsky YW, Litwin DE, Callery MP. The net immunologic advantage of laparoscopic surgery. Surg Endosc. 2004 Oct;18(10):1411–9.
63. Neuhaus SJ, Watson DI. Pneumoperitoneum and peritoneal surface changes: a review. Surg Endosc. 2004 Sep;18(9):1316–22.
64. Iwanaka T, Arkovitz MS, Arya G, Ziegler MM. Evaluation of operative stress and peritoneal macrophage function in minimally invasive operations. J Am Coll Surg. 1997 Apr;184(4):357–63.
65. McMasters KM, Cheadle WG. Regulation of macrophage TNF alpha, IL-1 beta, and ia (I-A alpha) mRNA expression during peritonitis is site dependent. J Surg Res. 1993 May;54(5):426–30.
66. Holzheimer RG, Schein M, Wittmann DH. Inflammatory response in peritoneal exudate and plasma of patients undergoing planned relaparotomy for severe secondary peritonitis. Arch Surg. 1995 Dec;130(12):1314–9; discussion 1319–20.
67. Redmond HP, Hofmann K, Shou J, Leon P, Kelly CJ, Daly JM. Effects of laparotomy on systemic macrophage function. Surgery. 1992 Jun;111(6):647–55.
68. Collet D, Vitale GC, Reynolds M, Klar E, Cheadle WG. Peritoneal host defenses are less impaired by laparoscopy than by open operation. Surg Endosc. 1995 Oct;9(10):1059–64.
69. Mathew G, Watson DI, Ellis TS, Jamieson GG, Rofe AM. The role of peritoneal immunity and the tumour-bearing state on the development of wound and peritoneal metastases after laparoscopy. Aust N Z J Surg. 1999 Jan;69(1):14–8.
70. Neuhaus SJ, Watson DI, Ellis T, Rofe AM, Mathew G, Jamieson GG. Influence of gases on intraperitoneal immunity during laparoscopy in tumor-bearing rats. World J Surg. 2000 Oct;24(10):1227–31.
71. Lee SW, Feingold DL, Carter JJ, Zhai C, Stapleton G, Gleason N, et al. Peritoneal macrophage and blood monocyte functions after open and laparoscopic-assisted cecectomy in rats. Surg Endosc. 2003 Dec;17(12): 1996–2002.
72. Rotstein OD. Peritoneal host defenses: modulation by carbon dioxide insufflation. Surg Infect (Larchmt). 2001 Summer;2(2):163–8; discussion 168–70.
73. Swallow CJ, Grinstein S, Sudsbury RA, Rotstein OD. Relative roles of Na+/H+ exchange and vacuolar-type H+ ATPases in regulating cytoplasmic pH and function in murine peritoneal macrophages. J Cell Physiol. 1993 Dec;157(3):453–60.
74. West MA, Hackam DJ, Baker J, Rodriguez JL, Bellingham J, Rotstein OD. Mechanism of decreased in vitro murine macrophage cytokine release after exposure to carbon dioxide: relevance to laparoscopic surgery. Ann Surg. 1997 Aug;226(2):179–90.
75. Kopernik G, Avinoach E, Grossman Y, Levy R, Yulzari R, Rogachev B, et al. The effect of a high partial pressure of

carbon dioxide environment on metabolism and immune functions of human peritoneal cells-relevance to carbon dioxide pneumoperitoneum. Am J Obstet Gynecol. 1998 Dec;179(6 Pt 1):1503–10.
76. Chekan EG, Nataraj C, Clary EM, Hayward TZ, Brody FJ, Stamat JC, et al. Intraperitoneal immunity and pneumoperitoneum. Surg Endosc. 1999 Nov;13(11): 1135–8.
77. Temple LK, Litwin DE, McLeod RS. A meta-analysis of laparoscopic versus open appendectomy in patients suspected of having acute appendicitis. Can J Surg. 1999 Oct;42(5):377–83.
78. Murthy MS, Travis JD, Scanlon EF. Factors influencing the growth and metastatic behavior of tumors. J Surg Oncol. 1987 May;35(1):44–9.
79. Rassweiler J, Tsivian A, Kumar AV, Lymberakis C, Schulze M, Seeman O, et al. Oncological safety of laparoscopic surgery for urological malignancy: experience with more than 1,000 operations. J Urol. 2003 Jun;169(6):2072–5.
80. Berti Riboli E, Terrizzi A, Arnulfo G, Bertoglio S. Immunosuppressive effect of surgery evaluated by the multitest cell-mediated immunity system. Can J Surg. 1984 Jan;27(1):60–3.
81. Southall JC, Lee SW, Allendorf JD, Bessler M, Whelan RL. Colon adenocarcinoma and B-16 melanoma grow larger following laparotomy vs. pneumoperitoneum in a murine model. Dis Colon Rectum. 1998 May;41(5): 564–9.
82. Da Costa ML, Redmond HP, Finnegan N, Flynn M, Bouchier-Hayes D. Laparotomy and laparoscopy differentially accelerate experimental flank tumour growth. Br J Surg. 1998 Oct;85(10):1439–42.
83. Chan DY, Cadeddu JA, Jarrett TW, Marshall FF, Kavoussi LR. Laparoscopic radical nephrectomy: cancer control for renal cell carcinoma. J Urol. 2001 Dec;166(6):2095–9; discussion 2099–100.
84. Makhoul B, De La Taille A, Vordos D, Salomon L, Sebe P, Audet JF, et al. Laparoscopic radical nephrectomy for T1 renal cancer: the gold standard? A comparison of laparoscopic vs. open nephrectomy. BJU Int. 2004 Jan;93(1): 67–70.
85. McNeill A, Oakley N, Tolley DA, Gill IS. Laparoscopic nephroureterectomy for upper tract transitional cell carcinoma: a critical appraisal. BJU Int. 2004 Aug;94(3): 259–63.
86. Tsivian A, Sidi AA. Port site metastases in urological laparoscopic surgery. J Urol. 2003 Apr;169(4): 1213–8.
87. Stolla V, Rossi D, Bladou F, Rattier C, Ayuso D, Serment G. Subcutaneous metastases after coelioscopic lymphadenectomy for vesical urothelial carcinoma. Eur Urol. 1994;26(4):342–3.
88. Bangma CH, Kirkels WJ, Chadha S, Schroder FH. Cutaneous metastasis following laparoscopic pelvic lymphadenectomy for prostatic carcinoma. J Urol. 1995 May;153(5):1635–6.
89. Dunn MD, Portis AJ, Shalhav AL, Elbahnasy AM, Heidorn C, McDougall EM, et al. Laparoscopic versus open radical nephrectomy: a 9-year experience. J Urol. 2000 Oct;164(4):1153–9.
90. Nduka CC, Monson JR, Menzies-Gow N, Darzi A. Abdominal wall metastases following laparoscopy. Br J Surg. 1994 May;81(5):648–52.
91. Kruitwagen RF, Swinkels BM, Keyser KG, Doesburg WH, Schijf CP. Incidence and effect on survival of abdominal wall metastases at trocar or puncture sites following laparoscopy or paracentesis in women with ovarian cancer. Gynecol Oncol. 1996 Feb;60(2): 233–7.
92. Uson AC. Tumor recurrence in the renal fossa and/or the abdominal wall after radical nephrectomy for renal cell carcinoma. Prog Clin Biol Res. 1982;100: 549–60.
93. Doudle M, King G, Thomas WM, Hewett P. The movement of mucosal cells of the gallbladder within the peritoneal cavity during laparoscopic cholecystectomy. Surg Endosc. 1996 Nov;10(11):1092–4.
94. Micali S, Celia A, Bove P, De Stefani S, Sighinolfi MC, Kavoussi LR, et al. Tumor seeding in urological laparoscopy: an international survey. J Urol. 2004 Jun;171(6 Pt 1):2151–4.
95. Castilho LN, Fugita OE, Mitre AI, Arap S. Port site tumor recurrences of renal cell carcinoma after videolaparoscopic radical nephrectomy. J Urol. 2001 Feb;165 (2):519.
96. Barrett PH, Fentie DD, Taranger LA. Laparoscopic radical nephrectomy with morcellation for renal cell carcinoma: the saskatoon experience. Urology. 1998 Jul;52(1): 23–8.
97. Uzzo RG, Novick AC. Nephron sparing surgery for renal tumors: indications, techniques and outcomes. J Urol. 2001 Jul;166(1):6–18.
98. Leibovich BC, Blute ML, Cheville JC, Lohse CM, Weaver AL, Zincke H. Nephron sparing surgery for appropriately selected renal cell carcinoma between 4 and 7 cm results in outcome similar to radical nephrectomy. J Urol. 2004 Mar;171(3):1066–70.
99. Huang WC, Levey AS, Serio AM, Snyder M, Vickers AJ, Raj GV, et al. Chronic kidney disease after nephrectomy in patients with renal cortical tumours: a retrospective cohort study. Lancet Oncol. 2006 Sep;7(9):735–40.
100. Godoy G, Ramanathan V, Kanofsky JA, O'Malley RL, Tareen BU, Taneja SS, et al. Effect of warm ischemia time during laparoscopic partial nephrectomy on early postoperative glomerular filtration rate. J Urol. 2009 Jun;181(6):2438–43; discussion 2443–5.
101. Nguyen MM, Gill IS. Halving ischemia time during laparoscopic partial nephrectomy. J Urol. 2008 Feb;179(2):627–32; discussion 632.
102. Bollens R, Rosenblatt A, Espinoza BP, De Groote A, Quackels T, Roumeguere T, et al. Laparoscopic partial nephrectomy with "on-demand" clamping reduces warm ischemia time. Eur Urol. 2007 Sep;52(3):804–9.
103. Lifshitz DA, Shikanov S, Jeldres C, Deklaj T, Karakiewicz PI, Zorn KC, et al. Laparoscopic partial nephrectomy: predictors of prolonged warm ischemia. J Urol. 2009 Sep;182(3):860–5.
104. Foyil KV, Ames CD, Ferguson GG, Weld KJ, Figenshau RS, Venkatesh R, et al. Longterm changes in creatinine clearance after laparoscopic renal surgery. J Am Coll Surg. 2008 Mar;206(3):511–5.

Positional and Neuromuscular Complications of Laparoscopic and Robotic Urologic Surgery

Ricardo A. Natalin and Jaime Landman

Keywords Injury · Neuromuscular · Complications · Laparoscopy

Introduction

Laparoscopic technique is being increasingly applied to urologic pathology. With the majority of urologic procedures, the laparoscopic approach provides our patients with excellent outcomes which are achieved with less pain and an expedited convalescence when compared to open surgery. Undoubtedly, with the increasing use of laparoscopy, we will also see an increase in the number of laparoscopic complications. Recently a large multicenter review of 2775 laparoscopic procedures reported that the most common laparoscopic complications included neurovascular injuries, vascular injuries, ileus, and injury to adjacent organs [1].

Although neuromuscular complications are rare, they represent very bothersome conditions that may lead to a substantial diminishment in patient's quality of life. Additionally, the majority of neuromuscular injuries are avoidable, and steps toward prevention are mandatory. These injuries arise from direct surgical trauma or from anatomic stress of improper positioning.

J. Landman (✉)
Department of Urology, Columbia Presbyterian Medical Center, 161 Fort Washington Ave., 11th Floor, New York, NY 10032, USA
e-mail: landman.jaime@gmail.com

The true incidence of neuromuscular injuries is probably underestimated due to the relatively low intensity of symptoms in most cases, and many of these injuries are likely attributed to normal postoperative healing. Of note, the decreased overall patient pain, and the higher patient expectations, associated with laparoscopic and robotic procedures may indeed cause a higher reported incidence of neuromuscular injuries.

The incidence of neuromuscular injuries during laparoscopic surgery is low. In a series with 2407 procedures Fahlenkamp and colleagues reported 4.4% of neural injuries. Direct trauma was the most common cause of neuromuscular injury in this report. The authors concluded that prevention of neuromuscular injury may be achieved by increased surgeon awareness of the anatomical course of relevant nerves. Additionally, the authors suggest that open conversion and nerve repair should be seriously considered if a nerve injury is appreciated intra-operatively [2].

In another recent report of complications on 1867 laparoscopic surgeries for urological cancer, approximately 1% of patients presented with muscular complications including one patient with laboratory-confirmed rhabdomyolysis and one patient with a compartment syndrome that required lower extremity fasciotomy [3].

Neuromuscular complications following laparoscopic and robotic surgery may be clinically detected as a patient's complaint of local or regional anesthesia, paresthesia, hypoesthesia, hyperesthesia, or pain. Major neuromuscular injury complications will present with association of paresis or paralysis of the affected muscle region.

The various injuries that may arise from laparoscopic or robotic surgery are included in Table 1. These injuries may result from patient positioning,

R. Ghavamian (ed.), *Complications of Laparoscopic and Robotic Urologic Surgery*,
DOI 10.1007/978-1-60761-676-4_4,

Table 1 Neuromuscular complications following laparoscopic and robotic surgeries

Abdominal wall neuralgia
Sensory deficit
Motor deficit
Rhabdomyolysis
Shoulder pain
Back spasms

incision sites (trocars), decreased peripheral perfusion, and direct nerve injury.

A recent survey on the neuromuscular injuries during laparoscopic surgery found longer hospital stay and more frequent extra office visits in the group of patients who developed some kind of this complications. Other findings from this survey are that older patients, men, and patients submitted to retroperitoneal procedures are at higher risk [4].

Mechanisms of Neuromuscular Injury-Associated Pain

Neuropathic pain mechanisms include a peripheral and a central pathway. The peripheral pathway is through sensitization of primary afferent nociceptors with numerous changes at the molecular level, including release of chemical substances (bradykinin, nerve growth factor, cytokines) leading to nociceptor sensitization. As a result of this sensitization patient presents with spontaneous nociceptor activity, decreased threshold, increased response to suprathreshold stimulation and recruitment of silent nociceptors contributing to pain hypersensitivity. The central pathway is based on increased afferent stimuli enabling exaggerated synaptic excitability and the generation of pain [5]. Besides the physiologic pathway there are psychological and environmental factors that are involved in perpetuating the pain [6].

Neuromuscular Injury Associated with Robotic Surgery

Standard laparoscopic urologic surgery is often performed in non-anatomic positions. Patient positioning may result in possible neuromuscular injury complications. Patient positions commonly used for laparoscopic urologic surgery are the flank position, lateral position, Trendelenburg position, and lithotomy position. The most commonly performed robotic surgical procedure (including non-urologic procedures) is robotic radical prostatectomy. For robotic radical prostatectomy the patient is positioned in the lithotomy position, often with associated steep Trendelenburg position. For renal and adrenal laparoscopic surgery with the use of the da Vinci robot, positioning varies little from open surgery and therefore we would expect the same type of neuromuscular complications [7].

Patient Positioning Considerations

Many urologic procedures of the adrenal gland, kidney, and ureter are commonly performed using a standard full flank or modified flank position. The flank position is commonly applied for both transperitoneal and retroperitoneal procedures. Some advantages of the flank position include the gravitationally facilitated displacement of the small bowel, colon, and other surrounding solid viscera.

There are various neuromuscular complications associated with the flank position including rhabdomyolysis of the thigh, gluteal, or paraspinous musculature, pain, upper and lower extremity neural lesions due to stretch injuries, paresthesia, and numbness. These complications are increased with the severity of the flank position, the degree of flexion, and with the application of the kidney rest.

The probability of sciatic nerve injury is increased under several conditions. Conditions that increase the risk for sciatic nerve injury include elevated opposite buttock (lateral positioning), patients with low BMI, contact of the patient with an unpadded hard table surface, and prolonged surgical time. The most common injury to the lower limbs during lateral positioning is peroneal nerve injury. The peroneal nerve is injured as a result of compression of the lower leg on the table mattress. In order to avoid this type of lesion it is required to protect the nerve with adequate padding.

Shoulder pain may arise from flank and lateral positions due to joint contusion or stretch nerve injury, most commonly to the suprascapular nerve.

These complications arise primarily from prolonged procedures with patients having muscle and nerve injury from the compression of tissue between the bone surface and the operating-table surface.

Deane and colleagues evaluated the pressure generated at the skin-to-table surface interface in men and women with BMIs >25 and <25 on various commonly used protective surfaces and with the operating table positioned as it would be for a standard laparoscopic approach to the kidney as well as the influence of the table flexion and use of the kidney rest. They found higher pressures with the use of full flank position, a fully flexed position, and with the elevation of the kidney rest. These pressures were higher for men and for patients with BMI >25, independently of their gender [8].

Another common neuromuscular injury results from overstretching of the brachial plexus. The majority of brachial plexus injuries are typically the result of extensive arm abduction, arm external rotation, and posterior shoulder displacement. Compression of the brachial plexus has also been implicated as possible causative of brachial plexus injury, especially when the patient rests in the lateral decubitus position where the plexus is compressed against the thorax by the humeral head. Both supine position and the flank position may induce these lesions if attention to arm and shoulder positions is not taken [9].

Pelvic surgery of prostate or pelvic lymph node dissection, either via standard or robotic-assisted laparoscopic technique, requires application of the Trendelenburg position in conjunction with lithotomy position and often with application of shoulder bars to prevent the patient from sliding cranially. An exaggerated lithotomy position for radical prostate surgery carries a particularly high risk of neuromuscular complication since the patient's legs are flexed and abducted for a prolonged period of time. The sciatic nerve is especially at risk in this position since maximal external rotation of the flexed thigh may damage the nerve by stretching.

In a urologic laparoscopic population database, obese population was reported by Mendoza and coworkers as 12% of all patients. Among these obese patients peripheral nerve injury was found in 2% of patients and was mostly common due to patient positioning. The authors suggested that careful positioning of the obese patient with use of adequate padding is of extreme importance because the obese patient population has been shown to manifest a higher neuromuscular complication rate which is likely due to extended operating times and the patient's own weight compressing his or her own body structures [10].

Rhabdomyolysis

Rhabdomyolysis is generally due to muscle trauma that leads to ischemia and death of muscle cells. Postoperative rhabdomyolysis has been associated with prolonged muscle compression due to surgical positioning, extended operative time, high patient body mass, and unstable anesthetic patient's condition that may result in muscle injury, edema, and subsequent ischemia due to elevated compartment pressure.

Patient positioning is associated to rhabdomyolysis development through areas of direct pressure between bone structures and operating table, leading to muscle compression, compartment syndrome, and tissue ischemia.

Tissue injury develops when local blood pressure are 10–30 mmHg below of the diastolic blood pressure leading to ischemia, what is intensified in the surgical setting where patients are usually with a lower blood pressure due to anesthesia. The degree of injury presents a direct relation to the time length of the tissue exposure having myonecrosis and myoglobinuria more prone to occur after 4 h of ischemia [11].

Clinically rhabdomyolysis typically presents with muscular pain, dark-brown urine due to the presence of myoglobin pigment in the urine (myoglobinuria), and some degree of renal impairment. The renal impairment is due to myoglobin deposition on renal tubules leading to obstruction contributing to prerenal acute renal failure and may occur in up to one-third of the patients with rhabdomyolysis [11]. Laboratory analysis usually reveals high serum level of creatinine kinase (CK) (>5000 U/L) in the immediate postoperative period [12].

Current treatment includes vigorous hydration, sodium bicarbonate urine alkalinization (increased solubility of myoglobin with higher pH), and intravenous mannitol administration. Forced diuresis with dopamine, furosemide, and mannitol has been shown to enhance renal function and patient recovery after hypoxic insult. Supportive care with dialysis and hemodynamic supportive therapy may be necessary until renal impairment is resolved [12].

Laparoscopic procedures have been associated with postoperative rhabdomyolysis, most notably after laparoscopic surgeries in obese patients [13]. In a retroprospective analysis Reisiger and colleagues investigated risk factors for rhabdomyolysis after laparoscopic surgery. The authors identified risk factors for rhabdomyolysis including the exaggerated intraoperative lateral position, patients with high muscle mass or morbid obesity, hypovolemia, extended operative time (over 5 h), as well as preexisting renal dysfunction, diabetes, and hypertension [12].

Compartment Syndrome

The well leg compartment syndrome (WLCS) is a specific designation for the compartment syndrome caused by abnormal positioning of the lower limb during surgery. This term is used to differentiate this condition from the one cause by a trauma or direct injury [14]. WLCS is mostly commonly the result of positioning during pelvic surgery when the patient positioned into the lithotomy or hemi-lithotomy position. These positions can result in compression and edema of the lower limbs which results in a higher pressure inside the muscle fascial boundaries which can result in ischemia and tissue injury. The superficial and deep branches of the peroneal nerve and the tibial and sural nerves course through these compartments and may suffer as well from the ischemic condition induced by the lower extremities being elevated and abducted while resting on leg support pads.

The identification of compartment syndrome is crucial to avoid the possible devastating sequela. A high index of clinical suspicion from the health-care personal is needed and is based on the typical presentation during the postoperative period including extreme unusual leg pain. The signs may often be subtle and are frequently neurological because the neural tissues are the most sensitive tissue to hypoxia. Associated possible findings are calf swelling, plantar hypoesthesia, weakness of toe flexion, and pain.

Risk factors associated with the development of WLCS include the following: extended surgical time (usually greater than 4 h); lower limb position in the lithotomy/hemi-lithotomy; Trendelenburg position with the ankles at elevated positioning (may be present at laparoscopic/robotic prostatectomy); patient with high body mass index; leg holder type and leg positioning causing direct calf compression; lower blood pressure during anesthesia; hypovolemia and concomitance of peripheral vascular disease.

Treatment of the WLCS involves correction of metabolic electrolytes, restoration of fluid volume, and decompressive fasciotomies of the affected limbs. Fasciotomy need to be performed immediately after the diagnosis is made to avoid further tissue injury, if it is not performed within 12 h of initial ischemia, there is little recovery of neuromuscular function. Occasionally amputation of the limb is required if there is extensive tissue necrosis which may be a life threatening condition [14].

Direct Nerve Injuries

Direct nerve transaction is rare during laparoscopic and robotic surgery. The majority of nerve injuries sustained during laparoscopic and robotic procedures are caused by stretching (neurapraxia), electrofulguration injury, and dissection injury. However, direct nerve injury may occur leading to specific damage and related symptoms that can be motor or sensory, including variable gait disturbance.

Obturator nerve lesion during pelvic lymph node dissection is rare accounting for 3.5% of the complications according to a review of 372 patients reported by Kavoussi and colleagues [15]. In the event that obturator nerve transection is noted during the procedure, microsurgical epineural end-to-end tension-free coaptation without twisting, or malalignment of fascicles is recommended. Nerve reconstruction can be done with open surgery. However, laparoscopic and robotic nerve repair have been reported [16, 17].

Surgeon's Neuromuscular Complications

Laparoscopic and robotic procedures have helped to facilitate patients' post-operatory comfort and have expedited patient recovery. However, contemporary laparoscopic surgery often requires the surgeon to operate in a non-ergonomic position. Various surgeon neuromuscular injuries have been reported in association with laparoscopic procedures.

Surgeon positioning during laparoscopic surgery is difficult and non-ergonomic due to several technical challenges. Trocars which are well positioned for the majority of a case may not be ideally suited for access to all parts of the operative field during some portions of the procedure and may result in difficult working angles of the instruments.

As a function of limitations of contemporary laparoscopic technology, the laparoscopist is often required to achieve body positions that result in a significant amount of shoulder strain, excessive wrist supination or flexion, and ulnar deviations. Often, laparoscopic surgical technique involves the performance of precise manual maneuvers while standing on one leg and activating foot pedals with the other. These technical challenges make tasks which may be relatively simple during open surgery into complex manipulations which require increased body muscle effort and greater concentration. It is due to these exaggerated technical demands that the laparoscopist may experience pain, numbness, fatigue, and even injury during and after laparoscopic surgery.

Robotic-assisted laparoscopic surgery provides potential advantages over the standard laparoscopic surgery technique. During robotic-assisted laparoscopic procedures, the surgeon remains in a comfortable operating position, a three-dimensional view with a stable camera platform, and up to 7° of freedom during instrument manipulation inside the body. These advantages could theoretically reduce the magnitude of the ergonomics problems associated with standard laparoscopy. It is clear that robotic-assisted laparoscopy provide surgeons with a more natural and ergonomic surgical procedure [18].

In a survey among urologic laparoscopic surgeons regarding the prevalence of neuromuscular complications including pain, numbness, fatigue, and injuries during and after laparoscopic urologic surgery the most common injury reported was paresthesia. Paresthesias of the thumb or middle finger were most common. Other prevalent reported complaints were shoulder pain, neck pain, and lower back pain. Surgeons' chance of sustaining the injury was positively associated with laparoscopic experience.

Surgeons regarded robotic-assisted laparoscopic procedures to be the least bothersome, while hand-assisted laparoscopic procedures were considered to be the most related to neuromuscular complaints [19].

Prevention

Patient positioning before laparoscopic surgery is crucial for neuromuscular complication prevention and requires an awareness of the potential dangers of the various surgical positions used. Careful patient positioning, the application of adequate padding for the extremities, and table cushioning all help to reduce the risk of neuromuscular complications associated to laparoscopic and robotic surgery.

Improvements in patient positioning and cushioning during surgery are crucial to achieve reduction of this kind of complications. Patient positioning evaluation on the operating table should be done at every surgical procedure. Care must be taken to avoid direct contact of body surfaces with hard table components which may result in high-pressure contact.

Several surfaces are routinely applied for patient protection during positioning to theoretically minimize the risk of pressure-induced injury. Materials that are commonly used include gel padding and egg crate over the patient operating-table surface.

In order to reduce neuromuscular complications, the recommendations during laparoscopic/robotic surgery are to consider using partial flank positioning if possible, limiting the duration and the elevation of the kidney rest, and to decrease the degree of table flexion used.

It has also been suggested that the application of shoulder braces in combination with a steep Trendelenburg position for pelvic laparoscopy may be associated with brachial plexus injuries. Brachial plexus lesions prevention must include arm abduction limited to 90° or less, even when using arm holders. Martin and colleagues described a novel and ergonomic position for laparoscopic kidney surgery. The authors suggested a mild flank position (30° body rotation), an absence of table flexion, and placing the upper arm in an ergonomic position resting on the mid chest. The authors reported no neuromuscular complications due to positioning on a series of 1040 laparoscopic cases [20].

Rhabdomyolysis prevention includes the recognition of high-risk patients. The condition must be suspected on patients presenting excessive muscular pain, dark-brown urine, and/or oliguria in the post-operatory period. Patients suspected of having rhabdomyolysis should have close clinical evaluation as well as serum creatinine and CK levels measured immediately after suspicion. Vigorous hydration must be started and specific care should be initiated as soon as the diagnosis is confirmed in order to prevent or reduce renal damage.

Compartment syndrome risk factors should be identified in all patients undergoing laparoscopic and robotic pelvic urologic surgery. Urologists and healthcare professional on the operating room need to have a working knowledge about the risk, presentation, diagnosis, and management of compartment syndrome. Careful patient lithotomy positioning is recommended, with minimal elevation of the ankles above heart level and avoiding the head down position. If an extended surgical procedure time is anticipated, the legs should be removed from supports every 2 h for a short period to prevent reperfusion injury. The anesthesiologist should make efforts to avoid hypotension, hypovolemia, and vasoconstrictor drugs, especially in patients with known cardiac and vascular disease. If there is even a low degree of suspicion, efforts should be made to exclude WLCS.

In order to prevent surgeon's neuromuscular complications during laparoscopic surgery the monitor should be placed in front of the surgeon at a height between the surgeon's head and elbows, in such a manner that the surgeon's head is flexed between 15° and 45°. Shoulder pain, numbness, and back pain may be avoided or reduced by lowering the operating table and/or using an adjustable standing support enabling a decrease in back straining during surgery.

Improvements in the design of laparoscopic instruments and attention to ergonomic principles during surgery will provide less restrictive and straining laparoscopic surgeon positioning, enabling improvement in comfort and neuromuscular symptoms during operative time [19].

Establishment of guidelines for proper preparation of the operating room before initiating laparoscopic and robotic surgical procedures may help to reduce neuromuscular complications by assuring adequate padding and patients better ergonomic positioning.

References

1. Permpongkosol S, Link RE, Su LM, Romero FR, Bagga HS, Pavlovich CP, Jarrett TW, Kavoussi LR. Complications of 2,775 urological laparoscopic procedures: 1993 to 2005. J Urol. 2007;177(2):580–5.
2. Fahlenkamp D, Rassweiler J, Fornara P, Frede T, Loening SA. Complications of laparoscopic procedures in urology: experience with 2,407 procedures at 4 German centers. J Urol. 1999;162(3 Pt 1):765–70.
3. Colombo JR Jr, Haber GP, Jelovsek JE, Nguyen M, Fergany A, Desai MM, Kaouk JH, Gill IS. Complications of laparoscopic surgery for urological cancer: a single institution analysis. J Urol. 2007;178(3 Pt 1):786–91.
4. Wolf JS Jr, Marcovich R, Gill IS, Sung GT, Kavoussi LR, Clayman RV, et al. Survey of neuromuscular injuries to the patient and surgeon during urologic laparoscopic surgery. Urology. 2000;55(6):831–6.
5. Shipton E. Post-surgical neuropathic pain. ANZ J Surg. 2008;78(7):548–55.
6. Cousins MJ. Persistent pain: a disease entity. J Pain Symptom Manage. 2007;33 Suppl 2:S4–10.
7. Aron M, Koenig P, Kaouk JH, Nguyen MM, Desai MM, Gill IS. Robotic and laparoscopic partial nephrectomy: a matched-pair comparison from a high-volume centre. BJU Int. 2008;102(1):86–92.
8. Deane LA, Lee HJ, Box GN, Abraham JB, Abdelshehid CS, Elchico ER, et al. Third place: Flank position is associated with higher skin-to-surface interface pressures in men versus women: implications for laparoscopic renal surgery and the risk of rhabdomyolysis. J Endourol. 2008;22(6):1147–51.
9. Sawyer RJ, Richmond MN, Hickey JD, Jarrratt JA. Peripheral nerve injuries associated with anaesthesia. Anaesthesia. 2000;55(10):980–91.
10. Mendoza D, Newman RC, Albala D, Cohen MS, Tewari A, Lingeman J, et al. Laparoscopic complications in markedly obese urologic patients (a multi-institutional review). Urology. 1996;48(4):562–7.
11. Shaikh S, Nabi G, McClinton S. Risk factors and prevention of rhabdomyolysis after laparoscopic nephrectomy. BJU Int. 2006;98(5):960–2.
12. Reisiger KE, Landman J, Kibel A, Clayman RV. Laparoscopic renal surgery and the risk of rhabdomyolysis: diagnosis and treatment. Urology. 2005; 66 Suppl 5: 29–35.
13. Rehman J, Boglia J, Chughtai B, Sukkarieh T, Khan SA, Lewis R, et al. High body mass index in muscular patients and flank position are risk factors for rhabdomyolysis: case report after laparoscopic live-donor nephrectomy. J Endourol. 2006;20(9):646–50.
14. Raza A, Byrne D, Townell N. Lower limb (well leg) compartment syndrome after urological pelvic surgery. J Urol. 2004;171(1):5–11.
15. Kavoussi LR, Sosa E, Chandhoke P, Chodak G, Clayman RV, Hadley HR, et al. Complications of laparoscopic pelvic lymph node dissection. J Urol. 1993;149(2): 322–5.
16. Spaliviero M, Steinberg AP, Kaouk JH, Desai MM, Hammert WC, Gill IS. Laparoscopic injury and repair

of obturator nerve during radical prostatectomy. Urology. 2004;64(5):1030.

17. Matsuyama T, Mackay M, Midha R. Peripheral nerve repair and grafting techniques: a review. Neurol Med Chir (Tokyo). 2000;40(4):187–99.
18. Renda A, Vallancien G. Principles and advantages of robotics in urologic surgery. Curr Urol Rep. 2003;4(2): 114–8.
19. Gofrit ON, Mikahail AA, Zorn KC, Zagaja GP, Steinberg GD, Shalhav AL. Surgeons' perceptions and injuries during and after urologic laparoscopic surgery. Urology. 2008;71(3):404–7.
20. Martin GL, Nunez RN, Martin AD, Andrews PE, Castle EP. A novel and ergonomic patient position for laparoscopic kidney surgery. Can J Urol. 2009;16(2): 4580–3.

Part II
Surgical Complications

Vascular Complications in Laparoscopic and Robotic Urologic Surgery

Daniel Tare, Pedro Maria, and Reza Ghavamian

Keywords Vascular injuries · Hemorrhage · Embolism · Laparoscopy · Robotics

Introduction

Vascular injuries are among the most common major complications associated with laparoscopic urology. They can be the most devastating complications leading to blood loss, conversion to open surgery, multiple organ failure, shock, or death. These injuries may occur during any part of the procedure, while gaining laparoscopic access, during tissue dissection or isolating and ligating vascular structures. They can be diagnosed both intraoperatively and postoperatively. The key in avoiding these injuries is careful attention to surgical technique and anatomy. When vascular injuries do occur, the key to management is early recognition and a timely, calm response. Specific vascular injuries that are prone to occur with specific procedures are discussed in procedure-specific chapters in this book. This chapter briefly addresses the incidence of intraoperative and postoperative vascular complications and their recognition and management. Furthermore, we discuss thromboembolic complications, the unique set of circumstances brought about by laparoscopy and their management.

Incidence and Literature Review

Vascular injuries occur in approximately 1.6–4.7% [1, 2] of laparoscopic urologic procedures. In contrast, vascular injury in nonurologic literature appears to be less frequent with rates as low as 0.05–0.9% [3, 4]. Many of the earlier urologic reports were focused primarily on laparoscopic nephrectomy. The majority of vascular injuries in urologic laparoscopy are dissection injuries, as urologic laparoscopic procedures such as nephrectomy require much more dissection around major vascular structures. They require isolation, clamping, and reconstruction of the kidney in the case of partial nephrectomy, a parenchymous organ with a rich blood supply. In contrast, the bulk of the vascular complications in the nonurologic literature is trocar-related injuries.

More recently there have been a number of reports in the literature of complications from large numbers of varied laparoscopic procedures. Colombo et al. [5] reviewed 1,867 laparoscopic cases performed for urologic malignancy. The most common intraoperative complication was hemorrhage occurring in 2.3% of patients. Postoperatively, hemorrhage was again the most common complication occurring in 2.7% of patients. Overall, intraoperative and postoperative hemorrhage accounted for 40% of all perioperative complications. Similarly, Permpongkosol et al. [6] reviewed complications in 2,775 laparoscopic urologic procedures and found that the two most common complications were intraoperative vascular injuries (1.98%) and postoperative bleeding requiring blood transfusion (1.76%). As expected, vascular injuries were more common in procedures requiring dissection around major vessels, such as laparoscopic retroperitoneal lymph node dissection.

R. Ghavamian (✉)
Department of Urology, Montefiore Medical Center, Albert Einstein College of Medicine, 3400 Bainbridge Ave, Bronx, NY 10708, USA
e-mail: rghavami@montefiore.org

R. Ghavamian (ed.), *Complications of Laparoscopic and Robotic Urologic Surgery*,
DOI 10.1007/978-1-60761-676-4_5, © Springer Science+Business Media, LLC 2010

Vascular injuries can be the most common reason for conversion to open surgery. These are mostly vascular dissection injuries which have been reported more commonly after urologic or gynecologic laparoscopy as they involve more dissection around major vessels. Parsons et al. [7] reported a rate of vascular injury of about 2.6% in 894 cases. Vascular injuries were responsible for 12 of the 13 open conversions in that series. The vessels injured included the renal artery and vein, inferior vena cava, and external iliac artery and vein. Fahlenkamp et al. [8] found that most of the complications occurred during dissection (2.9%) while trocar-related injuries occurred in 0.2% of complications. Meraney et al. [9] identified vascular injuries in 7 of 404 (1.7%) patients undergoing retroperitoneal laparoscopic renal and adrenal surgery. Again, five of these injuries were due to dissection and the other two were caused by an Endo-GIA stapler malfunction and the accidental dislodgement of a vascular clip. Previous major abdominal surgery was also a risk factor for complications. In this series, one patient was converted to an open procedure, two of the complications were managed through the extraction incision, and all the remaining injuries were managed laparoscopically. This reinforced previous findings [8] that the occurrence of complications and the rate of open conversion for these complications are directly related to surgeon experience.

Intraoperative Vascular Complications

Adequate knowledge of anatomy is essential in order to prevent any type of injury during surgery. Laparoscopy does not change the anatomy or the surgical procedure. During traditional open surgery sources of bleeding can be quickly controlled using forceps, clamps, or manual compression. While there have been numerous advances in laparoscopic instruments and improvements in suturing techniques, control of hemorrhage is more difficult in laparoscopic procedures. It is for this reason that careful preparation and meticulous technique are important for laparoscopic procedures. Careful inspection of preoperative imaging for anomalous vasculature is critical. Of course, every laparoscopic procedure should be performed in an operating room equipped to handle all aspects of open surgery.

Vascular Injury During Abdominal Access

Access and the creation of a pneumoperitoneum carry a significant risk of vascular injuries. The incidence of major vascular injuries from trocars and Veress needle insertion averages around 0.1% [10–14]. Access-related injuries to vascular structures are a rare but potentially devastating complication.

Approximately 75% of major vascular injuries associated with laparoscopy occur while obtaining access. Access-related vascular injuries account for 81% of the mortalities as reported to the FDA by the laparoscopic equipment manufacturers [15]. Vascular injuries can carry a mortality rate as high as 15% second only to anesthesia as a cause for mortality in laparoscopy [16]. A French study of 103,852 laparoscopic operations found the rate of serious trocar accidents to be 0.32% [3]. Blind insertions were responsible for 90% of the major injuries. Major vascular injuries occurred at a rate of 0.5% with 17% mortality (six patients). The aorta, vena cava, and iliac veins were the most commonly injured structures while the superior mesenteric vein, lumbar veins, greater omentum, and pelvic veins were injured less frequently. All the mortalities in this series were related to vascular injuries.

Kavoussi et al. reported 10 (2.7%) trocar-related injuries in 372 patients undergoing laparoscopic pelvic lymph node dissection [17]. Four of these injuries were laceration of the epigastric vessels and two were due to injury of superficial abdominal wall vessels. A review of 2,407 laparoscopic cases from four German centers found access-related complications rate was only 0.2% [8]. In a survey of pediatric urological laparoscopy, Peters noted that significantly more complications occurred in patients in whom the Veress needle was used compared to the open Hassan technique (2.55% vs. 1.2%) [18]. In this study experience of the practitioner was the most important factor in predicting complications.

As reported by Chandler et al. [19], data from the Physicians Insurers Association (1980–1999) and the FDA (1995–1997) reported 594 trocar-related injuries in 506 patients, of which 556 (94%) were caused by either the Veress needle or the primary trocar. This series included 239 major vascular injuries and 278 major visceral injuries, with a reported mortality of 13%. Logistic regression analysis showed that age >59 years, major visceral vessel injury, and a delay in diagnosis of injury >24 h were independent predictors of death.

Inadequate reporting of major injuries during laparoscopy underlies the difficulty in addressing the question of safety, highlighted by the number of vascular injuries reported to the FDA and the Physicians Insurers Association. It is important to note that the true incidence of vascular injury is unknown and undoubtedly higher than the literature suggests. This is in part due to medico-legal implications of reporting major vascular injuries. Most surgeons who report their data have greater experience and therefore may have lower complication rates. Furthermore, the exact reason of the injury may be mistakenly ascribed to the wrong etiology. For example, until the landmark paper by Levy and Soderstrom [20] in 1976, most bowel injuries during laparoscopy that were attributed to electrosurgery were actually the result of needles and trocars [21].

Multiple techniques have been developed to make laparoscopic access safer. There is no consensus as to which technique has the fewest overall complications. The Veress needle technique is the most commonly used but is considered to cause slightly more vascular accidents [22]. The open Hassan technique causes more visceral injuries but major vascular injuries have been reported and the open access method is not without its own complications [23]. Direct view trocars were designed to avoid injuries by allowing the surgeon to see the tissues as the trocar passes through them. However, major vascular injuries and even deaths have been reported to the FDA using these devices. Devices that help control axial force needed to penetrate the trocars have been developed. The most widely studied device uses an expandable sheath that neutralizes the axial force by countertraction on its outer flange. A cone-shaped dilator is pushed through the sheath while forward movement is controlled by the surgeon's nondominant hand. The sheath stretches and pushes away blood vessels and leaves a smaller wound. No major vascular injuries have been reported using this device.

Insufficient acquaintance with the relationships between anatomic landmarks, especially between the abdominal wall and retroperitoneal vascular structures, is a major cause of vascular injury during trocar placement. In a thin patient, the distance between the anterior abdominal wall and retroperitoneal structures can be as little as 2 cm [15]. A patient with a medium height has an average of 6 cm from skin to retroperitoneal vascular structures [24]. If the patient is placed in extreme Trendelenburg, this can bring the aortic bifurcation dangerously close to the skin [25]. The cephalo-caudal relationship between the aortic bifurcation and the umbilicus varies widely and is not considered to be a useful landmark for access. In one study, the position of the aortic bifurcation ranged from 5 cm cephalad to 3 cm caudal to the umbilicus in the supine position and from 3 cm cephalad to 3 cm caudal in the Trendelenburg position [26]. The umbilical base moves more caudally in relation to the aortic bifurcation with increasing body mass index (BMI) and thus is more likely to overlie the unbifurcated aorta in slimmer patients [24]. A study using post-contrast CT images found the relation of anterior superior iliac spine and the aortic bifurcation to be more consistent and recommended the ASIS plane in the midline as the ideal primary access point [27]. In most situations, with the aortic and the vena caval bifurcation at or near the umbilicus in general, the most likely vessel injured directly with an umbilical Veress needle or trocar is the left common iliac vein.

Veress needles should be placed at a 45° angle toward the pelvis in the midline. Once in the abdomen the needle should be aspirated to determine if there is an injury to a vessel or hollow viscus, i.e., for blood or bowel contents. If an injury is suspected the Veress needle should not be removed as it may aid in identifying the site of injury once access is established. Similarly if blood is seen filling a trocar it should not be removed as it may aid in tamponading the bleeding. The Veress needle or trocar should not be insufflated as this may cause a CO_2 embolus. CO_2 embolization presents as sudden hypotension, cyanosis of the head and upper extremities, elevated right heart pressures and central venous pressure. The insufflation should be immediately stopped and the patient placed in the left lateral decubitus position with the head down and the CO_2 aspirated through a central line.

Other factors that may lead to vascular injury include failure to place the patient in Trendelenburg position, placement of trocars on the wrong side of the patient, failure to elevate or stabilize the abdominal wall, and perpendicular insertion of the needle or trocar. Surgeon experience is believed to be a critical factor [3] as it relates to knowledge of the relevant anatomy and the amount of force to be used when placing the trocar. Once the abdomen is visualized vascular injuries may be recognized by direct visualizing of blood or a retroperitoneal hematoma. As soon as an injury is suspected the anesthesiologist should be notified so proper resuscitation can be initiated. Repair of the injury via laparoscopic or open technique will depend on the type of injury and the experience of the surgeon.

Injury to the epigastric vessels is the most common minor vascular injury. The incidence of this injury can be avoided by careful surgical technique. Placement of secondary trocars should be under direct vision with guided transillumination of the abdominal wall vessels. The inferior epigastric vessels lie on the lateralmost border of the rectus sheath. Trocars placed lateral to rectus sheath can still injure these vessels if placed obliquely towards the midline.

All cannula sites should be inspected at the end of the case as the trocars may tamponade any bleeding from injured epigastric vessels. A number of different methods are available to repair injured vessels. First, the trocar itself can be used to tamponade the bleeding with direct pressure. Some have reported using a Foley catheter to control the bleeding [21]. Once inserted through the trocar site the balloon is inflated and pulled up against the abdominal wall. This is at best a temporizing measure, as the surgeon optimizes exposure and prepares sutures for definitive repair. Open suture ligation via a cut-down technique or laparoscopic suture ligation or electrocautery can be employed. Continuous venous oozing can occur postoperatively necessitating transfusion and re-exploration (Figs. 1 and 2). Fascial closures devices can be used to control bleeding from an injured epigastric vessel. The Carter-Thomason device can be used under direct laparoscopic visualization, and a figure of eight suture can be applied with this device reliably controlling the epigastric vessels. This, in the authors' hands, is the most reliable method for controlling this injured vessel. It is quick and does not require a cut-down and difficult suture placements through a small trocar incision.

Injury to Major Blood Vessels

Injury to major blood vessels can occur during dissection as well as during trocar or Veress needle insertion. Timely recognition of a vascular injury is critical. Many injuries may be initially unrecognized but become apparent as the procedure progresses. For example, carbon dioxide insufflation may conceal venous bleeding. A mesenteric or retroperitoneal hematoma caused during trocar placement may take time to develop. Ligation of the superior mesenteric artery or splenic artery may cause bowel necrosis or splenic infarct which will not become readily apparent.

Once a vascular injury is identified the surgeon must immediately determine whether it can be managed laparoscopically or through an open conversion. When a dissection injury is encountered the surgeon should be quick to assess the etiology. There are difficulties with exposure in laparoscopy, and bleeding quickly further obscures the field. Direct manual

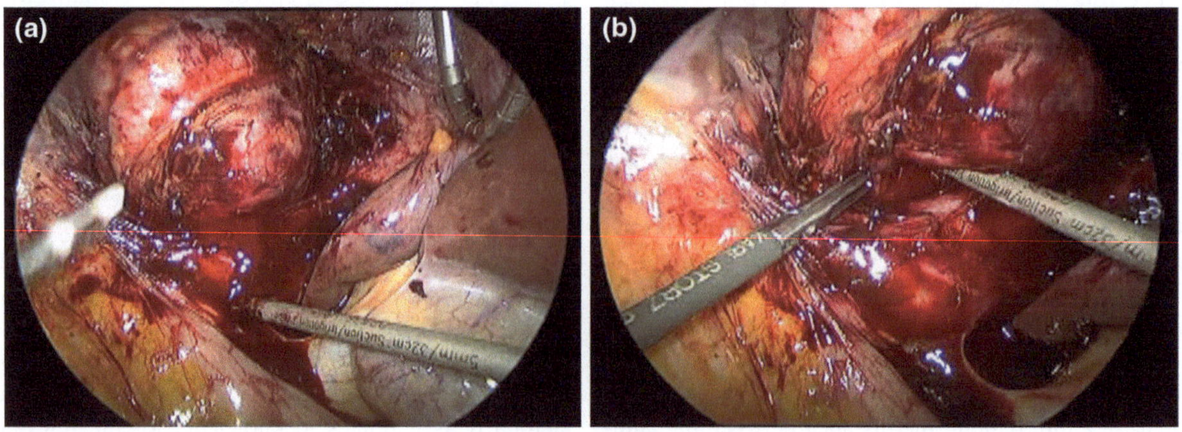

Fig. 1 (**a**) Bleeding from the medial aspect of the vena cava obscures the point of hemorrhage in a right-sided adrenalectomy for pheochromocytoma. (**b**) Exposure cannot be obtained for Ligasure use

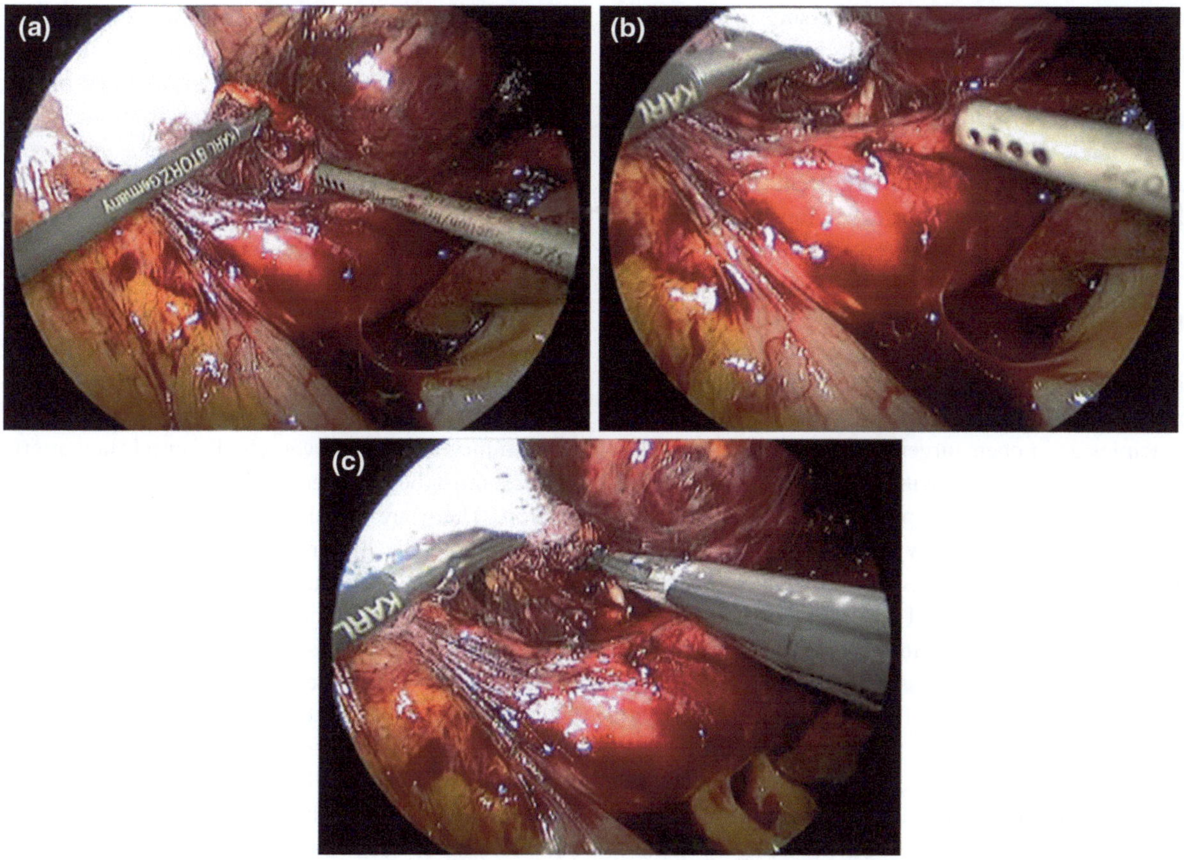

Fig. 2 (**a and b**) A rolled 4×4 sponge is applied laparoscopically. This aids in identification of bleeding medial vessel as it is held on stretch. (**c**) A laparoscopic clip applier is used to control the bleeding

pressure is difficult and laparoscopic suction devices rarely emulate blotting with laparotomy pads that can be performed with open surgery (Fig. 1). The pad is used to soak up excess blood allowing for better utilization of the suction device to delineate and control the bleeding vessel (Fig. 2). The management of individual vascular injuries will be determined by the patient's anatomy and collateral circulation. Major vessels such as the aorta, common iliac, and external iliac must obviously be repaired. If adequate collateral circulation exists consideration can be given to ligating certain injured vessels such as the celiac axis and inferior mesenteric artery [28]. Superior mesenteric artery injuries are almost universally repaired as its collateral circulation cannot be relied upon. Superior mesenteric trunk injuries have been reported after laparoscopic radical nephrectomy and can lead to devastating outcomes [1, 2].

If the renal artery is injured during partial nephrectomy or a solitary kidney, then it too must be repaired. During renal surgery injury to the renal hilum can occur by inadequate dissection prior to vascular control. In order to prevent bleeding from branches of major vessels during dissection it is recommended to use the right angle clamp for dissection. Additional tools in the laparoscopic surgeon's armamentarium include the use of the harmonic scalpel (Ethicon), Ligasure (Valley Lab), and bipolar coagulation forceps. Monopolar electrocautery and surgical clips may be used for hemostasis but care must be taken not to occlude important vessels. Also, nonjudicious placement of clips near the hilum may complicate placement of laparoscopic stapling devices. In order to control bleeding from renal hilum the surgeon may put traction on the hilum by elevating the kidney while further dissection to expose a bleeding vessel can occur.

Increasing the intra-abdominal pressure to 20 mmHg can slow down or stop any venous bleeding.

In general, if the surgeon is an experienced laparoscopist, attempts at repair of major or minor vessels can be made. Exposure is key in this situation. This is rarely the case with aortic or large vena caval injuries. However, some smaller vena caval injuries and venous injuries in general can be repaired laparoscopically. The suction device is an excellent means of pressure application and exposure. A surgical sponge rolled into a trocar can be expeditiously applied to the bleeding site to get exposure. Then the need for additional ports can be assessed and repair attempted with the same principles as in open surgery. The difference is that in laparoscopy, especially with repair of venous injuries, transient increases in the pneumoperitoneal pressures to around 20 mmHg allow for a decrease in bleeding and can aid in the repair. Attention should be made to a quick repair as increased abdominal pressures in the setting of a large defect in the vein can increase the risk for gas embolism. It is essential to have an open laparotomy tray available for immediate conversion if necessary.

The most common site of bleeding during prostatectomy is from the dorsal venous complex . Even with the advantage of magnification provided by laparoscopic surgery care must be taken during anterior and lateral dissection of the prostate. The dorsal venous complex is sutured with 2-0 or 3-0 vicryl. In some centers a second suture is placed at the anterior surface of the prostate at the level of the bladder neck to prevent backbleeding and to help achieve a secure ligation and "dry" transection. There are occasions when the suture at the dorsal venous complex can be loose which can cause gradual oozing. Increasing the pneumoperitoneum to 20 mmHg may slow down or stop the bleeding and allow time for appropriate suture repair. Levator ani muscles' attachments may tether these veins open exacerbating the bleeding. Bluntly dissecting these attachments may obviate the need for coagulation in this sensitive area. Another maneuver more specific to robotic-assisted laparoscopic prostatectomy is the utilization of the 4th arm to clamp the bleeding vessel while you prepare the needle holders and sutures for final repair. When performing adjunctive pelvic lymph node dissection care must be taken to avoid injury to the iliac vessels. External iliac arterial injuries must be repaired and necessitate open conversion. There are instances where a four-arm robot can aid in repair of large vascular defects. This is hard to emulate with pure laparoscopy. In this fashion, external iliac vein lacerations can be managed by suture repair. Even in cases where a large laceration is noted, in expert hands the defect can be repaired robotically (Fig. 3). This is because flow through the vein is sequential and it is decompressed with pneumoperitoneum. At the time of injury, increasing insufflation pressure and temporarily turning off the sequential compression devices on the legs can decrease bleeding and help the repair. The 4th arm and one of the dissecting robotic arms can be used to gain control while the suture is prepared (Fig. 4). The repair is then carried out under optimal control (Fig. 5). At the end of the repair, the sequential devices are turned on and the pneumoperitoneum is decreased. In cases where more than half the lumen of the blood vessel is narrowed,

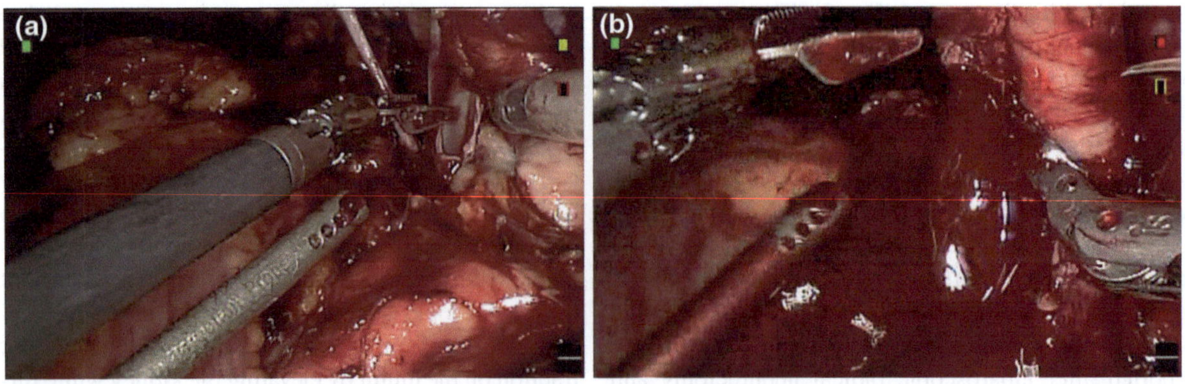

Fig. 3 (**a**) During a right robotic pelvic node dissection for bladder cancer, the external iliac vein is injured behind a tortuous external iliac artery. The endothelium of the vein can easily be appreciated. (**b**) Large bleeding is encountered with sequential venous pulsatile flow

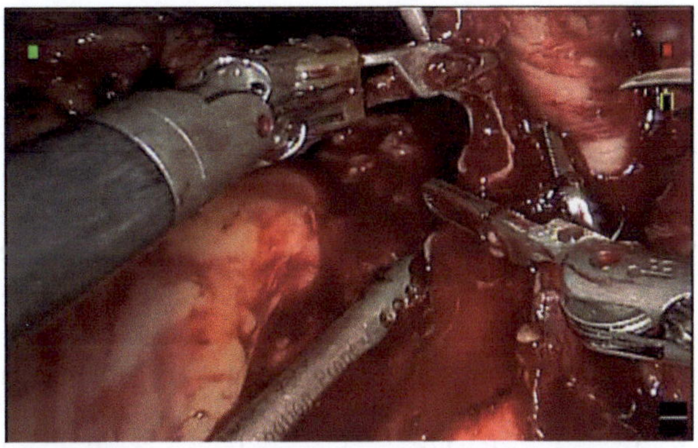

Fig. 4 The *left* dissecting arm and the 4th arm are utilized to obtain temporary control with this large defect

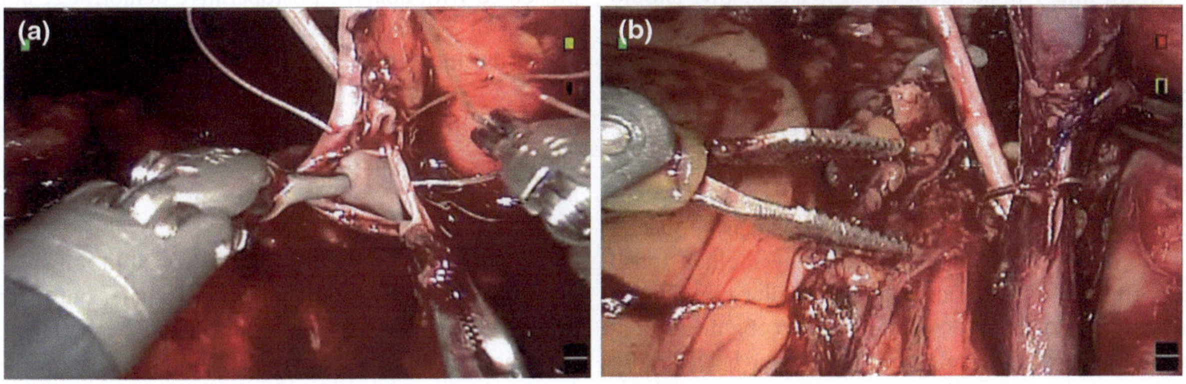

Fig. 5 (**a**) A running 5-0 prolene suture is used to repair the vessel under optimal control. (**b**) The completed repair with mild narrowing but obvious filling of the vein proximally and distally, confirming flow

consideration should be given to short-term, full anti-coagulation (1 month) postoperatively to decrease the chance of deep vein thrombosis. Postoperative duplex scanning can be performed to assess adequate flow. Internal iliac arterial injuries should be repaired if they are proximal to the superior gluteal artery. Ligation can be considered for more distal injuries if there is adequate collateral circulation.

Stapler Malfunction

Control and ligation of the renal hilum is a critical step during laparoscopic nephrectomy. Surgical staplers were developed for safe controlled ligation and division of the hilar vessels. However, reports of inadvertent stapling of the vena cava and aorta have been reported. In the later instance, the vena cava was mistaken for the right renal vein [29]. However, failure of the device can lead to significant complications including open conversion, hemorrhage, transfusion, and death. The majority of problems can be avoided with careful application of the device. If recognized early this potentially devastating complication can be managed judiciously without open conversion.

Staple malfunction is an uncommon event. Chan et al. [30] reported a malfunction rate of 1.7% in 565 cases with a primary device failure rate of 0.2%. Deng et al. [31] reported a malfunction rate of 1% in 460 cases with a primary device failure in 0.3%. In their series 60% of the malfunction required open conversion, one of which was for removal of the device. In a review of the Food and Drug Administration Manufacturer and User Facility Device Experience Database from 1992 to 2006, Hsi et al. [32] found 223 reported stapling device failures. Open surgery was required in 35% of patients and transfusion in 10%. There were three stapler-related fatalities although the exact mechanism of the malfunction was not reported.

Prevention and early recognition is the first step in the management of stapler malfunction. The device should be carefully inspected prior to application to ensure proper loading and alignment. In one case a stapler was found to be missing a proximal row of staples [30] and in another a surgeon fired a previously fired stapler [31], both of which necessitated open conversion. Judicious use of surgical clips around the hilum is important as it will reduce the risk of entrapping clips in the stapler's jaws. The use of Ligasure device (Valley Labs, Boulder, CO) or bipolar electrocautery for smaller vessels around the hilum can obviate the need for metallic clips. Proper placement of the device is critical to ensure complete transaction and to avoid injury to adjacent tissues. The stapler should not be deployed if the jaws do not close properly. Furthermore, excessive force should not be used which can override the lockout mechanism. If a misfire is suspected, a second stapler line or surgical clip can be placed prior to release of the first stapler. Bleeding can be controlled with further exposure and manual compression. Additional 10–12 mm trocar can be placed to aid in the management which may include intracorporeal suturing, placement of vascular clips, or an additional stapler if possible. Early recognition of a malfunction prior to releasing the stapler is critical in managing these complications laparoscopically. When applying the endoscopic stapler, it is best to apply the stapling device closer to the kidney, for example, rather than flush with the vena cava or the aorta to leave room for proximal application of a second stapler in case of a stapler jam or malfunction. Ultimately the decision to convert to open or to manage laparoscopically is dependent on the surgeon's expertise and comfort.

Postoperative Complications

With the limited field of view of laparoscopic surgery many injuries that occur during surgery may go unnoticed during the initial procedure. These injuries may cause delayed complications which require secondary intervention. Vascular complications contribute to a large share of the early postoperative complications after laparoscopic surgery [33]. There can be many reasons why recognition of a vascular injury may be delayed. Compressions by the pneumoperitoneum, vasospasm, or partial ligation are common reasons for delayed presentation. Unintentional ligation of an artery can lead to infarction and necrosis of its target organ and will usually present in a delayed fashion [1]. Some postoperative vascular complications are unique to laparoscopic urology. In a report by Ramani et al. [34] on laparoscopic partial nephrectomies most of the hemorrhagic complications occurred postoperatively and after the patient was discharged. Renal artery pseudoaneurysm and arteriovenous fistula (AVF) are two unique complications that may not arise until later in the postoperative period. Singh et al. reported a 1.7% incidence of pseudoaneurysm formation after laparoscopic partial nephrectomy [35]. These patients presented with delayed postoperative hemorrhage at a median of 12 days postoperatively. In another recent study, the incidence of renal artery pseudoaneurysms was 2.4% [36]. Arteriovenous fistulae and pseudoaneurysms form when proximate segmental arteries and veins are injured either during resection of renal masses or during suture repair of the parenchymal defect. The deeper the resection as is the case in endophytic tumors, the higher the probability of these complications. Each entity can exist alone, but often pseudoaneurysms and AVFs can co-exist. Several measures can be used to decrease the chance of pseudoaneurysms. Careful inspection of the resection bed and ligation of segmental branches when possible can help. In deep tumor resections, the tumor crater should be inspected and in the event of multiple segmental arterial transections, a hemostatic running intracorporeal suture at the crater should be employed with precise needle passes. Sutures for parenchymal repair should not be placed too deeply to risk segmental branch injury. Careful inspection of the repair before laparoscopic exit is mandatory. When clinically suspected and in the scenario of a precipitous decline in the hematocrit, computerized tomography (CT) is indicated. A characteristic blush during the arterial phase is seen (Fig. 6). The incidence and detailed management of these vascular complications are discussed in the complications of laparoscopic partial nephrectomy chapter in this book.

The incidence of delayed vascular complications is low and the symptoms may be nonspecific. A high index of suspicion is therefore needed to recognize and treat these potentially catastrophic complications. Possible symptoms of late vascular complications include but are not limited to general malaise, abdominal or flank pain, dizziness or syncope, hypotension, tachycardia, decreasing hemoglobin and hematocrit,

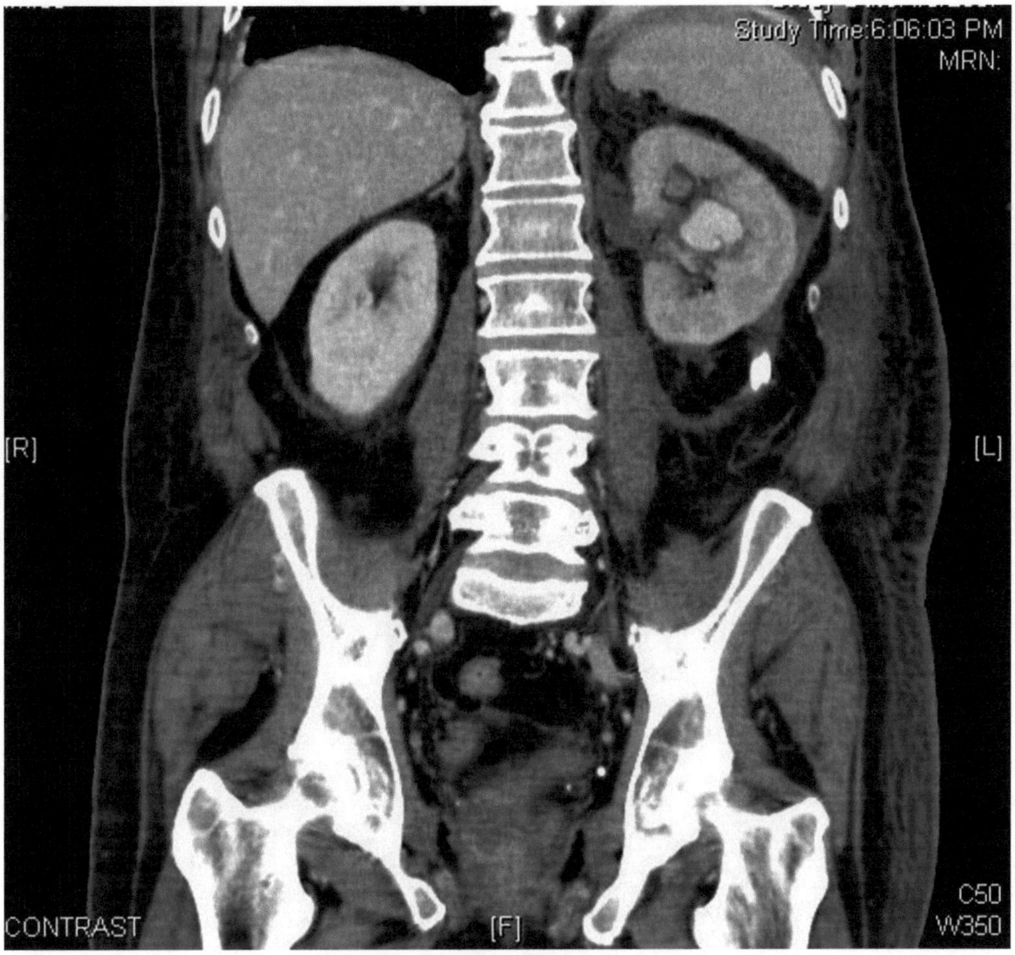

Fig. 6 Computed tomography 2 days after laparoscopic partial nephrectomy demonstrating a distinct blush during the arterial phase, characteristic of a segmental renal arterial pseudoaneurysm

gross hematuria, bloody drainage form drain site, nausea, vomiting, absent pulses, fever, and renal insufficiency [37]. In patients with suspicious clinical findings, a CT scan with intravenous contrast is the first study of choice and can fairly reliably localize the source of the bleeding. If active bleeding is suspected an angiography may provide additional information and adds the additional benefit of concomitant therapy via embolization.

If computed tomography shows a hematoma and the patient is hemodynamically stable conservative management with observation, serial monitoring of hemoglobin and hematocrit, and transfusion will often suffice. However, if hemodynamic stability is in doubt, and the situation allows, angiography, and possible embolization of the bleeding vessel, is the least invasive therapy and should be the first-line management. Selective angiographic embolization is the treatment of choice in managing renal artery pseudoaneurysms and arteriovenous fistulae (Fig. 7). If angiography is inappropriate or unsuccessful, then the next step is surgical intervention. A laparoscopic approach may be considered if the surgeon feels comfortable but is usually impractical in this setting. Patient safety is of primary concern and time should not be wasted in an attempt to manage this potentially catastrophic complication in a minimally invasive fashion. If an artery to an organ, for example, the superior mesenteric artery, has been ligated, immediate consultation with a vascular surgeon should be obtained in an attempt to revascularize the involved organ. One particular instant that should not be overlooked is venous oozing from trocar

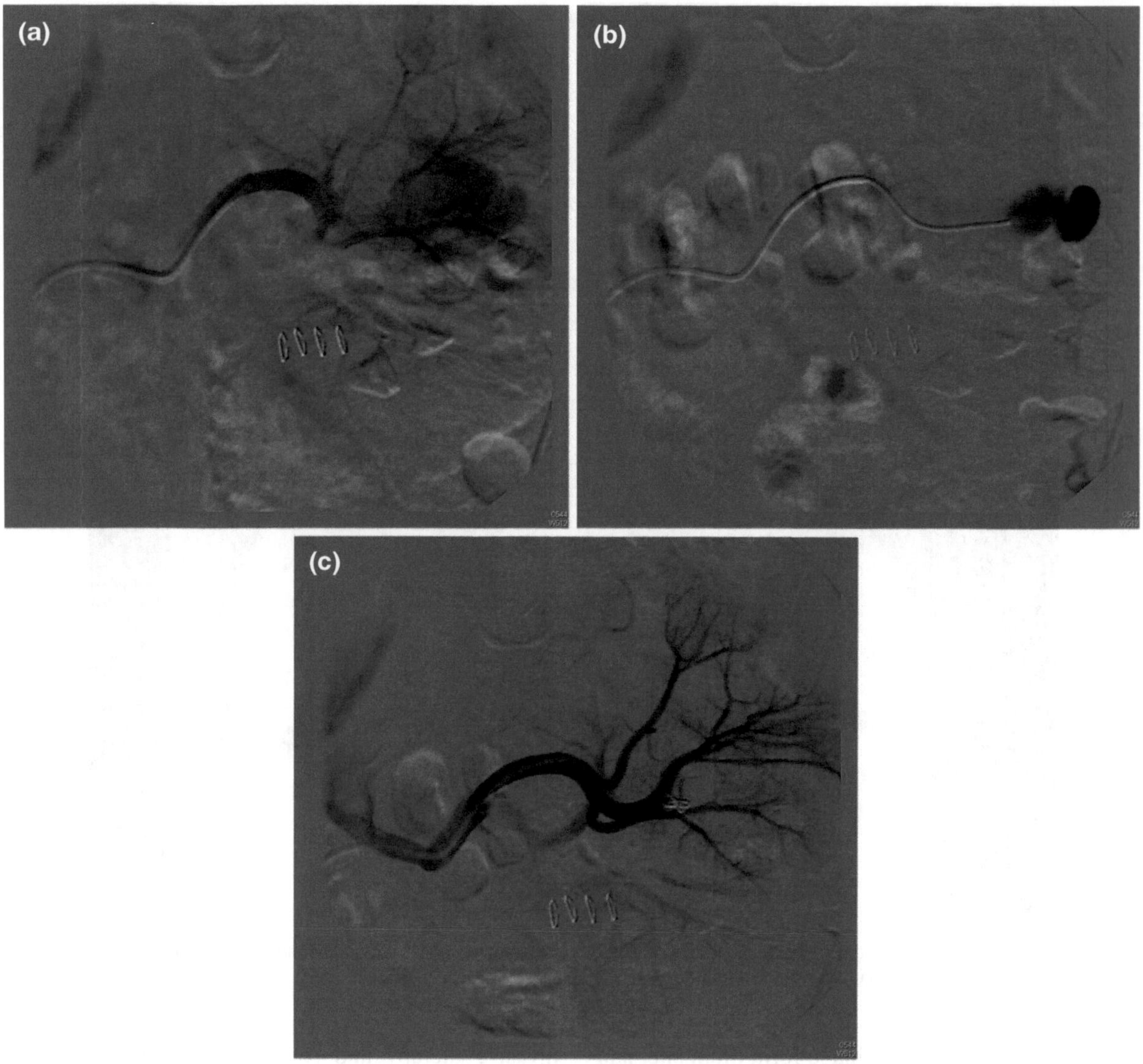

Fig. 7 Renal angiography for the patient in Fig. 6. (**a**) Arterial blush and extravasation with some venous filling is demonstrated consistent with pseudoaneurysm with delayed venous filling. (**b**) Selective cannulization accurately delineates the pseudoaneurysm. (**c**) Arterial angiogram demonstrates resolution of the pseudoaneurysm after selective arterial embolization

sites (Fig. 8). It is for these reasons that all trocar sites have to be meticulously inspected before laparoscopic exit.

Venous Thromboembolism

Surgery is a form of controlled trauma to the human body and when performed laparoscopically the cascade of benefits and complications may differ or be similar when compared to the open approach. Activation of the coagulation system, which could further lead to a thromboembolic event, is similar or slightly less with laparoscopic surgery [38–42]. It seems reasonable to assume that laparoscopic procedures may be associated with longer surgical times than comparable open procedures. Reverse Trendelenburg position and pneumoperitoneum reduce venous return from the legs creating venous stasis and possibly increasing the risk of deep venous thrombosis (DVT) in patients undergoing laparoscopy. Abdel-Meguid and Gomella [43] concluded that there

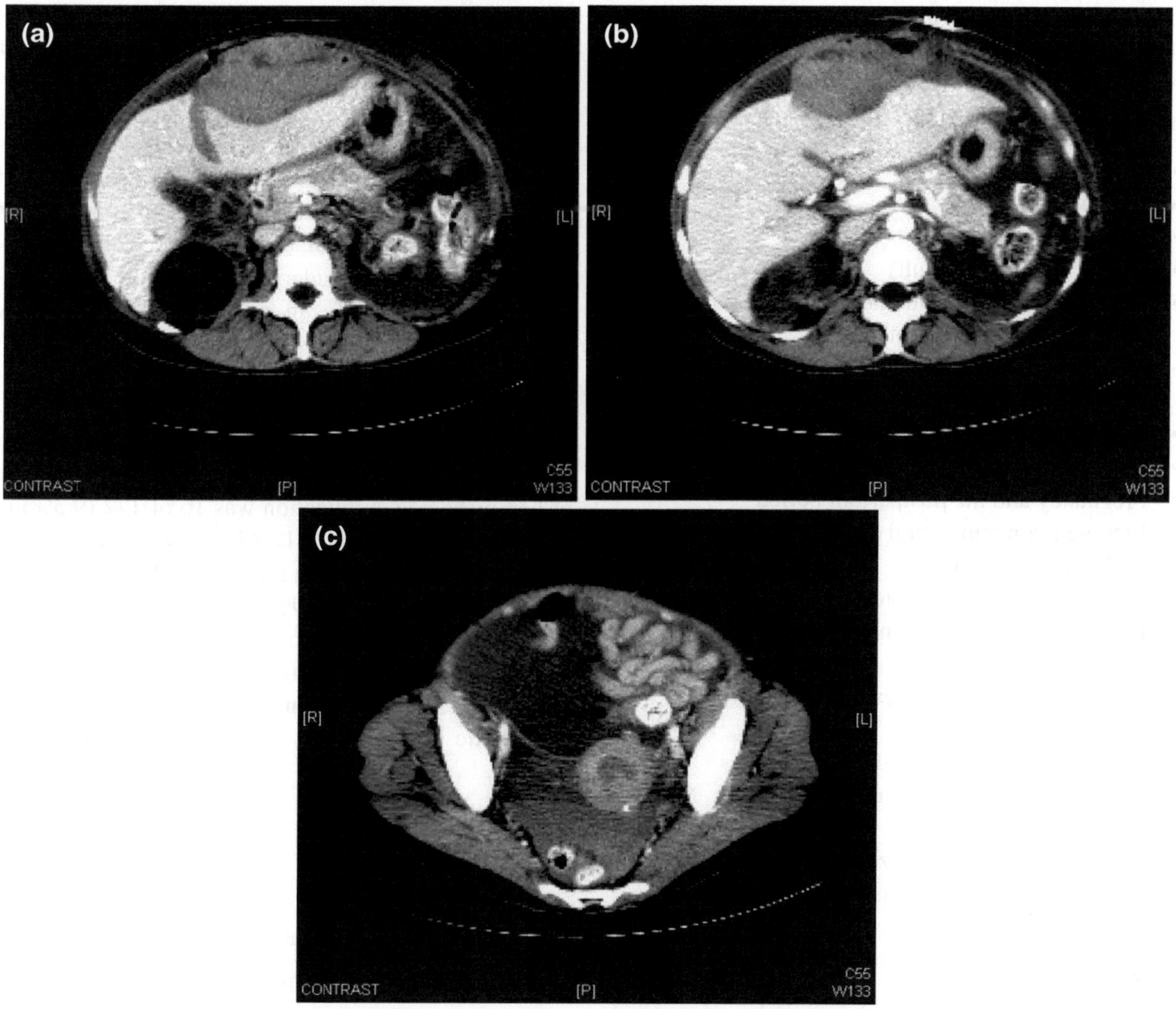

Fig. 8 (**a and b**) CT scan demonstrating a large hematoma anterior to the liver, under previous superior, medial trocar site of a laparoscopic radical nephrectomy in a patient with hemodynamic instability and decreasing hematocrit 4 h postop. Note staples on skin. (**c**) Large amounts of blood in the dependent pelvis

is no evidence of increasing incidence of this complication during laparoscopic surgery. The true incidence of DVT and pulmonary embolism (PE) in laparoscopic urological surgery is unknown. Secin and colleagues conducted a multi-institutional study of symptomatic DVT and PE in prostate cancer patients undergoing laparoscopic or robot-assisted laparoscopic radical prostatectomy [44]. The study included 5,951 patients treated with laparoscopic radical prostatectomy (LRP), with or without robotic assistance. Of the 5,951 patients in the study, 31 developed symptomatic VTE (0.5%), 22 (71%) had DVT only, 4 had PE without identified DVT, and 5 had both PE and DVT. Two patients died of PE. In univariate analysis, current tobacco smoking, large prostate volume, patient re-exploration, longer operative time, and longer hospital stay were associated with VTE.

Patients at Risk

Pulmonary embolism is one of the most common causes of hospital death [45]. Identifying risk factors can provide surgeons and other medical practitioners with the tools to prevent and adequately prophylactically treat those at risk. Geerts and colleagues [38] identified the following risk factors that would promote the development of DVT:

- Surgery
- Trauma
- Immobility
- Cancer (active or occult)
- Cancer therapy (hormonal, chemotherapy, angiogenesis inhibitors, radiotherapy)
- Venous compression (tumor, hematoma, arterial abnormality)
- Previous VTE
- Increasing age
- Pregnancy and the postpartum period
- Estrogen-containing oral contraceptives or hormone replacement therapy
- Selective estrogen receptor modulators
- Erythropoiesis-stimulating agents
- Acute medical illness
- Inflammatory bowel disease
- Nephrotic syndrome
- Myeloproliferative disorders
- Paroxysmal nocturnal hemoglobinuria
- Obesity
- Central venous catheterization
- Inherited or acquired thrombophilia

This group established a thromboembolism risk stratification to provide thromboprophylaxis in patients undergoing surgical procedures. It was based on the patient's individual risks for VTE, type of surgical procedure (minor and major), age (<40 years, 40–60 years, and >60 years), and patient's predisposing factors.

Minor risk: Minor surgery in mobile patients, minor surgery <40 years with no additional risk factors.

Moderate risk: Most general, open gynecologic or urologic surgery patients, minor surgery in patients with additional risk factors, and surgery in patients aged 40–60 years with no additional risk factors.

High risk: Surgery in patients >60 years, or age 40–60 with additional risk factors (see list). *Highest risk:* Surgery in patients with multiple risk factors (age >40 years, cancer, prior venous thromboembolism) [38].

When considering therapeutic options for thromboprophylaxis two types of therapies can be used, either alone or in combination: pharmacological therapies such as low-dose unfractionated heparin (LDUH) or low molecular weight heparin (LMWH) and nonpharmacological therapies, such as graduated compression stockings (GCS), intermittent pneumatic compression (IPC), and early ambulation. There is always risk of bleeding when considering pharmacological treatment to prevent VTE. In a study by Montgomery et al. [46], 344 patients were given either fractionated heparin (FH) or sequential compression devices (SCD) for venous thrombosis prophylaxis for urological laparoscopy [46]. In both groups the rate of thrombotic complication was 2 of 172 (1.2%). The rate of hemorrhagic complication was 16 of 172 (9.3%) in the FH group, of which 12 (7.0%) were major. The hemorrhagic complication rate was 6 of 172 (3.5%) on the SCD group, with 5 (2.9%) being major. The authors concluded that after urological laparoscopy, subcutaneous fractionated heparin is associated with increased hemorrhagic complications, without a reduction in thrombotic complications compared with sequential devices.

Recommendations

Based on the American College of Chest Physicians Evidence-Based clinical Practice guidelines the recommendations for prevention of venous thromboembolism during laparoscopic surgery are as follows [38]:

1. VTE prophylaxis is needed for all patients undergoing laparoscopic and robotic Urologic surgery except, those patients undergoing minor laparoscopic procedures who are also under the age of 40.
2. For patients with additional VTE risk factors, thromboprophylaxis with one or more of LMWH, LDUH, fondaparinux, IPC, or GCS is recommended based on their risk stratification.

Despite these recommendations most patients undergoing Urologic laparoscopy fall under the moderate and high risk category for which VTE prophylaxis is crucial. Consideration for double VTE prophylaxis has to be entertained at all times.

Summary

Vascular injuries are rare but still comprise the most common major complications in urologic laparoscopy. Most are due to dissection injuries and their management should be approached with composure, expediency, and decisiveness. Adjunctive hemostatic agents can be utilized. These include fibrin products, clips, and stapling devices. Exposure is key and the same principles of open surgery apply. If adequate exposure cannot be obtained, additional trocars can be placed. Especially in the scenario of major vascular injury, if optimal control cannot be obtained expeditiously, open conversion is mandatory. Great care should be employed from access to closure in order to avoid potentially devastating vascular injuries.

References

1. Gill IS, Kavoussi LR, et al. Complications of laparoscopic nephrectomy in 185 patients. A multiinstitutional review. J Urol. 1995;154:479.
2. Siqueira TM, Kuo Rl, Gardner TA, et al. Major complication in 213 laparoscopic nephrectomies: the Indianapolis experience. J Urol. 2002;168:1361.
3. Champault G, Cazacu F, Taffinder N. Serious Trocar injuries in laparoscopic surgery: a French survey of 103,852 operation. Surg Laparosc Endosc. 1996;6:367–70.
4. Roviaro GC, Varoli F, Saguatti L, Vergani C, Maciocco M, Scarduelli A. Major vascular injuries in laparoscopic surgery. Surg Endosc. 2002;16:1192.
5. Colombo JR Jr, Haber GP, Jelovsek JE, Nguyen M, Fergany A, Desai MM, Kaouk JH, Gill IS. Complications of laparoscopic surgery for urological cancer: a single institution analysis. J Urol. 2007;178:786–91.
6. Permpongkosol S, Link RE, Su LM, et al. Complications of 2,775 urological laparoscopic procedures: 1993 to 2005. J Urol. 2007;177:580–5.
7. Parsons JK, Varkarakis I, Rha KH, et al. Complications of abdominal urologic laparoscopy: longitudinal five-year analysis. Urology. 2004;63:27–32.
8. Fahlenkamp D, Rassweiler J, Fornara P, et al. Complications of laparoscopic procedures in urology: experience with 2407 procedures at 4 German centers. J Urol. 1999;162:765–70.
9. Meraney AM, Abd-El Samee A, Gill IS. Vascular and bowel complications during retroperitoneal laparoscopic surgery. J Urol. 2002;168:1941–4.
10. Härkki-Sirén P. The incidence of entry-related laparoscopic injuries in Finland. Gyn Endo. 1999;8:355.
11. Geers J, Holden C. Major vascular injury as a complication of laparoscopic surgery: a report of 3 cases and a review of the literature. Am Aurg. 1996;62:377–9.
12. Saville LE, Woods MS. Laparoscopy and major retroperitoneal vascular injuries. Surg Endosc. 1995;9: 1096–100.
13. Wherry DC, Marohn MR, Malanoski MP, et al. An external audit of laparoscopic cholecystectomy in the steady state performed in medical treatment facilities of the department of defense. Ann Surg. 1996;224:145–54.
14. Hashizume M, Sugimachi K. Needle and trocar injury during laparoscopic surgery in Japan. Surg Endosc. 1997;11:1198–201.
15. Bhoyrul S, et al. Trocar injuries in laparoscopic surgery. J Am Coll Surg. 2001 Jun;192(6):677–83.
16. Nordestgaard AG, Bodily KC, Osborne RW, Buttorff. Major vascular injuries during laparoscopic procedures. Am J Surg. 1995;169:543–5.
17. Kavoussi LR, Sosa E, Chandhoke P, Chodak G, Clayman RV, Hadley HR, et al. Complications of laparoscopic pelvic lymph node dissection. J Urol. 1993;149:322.
18. Peters CA. Complications in pediatric urological laparoscopy: results of a survey. J Urol. 1996;155:1070–3.
19. Chandler JG, Corson SL, Way LW. Three spectra of laparoscopic entry access injuries. J Am Coll Surg. 2001;192:478–91.
20. Levy BS, Soderstrom RM, Dail DH. Bowel injuries during laparoscopy gross anatomy and histology. J Reprod Med. 1985;30:168–75.
21. Philips PA, Amaral JF. Abdominal access complications in laparoscopic surgery. J Am Coll Surg. 2001;192:525.
22. Molloy D, Kaloo PD, Cooper M, Nguyen TV. Laparoscopic entry: a literature review and analysis of techniques and complications of primary port entry. Aust N Z J Obstet Gynaecol. 2002;42:246–5.
23. Hanney RM, Carmalt HL, Merrett N, et al. Use of the Hasson cannula producing major vascular injury at laparoscopy. Surg Endosc. 1999;12:1238–40.
24. Hurd WW, Bude RO, De Lancey JO, Pearl ML. The relationship of the umbilicus to aortic bifurcation: implications for laparoscopic technique. Obstet Gynecol. 1992;80: 48–51.
25. Soderstrom RM. Injuries to major blood vessels during endoscopy. J Am Assoc Gynecol Laparosc. 1997;4: 395–8.
26. Nezhat F, Brill AI, Nezhat CH, Nezhat A, Seidman DS, Nezhat C. Laparoscopic appraisal of the anatomic relationship of the umbilicus to the aortic bifurcation. J Am Assoc Gynecol Laparosc. 1998;5:135–40.
27. Sriprasad S, Yu DF, Muir GH, Poulsen J, Sidhu PS. Positional anatomy of vessels that may be damaged at laparoscopy: new access criteria based on CT and ultrasonography to avoid vascular injury. J Endourol. 2006;20(7):498–503.
28. Asensio JA. Visceral vascular injuries. Surg Clin North Am. 2002;82(1):1–20.
29. McAllister M, Bhayani SB, Ong A, et al. Vena caval transection during retroperitoneoscopic nephrectomy: report of the complication and review of the literature. J Urol. 2004;172:183–5.
30. Chan D, Bishoff JT, Ratner L, Kavoussi LR, Jarrett TW. Endovascular gastrointestinal stapler device malfunction during laparoscopic nephrectomy: early recognition and management. J Urol. 2000;164(2):319–21.

31. Deng DY, Meng MV, Nguyen HT, Bellman GC, Stoller ML. Laparoscopic linear cutting stapler failure. Urology. 2002;60(3):415–9.
32. Hsi R, Saint-Elie D, Zimmerman G, Baldwin D. Mechanisms of hemostatic failure during laparoscopic nephrectomy: review of food and drug administration database. Urology. 2007;70(5):888–92.
33. Yaycioglu O. Delayed complications. In: Ramakumar S, Jarrett T, editors. Complications of urologic laparoscopic surgery. Boca Raton: Taylor & Francis; 2005. p. 149.
34. Ramani A, Desai M, Steinberg A, et al. Complications of laparoscopic partial nephrectomy in 200 cases. J Urol. 2005;173:42–7.
35. Singh D, Gill IS. Renal artery pseudoaneurysm following laparoscopic partial nephrectomy. J Urol. 2005;174:2256.
36. Shapiro EY, Ari Hakimi A, Hyams ES, Cynamon J, Stifelman M, Ghavamian R. Renal artery pseudoaneurysm following laparoscopic partial nephrectomy. Urology. 2009 Oct;74(4):819–23.
37. Muntener M, Romero FR, Kavoussi R. Complications in laparoscopic surgery. In: Hohenfellner M, Santucci R, editors. Emergencies in urology. Springer; 2007. pp. 359–360.
38. Geerts WH, Pineo GF, Heit JA, et al. Prevention of venous thromboembolism: the Seventh ACCP Conference on Antithrombotic and Thrombolytic Therapy. Chest 2004;126:338S–400S.
39. Zacharoulis D, Kakkar AK. Venous thromboembolism in laparoscopic surgery. Curr Opin Pulm Med 2003;9: 356–61.
40. Ljungstrom KG. Is there a need for antithromboembolic prophylaxis during laparoscopic surgery? Not always. J Thromb Haemost 2005;3:212–3.
41. Rasmussen MS. Is there a need for antithrombotic prophylaxis during laparoscopic surgery? Always. J Thromb Haemos 2005;3:210–1.
42. Society of American Gastrointestinal and Endoscopic Surgeons. Deep venous thrombosis prophylaxis during laparoscopic surgery. Accessed 31 March 2008.
43. Abdel-Meguid TA, Gomella LG. Prevention and management of complications. In: Smith AD, Badlani GH, Bagley DH, et al., editors. Smith's textbook of endourology. St. Louis: Quality Medical; 1996. pp. 851–869.
44. Secin FP, Jiborn T, Bjartell AS, et al. Multi-institutional study of symptomatic deep venous thrombosis and pulmonary embolism in prostate cancer patients undergoing laparoscopic or robot-assisted laparoscopic radical prostatectomy. Eur Urol. 2008;53:134–45.
45. Shojania KG, Duncan BW, McDonald KM, et al. Making health care safer: a critical analysis of patient safety practices; evidence report/technology assessment No. 43 (prepared by the University of California at San Francisco-Stanford Evidence-Based Practice Center under contract No. 290–97-0013). AHRQ Publication No. 01-E058, Rockville, MD. Agency for Healthcare Research and Quality.
46. Montgomery JS, Wolf JS Jr. Venous thrombosis prophylaxis for urologic laparoscopy: fractionated heparin versus sequential compression devices. J Urol. 2005;173:1623–6.

Urinary and Urologic Complications of Laparoscopic and Robotic Urologic Procedures

Abraham Ari Hakimi and Reza Ghavamian

Keywords Laparoscopy · Robotic surgery · Urine leak · Complications

Introduction

Urinary complications are some of the more common complications of laparoscopic urologic surgery. The overall incidence of urinary tract injury following laparoscopy urologic surgery in large series is under 1% [1, 2]. These injuries can occur both in upper tract and in pelvic urologic laparoscopy. They include injures to the ureter, urinary leaks after extirpative and reconstructive procedures, bladder injuries, and anastomotic leaks. In general, urinary complications after robotic-assisted laparoscopic procedures is similar and is thus discussed together.

Urine leaks after upper tract surgery can occur with significant frequency after laparoscopic partial nephrectomy (LPN) as well as pyeloplasty. Anastomotic leaks occur after laparoscopic and robotic prostatectomy and can lead to significant morbidity and increased hospital stay. They can also occur after laparoscopic ureteral reimplantation and uretero-intestinal anastomosis in conjunction with laparoscopic or robotic cystectomy. Ureteral complications can occur in both upper and lower tract procedures. Urinary complications can be encountered, detected, and repaired intraoperatively. Detection is key, as significant morbidity can be avoided. Unfortunately, not all injuries are detected intraoperatively. There are delayed presentations of injuries and complications that manifest several days or weeks postoperatively.

R. Ghavamian (✉)
Department of Urology, Montefiore Medical Center, Albert Einstein College of Medicine, 3400 Bainbridge Ave, Bronx, NY 10467, USA
e-mail: rghavami@montefiore.org

Urine Leaks After Laparoscopic Upper Tract Surgery

Urinary leakage can occur after extirpative upper tract surgery (LPN) or after reconstructive procedures such as pyeloplasty. The ureter can also be injured during other urologic laparoscopic procedures involving the upper tract such as ureterolysis. There are similarities in presentation and management of this potentially morbid complication and each scenario will be discussed separately.

Urinary Leakage After Laparoscopic Partial Nephrectomy

As an entity, urine leak is the most common complication second to only hemorrhage that can occur after laparoscopic partial nephrectomy. The overall range of urine leak after LPN varies widely in the literature due to heterogeneity of definitions and reporting. As more complex tumors are tackled laparoscopically, the theoretical risks of urinary leakage increase. The reported incidence ranges from as low as 0.5% to a high of 21% [3–5]. Gill et al. recently reviewed the Cleveland

R. Ghavamian (ed.), *Complications of Laparoscopic and Robotic Urologic Surgery*,
DOI 10.1007/978-1-60761-676-4_6, © Springer Science+Business Media, LLC 2010

Clinic's experience with complications following 507 LPNs and found an overall urologic complication rate of 9.4%, with a leak-specific complication rate of 2.4% [12]. There were no specific predictors on multivariate analysis. Others have found increased leaks after larger tumors, endophytic masses, and those with collecting system entry [4]. Meeks et al. found that the volume of renal parenchyma removed was significantly associated with leaks after LPN [6]. A recent comparative review of the OPN and LPN literature by Porpglia et al. [7] found that OPN groups had a higher urologic complication rate compared to LPN, while LPN had increased hemorrhagic complications. One explanation could be that more complex, deeper endophytic tumors were tackled in the open group with more collecting system entry.

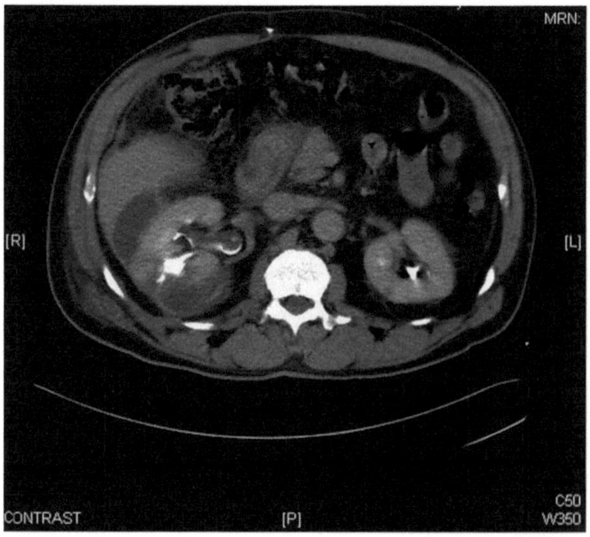

Fig. 1 Urinary extravasation after right laparoscopic partial nephrectomy

Diagnosis

Renal leak after LPN can present in both the immediate and the delayed postoperative setting. The immediate diagnosis is often made when increased drainage from the peri-renal drain is noted. The fluid can be sent for creatinine, which will be markedly elevated and helps distinguish it from serous fluid. Patients may have low-grade postoperative fevers and abdominal distention and/or ileus if the urine tracks into the peritoneum. As intraperitoneal laparoscopic approach is the most common approach utilized in LPN, the incidence of ileus is theoretically higher than open partial nephrectomy, where an extraperitoneal approach is utilized. Most small, non-obstructed renal leaks will resolve spontaneously. The urethral catheter is left indwelling and the surgical drain is typically left in for several days to prevent abscess or urinoma formation, and outputs are recorded. Often, the drain will be taken off suction if drainage persists based on the theory that the increased negative pressure prolongs the leak.

Delayed presentations can be variable. Again if the operated kidney is not obstructed, most leaks tend to resolve spontaneously. If an obstruction is present, the patient may develop increased drainage or nephrocutaneous fistulas often through the drain incision site. This can be confirmed through sampling of the fluid for creatinine or administration of indigo carmine. Most obstructions in the immediate postoperative period are due to postoperative bleeding into the collecting system with subsequent clot obstruction of the ureter and renal pelvis. Identification of obstruction usually occurs through cross-sectional imaging which typically shows perinephric fluid collections and surrounding tissue stranding. The ideal imaging modality is an intravenous contrast CT scan with delayed imaging which will help delineate the etiology of the fluid collection (Figs. 1 and 2). Left alone, many of the

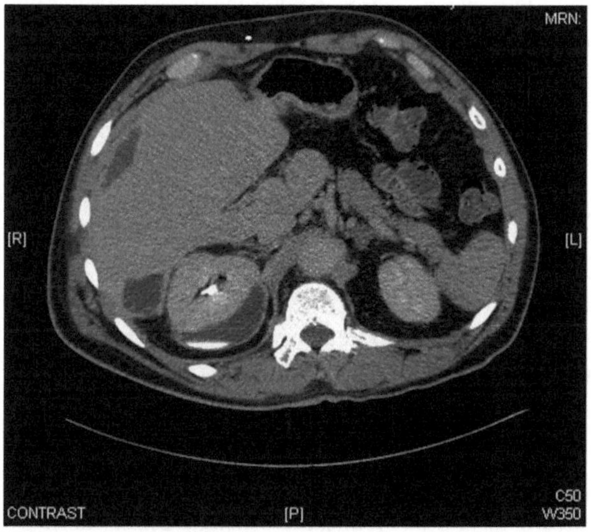

Fig. 2 Layering of contrast noted in the retroperitoneum after laparoscopic partial nephrectomy

larger collections can form urinomas or abscesses, in which case the patient will often present with urinary tract infections, fevers, abdominal distention, nausea, vomiting, and potentially sepsis.

Management of Urine Leaks

Meeks et al. reported on their experience with 21 patients who developed urine leaks after both OPN and LPN. In this series, 90% of the patients had ureteral stents placed before the actual partial nephrectomy. The mean duration of leakage was 53 days. About 80% of the patients presented with increased drain output while two presented with fever and two had wound infection after drain removal. In 62% of the patients urine leakage was managed only by prolonged percutaneous drainage. Eight patients (38%) required placement of a second ureteral stent for a urine leak, which was done a median of 25 days after the initial partial nephrectomy and which remained an average of 53 days. The drain was left a mean of 26 days in patients with a urine leak. Patient age at surgery was the only clinical factor associated with longer leak duration when patients were stratified into groups based on short (less than 30 days) and long (greater than 30 days) urine leaks. All patients with long urine leak duration required a ureteral stent. Overall median leak duration was significantly different between patients with long and short urine leaks (9 vs. 105 days, $p < 0.00001$). Median Jackson–Pratt drainage time was significantly different between patients with short and long urine leaks (9 vs. 28 days, $p < 0.02$). Two patients required multiple percutaneous and endoscopic procedures to resolve urine leaks with a median leakage duration of 163 days. No patient required open or laparoscopic reoperation.

Generally, the management of renal leaks after LPN is the same as in OPN. Most leaks can be managed conservatively, especially if the surgical drain remains in place. Many patients will require the drain for several days or even weeks in rare instances. Many surgeons will leave or reinsert a Foley catheter due to the theory that increased bladder pressures can lead to increased upper tract pressures, exacerbating the leak. Most patients who have failed conservative management can be managed with ureteral stent insertion. A concomitant retrograde pyelogram can help define the magnitude and location of the leak and its relation to the location of the drain. If stent insertion does not stop the leakage, the drain can be taken off suction. It should be noted that if the drain is close or abutting the fistula site, it will act as a siphon, keeping the fistula open even if the drain is off suction (Fig. 3). In this scenario, the drain can be retracted incrementally. A potential problem can arise from excess urinary drainage around the drain, which can soil and moisten the dressing and clothing and ultimately lead to skin breakdown. A novel method to manage this scenario is the application of a urostomy collection appliance around the drain. This allows for a clean and dry collection mechanism that is easily managed by the patient at home. The patient is instructed to keep a log of drainage from the drain site and the Foley catheter, until the leakage resolves and the drains and catheters are removed. Patients with perinephric abscesses or large urinomas may need additional percutaneous drainage usually performed by interventional radiology. This is in scenarios where the urinoma is not drained adequately by the indwelling drain or in situations where the drain was prematurely removed. In high output circumstances, some have reported placement of second ureteral catheters or percutaneous nephrostomy drainage.

It is very rare for patients not to resolve prolonged leakage with endoscopic or percutaneous drainage. Some novel case reports have utilized fibrin glue

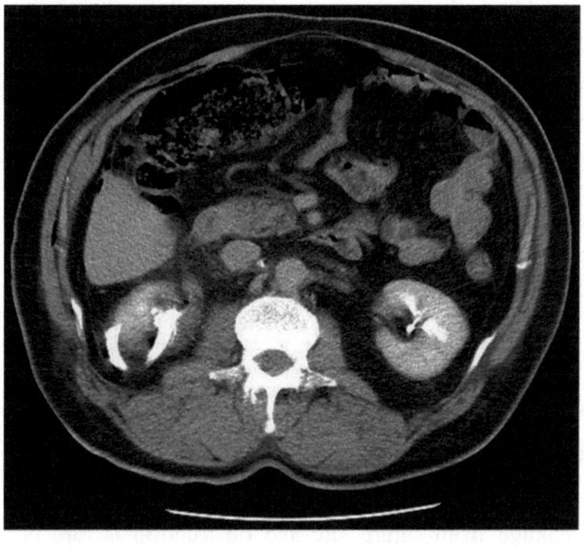

Fig. 3 The distal end of the Jackson–Pratt drain directly abuts the leak, acting as a siphon to keep leak open

both ureteroscopically and percutaneously to close refractory leaks [8, 9]. Isolated reports of the use of desmopressin are also described in the literature to decrease urinary outputs after other types of renal surgery, but its use has to be considered as a last resort [10]. Unresolved refractory leaks and subsequent resultant infections can mandate nephrectomy. This step is an absolute last resort.

Future Direction

Recently, there has been an increased interest in the use of Da Vinci surgical system for performing a laparoscopic partial nephrectomy. As pure LPN is a technically challenging procedure in particular, with specific reference to intracorporeal suturing, the speculation is that the robot can decrease the learning curve and actually lead to easier parenchymal and collecting system reconstruction. It is thought that more laparoscopically naive surgeons will employ the minimally invasive approach to partial nephrectomy utilizing the new technology. Many surgeons who have been facile with the pure LPN technique are adopting the robotic approach. Several early series using the da Vinci robot system to assist in LPN have been described. There is a theoretical advantage to the robot specifically for more challenging endophytic tumors in which suturing of the collecting system is necessary. Nonetheless, data are still too premature to assess whether the theoretic benefit of robotic assistance during renorrhaphy leads to decreased postoperative urinary leak or obstruction. Shapiro et al.'s review of the robotic literature still reported a leak rate of 1.5% in a review of several small series [11]. Whether the robotic approach actually leads to less leakage and better repair remains to be seen. This is best evaluated if expert laparoscopic surgeons who have adopted the robotic approach actually experience less urinary complications.

Urinary Complications After Laparoscopic Pyeloplasty

Leakage from suture site and obstruction is rare but well-documented complications following both open and laparoscopic pyeloplasties (LP). Rassweiler et al. [12] reviewed their series of 189 pyeloplasties and found an overall complication rate of 7.9% with a urinary complication rate of 3.1% including 4 urine leaks and 2 stent obstructions; 1 patient developed a stone upon late follow-up. Kavoussi et al. [13] reported an overall incidence of urine leak following LP of 2.33% finding it to be the most common Grade I complication.

The most likely explanation of immediate postoperative stent obstruction after LP is postoperative bleeding into the collecting system leading to clot formation. Meticulous hemostasis with bipolar coagulation is absolutely mandatory. Renal ultrasound is usually sufficient for diagnosis, and KUB can be performed to confirm appropriate stent placement. Management can be with either percutaneous nephrostomy or nephroureteral stent to augment drainage or possibly replace the double J stent. The use of continuous suturing may reduce the risk of this type of complication.

Urinary extravasation may occur early and may be due to the use of interrupted sutures. Alternatively, it can occur in the setting of insufficient tension on the continuous suture or if the double J stent is obstructed with clot or has migrated. The exchange of the JJ stent has to be performed using a hydrophilic guide-wire to minimize the trauma on the anastomosis under fluoroscopic guidance. Urinary leakage may also occur after Foley catheter removal due to transmitted voiding pressures. If the drain has been removed already it should be replaced percutaneously. For this reason, we routinely keep the drain in place upon withdrawal of the Foley catheter and strictly monitor output. The management of urinary leakage post-pyeloplasty is similar to laparoscopic partial nephrectomy. Maximum drainage is the key, utilizing JJ stents, drains, and Foley catheter drainage. In refractory cases nephroureteral or nephrostomy tube drainage can be employed.

The consequence of inappropriate management of excessive urinary extravasation after pyeloplasty is dense and extensive scarring that can result, compromising healing and ultimately drainage of the kidney. In cases where scarring has resulted in repeat obstruction, endourologic maneuvers such as endopyelotomy can be employed to correct the situation. A repeat pyeloplasty is usually difficult and ureterocalicostomy might be the procedure of choice in this setting.

With respect to the theoretic benefit of robotic assistance in pyeloplasty, Braga et al. [14] performed a meta-analysis of eight studies comparing robotic-assisted LP with conventional LP. Outcomes assessed included operative time, blood loss, hospital stay, and peri-operative and postoperative complications. Their review found no difference in terms of complications between the two approaches. The overall leak rate in the pooled meta-analysis was 5% (13/260).

Ureteral Injuries

Ureteral injuries are unfortunately a well-known complication of urologic surgery, and laparoscopy has been no exception. The urologist is far more likely to encounter a laparoscopically induced ureteral injury as a consultation from the other services, specifically gynecology and colorectal surgery. Gynecologic laparoscopy is associated with an overall incidence of urinary tract injury ranging from 0.5 to 4.8% with 80% of the injuries occurring to the bladder [3–15]. The urinary tract is at particular risk due to its proximity to the uterine and ovarian vascular supply. Risk factors for injury include prior pelvic radiation, malignancy, and pelvic adhesions. A recent review from Vakili et al. utilized intraoperative cystoscopy after hysterectomy and found a 4.8% incidence of urinary tract injury, of which 1.7% was ureteral. Nonetheless, only 12.5% of ureteral injuries were detected before cystoscopy. Ureteral injury most commonly occurs proximally at the pelvic brim during ligation of the infundibulopelvic ligament and distally during ligation of the uterine artery during hysterectomy. A review of all laparoscopic hysterectomies found a 0.3% incidence of ureteral injury, with all injuries occurring at the distal ureter at the level of the uterine artery or uterosacral ligament [16]. Up to 50% of cases of unilateral ureteral injury are asymptomatic postoperatively. Fortunately, ureteral injuries in the urologic laparoscopic literature are rare. Kavoussi et al. only reported 6 cases in a review of 2775 procedures, including 1 which was recognized intraoperatively and 5 postoperatively.

Early recognition is crucial to avoid the need for re-intervention. The best way to avoid ureteral injuries is to identify the ureter as early as possible, certainly before clamping critical pedicles. Mechanisms of ureteral injuries include division, ligation, and cauterization. Devascularization injury can lead to stricture formation or even delayed necrosis. Most complete ureteral divisions are often recognized intra-operatively whereas ligation and cautery injuries often present in a delayed fashion.

Intra-operative Management

A high index of suspicion is necessary to detect ureteral injuries intraoperatively. The surgeon should be cognizant of the proximity of the ureter to the surgical site and the locations at which potential injury can occur. In cases where identification is difficult, landmarks should be used for the identification of the ureter at all times. In the upper tract this includes the proximity of the gonadal vessels and the lower pole of the kidney. In the pelvis, the pelvic brim is an excellent landmark. The ureter crosses over the common iliac artery just proximal to the common iliac bifurcation. At this location, the excellent magnification of laparoscopy and robotics often allows visualization of the ureter and its peristalsis in the retroperitoneum especially in the non-obese patient. In cases where difficulty in ureteral identification is anticipated, a preoperative retrograde ureteral catheter inserted endoscopically can aid in its identification intraoperatively. This is especially useful in procedures where the ureter is involved with neoplastic or inflammatory intra-abdominal processes in close proximity. The ureter should be identified and tagged with a vessel loop to help with its mobilization away from the surgical site and to help with atraumatic manipulation. There are disease processes that make ureteral identification difficult. These include inflammatory retroperitoneal diseases such as retroperitoneal fibrosis and infection and previous urologic or intra-abdominal surgery.

If the ureter is injured with a suture, the suture can be removed and a stent is placed. If the ureter is partially transected a stent should be placed through the ureterostomy and should be left in place for 4–8 weeks. In the setting of a complete transaction recognized intraoperatively, management depends on the location of the injury. If a proximal or mid-ureteral injury is identified, a laparoscopic uretero-ureterostomy can be performed. The ureteral edges are trimmed and

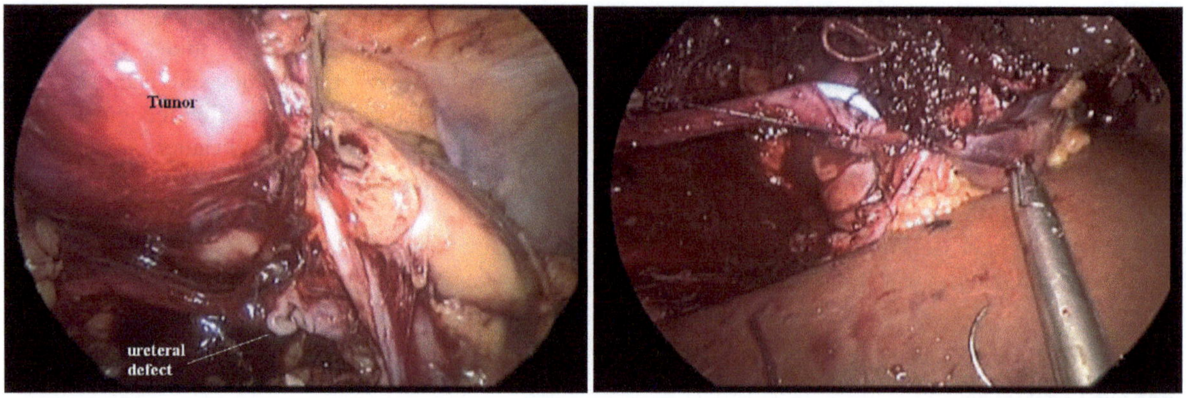

Fig. 4 (**a**) Proximal ureteral injury during a laparoscopic partial nephrectomy for a hilar renal tumor. (**b**) Tension-free repair over a stent placed through the ureteral defect laparoscopically

spatulated. An apical stitch using an absorbable suture is placed at the 12 o'clock position of the distal segment and placed in the proximal ureter at its corresponding 12 o'clock position. A suture is then applied in a similar fashion at the 6 o'clock position, followed by a running anastomosis. For distal ureteral injuries, an experienced laparoscopist can perform an ureteroneocystostomy often with a psoas hitch, or a Boari flap if necessary. Insertion of a ureteral stent is critical in the ultimate repair and healing of the traumatized ureter.

With increasing use of laparoscopic partial nephrectomy for more and more complex lesions, the risk of ureteral injury intraoperatively exists. In the event of such injury, if detected intraoperatively, the same principles of stented repair are utilized as in open surgery (Fig. 4). The ureter is repaired with a tension-free anastomosis and the surgical site is drained as is common practice with partial nephrectomy.

Postoperative Management

Delayed presentation of ureteral injuries is unfortunately a more common occurrence. Presentations can be variable and can present as flank pain, abdominal pain/distention with ileus, fever, nausea, vomiting, and/or hematuria. Fistulas can form to the surgical incision or to the vagina especially after abdominal hysterectomy. Patients that are initially left with surgical drains may have high fluid outputs which can be sent for creatinine. CT scan is the modality of choice and may show retroperitoneal fluid, urinary ascites, and possibly hydroureteronephrosis, depending on the location and severity of the injury. Ultrasound and Tc-99m mercaptotriacetylglycine (MAG3) renal scans have been utilized as well with a high degree of intraoperative correlation [17].

Once a leak is confirmed postoperatively, identification of the location and extent is critical. CT imaging is the preferred imaging modality. It confirms the presence of peri-renal fluid, its extent, and whether it should be drained (Fig. 5). It is specifically helpful as delayed images can confirm communication with the collecting system and contrast-enhanced fluid in the retroperitoneum (Fig. 6). Either retrograde or antegrade pyelography (in the setting of a nephrostomy tube) is generally the best method. If the injury is small and the extravasation is limited, a ureteral stent can usually be manipulated traversing the defect and left in situ for 4–8 weeks. It might be necessary to utilize a flexible ureteroscope to manipulate and negotiate a stent past the ureteral defect. Every attempt at endoscopic management should be performed prior to an open repair. It might not be possible to bridge the gap with a ureteral stent. In this scenario or if the extravasation of contrast on retrograde ureteropyelography is extensive, a percutaneous nephrostomy tube is necessary. The urinoma is then treated with a separate drain placed by interventional radiology for maximum drainage (Fig. 7). The patient can then undergo an elective open repair of the ureter at a later date when the inflammation has subsided, usually in 6 weeks. The consequence of delaying open repair can be dire. Even with optimal drainage further complications

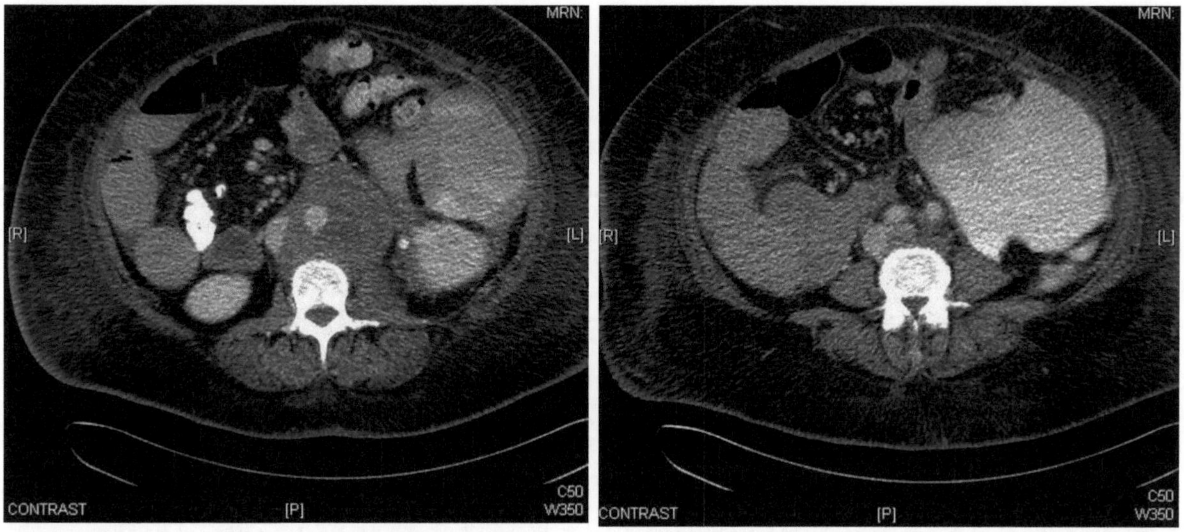

Fig. 5 (**a**) A patient with lymphoma who had recently undergone a laparoscopic biopsy of the para-aortic lymphadenopathy. Large urinoma anterior to the lower pole of the left kidney. A ureteral injury was suspected. (**b**) The urinoma is confirmed with the presence of contrast within the collection

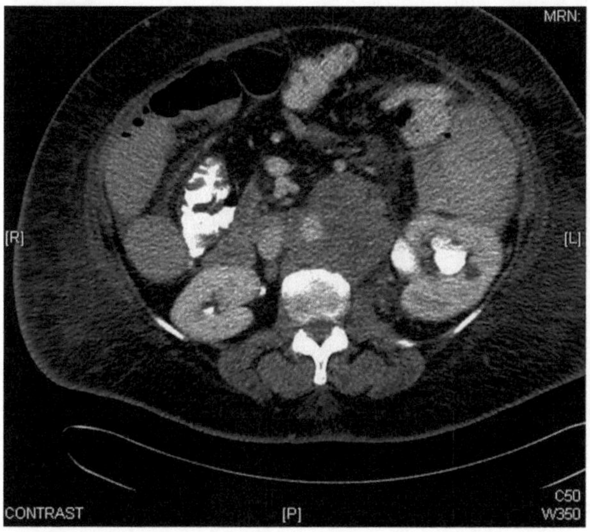

Fig. 6 The relationship of the collecting system and the collection is demonstrated

with these percutaneous drains are possible. Continued sepsis, non-optimal drainage, and ultimately colorenal fistulas can ensue, making definitive surgical repairs difficult and often resulting in nephrectomy (Fig. 8).

If the ureteral injury was detected in the early postoperative period an immediate open repair can be justified, as the inflammation might not be too extensive. The authors preference is early repair in the absence of a large urinoma within 1 week. In cases where a large collection is present or if the problem is detected after 7 days, a delayed exploration after temporary drainage and diversion is more prudent.

The techniques for repair of a proximal ureteral injury include mobilization of the kidney and upper ureter, mobilization of the lower ureter, and a tension-free uretero-ureterostomy. In cases where significant inflammation is present, an omental wrap is an excellent means of anastomotic coverage. For lower ureteral delayed ureteral injuries, the safest mode of repair is a formal ureteral reimplantation utilizing a psoas hitch. Extensive ureteral damaged segments can be repaired utilizing a Boari flap reserving an ileal ureter replacement as a last resort. In cases in which the ureteral fistula was successfully stented and ureteral leakage persists past the 6 week mark an open formal repair might be necessary.

A possible complication after initial successful management of intraoperative or delayed ureteral injury is ureteral stricture formation. These can often be managed endourologically depending on the size and location, with either incision utilizing holmium laser or balloon dilation. If conservative measures fail, operative intervention as described earlier is indicated. Recent studies have described feasibility of

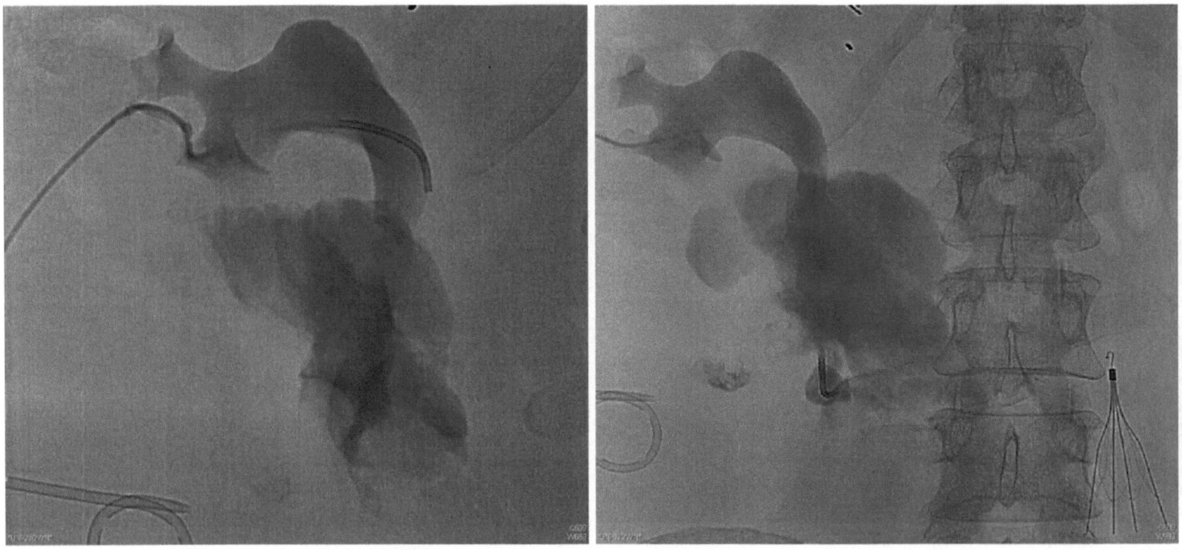

Fig. 7 (**a and b**) Same patient as in Figs. 4 and 5. Antegrade nephrostomy drainage is instituted and a peri-renal drain is placed

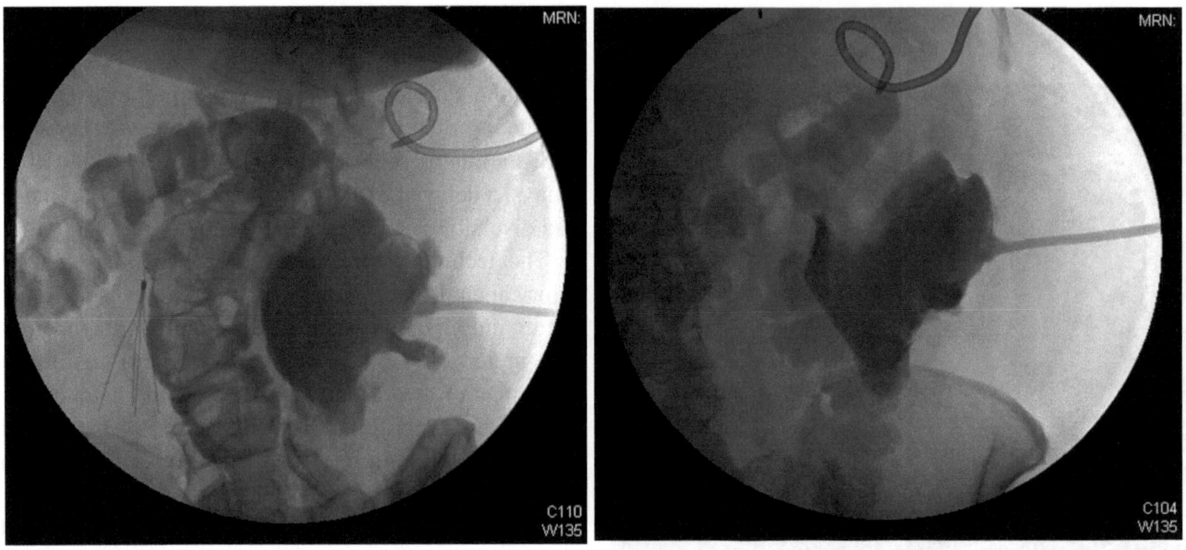

Fig. 8 (**a and b**) Colo-renal fistula with associated colo-cutaneous fistula as a late sequelae of prolonged urinoma and collecting system drainage

robotic-assisted laparoscopic reimplantation for distal ureteral strictures and ureterovaginal fistulas with a mean follow-up of 15.5 months [18].

The diagnosis of an ureterovaginal fistula can be made with several novel techniques. The patient may complain of persistent urinary incontinence. A "pad test" utilizes a sanitary pad placed within the vagina. The patient is then given intravenous methylene blue and staining of the pad will confirm the diagnosis. The diagnosis of vesicovaginal fistula is excluded in this scenario by utilizing a "double dye pad test." Here, the patient is given oral pyridium as well as intravesical methylene blue followed by clamping of the Foley catheter. Orange staining confirms a ureteral source, whereas blue staining suggests a vesicovaginal fistula.

Lower Tract Urinary Complications

Bladder Injuries

Fortunately, bladder injuries are extremely rare during laparoscopic/robotic urologic procedures. However, they are much more common during gynecologic surgery, particularly in patients with previous cesarean sections or with pelvic malignancy [19]. During laparoscopic abdominal hysterectomy, the bladder is at risk for injury during the creation of the bladder flap, at which time the bladder dome is dissected from the lower uterine segment. Intraoperative recognition warrants closure which can safely be performed laparoscopically in a two-layer closure with absorbable sutures. Extraperitoneal leaks can often be managed with Foley catheter drainage for 7–10 days.

Postoperative presentation may be similar to ureteral injuries. Patients may present with abdominal distention, ileus, fevers, and increased fluid drainage from pelvic drains. The emerging gold standard for imaging consists of a CT cystogram which offers better anatomic detail compared to conventional cystography [20]. If intraperitoneal leakage with urinary ascites is identified, management consists of an open two- or three-layer repair. The most common procedure in which bladder injuries can potentially occur is robotic or laparoscopic radical prostatectomy. This is a very rare occurrence for the expert robotic surgeon, but several factors such as previous pelvic or bladder surgery and previous hernia repair especially with mesh could be potential risk factors. Bladder repair is usually straightforward with a two-layer closure with absorbable sutures.

Anastomotic Leaks After Robotic or Laparoscopic Prostatectomy

Anastomotic leaks are a feared complication following radical prostatectomy. One of the greatest challenges of operating in the deep pelvis has been creating a water-tight urethro-vesical anastomosis. The actual incidence of leakage is difficult to fully assess as there tends to be varying definitions. The presence of significant extravasated urine may have several short- and long-term consequences. Patients may have prolonged postoperative ileus, fever, and urinary tract infection. They are also at long-term risk for development of bladder neck contractures which can lead to voiding difficulties and repeat incisions or dilatations. Significant scarring can occur, compromising appropriate sphincteric coaptation and support. If not in the immediate postoperative period, dense bladder neck contractures can involve the external sphincter mechanism during the healing phase and prevent its optimal coaptation and function. This exposes the patient to a lifelong battle with continence issues long after his battle with prostate cancer. This complication is discussed in more detail in the chapter on complications of RALP and will only be briefly discussed here.

The difficulty with quantifying anastomotic leakage after prostatectomy is that most asymptomatic patients are not routinely imaged upon catheter removal. In a novel study of robotic-assisted laparoscopic prostatectomy (RALP), Menon et al. retrospectively reviewed about 450 patients from 2004 to 2005 [21]. Patients routinely underwent cystography 7 days after robotic prostatectomy, while the Foley catheter was still in place. Standard scout radiograph, antero-posterior (AP) and shallow oblique views after retrograde instillation of approximately 125–250 cc of iodinated contrast, and a postvoid AP image were obtained in all imaged patients. All cases were retrospectively reviewed by two radiologists. Results were further classified as small extraperitoneal leaks adjacent to the urethrovesical anastomosis in the surgical bed, moderate extraperitoneal leak confined to the pelvis, or large combined extra/intraperitoneal leaks arising from the urethrovesical anastomosis. A total of 67 leaks were identified (15.2%). About 60% of the leaks were small, extraperitoneal, and confined to the surgical bed. Twenty-one patients had moderate sized leaks limited to the extraperitoneal space, 31% of all leaks or 4.2% of all patients. Six leaks were large, extending into the intraperitoneal space from the extraperitoneal space. Two of these six patients required CT-guided drainage for urinoma (<0.5% of all patients). One patient had a colo-vesical fistula requiring revision. Two cases demonstrated Grade I vesicoureteral reflux.

In the early first large series of peri-operative outcomes following laparoscopic radical prostatectomy (LRP) Guillonneau et al. reported an anastomotic leak of nearly 10%. Anastomotic leakage developed in 57 patients (10%) [22]. Anastomotic leakage was defined as persistent urine in the suction drain for more than 6 days, justifying the maintenance of bladder drainage. In 43 cases the fistula healed spontaneously by continuing suction drainage until cure and by prolonging bladder drainage for an average of 12 days, with 1 patient requiring reoperation due to a persistent urinary fistula. Two patients required percutaneous drain placement. In 11 cases anastomotic urine leakage was diagnosed after catheter removal in a context of acute pain, urinary retention, and peritoneal irritation. These patients were managed with continued bladder catheterization for another week. The mean duration of bladder catheterization in the series was about 6 days. Acute urinary retention developed as a function of the duration of catheterization in 26 cases (4.6%).

Menon et al. evaluated the effect of anastomotic leak on long-term continence by routinely obtaining cystography upon catheter removal [23]. The degree of leakage was graded and the patients were followed for 12 months using validated questionnaires. In their series 8.6% of patients had radiographic evidence of leaks of which the majority were minor. At 1 year, they found that patients with significant leaks had delayed time to continence, but ultimately achieved the same continence rate (94%) as those with no leak. They did, however, see a higher rate of bladder neck contractures.

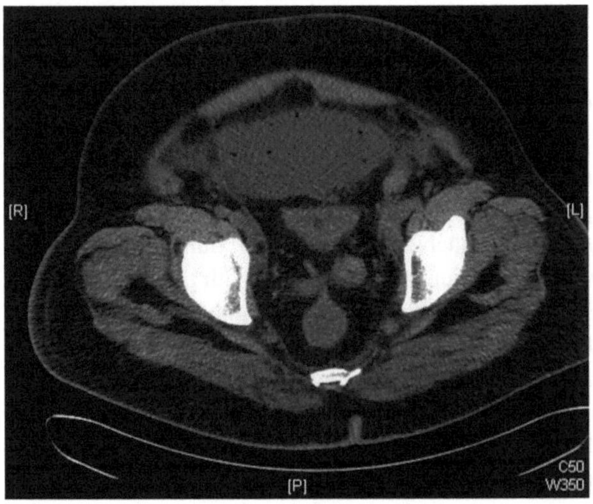

Fig. 9 CT scan of the pelvis reveals a large fluid collection anterior and superior to the bladder

Presentations of Anastomotic Leaks

Urine leak from the vesicourethral anastomosis can have a variable presentation ranging from transient increase in surgical drain output, to complete anastomotic disruption, to urethrocutaneous fistula. Most often patients will have persistent high outputs from the surgical drains, which will have high creatinine content. Some patients can present with delayed

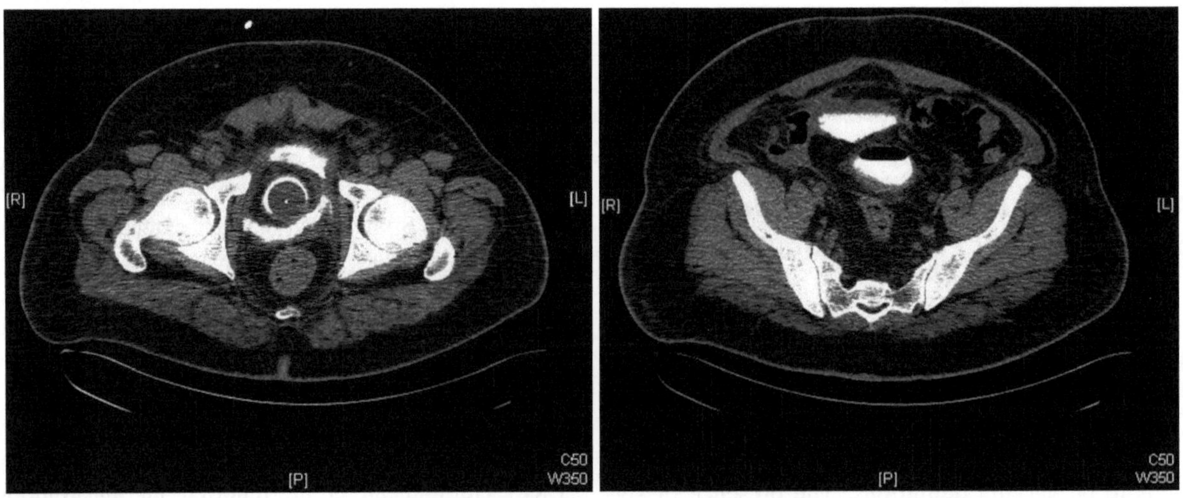

Fig. 10 (**a**) CT cystogram revealing urinary leak from the posterior aspect of the anastomosis tracking anteriorly. (**b**) Contrast in the dome of the bladder and extravasated contrast in the anterior fluid collection confirming the leak

leakage which can present with pelvic collections, ileus, fever, leukocytosis, and sepsis. A CT scan is critical in evaluation and delineation of the extent of the leak (Fig. 9). Specifically a CT cystogram is the preferred imaging modality (Figs. 10 and 11). It is crucial to ensure that the Foley catheter is adequately draining, as an obstructed catheter can jeopardize the anastomosis. Mild traction should not be employed as it can cause ischemic changes and risk contractures.

As with open radical prostatectomy, most anastomotic leaks following LRP or RALP can be managed conservatively with prolonged Foley catheterization and continued surgical drain placement. In cases in which the drain has been removed and the patient presents with a delayed leak, the urinoma if extensive has to be drained (Fig. 12). Prolonged

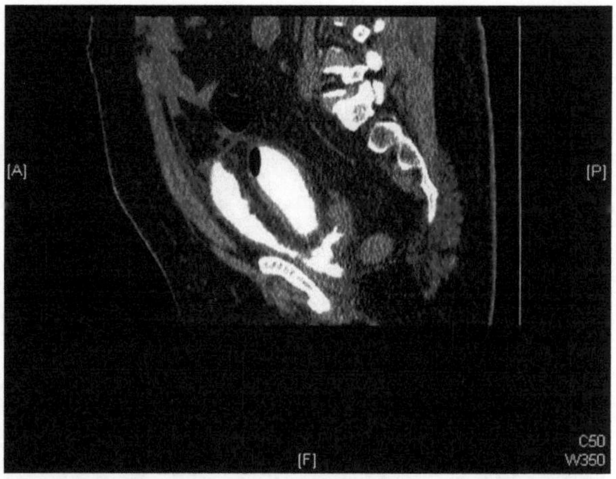

Fig. 11 Sagittal image of the patient in Fig. 9, showing the course of the urine leak

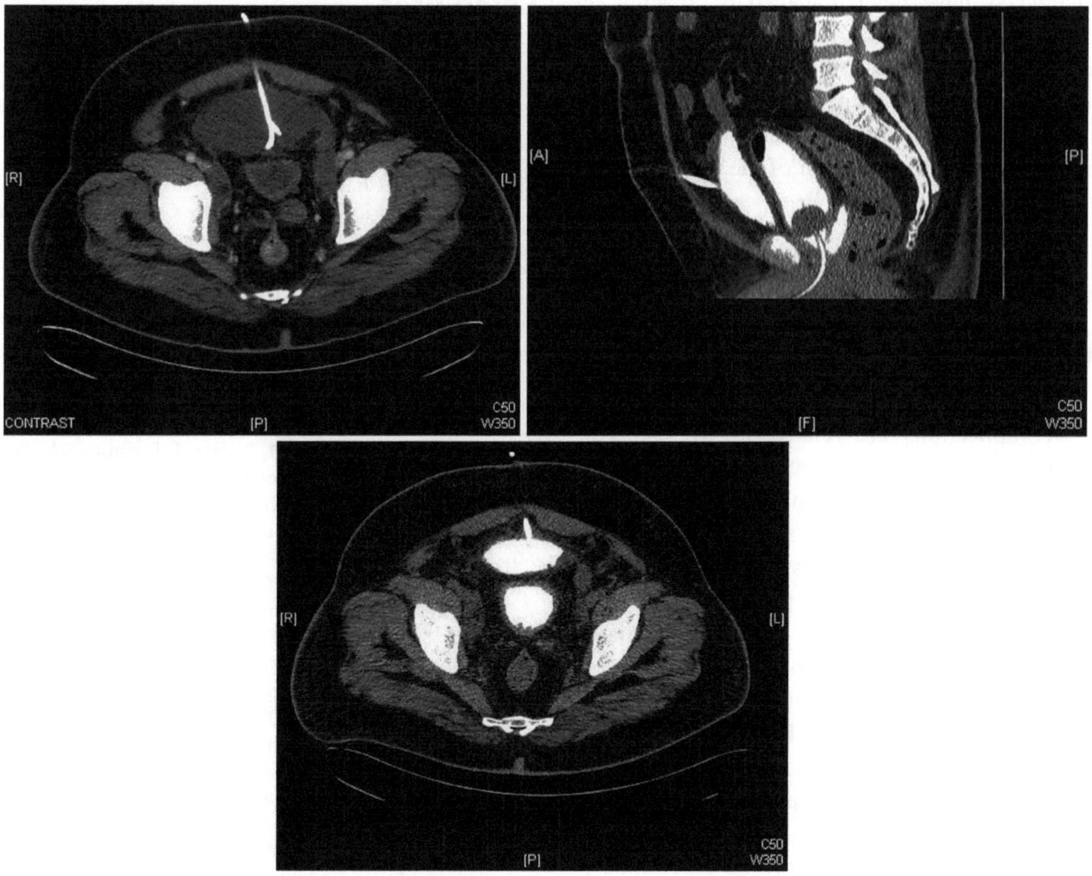

Fig. 12 (**a**) Noncontrast CT scan revealing drain placement. (**b**) Sagittal image revealing the bladder with a Foley catheter in the bladder and the drain in the collection. (**c**) Cross-sectional view

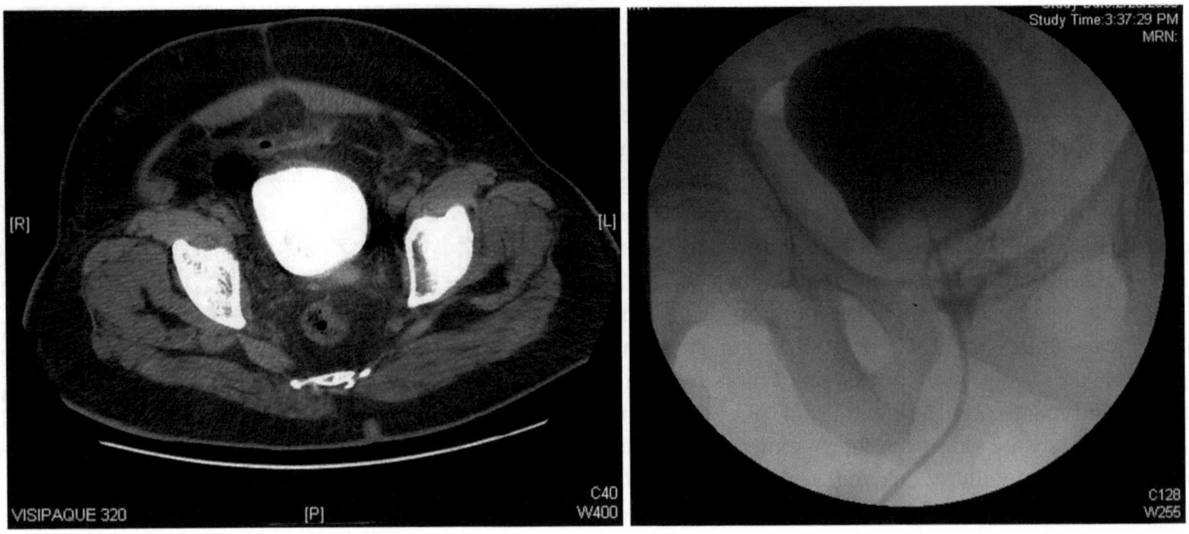

Fig. 13 (**a**) Follow-up CT cystogram of the patient in Fig. 10, revealing no leakage. (**b**) Fluoroscopic image of a cystogram revealing no leakage

extensive leaks have been managed by placing the Foley catheters on suction or placing additional percutaneous drains. Almost all leaks will eventually seal with conservative measures and optimal drainage (Fig. 13). Rarely, and only in extreme circumstances, patients require surgical revision of the vesicourethral anastomosis.

Conclusions

Urinary complications are relatively rare but well-described events following laparoscopic urologic surgery. Water-tight intracorporeal suturing and awareness of surrounding structures are key preventative measures to avoid these injuries. Prudent placement of surgical drains is critical postoperatively, and monitoring of drain outputs is crucial. The majority of leaks/injuries can be managed conservatively. Intervention, when needed, can often be accomplished through percutaneous or endourologic means.

Laparoscopic or open reconstructive repairs are reserved for injuries or complications that cannot be addressed by endourologic or conservative means. Extirpative procedures should only be performed as a last resort for injuries causing morbidity that are refractory to treatment and repair.

References

1. Permpongkosol S, Link RE, Su LM, Romero FR, Bagga HS, Pavlovich CP, Jarrett TW, Kavoussi LR. Complications of 2,775 urological laparoscopic procedures: 1993 to 2005. J Urol. 2007 Feb;177(2):580–5.
2. Colombo JR Jr, Haber GP, Jelovsek JE, Nguyen M, Fergany A, Desai MM, Kaouk JH, Gill IS. Complications of laparoscopic surgery for urological cancer: a single institution analysis. J Urol. 2007 Sep;178(3 Pt 1):786–91.
3. Simmons MN, Gill IS. Decreased complications of contemporary laparoscopic partial nephrectomy: use of a standardized reporting system. J Urol 2007;177:2067.
4. Campbell SC, Novick AC, Streem SB, Klein E, Licht M. Complications of nephron sparing surgery for renal tumors. J Urol. 1994;151:1177.
5. Wille AH, Tullmann M, Roigas J, Loening SA, Deger S. Laparoscopic partial nephrectomy in renal cell cancer – results and reproducibility by different surgeons in a high volume laparoscopic center. Eur Urol. 2006;49:337.
6. Meeks JJ, Zhao LC, Navai N, Perry KT Jr, Nadler RB, Smith ND. Risk factors and management of urine leaks after partial nephrectomy. J Urol. 2008 Dec;180(6): 2375–8.
7. Porpiglia F, Volpe A, Billia M, Scarpa RM. Laparoscopic versus open partial nephrectomy: analysis of the current literature. Eur Urol. 2008 Apr;53(4):732–42.
8. French DB, Marcovich R. Fibrin sealant for retrograde ureteroscopic closure of urine leak after partial nephrectomy. Urology. 2006 May;67(5):1085.e1–3.
9. Seo IY, Lee YH, Rim JS. Case report: percutaneous fibrin glue injection for urine leakage in laparoscopic partial nephrectomy. J Endourol. 2008 May;22(5):959–62.
10. Razzaghi MR, Rezaei A, Javanmard B, Lotfi B. Desmopressin as an alternative solution for urinary leakage

after ureterocaliceal surgeries. Urol J. 2009 Spring;6(2): 120–2.
11. Shapiro E, Benway BM, Wang AJ, Bhayani SB. The role of nephron-sparing robotic surgery in the management of renal malignancy. Curr Opin Urol. 2009 Jan;19(1):76–80.
12. Rassweiler JJ, Teber D, Frede T. Complications of laparoscopic pyeloplasty. World J Urol. 2008 Dec;26(6): 539–47.
13. Permpongkosol S, Link RE, Su LM, Romero FR, Bagga HS, Pavlovich CP, Jarrett TW, Kavoussi LR. Complications of 2,775 urological laparoscopic procedures: 1993 to 2005. J Urol. 2007 Feb;177(2):580–5.
14. Braga LH, Pace K, Demaria J, Lorenzo AJ. Systematic review and meta-analysis of robotic-assisted versus conventional laparoscopic pyeloplasty for patients with ureteropelvic junction obstruction: effect on operative time, length of hospital stay, postoperative complications, and success rate. Eur Urol. 2009 Apr 1.
15. Stany MP, Farley JH. Complications of gynecologic surgery. Surg Clin North Am. 2008 Apr;88(2):343–59.
16. Leonard F, Fotso A, Borghese B, et al. Ureteral complications from laparoscopic hysterectomy indicated for benign uterine pathologies: a 13-year experience in a continuous series of 1300 patients. Hum Reprod. 2007;22:2006–11.
17. Yaycioglu O, Ramakumar S, Kavoussi LR, Jarrett TW. Early repeated exploration after laparoscopic urologic surgery: comparison of clinical, radiologic, and surgical findings. Urology. 2002 Feb;59(2):190–4.
18. Patil NN, Mottrie A, Sundaram B, Patel VR. Robotic-assisted laparoscopic ureteral reimplantation with psoas hitch: a multi-institutional, multinational evaluation. Urology. 2008 Jul;72(1):47–50.
19. Boukerrou M, Lambaudie E, Collinet P, et al. A history of cesareans is a risk factor in vaginal hysterectomies. Acta Obstet Gynecol Scand. 2003;82:1135–9.
20. Chan DP, Abujudeh HH, Cushing GL Jr, Novelline RA. CT cystography with multiplanar reformation for suspected bladder rupture: experience in 234 cases. AJR Am J Roentgenol. 2006 Nov;187(5):1296–302.
21. Williams TR, Longoria OJ, Asselmeier S, Menon M. Incidence and imaging appearance of urethrovesical anastomotic urinary leaks following da Vinci robotic prostatectomy. Abdom Imaging. 2008 May–Jun;33(3):367–70.
22. Guillonneau B, Rozet F, Cathelineau X, Lay F, Barret E, Doublet JD, Baumert H, Vallancien G. Perioperative complications of laparoscopic radical prostatectomy: the Montsouris 3-year experience. J Urol. 2002 Jan;167(1): 51–6.
23. Patil N, Krane L, Javed K, Williams T, Bhandari M, Menon M. Evaluating and grading cystographic leakage: correlation with clinical outcomes in patients undergoing robotic prostatectomy. BJU Int. 2009 Apr;103(8):1108–10.

Visceral and Gastrointestinal Complications of Laparoscopic and Robotic Urologic Surgery

S. Scott Putman and Jay T. Bishoff

Keywords Injury · Complications · Bowel injury · Laparoscopy · Robotics

Introduction

The first laparoscopic procedures for urologic surgery were radical nephrectomy and a pelvic lymph node dissection for prostate cancer staging performed in 1991 [1, 2]. Since that time, laparoscopic and robot-assisted procedures have become commonplace in urologic surgery. Unfortunately, many different complications are seen in all types of laparoscopic and robot-assisted laparoscopic surgery. The focus of this chapter is on bowel and solid organ complications. Overall, bowel complications have been estimated to be 1.3/1,000 laparoscopic cases [3].

Patient Selection

Patients who have had intraperitoneal surgery are at an increased risk of forming intra-abdominal adhesions [4]. Although the presence of intraperitoneal adhesions can be daunting and add time to the procedure, there is no evidence that there is an increased incidence of bowel complications in patients undergoing laparoscopic or robot-assisted surgery. Several studies have shown that there is no increase in bowel complications in patients with previous abdominal surgery undergoing laparoscopic surgery compared with a controlled group that had not [5, 6]. Recently, Nazemi et al. evaluated this question and have shown that there is no increase in complications in patients undergoing robotic surgery who had undergone previous abdominal surgery compared with a controlled group that had not.

Anesthesia

An oro- or nasogastric tube is routinely placed to avoid bowel distention, especially during procedures involving the upper urinary tracts. Nitrous oxide is a useful inhalational anesthetic because of its analgesic effect, low cost, rapid onset of action, and ability to reduce the concentration of other anesthetic agents that may cause cardiorespiratory depression [7]. Unfortunately, the use of nitrous oxide is discouraged in laparoscopic and robotic surgery due to bowel distention, which can obscure the operative field. El-Galley et al. reported in a series of patients undergoing laparoscopic donor nephrectomy that 50% of the patients in the NO_2 group developed mild to moderate bowel distention compared to 6% in the control group. Furthermore, 25% of the NO_2 group developed severe bowel distention compared to 6% in the control group. Although there were no complications in either group, severe bowel distention may increase the risk of bowel injury and may increase post-operative bowel recovery. Accrual in this study was halted due to these findings [8].

S.S. Putman (✉)
Intermountain Urological Institute, 6159 South Cottonwood Stree, Suite 420, Murray, UT 84157, USA
e-mail: scott.putman@imail.org

R. Ghavamian (ed.), *Complications of Laparoscopic and Robotic Urologic Surgery*,
DOI 10.1007/978-1-60761-676-4_7,

Bowel Complications Associated with Access

Access to the peritoneal cavity or the retro/extraperitoneal space and insufflation is necessary to create a working space for laparoscopic and robotic surgery. There are several techniques that are used to gain access to the peritoneum and retroperitoneum, including Veress needle placement, the Hasson entry, direct trocar entry, and the STEP procedure (the rapidly expanding access system). Complications associated with access include minor complications such as extraperitoneal or subcutaneous insufflation and minor skin or subcutaneous bleeding. Major complications include vascular injury, gastrointestinal injury, ureteral or bladder injury, solid organ injury, and gas embolism. Major complications are rare and have been well studied. A meta-analysis of access techniques found bowel injuries to occur in 0.18% of cases and vascular injuries to occur in 0.09% of cases [9].

The Veress needle approach is one of the most common access techniques used. The Veress needle is a blunt needle with a spring-loaded obturator. The Veress needle is placed blindly into the peritoneal cavity. The needle is most often placed either infra- or supra-umbilically. The skin and subcutaneous tissue may be lifted with penetrating towel clips or a suture in order to create tension on the skin and create some distance between the bowel/vasculature and the peritoneal cavity. Once the Veress needle is placed, a saline drop test is performed. A 5 cc syringe half-filled with sterile normal saline is placed on the Veress needle and the contents are aspirated to check for succus or blood. If nothing is aspirated, the sterile saline is irrigated into the cavity. If this freely irrigates into the cavity, then peritoneal placement is likely. The abdomen is then insufflated with CO_2. If the placement is correct, then the initial intra-abdominal pressure should be low – less than 9 mmHg. This may be higher in morbidly obese patients where the pannus increases baseline intra-abdominal pressure. High initial pressures in a patient with a normal BMI indicate incorrect placement of the Veress needle. This is most likely subcutaneous or extraperitoneal placement. If blood returns when aspirating the drop test syringe, the Veress needle is removed and replaced until placed correctly. The vasculature and bowel mesentery is then checked for active bleeding or hematoma. If succus returns after aspiration, the needle is removed without using any torque and replaced correctly. The area of injury is inspected. If there are no obvious enterotomies with spillage of succus, the injury may be treated conservatively and the case may proceed. If there is a large injury or spillage of succus, the injury must be repaired, either in a laparoscopic or in an open fashion. Failure of the syringe to irrigate easily suggests subcutaneous or extraperitoneal placement of the Veress needle and replacement until a positive saline drop test occurs must be performed. To avoid failures, the Veress needle should be placed away from any areas of previous surgery. Paramedian (lateral to the rectus muscles) and right and left upper quadrant placements are acceptable as a primary placement or a secondary placement when midline or periumbilical scars are present.

The Hasson technique was developed in 1971 as a safe way to gain entrance to the peritoneal cavity [10]. Generally, a 10–12 mm skin incision is made through the skin and subcutaneous tissue until the fascia is encountered. A fascial closing suture may then be placed in a longitudinal fashion on either side of the proposed site of the incision and the incision is then made. The sutures have the dual purpose of lifting the fascia away from the peritoneal catheter and as preplaced fascial closure sutures. Once the fascia has been opened, the peritoneal cavity is inspected and a finger is used to sweep the edges of the fascia to ensure there are no adhesions near the incision. A blunt-tipped Hasson cannula is then placed directly in the peritoneum and secured with sutures. The Hasson technique is used as a primary technique by many laparoscopic and robotic surgeons. For those who primarily use the closed, Veress needle technique, the Hasson technique is used when the patient has had multiple previous abdominal operations and the risk of intra-abdominal adhesions is high. The Hasson technique is also useful in morbidly obese patients, when Veress needle placement can be unreliable. The Hasson technique is also used to gain access to the retroperitoneum, as the retroperitoneum is a potential space that must first be created bluntly with the finger and then with balloon dilation before visual inspection is possible.

The radially expanding access system (STEP™, InnerDyne, Sunnyvale, CA) was developed as an alternative to the Veress and Hasson techniques [11]. The STEP system uses a pneumoperitoneum needle with an outer, polymeric sleeve. Once the needle is correctly placed, much like the Veress needle, the inner needle is removed and the outer sleeve is dilated to the required size. In theory, there is less tissue trauma and less of a risk of bowel and vascular injuries.

The bladeless optical trocar is a multi-component, integrated system that uses a trocar with an inner sleeve-handle system that accommodates a 5 or 10 mm lens. The bladeless optical trocar is placed at the entry site in the desufflated abdomen and the surgeon is able to visualize the various tissue layers until the peritoneal cavity is identified and entered. The bladeless optical trocar was designed to save time, cause less tissue trauma, and decrease bowel and vascular injuries [12].

Complications during access make up over half of the total complications in some series [13]. There have been many retrospective and well-designed randomized controlled trials in an attempt to identify the safest access technique. Recently, a meta-analysis of 17 randomized, controlled trials with a total of 3,075 patients was conducted evaluating the various methods of access [14]. The meta-analysis showed no evidence of an advantage using any single technique in preventing major complications. It did show that extraperitoneal insufflation is less likely to occur with direct trocar entry (Hasson and bladeless optical trocar). The radially expanding access system showed less trocar site bleeding when compared to other techniques. An advantage was shown to not lifting the abdomen when obtaining access with the Veress needle in terms of avoiding extraperitoneal insufflation. Major complications involving access are rare but serious. There is no clear evidence that the open technique (Hasson) is superior to the closed technique (Veress needle, STEP, or bladeless optical access system) in the gynecological literature, but there is level one evidence that open access is safer than closed access [15].

Gastrointestinal and Solid Organ Injuries During Laparoscopic and Robotic Surgery

A bowel injury during laparoscopic or robotic surgery may be life-threatening if not recognized and repaired during the procedure (Tables 1 and 2). In the

Table 1 Summary of ten patients with laparoscopic bowel injury

Injuries recognized at the time of surgery

Patient No.	Procedure	Injury site	Injury type	Repair	Complication (post-op days to recognition)
1	Nephrectomy	Small bowel	Dissection abrasion	None	Abscess + fistula*
2	Pyeloplasty	Colon	Dissection abrasion	Oversewn	None
3	Pelvic lymph node dissection	Colon	Dissection abrasion	Oversewn	None
4	Pelvic lymph node dissection	Colon	Dissection abrasion	Oversewn	None
5	Pyeloplasty	Colon	Dissection abrasion	Oversewn	None
6	Pelvic lymph node dissection	Colon	Burn	Oversewn	None
7	Nephrectomy	Colon	Closure perforation	Drain	Enterocutaneous fistula (10)
8	Pelvic lymph node dissection	Colon	Scissor perforation	None	Sepsis, death (4)
9	Cholecystectomy	Duodenal	Scissor perforation	Laparotomy	Necrotizing fasciitis (3)
10	Pelvic lymph node dissection	Colon	Thermal perforation	Laparotomy	Sepsis, death (3)

*One patient who had a serosal abrasion considered insignificant at surgery presented with injuries 2 weeks later

Table 2 Location of injury, treatment, and outcome

References	Specialty	No. of patients	No. injuries: Bowel	Small intestine	Colon	Stomach	Recognized	Unrecognized	Treatment (No. of patients/total no.)	No. of deaths
Harkki-Siren and Kurki	Gynecology	70,607	44	26	16	2	8	36	All laparotomy	
Bateman et al.	Gynecology	2,324	6	3	2	1				
Wolfe et al.	General surgery	381	2	1	1	0	0	2		2
Deziel et al.	General surgery	77,604	109	69	35	5			Laparotomy (85/109)	5
Phillips et al.	General surgery	51	0							
Schrenk et al.	Gynecology, general surgery	4,672	10	6	4	0	6	4	Laparotomy (9/10)	1
Penfield	Gynecology	10,840	6				4	2	All laparotomy	
Loffer and Pent	Gynecology	32,719	64	44	11	9			Laparotomy (47/64)	
Kaali and Barad	Gynecology	4,532	4						All laparotomy	
Casey et al.	Gynecology	93	4	2	1	1	0	4	All laparotomy	
Davis et al.	Gynecology	40	1				0	1	All laparotomy	
Chapron et al.	Gynecology	1,191	8	1	7					
Present series	Urology	915	8	1	7		6	4		
Totals		205,969	266	153	84	18	24	53		8

post-operative period, the recognition of a bowel injury may be difficult until the patient is quite ill. The presentation of a laparoscopic or robotic bowel injury is unique to minimally invasive surgery and its early recognition must be a part of the laparoscopic and robotic surgeon's skill set.

Bowel injury requiring repair is a rare occurrence in laparoscopic and robotic surgery, occurring in 0.1% of cases [3]. Unfortunately, the majority of the injuries are unrecognized. Bowel injury that occurs during access and is recognized was discussed earlier in this chapter. A recognized bowel injury that occurs during dissection is treated in a similar fashion. A notable exception is a thermal injury caused by electrocautery (Figs. 1 and 2). If there is an enterotomy made by electrocautery, a wide section of tissue must be excised before

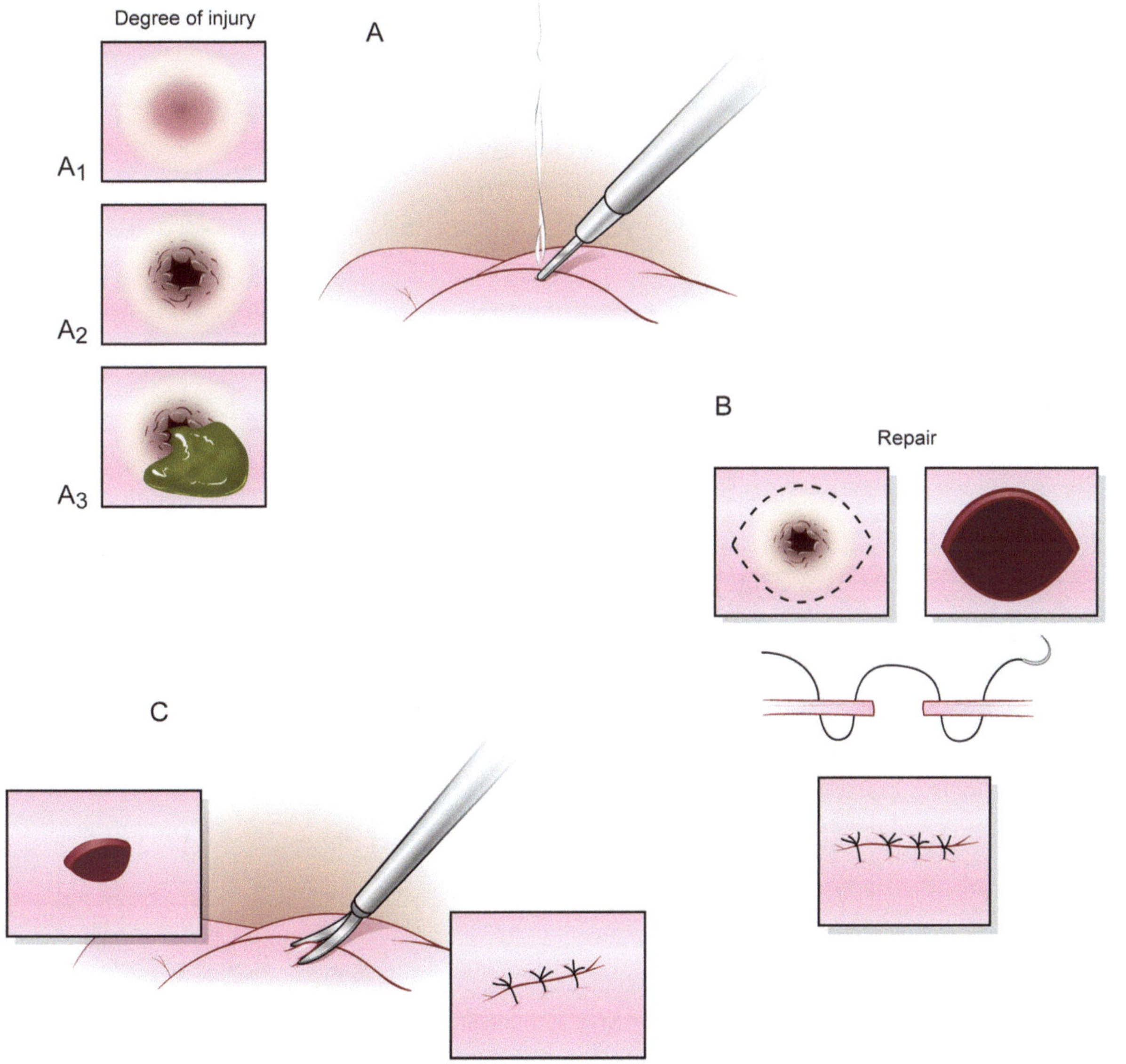

Fig. 1 Thermal and sharp injuries to the bowel during laparoscopic surgery. (**a**) Small thermal injury. The figures reveal the various appearances of thermal injuries. (A_1) The blanching apparent on the first panel may contain tissue that will ultimately undergo coagulation necrosis and sloughing. (A_2) The next panel shows a thermally induced enterotomy without spillage of succus and (A_3) the third panel shows a thermally induced enterotomy with spillage of succus. Repair of these injuries is necessary as shown in (b). (**b**) Repair of small, thermally induced bowel injuries requires excision to viable tissue and primary repair with Lembert suture. (**c**) Sharp enterotomy: This may be closed primarily, in most cases

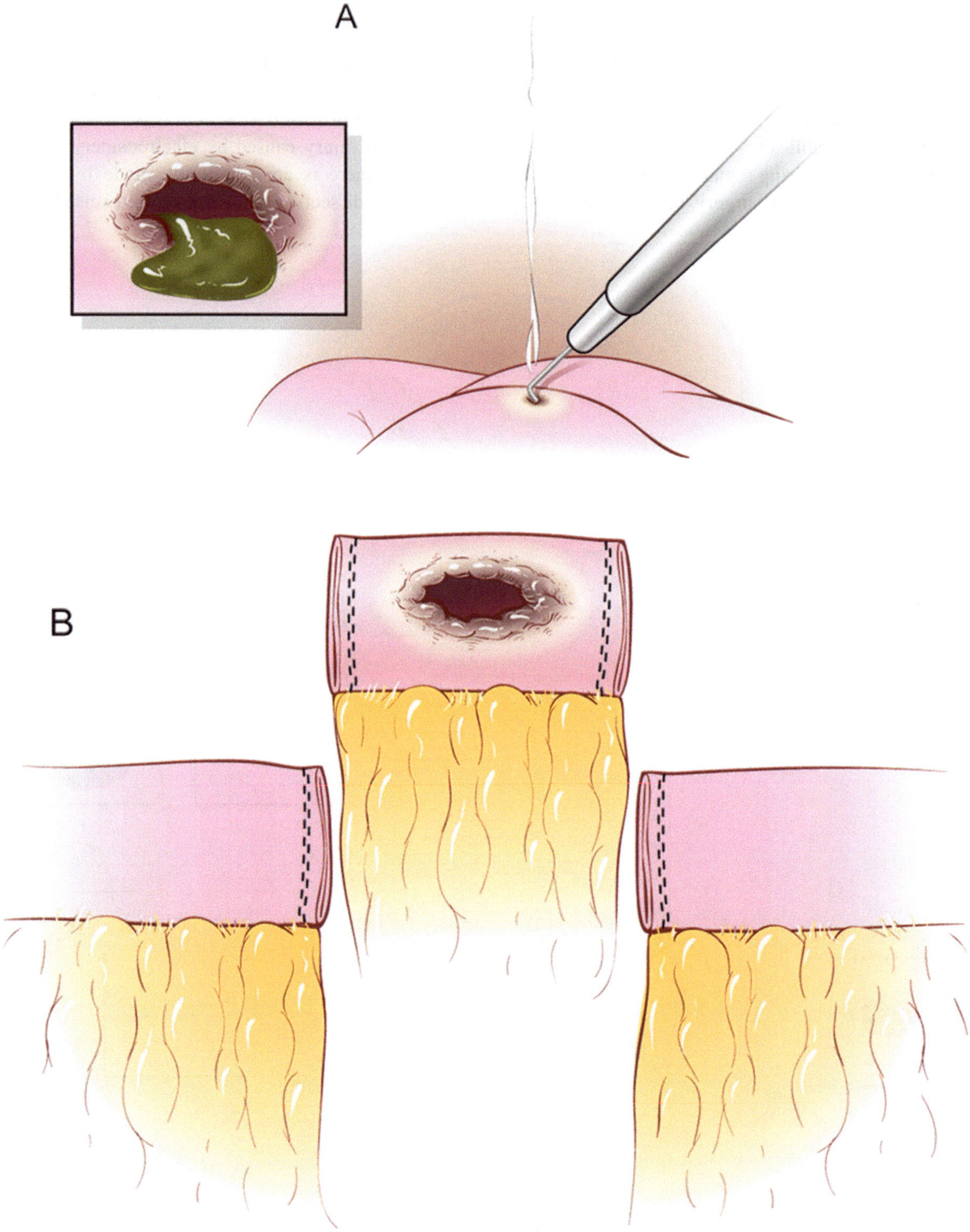

Fig. 2 Large, thermally induced bowel injury (**A**). Larger injuries may require bowel resection (**B**)

primary repair. If the area is blanched, but there is no enterotomy or there appears to be only a superficial serosal injury, the area must be excised until viable tissue is encountered and only then is it oversewn.

The unrecognized bowel injury in laparoscopic and robotic surgery is unique in its presentation (Table 3). The traditional recognition of a bowel injury in the patient who either underwent surgery or is seen in the emergency department includes ileus and exquisite abdominal pain with rigidity. The patient often has fever and leukocytosis and requires aggressive resuscitation. Bishoff and colleagues evaluated a series of laparoscopic surgeries and found the presentation to be quite different from that of a traditional acute abdomen caused by bowel injury. All but one of the patients who had an unrecognized bowel injury had a leukocytosis. Many of the patients had a low-grade fever. Furthermore, ileus is uncommon as is nausea and vomiting. Many times, the patient will have bowel sounds, no peritoneal signs, and diarrhea. There is often exquisite tenderness at the trocar site nearest to the bowel injury. If there is a high index of suspicion, the patient should be taken to the operating room immediately for exploratory laparotomy, washout, and repair. A computed tomography with oral contrast may be obtained if the diagnosis is less clear [3].

Injury to the pancreas, spleen, and liver also occurs in laparoscopic and robotic surgery. Most of these injuries may be managed conservatively. Injury to the pancreas is uncommon but can have significant morbidity. This most often occurs with laparoscopic left adrenalectomy, nephrectomy, and partial nephrectomy. In the urologic literature a rate of 0.2% has been reported [16]. These injuries are most commonly discovered post-operatively. If discovered intraoperatively, a GIA stapler can be used to repair the injury. If the injury is not discovered intraoperatively, there is usually a delay in diagnosis, and because of the rapid recovery of patients who have undergone laparoscopic surgery, the patient is often at home when the symptoms begin. The patient complains of pain out of proportion to the procedure, epigastric pain radiating to the back, nausea, and vomiting. The patient will have leukocytosis and an elevated serum amylase. Intravenous fluid hydration, nasogastric tube, parenteral nutrition, administration of somatostatin, and drainage may be required. If the surgeon has a high index of suspicion, a drain can be placed intraoperatively and the fluid can be sent for amylase if the patient develops symptoms. The drain can be removed when the output is less than 50 cc every 24 h and the patient can then be started on a low-fat diet [17]. A pancreatic fistula may develop and may take as long as 3 weeks to heal [18]. Splenic injuries occur in 0.3% of laparoscopic procedures [4]. Splenic injuries occur most often while mobilizing the splenic flexure to expose the retroperitoneum. There is an increased risk if the patient has adhesions. A splenic injury is most often managed with simple fulguration if minor. If the bleeding is more difficult to control, an argon beam coagulator can be used. Biocompatible liquid polymers have also been used to control splenic bleeding [19]. Splenectomy due to a large injury and excessive bleeding is rare, but has been reported [20]. Hepatic injury does not often occur and is treated much like a splenic injury. It is difficult to estimate the rate of hepatic injury as these are mostly incidental and controlled with electrocautery. Like a splenic injury, an argon beam coagulator may be necessary to control more excessive bleeding from hepatic injuries. Difficult to control bleeding may require placing a figure of eight suture at the site of the injury.

Table 3 Presenting signs and symptoms of unrecognized laparoscopic bowel injuries

	Patient No.				
	1	7	8	9	10
Trocar pain	Yes	Yes	Yes	Yes	Yes
Abdominal distention	Yes	Yes	Yes	Yes	Yes
Leukopenia	Yes	No	Yes	Yes	Yes
Diarrhea	Yes	No	Yes	Yes	Yes
Cardiovascular collapse	No	No	Yes	Yes	Yes
Ileus	No	No	No	No	Yes
Abdominal pain	No	No	No	No	No
Leukocytosis	No	No	No	No	No
Fever greater than 101 F	No	No	No	Yes	No
Nausea	Yes	No	No	Yes	Yes
Vomiting	No	No	No	Yes	Yes

Trocar Site and Incisional Hernias in Laparoscopic and Robotic Surgery

Herniation of bowel through a trocar site is an uncommon occurrence in laparoscopic and robotic surgery (Fig. 3). The first trocar site hernia was reported in

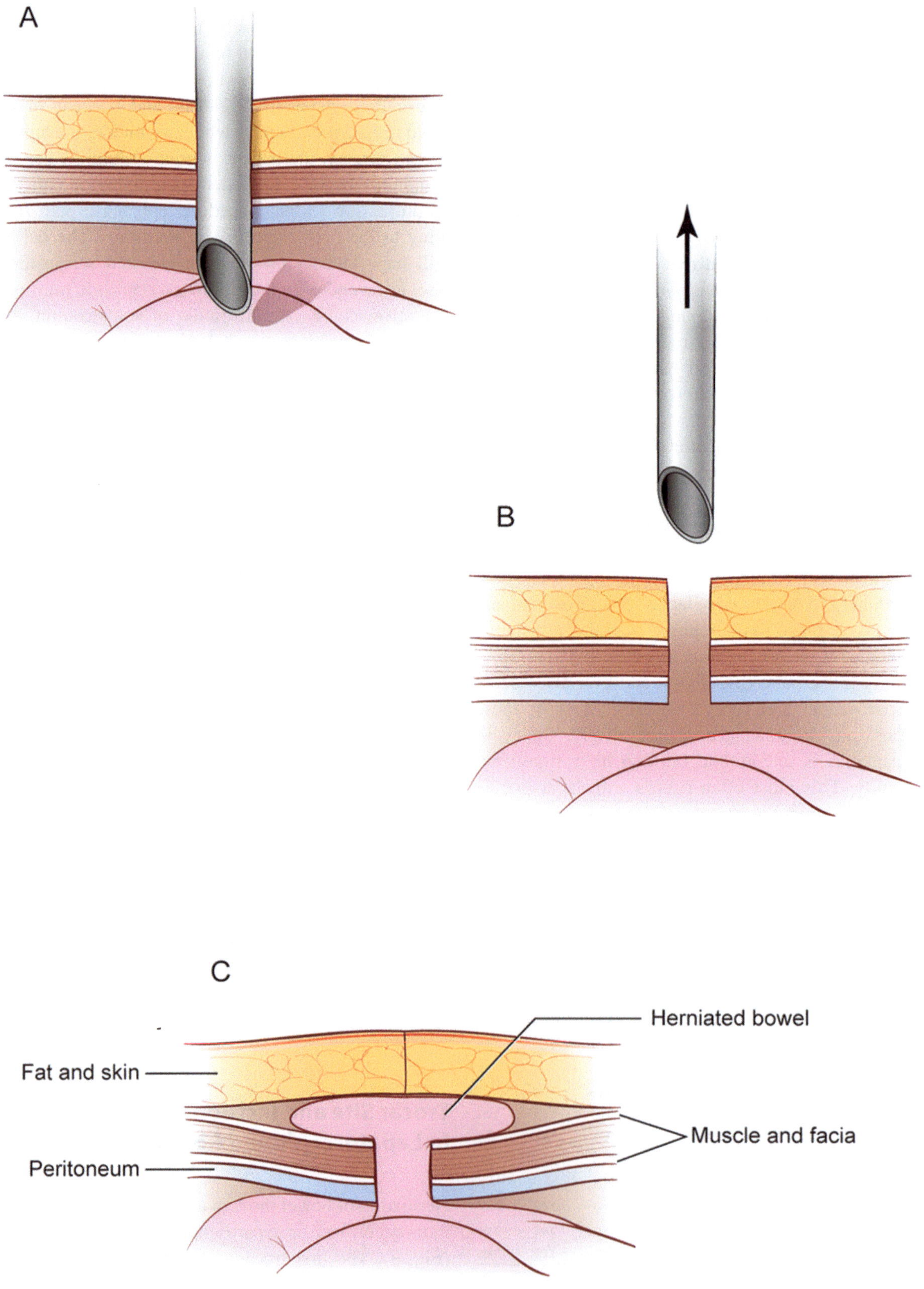

Fig. 3 Evolution of a trocar site hernia: The trocar is placed (**A**). The trocar is then removed after the completion of the laparoscopic portion of the case (**B**). The fascial defect was not closed and the bowel herniates through the fascial defect (**C**)

the gynecologic literature in a large series of diagnostic procedures in 1968 [21]. Since that time, there have been many reports of trocar site hernias. The incidence ranges from 0.65 to 2.8% in the general surgery literature [22, 23]. The true incidence of trocar site hernias may be higher due to underreporting. Larger trocars are predictably more prone to hernia formation, whether the fascial defect is closed or not. In the gynecologic literature, 86.3% of trocar site hernias were found in defects larger than 10 mm, 10.9% in defects at least 8 mm in length, and 2.7% in those 5 mm or less [24]. The overall incidence of trocar site hernias in ports 5 mm or less has been reported to be 0.056% [25, 26].

There is a question of whether to close the fascial defects after the trocar removal and whether trocar sites of a certain size should be closed is a debated subject. It has been reported that the incidence of bowel adhesions and incarcerations that occur after the defect is closed or left open is similar [27]. Many suggest that a trocar site hernia after closure of the fascial defect is a result of partial closure and improper suturing technique. The gynecologic literature has shown that closing the fascial defect of a 12 mm incision significantly reduces development of a trocar site hernia [25]. It has also been noted that closed laparoscopy has a higher trocar site hernia incidence than open (Hasson) laparoscopy and this has been attributed to a higher rate of wound infection in the closed series [28].

The paraumbilical region has been shown in many studies to be the area where most hernias develop and this has been attributed to the inherent weakness of the area and a lack of a posterior fascial covering with intervening muscle between the anterior fascial leaves [29]. Using the umbilical and paraumbilical region as the extraction site, which leads to stretching of the fascia and possibly extending the fascial incision, has also been found to increase the incidence of trocar site hernias [14].

Host factors have been attributed to an increase in trocar site hernia formation and these include obesity, poor nutrition, diabetes mellitus, steroid use, and concomitant wound infection, although these factors did not reach statistical significance when evaluated [28].

There have been recent reports of trocar site herniation of bowel contents after using the 8 mm DaVinci (Intuitive Surgical, Sunnydale, CA) trocar [30]. Although it is generally accepted that these fascial defects do not have to be closed, as these reports gather, they may suggest a benefit to closing 8 mm fascial defects (Fig. 4).

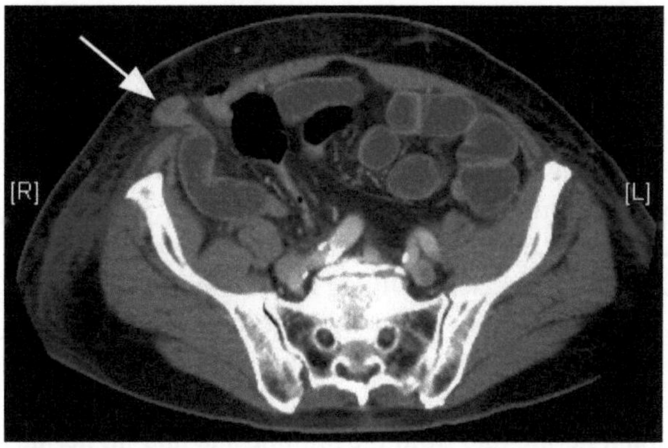

Fig. 4 A trocar site hernia that occurred from an 8 mm robotic trocar

Trocar site hernias usually present as abdominal pain at the trocar site and small bowel obstruction. A portion of patients are asymptomatic. All trocar site hernias must be recognized and repaired immediately to prevent small bowel obstruction or incarceration and bowel necrosis.

Incisional or extraction site hernias can occur in laparoscopic and robot-assisted laparoscopic surgery (Fig. 5). There is generally a loss of fascial integrity that occurs during or after healing. In general, the incidence of incisional hernia formation after surgery is 5–15% [31]. Risk factors associated with formation of incisional hernia include previous abdominal surgery, obesity, renal insufficiency, renal failure, postoperative respiratory tract infection, diabetes, age older

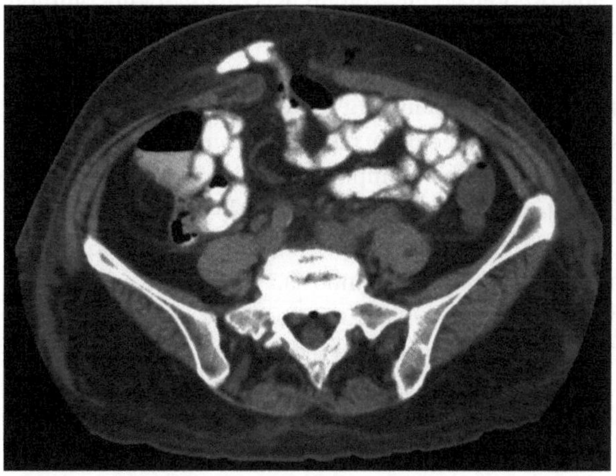

Fig. 5 Extraction site hernia after laparoscopic radical nephrectomy

than 50 years, metastatic disease, and impaired nutrition [32]. Most of the literature looking at extraction site hernias evaluates hand-assisted and pure laparoscopic radical nephrectomy or nephroureterectomy. Hand-assisted laparoscopic radical nephrectomy has been reported in a series to have an incisional hernia rate of 6% when the extraction site was either the midline or a muscle-splitting right lower quadrant incision [32]. Midline extraction site versus Pfannenstiel extraction site was compared to evaluate pain in one study; however, it was noted that there was a 2.9% incisional hernia rate from the midline site and no hernias developed after extraction from the Pfannenstiel site [33]. Another study compared midline with paramedian extraction sites and the midline extraction site to have a higher rate of hernia formation than the paramedian extraction site [34]. This has also been noted in the general surgery literature for laparoscopic colectomy [35]. Bird et al. performed an excellent study evaluating the location of the extraction site specifically as a primary end point and found a paramedian incision in someone with a high BMI to be the highest risk factor for incisional hernia formation [36].

Bowel Complications in Specific Procedures

Complications of Laparoscopic and Robot-Assisted Adrenalectomy

Laparoscopic adrenalectomy is a relatively uncommon procedure and makes up only 2% of the procedures in an academic laparoscopic program [7]. The largest series to date evaluating the complications of laparoscopic adrenalectomy reports a complication rate of 7.5% [37]. The complications included hematoma formation (the most common), splenic injury, pancreatic injury, intraoperative bleeding, pneumothorax, and deep venous thrombosis. Open conversion was required in 5% of the cases. There were no bowel complications reported in these larger series.

There is a paucity of data regarding robot-assisted laparoscopic adrenalectomy. Two studies have compared the two procedures and shown them to be equivalent in complication rate. The only significant differences between the two procedures are a longer operative time and more expense for the robot-assisted laparoscopic adrenalectomy [38, 39] (Tables 4 and 5).

Complications of Laparoscopic and Robot-Assisted Nephrectomy

Laparoscopic renal surgery has been growing in its use and indications since Clayman performed the first laparoscopic nephrectomy in 1990 [40]. The laparoscopic nephrectomy has been one of the most commonly performed laparoscopic cases in urology. Recently, a meta-analysis was performed to evaluate the complications of the laparoscopic renal surgery and the hand-assisted laparoscopic renal surgery (HALRN) [41]. LRN and HALRN have a major and minor complication rate of 13%. The major complication rate of LRN and HALRN is 3% and the minor complication rate is 10%. LRN had a small bowel complication rate of 0.6% and colonic injury incidence of 1.5%. The meta-analysis of HALRN revealed a small intestinal injury of 0.5% and an incisional hernia rate of 0.5%. It should be noted that the meta-analysis of LRN reported no incidents of incisional hernia.

The robotic radical nephrectomy has been evaluated at several centers for safety, efficacy, and feasibility [42]. A series of 43 patients show the robotic radical nephrectomy to be a safe procedure that is not significantly different than LRN or HALRN. There were no major complications and one minor complication (2.6%) which was a morbidly obese patient who developed a wound dehiscence. No bowel injuries have been reported in robot-assisted laparoscopic nephrectomies. Select academic centers studying robotic technology need to develop a larger series in order to evaluate the nature and incidence of complications of robot-assisted laparoscopic nephrectomy before a true comparison with LRN and HALRN can be made.

The transperitoneal and retroperitoneal approaches have been evaluated by Gill and colleagues [43]. The transperitoneal approach provides a larger working space and familiar anatomic landmarks whereas the retroperitoneal approach has a theoretic advantage of a faster return to full bowel function by avoiding the peritoneal cavity. Another advantage of retroperitoneoscopic surgery may be avoiding the peritoneal cavity in patients with multiple prior

Table 4 Laparoscopic bowel complications

Procedure	Overall incidence of bowel complications	Ileus	Small bowel injury	Large bowel injury	Rectal injury	Port-site hernia	Incisional/extraction site hernia	Small bowel obstruction
Adrenalectomy	None reported	–	–	–	–	–	–	–
Nephrectomy	2.1%		0.6%	1.5%	–	–	–	–
HALRN	1%		0.5%	–	–	–	0.5%	–
Partial nephrectomy	None reported	–	–	–	–	–	–	–
HALPN	None reported	–	–	–	–	–	–	–
Nephroureterectomy	3.9%	–	2.3%	0.8%	–	–	0.8%	–
Pyeloplasty	0.6%	–	–	0.6%	–	–	–	–
RPLND	0.65%	–	0.65%	–	–	–	–	–
Cystectomy	7%	6%	–	–	0.5%	–	0.5%	–
Prostatectomy		5.3%	–	0.3%	1.5–2.5%	–	–	–

Table 5 Bowel complications of robot-assisted laparoscopic surgery

Procedure	Overall incidence of bowel complications	Ileus	Small bowel injury	Large bowel injury	Rectal injury	Port-site hernia	Incisional/extraction site hernia	Small bowel obstruction
Adrenalectomy	None reported	–	–	–	–	–	–	–
Nephrectomy	2.6%	–	–	–	–	–	2.6%	–
Partial nephrectomy	Yes	Yes	–	–	–	–	–	–
Nephroureterectomy	None reported	–	–	–	–	–	–	–
Pyeloplasty	None reported	–	–	–	–	–	–	–
RPLND	None reported							
Cystectomy	8.2%	5.7%	1% (enterocutaneous fistula)	–	1%	1% (parastomal)	–	–
Prostatectomy	0.85%	0.2%	0.14%	-	0.1%	0.14%	0.2%	0.06%

surgeries. In Gill's study there were no statistically significant differences in the incidences of complications. In the transperitoneal group, there was an overall complication rate of 10% with one minor bowel injury. The retroperitoneal group had an overall complication rate of 7.7% with no bowel injuries. Although one bowel injury occurred in the transperitoneal group, the difference between the groups is not statistically significant (Tables 4 and 5).

Laparoscopic and Robot-Assisted Laparoscopic Partial Nephrectomy

The laparoscopic partial nephrectomy is one of the most challenging commonly performed cases in urology. There are several steps in the procedure that make it quite difficult. The renal hilum must be dissected meticulously to allow placement of vascular clamps for bleeding control. The position of the mass may make it very difficult to excise the mass and close the defect. Unfortunately, this must be done as quickly as possible to save the nephrons of the kidney. A meta-analysis of laparoscopic partial nephrectomy (LPN) and hand-assisted laparoscopic partial nephrectomy (HALPN) showed a significantly higher rate of major complications in the LPN group (21 versus 3.3%). However, it must be noted that the size of the groups was not equal in this retrospective comparison. The common major complications of LPN are blood transfusion (4.4%), urinoma (3.9%), and arterial bleeding (1.7%). The most common complication of HALPN is urinoma (3.3%). Notably, there was no report of bowel injuries in this meta-analysis.

The robot-assisted laparoscopic partial nephrectomy is seen as being well suited to the robotic procedure as compared to the RALRN mainly because of the surgeon's ability to control the kidney with the fourth arm and the greater degrees of freedom of the robotic instruments that allow a theoretically faster reconstruction of the renal defect and therefore a shorter ischemic time. A multi-institutional analysis of the RALPN evaluated 143 patients [44]. The complication rate was 6.1% and included a hematoma requiring drainage, ileus, pulmonary embolus, urinoma, and rhabdomyolysis. Two procedures were converted to an open procedure. One patient was morbidly obese and the other had a prior open ureterolithotomy. There were no bowel injuries reported in this series (Tables 4 and 5).

Laparoscopic and Robot-Assisted Laparoscopic Nephroureterectomy

Laparoscopic nephroureterectomy (LNU) and hand-assisted laparoscopic nephroureterectomy (HALNU) are a standard minimally invasive procedure for the treatment of transitional cell carcinoma of the upper urinary tract. It is accepted that complete excision of the ureter is a necessary part of the operation [45]. In the traditional operation, either a long midline incision or two separate incisions were made to accomplish this task. Laparoscopy allows the surgeon to make at the most a small Gibson or partial Pfannenstiel incision to complete the excision of the distal ureters and many complete this by using endoscopic methods [46]. LNU has a 19% major and 2% minor complication rate. The most common complication of LNU is hernia at the extraction site. This may be a result of using a paramedian incision in order to address the distal ureter through the extraction site. Wolf and colleagues have reported their complication rate with HALNU. There is an overall 37% complication rate [47]. Major complications represent 19% and minor complications represent 39%. The most common major complication was development of an incisional hernia at the hand port site. Blood transfusion was required in 17% of patients.

The robot-assisted laparoscopic nephroureterectomy is a new procedure that has scant data reporting complications. The largest series has been reported by Nanigian and colleagues [15]. They reported no significant complications in this small group of patients (Tables 4 and 5).

Laparoscopic and Robot-Assisted Laparoscopic Pyeloplasty

Laparoscopic pyeloplasty has become the gold standard for excision and reconstruction of the ureteropelvic junction. It has been proven to have similar functional outcomes as compared to the open procedure [48]. Rassweiler and colleagues took their experience of 189 laparoscopic pyeloplasties and created a meta-analysis of several other large series to develop a group of 601 patients that had undergone laparoscopic pyeloplasties at high-volume institutions and subjected this cohort to the Clavien classification for complications. Intraoperative complications occurred in 2.3% of the cases and these complications were variable. Conversion to an open operation occurred in 0.5–5.5% of cases as the result of an inability to access the UPJ or finish the anastomosis. Post-operative complications ranged from 5.4 to 15% and represented urine leak, hematoma, bowel injury, and stone formation. Out of the 601 patients, 4 had colonic injuries. Recurrent UPJ obstruction occurred in 3.5–4.8% of cases. It should be noted that the majority of these complications took place during the learning curve.

Robot-assisted laparoscopic pyeloplasty has gained popularity due to its extra degrees of freedom which aid during reconstruction of the UPJ. Mufarrij and associates in a multi-institutional analysis report a 7.1% major and a 2.9% minor complication rate [49]. The most common major complication was stent migration requiring repositioning or replacement. Other major complications included gluteal compartment syndrome, splenic injury, and pyelonephritis requiring stent exchange. Minor complications included urinary tract infection and prolonged urine leak. No bowel injuries were reported in this series. Recurrent ureteropelvic junction obstruction occurred in 4.3% of patients, which is similar to Rassweiler's meta-analysis of laparoscopic pyeloplasty (Tables 4 and 5).

Laparoscopic and Robot-Assisted Retroperitoneal Lymph Node Dissection

Laparoscopic retroperitoneal lymph node dissection (LRPLND) has been making inroads in recent years for the treatment of stage I non-seminomatous germ cell tumors, although it remains controversial. Steiner and associates reviewed the long-term results of LRPLND [50]. The major complication rate of 1.1% included a recognized colon injury and injury to the renal artery. Minor complications included lymphocele (8.5%) and chylous ascites (4.8%). Transfusion was required in 1.3% of patients, and 2.6% of procedures were converted to an open procedure for bleeding. The complication rate for a post-chemotherapy LPRLND is higher and has been estimated to be almost 50% in some series [51]. Most of those complications are intraoperative and are a result of bleeding. There have been several case reports and some small series evaluating the safety and efficacy of RALRPLND. RALRPLND is safe and there have been no major complications in these reports, but further study is needed (Tables 4 and 5).

Laparoscopic and Robotic Radical Cystectomy

The first laparoscopic cystectomy was performed in 1992 followed by only sporadic attempts at this technically difficult procedure with limited instrumentation [52]. Since that time, with increased experience in laparoscopic techniques and improved instrumentation, laparoscopic, and now robot-assisted laparoscopic, radical cystectomy has become an accepted procedure with the potential benefits of lower blood loss, less pain, and quicker time to recovery. However, open radical cystectomy remains the gold standard for the treatment of muscle invasive transitional cell carcinoma of the bladder. Several larger series of laparoscopic radical cystectomy have evaluated their complications [53–57]. Although various techniques were used, such as extracorporeal suturing in some and different diversions in other series, the results have been pooled to look at the bowel complications. These series evaluate a total of 211 patients that underwent laparoscopic radical cystectomy. The most common bowel complication is ileus, which occurred in 6% of patients. Rectal injury and bowel herniation were encountered in less than 1% of cases. There are a growing number of series that have evaluated robot-assisted laparoscopic radical cystectomy [53, 58–61]. A pooled analysis of these series produces 175 patients undergoing robot-assisted laparoscopic radical cystectomy. The most common complication was formation of an ileus, which occurred in 5.7% of cases. Other bowel complications include rectal injury, which had an incidence of about 1%, as well as parastomal hernia, which also had an incidence of about 1%; enterocutaneous fistula occurred in less than 1% of cases. These analyses serve only to estimate the complication rate. A large-scale study needs to be performed in order to compare these outcomes to those of open radical cystectomy, although there is a suggestion that the bowel complication rate is comparable or even lower than those in the open series [62] (Tables 4 and 5).

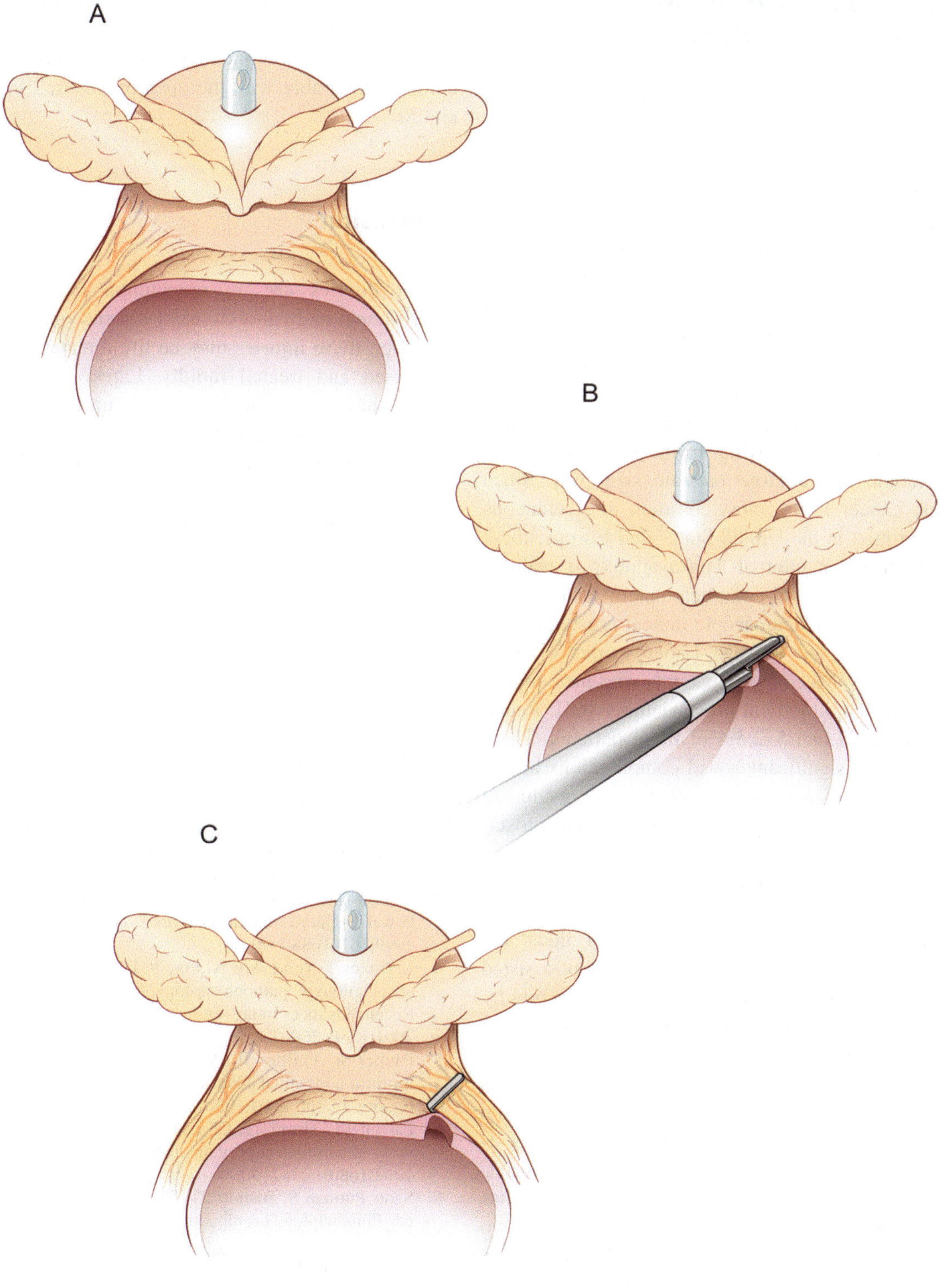

Fig. 6 Rectal injury during laparoscopic radical prostatectomy or robot-assisted laparoscopic radical prostatectomy. (**a**) The bladder neck has been dissected off of the prostate and the rectum has been dissected off of the pedicles of the prostate. (**b**) The rectum is adherent to the right pedicle of the prostate and the right pedicle is about to be transected. (**c**) The rectal injury has occurred and must be repaired in primary fashion, with or without diversion

Laparoscopic and Robot-Assisted Laparoscopic Radical Prostatectomy

The open radical prostatectomy is the gold standard for the treatment of localized adenocarcinoma of the prostate; however, over the last 10 years, minimally invasive approaches to the treatment of prostate cancer have made significant inroads. It is estimated that over 70% of laparoscopic radical prostatectomies were performed with robotic assistance in 2009 [63]. The most common and feared bowel complication related to the open, laparoscopic, and robot-assisted radical prostatectomy is the rectal injury, as it is separated by the two layers of Denonvillier's fascia and the perirectal fat. Risk factors for rectal injuries include previous radiation, scarring from previous surgery or infection, and a large prostate size [64]. Since prostate cancer is the most common non-cutaneous cancer in men in the United States and Europe, there is a significant amount of data available to evaluate the incidence of bowel complications of laparoscopic and robot-assisted laparoscopic radical prostatectomy. Rassweiler and the German Laparoscopic Working Group have evaluated 5,824 patients who have undergone laparoscopic radical prostatectomy [65]. Rectal injury occurred in 1.5–2.5% of these patients. There were no other significant bowel complications in this large number of patients. Hu et al. have evaluated 358 patients undergoing laparoscopic radical prostatectomy [66]. They report a 1.9% incidence in rectal injuries with a resultant 1.9% incidence of rectourethral fistulae. Other bowel complications from this series include a 5.3% incidence of ileus and a 0.3% incidence of colonic injury. Robot-assisted laparoscopic prostatectomy (RALRP) has been rapidly accepted and there are several large series that have well documented their complications. Menon and colleagues have a series of 2,766 RALRPs [67]. In this series there were four bowel injuries and four port-site hernias, for an incidence of 0.1%. It is not specified whether these bowel injuries were rectal injuries. There was one case of prolonged ileus. Patel has reported on 1,500 consecutive RALRPs [68]. Two rectal injuries (0.1%) were encountered and repaired intraoperatively. Three incisional hernias and three cases of ileus were noted (0.2%). There was one port-site hernia and one case of a small bowel obstruction (0.06%). Rectal injuries, when recognized, were repaired primarily in two layers without consequence in all cases reported (see Fig. 6). LRP and RALRP appear to have a low incidence of bowel injuries that compare favorably with the open procedure (Tables 4 and 5).

Conclusion

Bowel injuries are an uncommon occurrence in laparoscopic and robot-assisted laparoscopic surgery. However, these injuries may be life-threatening if not diagnosed and treated rapidly. Laparoscopic bowel injuries have a presentation that is unique compared to bowel injuries encountered during open surgery. It is imperative to understand and recognize this presentation in order to treat the bowel injury in an expeditious manner. The overall incidence, on a procedure per procedure basis, compares favorably with open surgery.

References

1. Clayman RV. Visceral and gastrointestinal complications of laparoscopic and robotic urologic surgery. N Engl J Med. 1991 May;324(19):1370–1.
2. Schuessler WW, Vancaillie TG, Reich H, et al. Transperitoneal endosurgical lymphadenectomy in patients with localized prostate cancer. J Urol. 1991;145:988–91.
3. Bishoff JT, Allaf ME, Kirkels W, et al. Laparoscopic bowel injury: incidence and clinical presentation. 1999;161(3):887–90.
4. Liakakos T, Thomakos N, Fine PM, et al. Peritoneal adhesions: etiology, pathophysiology, and clinical significance. Recent advances in prevention and management. Dig Surg. 2001;18(4):260–73.
5. Paulter Se, Phillips JL, Walther MM. Assessment of risk for intra-abdominal adhesions at laparoscopy for urological tumors. J Urol. 2002;168(6):2391–4.
6. Parson JK, Jarrett TJ, Chow GK, et al. The effect of previous abdominal surgery on urological laparoscopy. J Urol. 2002;168(6):2387–90.
7. Scott Putman S, Bishoff JT. Clinical anaesthesiology. 5th ed. Philadelphia: Lippincott Williams and Wilkins; 2006. p. 396.
8. El-Galley R, Hammontree L, Urban D, et al. Anesthesia for laparoscopic donor nephrectomy: is nitrous oxide contraindicated? J Urol. 2007;178(1):255–7.
9. Ahmad G, Duffy JM, Phillips K, et al. Laparoscopic entry techniques. Cochrane Database Syst Rev. 2008;16(2):CD006583.

10. Hasson HM. A modified instrument and method for laparoscopy. Am J Obstet Gynecol. 1971;110:886–7.
11. Ternamian AM. Laparoscopy without trocars. Surg Endosc. 1997;11(8):815–8.
12. Minervini A, Davenport K, Pefanis G, et al. Prospective study comparing the bladeless optical access trocar versus Hasson open trocar for the establishment of pneumoperitoneum in laparoscopic renal procedures. Arch Ital Urol Androl. 2008;80(3)95–8.
13. Neudecker J, Sauerland S, Neugebauer E, et al. The European Association for Endoscopic Surgery clinical practice guideline on the pneumoperitoneum for laparoscopic surgery. Surg Endosc. 2002;16(7):1121–43.
14. Nassar AH, Ashkar KA, Rashed AA, et al. Laparoscopic cholecystectomy and the umbilicus. Br J Surg. 1997;84:630–33.
15. Nanigian DK, Smith W, Ellison LM. Robot-assisted laparoscopic nephroureterectomy. J Endourol. 2006;20(7):463–5.
16. Fahlenkamp D, Rassweiler J, Fornara P, et al. Complications of laparoscopic procedures in urology: experience with 2.407 procedures at 4 German centers. J Urol. 1999;162(3 Pt 1):765–70.
17. Varkarakis IM, Allaf ME, Ghayani SB, et al. Pancreatic injuries during laparoscopic urologic surgery. Urology 2004;64(6):1089–93.
18. Penfield AJ. How to prevent complications of open laparoscopy. J Reprod Med. 1985;30(9):660–3.
19. Biggs G, Hafron J, Feliciano J, et al. Treatment of splenic injury during laparoscopic nephrectomy with BioGlue, a surgical adhesive. Urology 2005;66(4):882.
20. Gill IS, Kavoussi LR, Clayman RV, et al. Complications of laparoscopic nephrectomy in 185 patients: a multi-institutional review. J Urol. 1995;154:479–83.
21. Fear RE. Laparoscopy: a valuable aid in gynecologic diagnosis. Obstet Gynecol. 1968;31:297–309.
22. Susmallian S, Ezri T, Charuzi I. Laparoscopic repair of access port site hernia after Lap-Band system implantation. Obes Surg. 2002;12:682–4.
23. Bowrey DJ, Blom D, Crookes PF, et al. Risk factors and the prevalence of trocar site herniation after laparoscopic fundoplication. Surg Endosc. 2001;15:663–6.
24. Montz FJ, Holschneider CH, Munro MG. Incisional hernia following laparoscopy: a survey of the American Association of Gynecologic Laparoscopists. Obstet Gynecol. 1994;84:881–4.
25. Kadar N, Reich H, Liu CY, et al. Incisional hernia after major laparoscopic gynecologic procedures. Am J Obstet Gynecol. 1993;168:1493–5.
26. Nezhat C, Nezhat F, Seidman DS, et al. Incisional hernias after operative laparoscopy. J Laparoendosc Adv Surg Tech A. 1997;7:111–5.
27. Duron JJ, Hay JM, Msika S, et al. Prevalence and mechanisms of small intestinal obstruction following laparoscopic abdominal surgery: a retrospective multicenter study. Arch Surg. 2000;135:208–12.
28. Mayol J, Garcia-Aguilar J, Ortiz-Oshiro E, et al. Risks of the minimal access approach for laparoscopic surgery: multivariate analysis of morbidity related to umbilical trocar insertion. World J Surg. 1997;21:529–33.
29. Azurin DJ, Go LS, Arroyo LR, Kirkland ML. Trocar site herniation following laparoscopic cholecystectomy and the significance of an incidental preexisting umbilical hernia. Am Surg. 1995;61:718–20.
30. Seamon LG, Backes F, Resnick K, et al. Robotic trocar site small bowel evisceration after gynecologic cancer surgery. Obstet Gynecol. 2008;112(2):462–64.
31. Irvin TT, Stoddard CJ, Greaney MG, Duthie HL. Abdominal wound healing: a prospective clinical study. Br Med J. 1977;2:351–2.
32. Troxel SA, Das D. Incisional hernia following hand-assisted laparoscopic surgery for renal cell cancer. JSLS. 2005;9(2):196–8.
33. Tisdale BE, Kapoor A, Hussain A, Piercey K, Whelan JP. Intact specimen extraction in laparoscopic nephrectomy procedures: Pfannenstiel versus expanded port site incisions. Urology. 2007;69(2):241–4.
34. Camargo AH, Rubenstein JN, Ershoff BD, et al. The effect of kidney morcellation on operative time, incision complications, and postoperative analgesia after laparoscopic nephrectomy. Int Braz J Urol. 2006; 32(2):273.
35. Singh R, Omiccioli A, Hegge S, McKinley C. Does the extraction site location in laparoscopic colorectal surgery have an impact on incisional hernia rates? Surg Endosc. 2008;22(12):2596–600.
36. Bird VG. Comparison of different extraction sites used during laparoscopic radical nephrectomy. J Urol. 2009;181(4):1565–70.
37. Henry JF, Defechereux T, Raffaelli M, et al. Complications of laparoscopic adrenalectomy: results of 169 consecutive procedures. World J Surg. 2000;24:1342–46.
38. Wu JC, Wu HS, Lin MS, et al. Comparison of robot-assisted laparoscopic adrenalectomy with traditional laparoscopic adrenalectomy – 1 year follow-up. Surg Endosc. 2008;22(2):463–6. Epub 2007 Aug 18.
39. Morino M, Beninca G, Giraudo G, et al. Robot-assisted vs. laparoscopic adrenalectomy: a prospective randomized controlled trial. Surg Endosc. 2004;18(12):1742–6. Epub 2004 Oct 26.
40. Clayman RV, Kavoussi LR, Soper NJ, Dierks SM, et al. Laparoscopic nephrectomy: initial case report. J Urol 1991;146(2):278–82.
41. Pareek G, Hedican SP, Gee JR, et al. Meta-analysis of the complications of laparoscopic renal surgery: comparison of procedures and techniques. J Urol. 2006;175(4): 1208–13.
42. Rogers C, Launqani R, Krane LS, et al. Robotic nephrectomy for the treatment of benign and malignant disease. BJU Int. 2008;102(11):1660–5. Epub 2008 Jul 29.
43. Desai MM, Strzempkowski B, Matin SF, et al. Prospective randomized comparison of transperitoneal versus retroperitoneal laparoscopic radical nephrectomy. J Urol. 2005;173(1):38–41.
44. Rogers MM, Menon M, Weise ES, et al. Robotic partial nephrectomy: a multi-institutional analysis. J Robotic Surg. 2008;2(3), 141–3.
45. Hall MC, Womack S, Sagalowsky AI, et al. Prognostic factors, recurrence, and survival in transitional cell carcinoma of the upper urinary tract: a 30-year experience in 252 patients. Urology. 1998;52(4):594–601.
46. Matin SF, Gill IS. Recurrence and survival following laparoscopic radical nephroureterectomy with vari-

ous forms of bladder cuff control. J Urol. 2005;173(2):395–400.
47. Wolf JS, Dash BK, Hollenbeck WK, et al. Intermediate followup of hand assisted laparoscopic nephroureterectomy for urothelial carcinoma: Factors associated with outcomes. J Urol. 2005;173(4):1102–7.
48. Moon DA, El-shazly MA, Chang CM, et al. Laparoscopic pyeloplasty: evolution of a new gold standard. Urology. 2006;67(5):932–6. Epub 2006 Apr 25.
49. Mufarrij PW, Woods M, Shah OD, et al. Robotic dismembered pyeloplasty: a 6-year, multi-institutional experience. J Urol. 2008;180(4):1391–6. Epub 2008 Aug 15.
50. Steiner H, Peschel R, Janetschek G, et al. Long-term results of laparoscopic retroperitoneal lymph node dissection: a single-center 10-year experience. Urology. 2004;63(3):550–5.
51. Permponqkosol S, Lima GC, Warlick CA, et al. Postchemotherapy laparoscopic retroperitoneal lymph node dissection: evaluation of complications. Urology. 2007;69(2):361–5.
52. Parra RO, Andrus CH, Jones JP, et al. Laparoscopic cystectomy: initial report on a new treatment for the retained bladder. J Urol. 1992;148(4):1140–4.
53. Abraham JB, Young JL, Box GN, et al. Comparative analysis of laparoscopic and robot-assisted radical cystectomy with ileal conduit urinary division. J Endourol. 2007;21(12):1473–80.
54. Guillotreau J, Gamé X, Mouzin M, et al. Radical cystectomy for bladder cancer: morbidity of laparoscopic versus open surgery. J Urol. 2009;181(2):554–9.
55. Haber GP, Crouzet S, Gill IS. Laparoscopic and robotic assisted radical cystectomy for bladder cancer: a critical analysis. Eur Urol. 2008:54(1):54–62.
56. Huang J, Lin T, Xu K, et al. Laparoscopic radical cystectomy with orthotopic ileal neobladder: a report of 85 cases. J Endourol. 2008;22(5):939–46.
57. Hemal AK, Kolla SB. Comparison of laparoscopic and open radical cystoprostatectomy for localized bladder cancer with 3-year oncological followup: a single surgeon experience. J Urol. 2007;178(6):2340–3.
58. Butt ZM, Perlmutter AE, Piacente PM, et al. Impact of body mass index on robot-assisted radical cystectomy. JSLS. 2008;12(3):241–5.
59. Pruthi RS, Wallen EM. Robotic-assisted laparoscopic radical cystoprostatectomy. Eur Urol. 2008;53(2):310–22.
60. Murphy DG, Challacombe BJ, Elhage O, et al. Robotic-assisted laparoscopic radical cystectomy with extracorporeal urinary diversion: initial experience. Eur Urol. 2008;54(3):570–80.
61. Wang GJ, Carocas DA, Raman JD, et al. Robotic vs. open radical cystectomy: prospective comparison of perioperative outcomes and pathological measures of early oncological efficacy. BJU Int. 2008;101(1):89–93.
62. Hollenbeck BK, Miller DC, Taub D, et al. Identifying risk factors for potentially avoidable complications following radical cystectomy. J Urol. 2005;174:1231–7.
63. Based on procedures performed against a surgical number of 90,000 procedures from Thompson Healthcare Solucient® data of 2007.
64. Harpster LE, Rommel FM, Sieber PR, et al. The incidence and management of rectal injury associated with radical prostatectomy in a community based urology practice. J Urol. 1995;154(4):1435–8.
65. Rassweiler J, Stolzenburg J, Sulser T, et al. Laparoscopic radical prostatectomy – the experience of the German Laparoscopic Working Group. Eur Urol. 2006;49(1):113–9.
66. Hu JC, Nelson RA, Wilson TG, et al. Perioperative complications of laparoscopic and robotic assisted laparoscopic radical prostatectomy. J Urol. 2006;175(2):541–6.
67. Badani KK, Kaul S, Menon M. Evolution of robotic radical prostatectomy: assessment after 2766 procedures. Cancer. 2007;110(9):1951–8.
68. Patel VR, Palmer KJ, Coughlin G, et al. Robot-assisted laparoscopic radical prostatectomy: perioperative outcomes of 1500 cases. J Endourol. 2008;22(10):2299–305.

Complications of Robotic-Assisted Laparoscopic Surgery: Iatrogenic and Doulogenic

John L. Phillips, Erin C. Grantham, and Bobby S. Alexander

Keywords Robotics · Malfunction · Complications · Laparoscopy

Introduction

Robotic surgery has greatly increased the ability of surgeons to apply laparoscopic techniques to challenging operations. As with any surgical procedure, unforeseen complications may occur in even the best of scenarios; it is knowledge of these complications, and the avoidance and correction of them, which will aid surgeons and their patients. A standardized approach to complications in laparoscopy has been proposed using the Clavien classification system, an ordinal grading scale encompassing the most minor to the most major, of life-threatening complications [1, 2] (Table 1). While the vast majority of reported complications in robotic laparoscopy are minor, level I events, this chapter will serve to review the range of complications of robotics as a distinct subset of those seen in standard laparoscopic approaches to urologic surgery.

Table 1 Clavien classification of surgical complications

Grade	Definition
Grade I	Any deviation from the normal post-op course without need for pharmacological treatment or surgical, endoscopic, and radiologic interventions; allowed therapeutic regimens are drugs (i.e., antiemetics, antipyretics, analgesics, diuretics, and electrolytes) and physiotherapy. This grade also includes wound infections opened at the bedside
Grade II	Requiring pharmacological treatment with drugs other than those allowed for grade I complications. Blood transfusions and TPN are also included
Grade III	Requiring surgical, endoscopic, or radiologic intervention
Grade IIIa	Intervention not under general anesthesia
Grade IIIb	Intervention under general anesthesia
Grade IV	Life-threatening complication requiring ICU management
Grade IVa	Single-organ dysfunction (including dialysis)
Grade IVb	Multi-organ dysfunction
Grade V	Death of a patient

Source: Dindo D, Demartines N, Clavien P-A. Classification of surgical complications: A new proposal with evaluation in a cohort of 6336 patients and results of a survey. Ann Surg. 2004;240:205–13

Technical Terms

An important aspect of robotic surgery is its technical complexity, both for the nursing and physician staffs and for the patient population who are to be educated by their physician what precisely "robotic surgery" is and what it is not. The term "robotic" has been applied to any mechanical device that has some apparent animation capability, i.e., movement. Surgical robots, as

J.L. Phillips (✉)
Department of Urology, New York Medical College, Valhalla, NY 10591, USA
e-mail: john_phillips@nymc.edu

R. Ghavamian (ed.), *Complications of Laparoscopic and Robotic Urologic Surgery*,
DOI 10.1007/978-1-60761-676-4_8, © Springer Science+Business Media, LLC 2010

most popularly used in the da Vinci telesurgical system, are more correctly termed *marginal manipulators*: the surgeon controls each movement of the robotic system from a distance as defined by the technological interface, e.g., cable length [3]. The terms "master" and "slave," while historically barbed, have popularly been used to refer to the surgeon at the console, or the *executor*, and the robotic device itself, or the *effector*, respectively. For simplicity, this chapter refers to the executor unit as the "console" and the effector unit as the "patient side cart." The power source and its monitor system is the "vision tower." Complications, or adverse events (AEs), associated with robotic surgery include any event which occurs as a result of the surgeon's activities and these should be referred to as *iatrogenic* complications irrespective of whether or not a robotic instrument is being handled. Complications related solely to console, patient side cart, or vision tower malfunction and which would not ordinarily be encountered in a non-robotic environment will be referred to as *doulogenic* (*Gk: doulos*, slave) complications (Table 2). Accidents refer to AEs which pose a risk to the caregivers in the robotic environment.

The surgeon's console, or the executor, includes the optics for binocular vision or "stereo viewer" that are individually served to the left and right eye. The hand pieces, or master tool manipulators, left and right (MTM-L and MTM-R, respectively), enable 270° of freedom and are disabled when the surgeon's head is removed from the stereo viewer, unbreaking an infrared safety switch. Tremor-corrected signals from the executor are relayed to the patient side cart where encoders (i.e., primary control sensor) and potentiometers (i.e., secondary control sensors) reconstruct the *xyz* grid and enable telerobotic marginal manipulation of the arms. Thus, the robotic arms are known as left and right "patient side manipulators" (PSM-L and PSM-R, respectively) and the camera arm is known as the "endoscopic camera manipulator" or ECM.

The user should also have some familiarity with errors and fault types in robotic surgery. In general, faults, or system errors, are usually detected during robotic setup. Most system errors involving the ECM or PSMs occur when the da Vinci safety system determines that the angular position of one or more robotic joints, as measured by the encoder or potentiometer, is out of a specified tolerance for agreement. Often, bumping, jarring, mishandling, or forced clutching of either the ECM or PSMs will result in fault errors and the freezing of the system. These are recoverable errors and an override can usually be obtained with disengagement of the fault switch at the console or rebooting of the system. In contrast, unrecoverable errors usually

Table 2 Technical terms associated with the da Vinci Surgical System^{TM}, a type of marginal manipulator telerobotic platform

I. *Complication* – an adverse event (AE) that poses a risk to the patient
  a. *Iatrogenic* – an AE as a result of physician activity
  b. *Doulogenic* – an AE as a result of robotic platform or instrument failure

II. *Accident* – an adverse event that poses a risk to the caregiver

III. *Executor* – the agent or the platform from which a robotic command originates, e.g., the surgical console

IV. *Effector* – the platform which carries out the commands of the executor, e.g., the patient side cart

V. *Marginal manipulator* – a robotic device in which the effector simulates movements of the executor from a prescribed distance, e.g., the da Vinci Surgical System (Intuitive Surgical, Sunnyvale, CA)

VI. *Manipulators* – the robotic devices of the effector unit which carry out the commands of the executor
  c. *Endoscopic camera manipulator* (ECM), i.e., the camera arm
  d. *Patient side manipulator* (PSM), i.e., the multiple robotic arms attached to the patient side cart
  e. *Master tool manipulator* (MTM) – the "hand pieces" of the surgical console through which the surgeon executes movement commands

VII. *Encoder* – a primary control sensor in each manipulator

VIII. *Potentiometer* – a secondary control sensor

IX. *Recoverable error* – a safety fault that can be corrected (e.g., excess jarring or pressure on the ECM or PSMs

X. *Unrecoverable error* – a safety fault due to fatal device failure requiring replacement (e.g., blown or damaged potentiometer in the ECM)

XI. *Malfunction* – failure of the patient side cart due to a detection safety limit breech

XII. *Breakage* – damage of any hardware or instrument of the robotic platform (e.g., ruptured cable, unscrewed MTM joint, needle driver jaw loss)

include encoder or potentiometer failure which results in a manipulator freeze that requires replacement of the offending device. A completed homing, draping, and vision testing at the console should therefore be done prior to a patient's entrance into the operating room. Hardware malfunction or unrecoverable errors requiring part replacement can thus allow postponement of a case prior to the patient receiving anesthetic medication.

Complications: Iatrogenic and Doulogenic

The minimally invasive surgery revolution of the early 1990s ushered in the robotic era when the US Food and Drug Administration cleared the use of the da Vinci Surgical System (Intuitive surgical, Sunny Valley, California) in 1998 for use in laparoscopic cholecystectomy. FDA approval of a medical device occurs only when the mechanical aspects of safety, hazards, and utility meet a certain standard for market application; FDA approval does not address physician-dependent complications after instrument deployment in the market place. The advantages of the robotic platform typically include unique hand-like dexterity and enhanced precision, three-dimensional magnified visualization of the operating field, a seven-degree range of motion, tremor filtration, and comfortably seated ergonomic operating posture [4, 5]. The disadvantages of the robot include the lack of haptic or tactile feedback while operating, the inability to switch instruments and operating field conveniently, the large size of the robot with bulky arms, and the high cost of the technology [6, 7]. Robotic-assisted laparoscopic radical prostatectomy (RALP) has been available to the urologic community since its first use in Germany in 2001 [8]. Robotic-assisted laparoscopic partial nephrectomy, adrenalectomy, cystectomy, and retroperitoneal node dissection have also been well described in the urologic literature [9–11]. Procedures in gynecologic, endocrine, bariatric, head and neck, intestinal, thoracic, and cardiac surgery have also had increasing appeal [12–14]. With the widespread application of robotic technology into the domain of clinical surgery, two distinct classes of complications have emerged: iatrogenic and doulogenic. As shown in Table 3, iatrogenic complications of RALP, for example, would include those encountered during any radical prostatectomy, e.g., DVT or hemorrhage; those seen in other laparoscopic procedures, e.g., port site hernia; and those which occur because of the precise nuances of robotic surgery, e.g., lack of tactile feedback causing vascular injury. In contrast, purely doulogenic complications are only those encountered because of device malfunction (e.g., ECM failure). Doulogenic complications are important to understand as many can be prevented and, if properly identified and understood, resolved without clinical sequelae.

Complications: Iatrogenic

Robotic surgery is among the most technically demanding aspects of minimally invasive surgery. No engineer, electrician, or software manager is typically present at the bedside; the surgeon must therefore be "baker, butcher, and basket maker" – he/she must maintain the standards of safety in the operating room, troubleshoot and identify problems before and during the procedure, and fix or repair instrument difficulties during critical portions of the operation. Complications of specific robotic procedures are addressed elsewhere in this textbook and include intra-operative events (hemorrhage, visceral injury, and anesthesia-related complications) and post-operative sequelae of these events (incontinence, impotence, DVT, etc.).

Iatrogenic complications unique to robotic surgery are unusual as many, e.g., hemorrhage, are problems of open surgery as well and others, e.g., port site hematoma, are seen in other laparoscopic procedures. Purely robotic iatrogenic complications would include those which occur because of the robotic environment: maloccurrence due to loss of haptic feedback and spatial awareness; arm, instrument, or console misuse; poor patient or robotic arm positioning; loss of spatial awareness; and surgical inability. Inappropriate resolve, or the prolonged desire to continue a robotic procedure despite clinical evidence to pursue an alternative course, is an important aspect of iatrogenic robotic events that may lead to adverse events, or injury.

Large series of robotic surgery often have low complication rates and it is from these high-volume, outlier series that a majority of published literature

Table 3 Types of complications encountered in robotic-assisted laparoscopic prostatectomy (RALP).

I. *Iatrogenic* (i.e., due to physician)
  a. General (common to all surgical procedures)
    i. Intraoperative (e.g., anesthesia, hemorrhage, injury)
    ii. Post-operative (e.g., infection, wound, pain)
  b. Laparoscopic, general (common to laparoscopic approaches)
    i. Access (e.g., port site ecchymosis, hematoma, hernia)
    ii. Innocent bystander injury (e.g., visceral, vascular)
    iii. Maloccurrence due to loss of tactile feedback
  c. Laparoscopic, robotic (i.e., encountered only in robotic approaches)
    i. Patient cart positioning injuries
    ii. PSM or ECM mishandling
    iii. Instrument misuse
    iv. Inappropriate resolve
    v. Maloccurrence due to loss of haptic feedback

II. *Doulogenic* (i.e., due to device)
  a. Malfunction
    i. Potentiometer or encoder failure
    ii. Stereo viewer failure
    iii. MTM failure
  b. Breakage
    i. Robotic instruments
    ii. ECM or PSM
    iii. MTMs
  c. Electrical events
    i. Bulb explosion
    ii. Power failure
    iii. Surge protection failure
  d. Burns
    i. Bifurcated light cord or insulation failure
    ii. Port conduction

Doulogenic (*Gk: doulos,* slave) complications are those due solely to robot malfunction; misuse or maloccurrence of robotic instruments are *iatrogenic (Gk: iatros,* physician) complications

regarding the efficacy, risks, and benefits of robotic surgery derives [15, 16]. Complications which arise from much smaller series, or even individual cases, may go unpublished but can hold valuable utility for the practitioner [17]. One source of such information is the FDA which has a publicly accessible collection of over 12 databases covering premarket approvals, clinical laboratory amendments, drug events, radiation emission warnings, and reports of experiences with FDA-approved products. MAUDE (Manufacturer and User Facility Device Experience) has proven useful to survey the range of complications of over 1500 medical and surgical devices from 1993 to the present, with an ability to screen for complications which arise from the device itself, maloccurrences with the device, or user mishandling of the device (URL: www.fda.gov, then search function). A limitation of MAUDE is that it is voluntary and only those events which are reported are available for inquiry. Thus no numerator [i.e., number of adverse events (AEs)] or denominator (i.e., total number of robotic cases) is available to consider frequency rates or maloccurrence prevalence trends. Still, MAUDE data can provide some experiential information that may have interdisciplinary benefit. The MAUDE database includes access to AEs from all robotic fields including cardiac surgery, gynecology, urology, and general surgery; date of AE, robotic model number, manufacturer, and trade name; a brief description of the AE from a surgical and engineering point of view; and event type: death, malfunction, injury, or other. Andonian et al. [18] used MAUDE to survey Zeus- and da Vinci-related AEs over a 7-year time frame with the presumption that not all AEs are ever reported to the FDA. Of an estimated 50,000 robotic surgery procedures nationwide, 168 (0.5%) were associated with an AE, 104 (62%) of which were system malfunctions; 9 (4.8%) were associated with patient injury including the minor (e.g., port site hematoma due to PSM hyper movement) or major vascular, atrial, or visceral injury due to faulty device or instrument misuse.

In a separate survey of FDA MAUDE for this manuscript, 21 of 125 (16.8%) AEs from 2002 to 2009 were user or iatrogenic events, 9 of which could be explained as due to the robotic environment (e.g., loss of haptic feedback). In one, the user disengaged the hands from the MTMs at the console without disengaging the head: the PSMs at the bedside dropped and a ureteral injury occurred which required conversion for repair. Two AEs were reported in which the monopolar scissors were engaged below or outside the vision field causing a ureteral injury in one and a combined ureteral and iliac artery injury in another. Two bowel injuries as well as burns due to monopolar engagement using the wrong pedal at the console were similarly reported. Two cardiac AEs were reported in which atrial injuries resulted from third PSM "drift" outside the vision field. One death during robotic nephrectomy occurred from hilar avulsion during dissection with the first and second PSMs. Of the remaining eight deaths reported to the FDA, none were associated with the robotic environment per se: clipping of the superior mesenteric artery (1), pulmonary failure (2), cardiac failure (3), and sepsis from delayed bowel injury (2).

Non-injurious iatrogenic complications reported to FDA MAUDE have included damage to an MTM or a PSM due to excess handling, rough handling without unclutching, or, in one, shorting of the main power cord due to trapping under the wheels of the patient side cart. The remaining AEs associated with patient injury in da Vinci robotic surgery in MAUDE are also seen in other non-robotic laparoscopic techniques and include unilateral or bilateral nerve palsy port site hematoma and hemorrhage. While statistical precautions must be considered in extrapolating implications from FDA MAUDE information, the data do give the impression that complications due to the surgeon in a robotic environment are uncommon. Furthermore, most if not all AEs are avoidable using a circumspective, wide-angled approach to instrument use, using visual cues for tissue and knot tension to compensate for the loss of haptic feedback, and by continual communication between the surgeon at the console and the assistant at the bedside.

Similar conclusions about the small prevalence of iatrogenic complications can also be drawn from the larger published series of urologic robotic procedures [8, 8, 15, 16, 19–21]. These and other authors describe a total perioperative complication rate of ~5% when including all levels of Clavien adverse events from perioperative ileus, prolonged drainage, or wound hematoma (1–4%) to reoperation and visceral or vascular injury (0.1–0.3%). None of these large series report Clavien IV or V level complications and thus are not the sources of such AE information reported to FDA MAUDE.

Complications: Doulogenic

Doulogenic complications are those AEs which occur because of device malfunction, breakage, or failure and may occur independent of surgeon activity. Complications may have little to no clinical sequelae, such as a case postponement or delay under anesthesia (DUA), to highly negative outcomes, such as great vessel injury or death. The MAUDE database has revealed that of the reported AEs associated with the da Vinci system, almost all are related to malfunction of the robotic arms, breakage of the robotic instruments near or in the patient, software failure, light source or electrical failure, or heat/burn AEs. As shown in Table 4, of the 123 reported AEs, 69 (57%) were due to system malfunction, 23 (19%) due to breakage of any robotic instrument, and 10 (12%) due to electrical or burn-related events. Doulogenic complications therefore represent 102 of 121 (84%) surveyed AEs. The prevalence of doulogenic complications may be low, given the large volume of robotic procedures that are currently performed. Zorn et al. [22] evaluated 725 RALPs and found a device failure leading to case abortion of only 0.5%, all of which were determined prior to induction of anesthesia. A meta-analysis by Lavery et al. [23] included 8,240 robotic cases from 11 institutions and found a 0.3% robotic failure rate. Of 34 cases, 10 (29%) required conversion after anesthesia; the remainder were cancelled after robotic failure was detected during setup. The majority of reported failures were due to the ECM or the PSM. This compares with a doulogenic failure rate of 2.6% in a series of 350 cases by Borden et al. and of 4.6% in the 130 cases of Kozlowksi et al. [17, 24].

Table 4 Survey of adverse events reported to the FDA MAUDE (Manufacturer and User Facility Device Experience) database associated with the use of the da Vinci Surgical System by Intuitive Surgical (Sunnyvale, CA) from 2002 to 2009

		Outcome type						
	Total	Death	Injury	DUA	Conversion	Abort	None	Others
Malfunction	69	0	3	3	44	15	1	3
Breakage	23	0	0	7	0	0	8	8
Heat	4	0	3	0	0	0	0	1
Electrical	6	0	3	0	0	0	3	0
User related	13	1	7	0	5	1	0	0
Unknown	8	8	0	0	0	0	0	0
Totals	123	9	16	10	49	16	12	12

The FDA MAUDE is an online searchable resource for all surgical fields which use any FDA-approved medical device (www.fda.gov). These data do not represent the population of unreported AEs nor is there an accounting for the total number of robotic procedures performed

Malfunction. The majority of doulogenic complications occur due to ECM or PSM malfunction: the relay of MTM activity at the console to the PSM and ECM at the bedside depends on potentiometers and encoders which, after homing, detect cable tension, arm freedom, and resistance to movement. Any deviation from a set limit of resistance or movement data will result in one of the several types of fault errors: 20008, 20009, 200013, or 20023 (Table 2). Malfunction of the cable units, the potentiometers themselves, the circuit boards, or, rarely, the software used to relay these signals can all result in a fault error that will "freeze" the system. These are recoverable errors if artificial limitations have been placed on PSM or ECM freedom, such as a sterile bag that is too tight, vision tower or PSM bumping of another PSM, or rough handling of the ECM or the PSM. Most interrogations of these errors require the surgeon to inspect the robotic arms and ensure their lack of confinement, and a stepwise shutdown and startup of the robotic system. In some cases, the errors are internal and have resulted from blown potentiometers, ruptured cables, screw joint misalignment, damage of an MTM, or software defects [17, 18, 22]. These, in contrast to arm limitation or jarring phenomenon, are often unrecoverable errors and require identification and replacement of the defective part, and system shutdown. In 69 reported malfunctions of this type in FDA MAUDE, 44 conversions to non-robotic surgery and 15 case aborts were documented. Of the case aborts, 12 occurred after the induction of anesthesia and placement of the robotic ports. In their evaluation of FDA MAUDE in 2007, Andonian et al. [18] found that of 108 conversions from robotic to non-robotic surgery (i.e., open or laparoscopic), 104 (96%) were due to system error malfunctions; only 4 were due to hardware breakage of one or more of the PSMs.

Breakage. Breakage refers to any event associated with the robotic instruments, hardware (e.g., cables, pulleys, master tool screws) or electrical (e.g., bulb), which requires the instrument to become nonfunctional. Graphite chips flaking off the end of an EndoWrist™ device, jaw loss from a needle driver, and dislodgement of a component of a master tool manipulator are all aspects of user-dependent "wear and tear" that can result in breakage and patient injury. Of the 23 occurrences of a breakage-type AE in FDA MAUDE, 7 resulted in a delay under anesthesia (DUA) in repairing or replacing the offending device. Missing needle driver components, frayed cables, and fragments of insulation require retrieval of all lost materials and inspection of visceral structures to ensure no bystander injury.

Electrical. Electrical events are an important, though rare, doulogenic complication, the most serious of which are burns and electrical injury. The monopolar scissors and EndoWrist™ are protected by an insulation sheath that, when missing or corroded, can expose bystander tissue to monopolar electrical injury. One case in FDA MAUDE reported port site burns due to conduction of the monopolar current up the metallic sheath of the robotic port. Burns associated with the bifurcated light cord, and one case of surgical drape fire in FDA MAUDE, demonstrate the extreme diligence and care the surgical team must have in handling the light and power cords associated with the robotic platform.

The da Vinci system requires a 240-V source and draws upward of a kilowatt of power for the multiple servo motors on the 1,180-pound patient side cart. Although the da Vinci device can remain on battery power for up to 6 h, sudden unplugging of the device could expose the worker or the patient to electrical injury. The plug units must be kept secured and protected to avoid tripping, entrapment, or damage. Damage of the cable insulators can occur during the rolling procedure and must be prevented, or at least detected, at all costs.

The xenon light source contains a 2000-lumen 300-W Cermax white light bulb that emits photons at 5050 K in a partial bulb vacuum whose surface temperature approaches 200°C. While a typical life span of these bulbs reaches 1,000 h, breakage of the bulb or damage of the filaments from use can result in sudden bulb rupture, a sometime explosive event that can result in equipment and bodily injury. In one FDA MAUDE case of a bulb explosion, fragments of glass could be detected in various parts of the operating room theatre. The bulb itself is housed in a ceramic alloy casing which is replaced with the bulb; spare bulbs cannot be simply rotated into place. Attention must be paid, therefore, to bulb's life span before each case so that bulb replacement can occur on a set, safe schedule, preferably far short of the maximum published life span of the bulb.

Burns. The bifurcated light cord used for the robotic procedure is well insulated along its 15 ft length. While the endoscopic lens tip generates a heat of 40°C up to 1 cm away, the end of the light cord itself may be injuriously hot upward of 110°C and can easily burn through drapes, surgical gloves, and skin. These components must be used with utmost care at all times to avoid potentially catastrophic fire, personal injury, and equipment damage. The nursing staff may be instructed to close the xenon light source filter whenever the cables themselves are disconnected from the LCD camera. This will ensure a margin of safety when resting the unconnected cables but does require absolute communication between the bedside and the staff during these maneuvers.

Robotic Accidents

Robotics has been used in industry since the 1950s but the rapid expansion of fixed sequence welding, heavy torque devices in the automotive industry prompted the United States government to standardize worker-related hazards via OSHA [3]. Most guidelines are classified into types of accidents and types of hazards, both of which have applications in robotic surgery. Doulogenic accidents fall into the four categories typically observed in the industrial setting (impact or collision events, crushing or trapping events, mechanical part accidents, and electrical/burn accidents) as well as the unique events which occur due to surgical robotic part malfunction described above.

Impact or collision accidents may occur during movement of the effector or patient side cart unit to or from the bedside, i.e., "docking" and "undocking." During the procedure itself, the surgeon will be unaware of the size of environment required for arm movement to execute even small maneuvers in the abdominal or the pelvic space. In two cases in FDA MAUDE, lack of appropriate spacing of the 4th PSM resulted in atrial injury and thoracic conversion. Bedside assistant injury can occur to the head, face, eye, or upper extremity if struck by an arm of the effector unit. Attention must be paid to arm movement when the assistant moves closely into the operative field to inspect ports, or manipulate sutures, lines, and devices.

Crushing and trapping accidents may be sustained by the patient if effector unit or arm positioning maintains pressure on an exposed body area. Extreme care must be taken to ensure non-pressured leg positioning in stirrups, that adequate space exists between the effector arms and lower extremities, and that the surgeon personally inspects the patient's upper and lower limbs, hands, and fingers for a "clenched fist safety margin" prior to sitting down at the executor console. The bed cannot be repositioned after docking of the effector unit – potentially catastrophic entrapment or abdominal wall injury could occur [18]. Unplugging of the bedside movement control apparatus has been advocated until the effector device is undocked. Excessive mechanical force applied to the grasping part of the large needle driver may cause it to shear off and break. In general, broken instruments can be seen and easily retrieved [22, 25]. Grasping of stents with in-dwelling wire coils by robotic needle drivers can lead to crushing and stent malfunction (Silhouette, Applied Medical, Rancho Santa Margarita, CA).

Mechanical part accidents refer to injuries that may occur due to the actual da Vinci surgical components themselves that are not handled properly, have become broken, and are faulty. These are rare and the da Vinci system has safe guards which do not allow effector deployment of faulty instruments, i.e., they do not "register" once deployed and cannot be used. However, attention must be paid to the sharp ends of the monopolar scissor arm, Potts scissor arm, and the exposed mechanical portions of the devices during handling, deployment, removal, and sterilization.

Conclusions

Robotic surgery has been performed over 250,000 times worldwide since its inception and first use in abdominal surgery nearly a decade ago [26]. Complications from robotic urologic procedures are, like any surgical procedure, expected to occur but due diligence and great attention to patient positioning, port placement, variations in pelvic characteristics, a careful, stepwise anatomic dissection, and vascular control can usually prevent the few complications that have been reported to occur. Verily, few complications are unique to robotics; indeed, most untoward events such as hemorrhage, anastomotic leaks, bladder neck contracture, vascular and ureteral injury, ophthalmic events, and anesthesia are well-recognized complications in open and laparoscopic prostatectomy [21, 27, 28–31]. Robotics may decrease these complications further still in that the robotic interface may allow the physician to accomplish laparoscopic prostatectomy with greater ergonomic efficiency, magnification, and surgical efficacy rather than relying on non-robotic, laparoscopic techniques. Most complications are iatrogenic; very few, $\sim$1%, are purely "doulogenic," that is, due to mechanical failure. The onus is, and will always remain, therefore, on the surgeon to avoid complications. Robotics is a mechanical interface and does not replace or minimize the need for surgical acuity, judgment, and alacrity in recognizing intra-operative problems. Patients should be counseled pre-operatively that while robotics and telesurgery can greatly enhance their clinical experience as a patient, it will not preclude unforeseen complications, however small that risk may be. An open discussion of the benefits of robotic-assisted laparoscopic prostatectomy should only by performed with an equal attention to the risks inherent in surgery in general and those few additional risks seen in the laparoscopic and robotic environment.

References

1. Clavien PA, Camargo CA Jr, Croxford R, Langer B, Levy GA, Greig PD. Definition and classification of negative outcomes in solid organ transplantation. Application in liver transplantation. Ann Surg. 1994;220:109.
2. Constantinides CA, Tyritzis SI, Skolarikos A, Liatsikos E, Zervas A, Deliveliotis C. Short- and long-term complications of open radical prostatectomy according to the Clavien classification system. BJU Int. 2009;103:336.
3. Colestock H. Industrial robotics: selection, design, and maintenance. 2005;211.
4. Wiklund NP. Technology Insight: surgical robots – expensive toys or the future of urologic surgery? Nat Clin Pract Urol. 2004;1:97.
5. Stefanidis D, Wang F, Korndorffer JR Jr, Dunne JB, Scott DJ. Robotic assistance improves intracorporeal suturing performance and safety in the operating room while decreasing operator workload. Surg Endosc. 2009;24(2):377–82.
6. Amodeo A, Linares Quevedo A, Joseph JV, Belgrano E, Patel HR. Robotic laparoscopic surgery: cost and training. Minerva Urol Nefrol. 2009;61:121.
7. Chin JL, Luke PP, Pautler SE. Initial experience with robotic-assisted laparoscopic radical prostatectomy in the Canadian health care system. Can Urol Assoc J. 2007; 1:97.
8. Binder J, Kramer W. Robotically-assisted laparoscopic radical prostatectomy. BJU Int. 2001;87:408.
9. Mottrie A, Schatteman P, Fonteyne E, Rotering J, Stockle M, Siemer S. Robot-assisted laparoscopic radical cystectomy. Urologe A. 2008;47:414, 416.
10. Aron M, Koenig P, Kaouk JH, Nguyen MM, Desai MM, Gill IS. Robotic and laparoscopic partial nephrectomy: a matched-pair comparison from a high-volume centre. BJU Int. 2008;102:86.
11. Schimpf MO, Wagner JR. Robot-assisted laparoscopic distal ureteral surgery. JSLS. 2009;13:44.
12. Augustin F, Schmid T, Bodner J. The robotic approach for mediastinal lesions. Int J Med Robot. 2006;2:262.
13. Nezhat C, Saberi NS, Shahmohamady B, Nezhat F. Robotic-assisted laparoscopy in gynecological surgery. JSLS. 2006;10:317.
14. Turner WF Jr, Sloan JH. Robotic-assisted coronary artery bypass on a beating heart: initial experience and implications for the future. Ann Thorac Surg. 2006;82:790.
15. Bhandari A, McIntire L, Kaul SA, Hemal AK, Peabody JO, Menon M. Perioperative complications of robotic radical prostatectomy after the learning curve. J Urol. 2005;174:915.
16. Fischer B, Engel N, Fehr JL, John H. Complications of robotic assisted radical prostatectomy. World J Urol. 2008;26:595.
17. Ham WS, Park SY, Yu HS, Choi YD, Hong SJ, Rha KH. Malfunction of da Vinci robotic system – disassembled surgeon's console hand piece: case report and review of the literature. Urology. 2009;73:209.e7.
18. Andonian S, Okeke Z, Okeke DA, Rastinehad A, Vanderbrink BA, Richstone L, et al. Device failures associated with patient injuries during robot-assisted laparo-

scopic surgeries: a comprehensive review of FDA MAUDE database. Can J Urol. 2008;15:3912.
19. Bhandari M, Menon M. Vattikuti Institute prostatectomy (VIP) and current results. Arch Esp Urol. 2007;60:397.
20. Hu JC, Nelson RA, Wilson TG, Kawachi MH, Ramin SA, Lau C, et al. Perioperative complications of laparoscopic and robotic assisted laparoscopic radical prostatectomy. J Urol. 2006;175:541.
21. Patel VR, Palmer KJ, Coughlin G, Samavedi S. Robot-assisted laparoscopic radical prostatectomy: perioperative outcomes of 1500 cases. J Endourol. 2008;22:2299.
22. Zorn KC, Gofrit ON, Orvieto MA, Mikhail AA, Galocy RM, Shalhav AL, et al. Da Vinci robot error and failure rates: single institution experience on a single three-arm robot unit of more than 700 consecutive robot-assisted laparoscopic radical prostatectomies. J Endourol. 2007;21:1341.
23. Lavery HJ, Thaly R, Albala D, Ahlering T, Shalhav A, Lee D, et al. Robotic equipment malfunction during robotic prostatectomy: a multi-institutional study. J Endourol. 2008;22:2165.
24. Borden LS Jr, Kozlowski PM, Porter CR, Corman JM. Mechanical failure rate of da Vinci robotic system. Can J Urol. 2007;14:3499.
25. Park SY, Cho KS, Lee SW, Soh BH, Rha KH. Intraoperative breakage of needle driver jaw during robotic-assisted laparoscopic radical prostatectomy. Urology. 2008;71:168.e5.
26. Box GN, Ahlering TE. Robotic radical prostatectomy: long-term outcomes. Curr Opin Urol. 2008;18:173.
27. Pierini P, Baldassarre E, Lillaz B, Vigano M, Merlo F. Robotic-assisted laparoscopic prostatectomy in Italy: perioperative data on the first 150 patients. Int J Med Robot. 2008;4:381.
28. Awad H, Santilli S, Ohr M, Roth A, Yan W, Fernandez S, et al. The effects of steep Trendelenburg positioning on intraocular pressure during robotic radical prostatectomy. Anesth Analg. 2009;109:473.
29. Brown JA, Garlitz C, Gomella LG, McGinnis DE, Diamond SM, Strup SE. Perioperative morbidity of laparoscopic radical prostatectomy compared with open radical retropubic prostatectomy. Urol Oncol. 2004;22:102.
30. Dinlenc CZ, Gerber E, Wagner JR. Ureteral reimplantation during robot assisted laparoscopic radical prostatectomy. J Urol. 2004;172:905.
31. Safi KC, Teber D, Moazen M, Anghel G, Maldonado RV, Rassweiler JJ. Laparoscopic repair of external iliac-artery transection during laparoscopic radical prostatectomy. J Endourol. 2006;20:237.

Part III
Procedure-Specific Complications

Complications of Laparoscopic and Robotic Adrenal Surgery

Jayant Uberoi and Ravi Munver

Keywords Adrenal · Surgery · Laparoscopy · Complications

Introduction

The continuing evolution of minimally invasive surgical approaches has led to the increasing popularity of laparoscopic adrenalectomy over the past two decades. Since its initial report in 1992 [1], laparoscopic adrenal surgery has spread to numerous centers worldwide and is now considered the standard of care for the management of benign tumors of the adrenal gland. The utilization of the laparoscopic approach for adrenal surgery stems from its ability to achieve similar results as traditional open surgery while minimizing patient discomfort, length of hospital stay, and time to recovery. With increasing experience and favorable outcomes, the technique has also been reported for small- and moderate-sized malignant tumors as well as metastases to the adrenal gland [2, 3].

Similar to open adrenalectomy, the laparoscopic approach remains challenging due to the relative vascularity of the adrenal gland as well as the intimate anatomic relationship to surrounding structures. The most commonly utilized laparoscopic approach to the adrenal gland, the lateral transperitoneal approach, places the liver, spleen, pancreas, bowel, and great vessels at risk for injury. Furthermore, adrenal surgery can be more complicated for larger tumors and also by the nature of the adrenal pathology, as witnessed by a distinct set of potential complications in patients with pheochromocytoma.

As in other laparoscopic urologic procedures, surgeons have recently utilized the three-dimensional magnification, improved dexterity, and tremor filtering afforded by robotic-assisted surgery in performing adrenal surgery. While the tenets of the robotic approach remain similar to pure laparoscopic adrenalectomy, some believe that robotic assistance allows for more precise dissection which may reduce perioperative complication rates.

This chapter reviews the indications for laparoscopic and robotic-assisted adrenal surgery as well as the diagnosis and treatment of potential complications.

Indications and Techniques for Laparoscopic and Robotic Adrenal Surgery

The indications for laparoscopic adrenalectomy may be classified into several categories. These include benign functional tumors, benign non-functional symptomatic tumors, indeterminant cystic lesions, solitary metastatic lesions, malignant tumors, and incidental adrenal lesions with features such as large size, rapid growth rate, and indeterminant radiographic characteristics.

R. Munver (✉)
Department of Urology, Hackensack University Medical Center, Touro University College of Medicine, 360 Essex Street, Suite 403, Hackensack, NJ 07601, USA
e-mail: rmunver@humed.com

R. Ghavamian (ed.), *Complications of Laparoscopic and Robotic Urologic Surgery*,
DOI 10.1007/978-1-60761-676-4_9, © Springer Science+Business Media, LLC 2010

Functional adrenal adenomas that secrete hormones such as aldosterone and cortisol are among the most common indications for surgical excision of the adrenal gland. These benign lesions are optimal for laparoscopic excision due to their location and small size. While the exact size of an adrenal lesion prompting surgical exploration is controversial, most authorities agree that lesions larger than 6 cm should be removed because of the higher likelihood of malignancy. Smaller lesions are more commonly benign and thus are often followed radiographically.

Laparoscopic excision of adrenal lesions larger than 10 cm, or adrenal carcinomas, remains controversial. While experienced surgeons have approached these lesions laparoscopically, many authorities consider these to be contraindications for laparoscopic adrenalectomy [4]. These cases can be exceedingly complex, with high complication rates and more frequent conversion to an open procedure. As such, large lesions or those with potential for local invasion may be better suited for an open approach.

Relative contraindications to laparoscopic adrenalectomy include extensive adhesions from prior surgery, morbid obesity, uncorrected coagulopathy, and cardiopulmonary disease that precludes hypercapnea that is associated with pneumoperitoneum. These cases must be evaluated on an individual basis, and the surgeon's experience and comfort level must be taken into consideration.

Operative Approaches

The adrenal gland can be removed laparoscopically by a variety of approaches. These include the lateral transperitoneal, anterior transperitoneal, lateral retroperitoneal, posterior retroperitoneal, and transthoracic approach. The majority of laparoscopic adrenalectomies are performed using the lateral transperitoneal technique [4]. The robotic approach utilizing the da Vinci^{TM} Surgical System (Intuitive Surgical – Sunnyvale, CA) utilizes a three- or four-arm robot which is controlled at the robotic console by the operating surgeon, while a bedside first assistant uses an accessory port for clip placement, suction, and additional maneuvers as needed.

Right Transperitoneal Laparoscopic/Robotic Adrenalectomy

Patients are placed in the lateral decubitus position with the right side up and the right arm extended and elevated. Trocar positioning for the laparoscopic and robotic approaches differs in that the robotic trocars must be placed sufficiently away from each other to prevent robotic arm collisions outside the patient. For the laparoscopic approach, the initial trocar is placed superior and lateral to the umbilicus. Additional trocars are placed based on surgeon preference. A liver retractor is essential for right-sided procedures. For the robotic approach, the initial 12-mm trocar is placed periumbilically. Two additional 8-mm robotic trocars are placed in a triangulated configuration. The fourth arm trocar is optional and is placed laterally.

The right triangular ligament is divided in order to mobilize the liver adequately for exposure of the adrenal gland. The posterior peritoneum is divided close to the liver edge and this incision is carried from the inferior vena cava to the abdominal side wall. Extensive liver mobilization is required such that the superior aspect of the adrenal gland is visible. Mobilization of the colon is rarely needed. A Kocher maneuver is performed to mobilize the duodenum medially to further expose the inferior vena cava. Exposure of the inferior vena cava is essential, as its medial border can be traced cephalad to identify the adrenal vein.

The upper pole of the kidney is identified and Gerota's fascia is entered. The adrenal gland is localized along the superomedial aspect of the kidney. Dissection begins at the medial aspect of the adrenal gland, lateral to the inferior vena cava. If inferior phrenic arterial branches are encountered, they are clipped and divided or can be controlled using a bipolar vessel-sealing device. The right adrenal vein is identified, dissected from surrounding tissues, ligated with clips, and divided. Alternatively, the adrenal vein can be ligated and divided with a vessel-sealing device. Care must be taken when manipulating the right adrenal vein due to its short length and insertion into the inferior vena cava.

Dissection continues circumferentially around the adrenal gland. As bleeding is easily encountered, this dissection is best accomplished using clips or a thermal energy device. Once the gland is completely dissected from surrounding structures, it is placed into a laparoscopic retrieval bag. The pneumoperitoneum pressure is lowered to 5 mmHg and the area is inspected for bleeding. The specimen is removed by enlarging a trocar site as necessary.

Left Transperitoneal Laparoscopic/Robotic Adrenalectomy

Patient positioning and operating room setup are the mirror image of the right-sided procedure. Trocar placement for the robotic trocars is similar to that for the laparoscopic approach. The initial trocar is placed superior to the umbilicus and to the left of the midline. Additional trocars are placed based on surgeon preference. An accessory trocar may be placed at the anterior axillary line below the costal margin for use by an assistant or the fourth robotic arm.

The descending colon is mobilized along the white line of Toldt. The superficial peritoneal attachments between the colon and lateral sidewall should be released initially. Lateral renal attachments to the sidewall should not be released as this will result in medial displacement of the kidney. This maneuver will obscure the renal hilum and interfere with further dissection. The colon is further dissected medially to expose the plane between the colonic mesentery and Gerota's fascia. Recognition of this plane is important, as inadvertent entry into the mesentery can lead to bleeding as well as mesenteric defects with potential for internal herniation. Premature entry into Gerota's fascia can create bleeding and limit visualization of the renal hilum. The dissection is carried cephalad toward the upper pole of the kidney. Extensive splenic mobilization is required to provide adequate exposure of the upper pole of the kidney and adrenal gland. This is one of the most critical parts of the operation, and with adequate mobilization, the spleen should fall medially without requiring active retraction.

Following splenic mobilization, some surgeons elect to approach the adrenal gland at its superomedial aspect and then proceed inferiorly along its lateral border. An alternative preference is to begin dissection at the inferomedial aspect. The renal hilum is identified, along with the insertion of the left adrenal vein into the renal vein. The left adrenal vein is dissected free from surrounding structures and is ligated with hemostatic clips and divided. Alternatively, the adrenal vein can be ligated and divided with a bipolar vessel-sealing device.

Once the adrenal vein is divided, the adrenal gland is gently retracted medially and meticulous dissection between the adrenal gland and the upper pole of the kidney is carried out. The use of clips or a thermal energy device is beneficial in this area due to the highly vascular nature of the adrenal gland. If bleeding is encountered in this area, the application of gentle pressure is usually effective in obtaining hemostasis. If inferior phrenic arterial branches are encountered, they are clipped and divided. In addition, renal arterial branches between the upper pole of the kidney and adrenal gland are not uncommonly encountered during this portion of the dissection, and one must exercise caution to avoid inadvertent vascular injury. The remaining attachments are divided superiorly and the specimen is placed into a laparoscopic retrieval bag. The pneumoperitoneum pressure is lowered to 5 mmHg and the area is inspected for bleeding. The specimen is removed by enlarging a trocar site as necessary.

Retroperitoneal Approach

A 1.5 cm skin incision is made in the midaxillary line 2 cm below the costal margin. The underlying muscles are split bluntly to access the retroperitoneum. Digital dissection is used to create a small space by retracting the peritoneum medially. The retroperitoneal space is developed in an atraumatic fashion with blunt dissection or by employing a commercially available dissecting balloon. On occasion, small perforating vessels that enter from the posterior side wall may be disrupted during this dissection. These vessels can easily be controlled with electrocautery or alternative thermal energy device. Additional trocars are placed under direct vision or with digital guidance. A variety of trocar configurations may be used and are based on surgeon preference.

The retroperitoneal approach is more difficult than its transperitoneal counterpart due to the paucity of anatomic landmarks and abundance of retroperitoneal adipose tissue. Reflecting the peritoneum medially is a critical maneuver that allows medial reflection of the liver and ascending colon during right adrenalectomy and of the spleen and descending colon during left adrenalectomy. Moreover, this maneuver exposes the psoas muscle and develops the working space. The renal hilum, located medial to the psoas muscle, is often identified by the pulsation of the renal artery. Surgical dissection is performed with minimal manipulation of the adrenal gland. Identification and control of the adrenal vein prior to mobilization of the adrenal gland is of critical importance. This is especially crucial for pheochromocytoma, although some authors have reported obtaining control of the vein at the end of the dissection without adverse sequelae [5, 6].

Right Retroperitoneal Laparoscopic Adrenalectomy

Removal of the right adrenal gland begins with identification of the psoas muscle and inferior vena cava, located medial to the psoas muscle. Blunt dissection of the posterolateral aspect of the vena cava leads to identification of the main adrenal vein which is meticulously isolated, ligated, and divided. Anomalous vessels that are encountered must be controlled and divided. The medial and inferior surfaces of the adrenal gland are dissected off the renal vein and the vena cava. If inferior phrenic vessels are encountered, they are clipped and divided. The inferior surface of the adrenal gland is dissected off the upper pole of the kidney. The lateral surface is the final portion that is dissected. Once the specimen is completely free from its surrounding tissues, it is placed into a laparoscopic retrieval bag. The specimen is removed by enlarging a trocar site as necessary.

Left Retroperitoneal Laparoscopic Adrenalectomy

Removal of the left adrenal gland begins with the identification of the renal hilum. Blunt dissection and caudal retraction of the left renal artery leads to identification of the left adrenal vein, which is meticulously isolated, ligated, and divided. The superior aspect of the adrenal gland is dissected from the diaphragm. Inferior phrenic vessels, if encountered, require vascular control. The lateral surface of the adrenal gland is then dissected off the kidney. Cephalad retraction allows dissection of the inferior surface. The medial surface of the adrenal gland is the final portion that is dissected. Once the specimen is completely free from its surrounding tissues, it is placed into a laparoscopic retrieval bag. The specimen is removed by enlarging a trocar site as necessary.

Complications of Laparoscopic and Robotic Adrenal Surgery

Laparoscopic adrenalectomy is safe and effective, with the benefits of less postoperative discomfort, decreased hospital stay, and shorter recovery time compared to open adrenalectomy [7, 8]. Recent series have reported that the minimally invasive approach has fewer complications than open surgery [9, 10]. Robotic technology is currently being employed in certain centers for adrenal surgery, and the types of complications are similar to those encountered in the conventional laparoscopic approach. Among the vast spectrum of complications reported, intraoperative and postoperative hemorrhagic complications are the most common.

Access-Related Complications

Obtaining safe intraabdominal access is of paramount importance during laparoscopic surgery. Access-related complications can be caused during insertion of the Veress needle or during placement of the initial trocar. Injury to the liver, spleen, pancreas, bowel, and great vessels are the most commonly encountered injuries. In the transperitoneal approach, the liver and the spleen are at higher risk for entry-related complications due to their location in the upper abdomen. Initial access in a periumbilical location can assist in avoiding injury to these organs. An open access technique may result in safer entry as compared to a closed technique. However, there is no definitive data that supports the use of an open pneumoperitoneum technique as a method to reduce access-related complications [11, 12].

Vascular Complications

Vascular injuries may be either access related or may occur during dissection of the adrenal gland and are the most common complications noted during minimally invasive adrenal surgery [13]. The potential for bleeding complications is not surprising based on the profuse vascularity of the adrenal gland and its proximity to major vessels. The adrenal is supplied by a cascade of arterial branches that can vary dramatically between individuals. In addition, venous anomalies are not uncommon. The rate of hemorrhage ranges from 0.7 to 5.4% [14], although major vascular injuries are rare. In right-sided adrenal surgery, meticulous dissection and early control of the short right adrenal vein is important in preventing major hemorrhage and inadvertent injury to the inferior vena cava. In left-sided adrenal surgery, major bleeding can result from injury to the left renal vein during dissection of the adrenal vein.

The adrenal vein can be ligated and transected using various modalities, including titanium or polymer clips, thermal energy vessel-sealing devices, or vascular stapling devices. Each of these methods is associated with distinct complications. Most surgeons prefer to place multiple clips on large vessels due to the risk of clip dislodgement, which can lead to life-threatening hemorrhage if displaced from insertion into the inferior vena cava or the renal vein. Clips that are not properly placed can puncture or avulse the adrenal vein, and as a result, vessel-sealing instruments have become a popular alternative during adrenalectomy [15, 16]. It must be noted, however, that bipolar vessel-sealing devices can potentially injure nearby tissues due to thermal spread (Fig. 1). Vascular stapling devices are also an option for ligation of the adrenal vein and have been reported to misfire or malfunction. Each of these complications may be due to faulty instrumentation or a result of surgeon error.

Blood transfusion rates can be used as a surrogate marker for significant intra- and postoperative hemorrhage. The reported rate of transfusion after minimally invasive adrenalectomy ranges from 2 to 10% [17, 18]. Delayed postoperative bleeding is rare after adrenalectomy and can be diagnosed based on serum laboratories as well as by clinical signs and symptoms. Early detection is imperative and abdominal imaging studies can be diagnostic.

Prevention of significant vascular injury requires thorough knowledge of the vascular anatomy of the adrenal gland and the more common variations. The main right adrenal vein exits the superior pole of the adrenal gland and enters directly into the posterolateral aspect of the inferior vena cava. In contrast, the left adrenal gland is drained by a narrow and longer main adrenal vein that inserts into the superior aspect of the left renal vein. Its insertion is usually more medial than the insertion of the left gonadal vein, which inserts at the inferior aspect of the left renal vein. Adrenal vein anatomy can demonstrate significant variability in as much as 8–22% of the population [19, 20]. The most common variations of the right adrenal vein include a common insertion of the adrenal vein with an accessory hepatic vein into the inferior vena cava, or insertion of the adrenal vein into the right renal vein. Alternatively, multiple adrenal veins may be encountered on either side. Occasionally preoperative imaging studies can aid in identifying variations in adrenal vascular anatomy; however, meticulous intraoperative dissection is imperative for identifying anomalies and preventing complications.

Management options for intraoperative bleeding range from applying temporary pressure to the bleeding area to emergent open conversion. As in open surgery, exposure of the area of bleeding is paramount to achieving hemostatic control. The initial step when encountering hemorrhage is to apply gentle constant pressure to the affected area. This can be accomplished using a gauze sponge or an oxidized cellulose product that is introduced through a trocar. An additional maneuver that may be helpful in the setting of venous bleeding is to increase the pneumoperitoneum pressure to 20–25 mmHg. Once pooled blood has been evacuated from the field, efforts can be focused on identification of the specific etiology of the bleed. Minor venous bleeding may cease with pressure alone, while larger vessels may require thermal energy or ligation with clips. In placing clips, the bleeding vessel must be well dissected and care must be taken to not include surrounding tissues within the clip. Other devices that can assist with bleeding include ultrasonic devices and bipolar vessel-sealing devices [e.g., LigaSure™ (Valleylab, Boulder, CO) or EnSeal™ (Ethicon, Cincinnati, OH)].

More significant bleeding that cannot be controlled with the above methods can result from injuries to the vena cava or the renal hilum. Laparoscopic suturing of

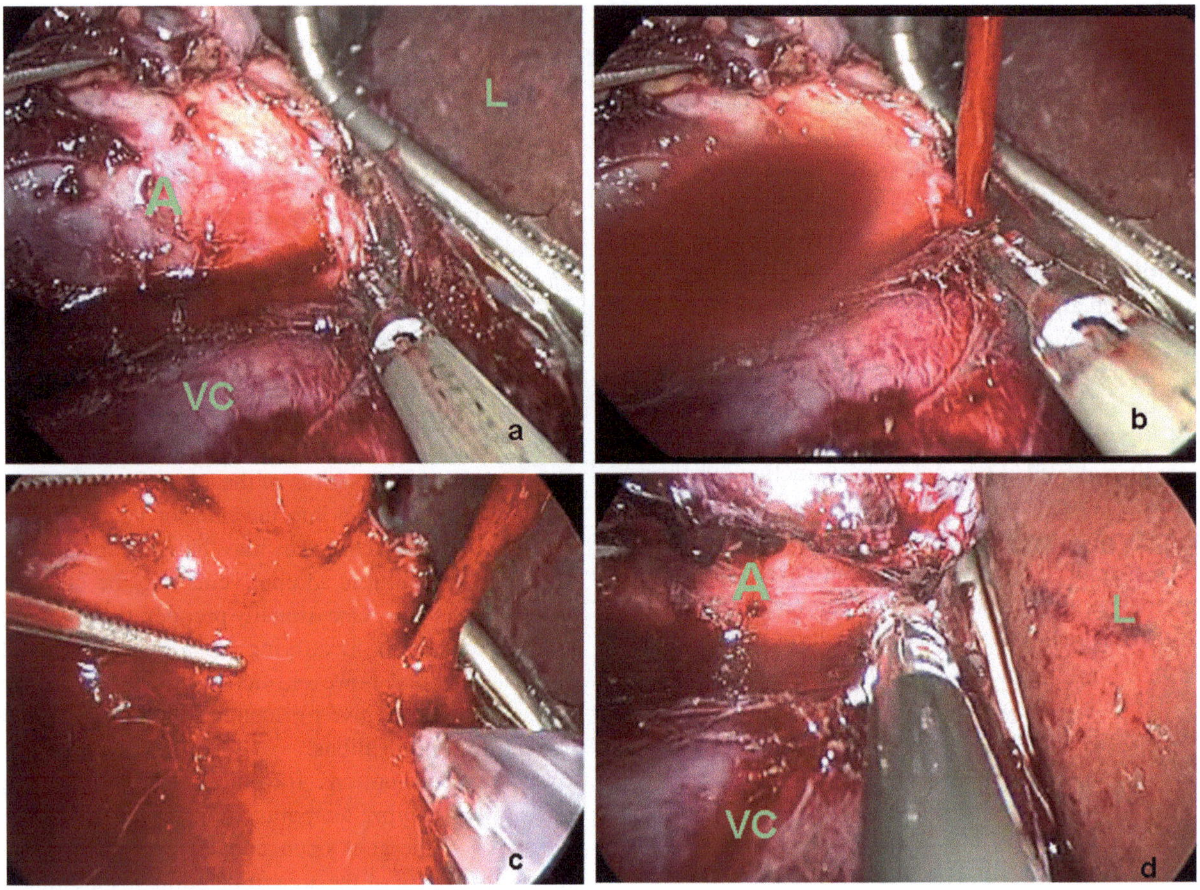

Fig. 1 Injury to the inferior vena cava at junction of right adrenal vein during right laparoscopic transperitoneal adrenalectomy. (**a**) Adrenal vein dissection using the Harmonic scalpel (Ethicon, Cincinnati, OH). (**b**) and (**c**) Hemorrhage from vena cava attempted to be managed by clip placement. (**d**) Bleeding controlled with a bipolar vessel-sealing instrument. VC, vena cava; L, liver (images courtesy of Reza Ghavamian MD)

an injured vessel can be successful when performed by experienced surgeons. Repair usually involves nonabsorbable sutures (4-0 or 5-0 monofilament) with or without the use of absorbable clips (Lapra-Ty; Ethicon, Cincinnati, OH) placed at the end of the suture (Fig. 2). The surgeon should not hesitate to place additional trocars to facilitate suturing. If these methods are unsuccessful, conversion to an open procedure must be considered for definitive management.

Bowel Injuries

Bowel injuries are more common than other organ injuries during laparoscopic surgery and are often not recognized intraoperatively, thereby increasing morbidity and mortality from these events. Prior reports have noted that only one in three bowel injuries is recognized intraoperatively [21]. Of the delayed injuries, one in four patients will expire as a result of this complication [22, 23]. Aside from access-related injury, bowel injury is most likely to occur during initial dissection around the adrenal gland. Patients with prior intraabdominal surgery are at increased risk for bowel injury, and a retroperitoneal approach may be favored in this instance. However, a retroperitoneal approach does not definitively preclude bowel injury [24].

The most common bowel injuries encountered during adrenalectomy include duodenal and colon injury. During mobilization of the duodenum, judicious use of

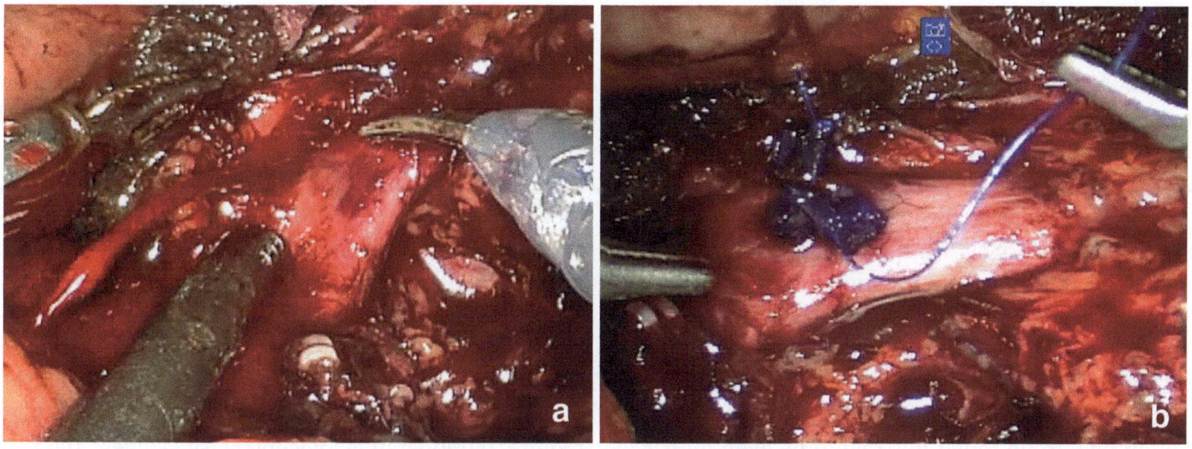

Fig. 2 Injury to the left renal vein during robotic-assisted laparoscopic left adrenalectomy. (**a**) Hemorrhage seen from the superior portion of the vein near the insertion of the left adrenal vein. (**b**) Left renal vein after suture repair using Lapra-Ty clips

cautery must be employed. Duodenal injury can also occur from excessive traction that can result in serosal tears and hematomas, or when the duodenum is mistaken for the inferior vena cava. The bowel can also be injured during manipulation of instruments outside of the field of view.

The left colon is at risk for injury during splenic flexure mobilization during the initial steps of left laparoscopic adrenalectomy. Judicious use of cautery and avoidance of excessive traction are important in preventing injury.

If recognized intraoperatively, bowel injuries can often be managed laparoscopically. These include instances in which the bowel wall has been damaged by an instrument without the use of cautery. In these cases the serosal edges can be approximated with nonabsorbable suture. If concern over the integrity of the repair exists, open repair with possible segmental bowel resection may be required. Cautery injuries to the bowel can cause significant morbidity as the extent of thermal injury is usually not immediately evident. Unrecognized bowel injuries must be suspected in the postoperative period in patients that have fever, abdominal pain, leukocytosis, or leukopenia.

Liver, Pancreas, and Splenic Injury

Adjacent organ injuries have been noted to occur during laparoscopic adrenal surgery and include the liver, pancreas, and spleen. Perihepatic ligaments should be released during right laparoscopic adrenalectomy, as cephalad retraction of the liver is necessary to expose the adrenal gland. In retracting the liver, care must be taken to use blunt instruments with examination of the retraction site to avoid capsular or parenchymal tears. The resection of larger tumors carries a higher risk of liver injury, as greater retraction and mobilization of the liver may be necessary [25]. Most liver injuries will be evident during the course of the operation, although delayed diagnosis of liver injury has also been reported [26]. Some authors have hypothesized that obese patients with larger livers are more at risk for retraction injury [26]. Regardless, liver injury may be avoided by periodic visual inspection of the liver during the procedure, noting excessive traction or signs of venous congestion.

Small capsular tears can be managed with direct pressure or oxidized cellulose. The argon beam coagulator or monopolar electrocautery may be used if conservative measures fail. Other types of liver injuries include puncture from a surgical instrument or thermal injuries from nearby use of cautery or other heat generating instruments. These injuries may be managed with hemostatic agents such as FloSeal^{TM} (Baxter International, Deerfield, IL). If bleeding persists despite these measures, a general surgical consultation is advised.

The mechanism of injury to the spleen is similar to that of liver injuries, in that many are either access related or due to excessive retraction. Care must be taken in releasing the splenocolic attachments as well as the splenorenal ligaments to avoid injury to the spleen. A similar management approach is used for injuries to the spleen during left-sided procedures, with liberal use of pressure, oxidized cellulose products, and the argon beam coagulator. Puncture injuries to the spleen may be managed with application of hemostatic agents such as FloSeal™. If bleeding is excessive and uncontrolled, surgical consultation is advised.

Injury to the tail of the pancreas has been reported during left-sided adrenalectomy. The quoted rate in the literature for pancreatic injuries during left radical nephrectomy or adrenalectomy is 0.2% [27, 28], though one group found this rate to be even higher in a small series of adrenalectomies [29]. The tail of the pancreas can be confused with the adrenal gland due to their similar color and consistency, as well as proximity. Diagnosis of a pancreatic injury is most commonly made in the postoperative period by a patient's symptoms. Measurement of serum amylase and concentration in drain fluid can be diagnostic. Radiographic characteristics in a patient with a clinical picture of pancreatitis are also diagnostic. If recognized intraoperatively, surgical consultation is advised. Deployment of a vascular stapler across the distal end of the pancreas is a treatment of choice. Patients diagnosed with pancreatic injury in the postoperative period should be placed on bowel rest with nasogastric aspiration and parenteral nutrition as needed. Abdominal imaging to assess for presence of an intraabdominal collection or abscess is of importance. Patients with pancreatic injuries can become quite ill, and constant monitoring of fluid status and clinical hemodynamic state is vital.

Diaphragmatic/Pleural Injuries

Injury to the diaphragm is uncommon in abdominal laparoscopy for renal or adrenal pathology [30]. Injuries are typically small and unrecognized intraoperatively. Certain indicators that can be used include a rise in airway pressure and end-tidal CO_2. The floppy diaphragm sign may be noted in which billowing of the diaphragm is observed during ventilation. The surgeon must assess the hemodynamic stability of the patient prior to continuing with the operation, as tension pneumothorax can result if the chest cavity is breached. Small holes in the diaphragm can be repaired laparoscopically by suturing the defect (Fig. 3) and suctioning the CO_2 from the chest in conjunction with hyperinflation [30]. With this type of repair, a chest tube may not be required. A postoperative chest x-ray should be obtained to determine if pneumothorax exists. Small pneumothoraces (<30%) can typically be observed. There is also evidence that pneumothorax with carbon dioxide will reabsorb faster due to the increased solubility of carbon dioxide gas [31]. Larger defects that cannot be adequately repaired may require intraoperative placement of a chest tube. If the patient remains hemodynamically stable, it may be possible to continue with the operation. A chest tube should also be placed if there is evidence of lung injury due to the risk of pulmonary compromise from a hemothorax.

Postoperative Hormonal Complications

Even though most adrenalectomies are performed for hormonally active lesions, the rate of postoperative complications due to hormonal problems is only approximately 1% [4]. This is likely a result of symptomatic patients achieving preoperative control of abnormal metabolic parameters such as hypokalemia, metabolic alkalosis, or hyperglycemia. Care must be taken to provide adequate steroid replacement in patients that undergo bilateral adrenalectomy. Inadequate replacement can result in hypotension, abdominal pain, nausea, vomiting, fever, or confusion. Plasma cortisol levels should be closely monitored in these patients.

Patients that have undergone pheochromocytoma resection also must be closely monitored postoperatively. Hypotension can result from continued alpha-adrenergic blockade and should be treated with fluid resuscitation and alpha agonists as needed. Preoperative evaluation of serum and urine hormone levels is of paramount importance in identification of these patients in order to prevent these complications.

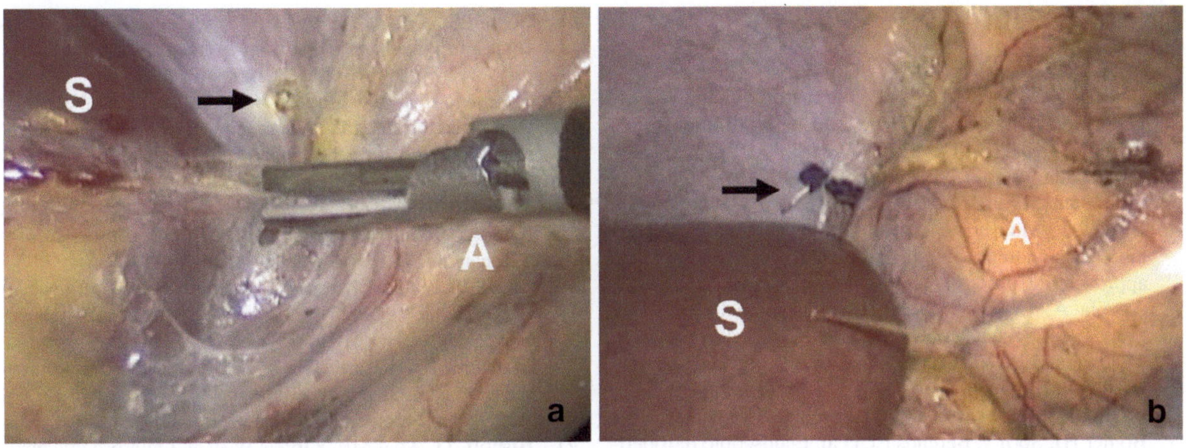

Fig. 3 Diaphragmatic injury during left laparoscopic transperitoneal adrenalectomy. (**a**) Injury was incurred during release of splenic attachments. (**b**) Completed suture repair of diaphragm. S, spleen; A, adrenal gland

Complications of Retroperitoneal Laparoscopic Adrenalectomy

Retroperitoneal laparoscopic adrenalectomy is associated with specific complications compared to transperitoneal laparoscopic adrenalectomy. While the retroperitoneal approach offers diminished risk to intraperitoneal organs, this approach is limited by a small working space, especially in obese individuals. In a large series of retroperitoneal laparoscopic adrenalectomies, Walz and colleagues reported their most common complications resulting in conversion to an open procedure [18]. These authors also reported an 8.5% rate of hypothesia or relaxation of the abdominal wall after retroperitoneal laparoscopic adrenalectomy. For these reasons, relative contraindications of the retroperitoneal approach include tumors larger than 6 cm and morbid obesity.

Complications of Robotic-Assisted Adrenalectomy

While robotic-assisted adrenalectomy shares the same potential complications as conventional laparoscopic adrenalectomy, there are a few potential hazards unique to the robotic approach. Collisions of the robotic arms outside of the body can limit the maneuverability of instruments within the surgical field, and therefore robotic trocars should be sufficiently distanced to avoid this problem. Additionally, there is currently no vessel-sealing instrument available for the da Vinci™ robotic platform, leaving the operating surgeon to utilize only mono- and bipolar energy during dissection of vascular adrenal attachments. If a vessel-sealing instrument is desired, this instrument can be introduced by the bedside assistant during the robotic approach. Lastly, robotic-assisted adrenalectomy necessitates an assistant that is comfortable with laparoscopic surgery.

Conclusions

Compared with open adrenalectomy, laparoscopic adrenalectomy has been shown to have been associated with fewer complications and improved perioperative parameters for patient care, without sacrificing the goals of the operation. Hemorrhagic complications remain the most common and comprise nearly half of the complications reported. Additionally, intraoperative hemorrhage can lead to other complications, such as vascular or organ injury, thereby increasing morbidity. With experience, a detailed understanding of adrenal anatomy, and meticulous laparoscopic dissection, surgeons may further reduce complications associated with laparoscopic- and robotic-assisted adrenalectomy.

References

1. Gagner, M, Lacroix A, Bolte E. Laparoscopic adrenalectomy in Cushing's syndrome and pheochromocytoma. N Engl J Med. 1992 Oct 1;327(14):1033.
2. Moinzadeh A, Gill IS. Laparoscopic radical adrenalectomy for malignancy in 31 patients. J Urol. 2005; 173(2):519–25.
3. Uberoi J, Munver R. Surgical management of metastases to the adrenal gland: open, laparoscopic and ablative approaches. Curr Urol Rep. 2009;10(1):67–72.
4. Assalia A, Gagner M. Laparoscopic adrenalectomy. In: Wetter PA, Kavic MS, Levinson CJ, Kelley WE Jr, McDougall EM, Nezhat C, editors. Prevention and management of laparoendoscopic surgical complications. 2nd ed. Miami, FL: Society of Laparoendoscopic Surgeons; 2005.
5. Bonjer HJ, Sorn V, Berends FJ, et al. Endoscopic retroperitoneal adrenalectomy: lessons learned from 111 consecutive cases. Ann Surg. 2000;232(6):796–803.
6. Vassiliou MC, Laycock WS. Laparoscopic adrenalectomy for pheochromocytoma: take the vein last? Surg Endosc. 2009;23:965–8.
7. Jacobs JK, Goldstein RE, Geer RJ. Laparoscopic adrenalectomy: a new standard of care. Ann Surg. 1997;225(5): 495–502.
8. Imai T, Kikumore R, Ohiwa M. A case-controlled study of laparoscopic compared with open lateral adrenalectomy. Am J Surg. 1999;178:50–4.
9. Brunt LM, Doherty GM, Norton JA, Soper NJ, Quasebarth MA, et al. Laparoscopic adrenalectomy compared to open adrenalectomy for benign adrenal neoplasms. J Am Coll Surg. 1996;183:1.
10. Thompson GB, Grant CS, Van Heerden JA, et al. Laparoscopic versus open posterior adrenalectomy: a case-control study of 100 patients. Surgery. 1997;122:1132.
11. Melin EL, Hiller JE, Jamieson GG, Brown AR, Kolbe A. Systematic review of the safety and effectiveness of methods used to establish pneumoperitoneum in laparoscopic surgery. Br J Surg. 2003;90:668–79.
12. Perunovic RM, Seepanovic RP, Stevanovic PD, Ceranic MS. Complications during the establishment of laparoscopic pneumoperitoneum. J Laparoendosc Adv Surg Tech. 2009 Feb;19(1):1–6.
13. Henry JF, Defechereux T, Raffaelli M, et al. Complications of laparoscopic adrenalectomy: results of 169 consecutive procedures. World J Surg. 2000;24:1342–6.
14. Permpongkosol S, Link RE, Su LM, Romero FR, Bagga HS, Pavlovich CP, Jarrett TW, Kavoussi LR. Complications of 2,775 urological laparoscopic procedures: 1993 to 2005. J Urol. 2007;177(2):580–5.
15. Guerrieri M, Crosta F, De Sanctis A, et al. Use of the electrothermal bipolar vessel system in laparoscopic adrenalectomy: a prospective study. Surg Endosc. 2008;22:141–5.
16. Soon PS, Yeh MY, Sywak MS, Sidhu SB. Use of the LigaSure vessel sealing system in laparoscopic adrenalectomy. ANZ J Surg. 2006;76(9):850–2.
17. Rosevear HM, Montgomery JS, Roberts WW, Wolf JS Jr. Characterization and management of postoperative hemorrhage following upper retroperitoneal laparoscopic surgery. J Urol. 2006;176(4 Pt 1):1458–62.
18. Walz MK, Alesina PF, Wenger FA, et al. Posterior retroperitoneoscopic adrenalectomy – results of 560 procedures in 520 patients. Surgery. 2006;140(6):943–8.
19. MacGillivray DC, Khwaja K, Shickman SJ. Confluence of the right adrenal vein with the accessory right hepatic veins. Surg Endosc. 1996;10:1095–6.
20. Matsuura T, Takase K, Ota H, et al. Radiologic anatomy of the right adrenal vein: preliminary experience with MDCT. AJR Am J Roentgenol. 2008;191(2):402–8.
21. Bishoff, JT, Allaf ME, Kirkels W, et al. Laparoscopic bowel injury: incidence and unique clinical presentation. J Urol. 1999;161(3):887–90.
22. Chandler JG, Corson SL, Way LW. Three spectra of laparoscopic entry access injuries. J Am Coll Surg. 2001;192(4):478–90.
23. O'Boyle CJ, Kapadia CR, Sedman PC et al. Laparoscopic transperitoneal adrenalectomy. Surg Endosc. 2003;17(12):1905–9.
24. Meraney AM, Samee AA, Gill IS. Vascular and bowel complications during retroperitoneal laparoscopic surgery. J Urol. 2002;168(5):1941–4.
25. Kim AW, Quiros RM, Maxhimer JB, El-Ganzouri AR, Prinz RA. Outcome of laparoscopic adrenalectomy for pheochromocytomas vs aldosteronomas. Arch Surg. 2004;139:526–31.
26. Yoon GH, Dunn MD. Subcapsular hepatic hematoma: retraction injury during laparoscopic adrenalectomy. J Endourol. 2006;20:127–9.
27. Fahlenkamp D, Rasseiler J, Fornara P, et al. Complications of laparoscopic procedures in urology: experience with 2,407 procedures at 4 German centers. J Urol. 1999;162:765–70.
28. Gill IS, Clayman RV, Albala DM, et al. Retroperitoneal and pelvic extraperitoneal laparoscopy: an international perspective. Urology. 1998;52:566–71.
29. Varkarakis IM, Allaf ME, Bhayani SB, et al. Pancreatic injuries during laparoscopic urologic surgery. Urology. 2004;64:1089–93.
30. Aron M, Colombo JR Jr, Turna B, Stein RJ, Huber GP, Gill IS. Diaphragmatic repair and/or reconstruction during abdominal urological laparoscopy. J Urol. 2007;178(6):2444–50.
31. Venkatesh R, Kibel AS, Lee D, et al. Rapid resolution of carbon dioxide pneumothorax (capnothorax) resulting from diaphragmatic injury during laparoscopic nephrectomy. J Urol. 2002;167:1387.

Complications of Laparoscopic Radical Nephrectomy and Nephroureterectomy

David A. Green and Michael Grasso III

Keywords Laparoscopy · Nephrectomy · Nephroureterectomy · Kidney Cancer

Introduction

Laparoscopic nephrectomy was first described almost 20 years ago by Clayman et al. [1]. Since then, laparoscopic surgical acumen has evolved, and the complexity of operations undertaken has grown in parallel. A body of literature has developed which sheds light on both the many advantages and the potential pitfalls of urologic laparoscopy for malignant disease of the kidney. It is, of course, this angle that we set out to explore in this chapter.

We will begin by describing the steps of laparoscopic radical nephrectomy and nephroureterectomy and then move on to review many of the larger series that have included their specific relevant experiences (Table 1). From there we will describe in detail the identification and treatment of intra-operative and post-operative complications (Table 2) and those associated with oncologic outcome. We have divided intra-operative complications into four categories: those associated with prolonged operative time, port site injuries, injury to vascular structures, and injury to adjacent bowel and viscera. Post-operative complications are described as surgical or medical, although the appropriate category is not always clear as in the case of ileus, for example.

What will be accomplished in this discussion of radical nephrectomy and nephroureterectomy is a presentation of the breadth of adverse events and complications that have occurred over the past two decades. These multi-step procedures constitute an orchestra of events where at any point from the moment the patient is positioned on the table, exquisite care must be taken to optimize outcome.

Surgical Approach

Laparoscopic radical nephrectomy (LRN) can be performed through a transperitoneal or a retroperitoneal approach and these two techniques will be described. Generally, the renal dissection performed with laparoscopic nephroureterectomy (LNU) is the same as radical nephrectomy with the modification that the ureteral dissection is carried further into the pelvis past the iliac bifurcation, including the distal ureter.

Transperitoneal

For transperitoneal laparoscopic radical nephrectomy, the patient is positioned in a modified flank or semi-lateral position and primary port placement is accomplished 3 cm below the umbilicus in the midclavicular line. Pneumoperitoneum at a pressure of 14 mmHg is obtained through this port and a 10-mm laparoscope is inserted. Under direct laparoscopic vision, two 12-mm

M. Grasso III (✉)
Department of Urology, Saint Vincent's Medical Center, New York Medical College, New York, NY, USA
e-mail: mgrasso3@earthlink.net

R. Ghavamian (ed.), *Complications of Laparoscopic and Robotic Urologic Surgery*,
DOI 10.1007/978-1-60761-676-4_10,

Table 1 Laparoscopic radical nephrectomy and nephroureterectomy series

Study	No. of cases (Total)	No. of cases (LRN or LNU)	No. of complications (LRN or LNU) (%)	No. of conversions (%)	No. of conversions (LRN/LNU)	
					Elective	Emergent
Gill et al. [13]	185	32	11 (34)	5 (16)	4	1
Rassweiler et al. [14]	482	38	NA	NA		
Fahlenkamp et al. [16]	2400	NA				
Ono et al. [2]	60	60	NA	1 (1.7)		1
Gill, Schweizer, et al. [3]	47	47	10 (13)*	2 (4.3)		2
Gill, Sung, et al. [8]**	42	42	5(12)	2 (4.7)	1	1
Shalhav et al. [10]	25	25	2 (8)	1		1
Soulie et al. [17]	350	NA	1	1		1
Vallancien et al. [26]	1311	116	NA	2 (1.7)		2
Siqueira et al. [27]	213	74	7 (9.5); all major	2 (2.7)		2
Simon et al. [7]	285	134	NA	NA	4	
Parsons et al. [18]	896	178	NA	NA		1
Berger et al. [20]**	100	100	NA	3 (3)	1	2

NA Not available

*Study reported eight minor complications and two major complications in total. Also reported overall complication rate was 13%. Likely that some patients experienced more than one complication

**Study patients in citation [8] are subset of [20].

trocars are then placed, one just below the costal margin in the midclavicular line and another 1 cm below the umbilicus in the anterior axillary line. The camera port flanked by these two initial working ports gives triangulating access to the area of dissection. A 5-mm trocar is then placed at the costal margin in the posterior axillary line to complete port placement and is employed for retraction of either the liver or the spleen [2].

Depending upon laterality, dissection of the kidney begins with an incision in the peritoneum at the level of the liver or the spleen which is subsequently carried down along the line of Toldt to 6–8 cm below the lower pole of the kidney. Dissection of Gerota's fascia is then performed along the posterior and anterior aspects after medial retraction of the ascending or the descending colon. Posteriorly, Gerota's fascia is dissected from the underlying psoas muscle. The ureter can be identified from this dissection and for radical nephrectomy it is clipped and ligated several centimeters below the lower pole of the kidney. On the right side, medial reflection of the duodenum exposes the inferior vena cava (IVC) anteriorly and laterally at an infrarenal location. By dissecting along the IVC moving superiorly, the renal vein as well as the renal artery is safely identified. At this point the renal artery can be clipped and divided, followed by stapling of the renal vein with a vascular Endo-GIA stapler. With the renal hilum controlled, the anterior surface of Gerota's fascia is dissected from the peritoneum by retracting the peritoneum medially, providing access to the adrenal gland and the suprarenal IVC. The adrenal vein is carefully identified, clipped, and divided, completing the cephalad dissection.

Left nephrectomy proceeds in a similar fashion with medial retraction of the descending colon, giving access to the anterior surface of Gerota's fascia and the anterior surface of the aorta. As in the right-sided procedure, early identification and control of the renal hilum is paramount. Dissecting along the posterior surface of Gerota's fascia and freeing it from the underlying psoas muscle gives access to the renal vessels. The adrenal gland is freed from the tail of the pancreas as care is taken to avoid the superior mesenteric artery (SMA), with Gerota's fascia dissected anteriorly from the peritoneal edge.

Table 2 Intra-operative and post-operative complications

Study	Incidence of intra-operative complications				Incidence of post-operative complications	
	Associated with prolonged operative time	Abdominal wall	Vascular	Bowel/viscera	Surgical	Medical
Gill et al. [13]	Post-op MI (1), brachial plexus palsy (1), lateral thigh compartment syndrome (1), acute CHF (NA)	Trocar site hernia (2)	Superior mesenteric artery (SMA) (1)	Splenic laceration (1)		
Rassweiler et al. [14]						
Fahlenkamp et al. [16]					Retroperitoneal bleed (1)	
Ono et al. [2]			Left renal artery (1), adrenal hemorrhage (1), periureteral vessels (1)	Duodenal injury (1), splenic injury (1)	Ileus (2)	
Gill, Schweizer, et al. [3]			Renal artery (1)		Hematoma (2), cutaneous hyperesthesia (2), port site infection (2), ileus (2)	Atelectasis (2), skin rash (2)
Gill, Sung, et al. [8]**			Renal vein hemorrhage (1)			
Shalhav et al. [10]			Adrenal hemorrhage (1)		Urine leak (1)	
Soulie et al. [17]			Vena cava hemorrhage (1)			
Vallancien et al. [26]		Skin burn from saline used to clean laparoscope (1)			Wound infection (2), bowel obstruction (1)	Pneumonia (2), urinary retention (2)
Siqueira et al. [27]		Inferior epigastric injury from secondary port placement (1)	Right lower pole artery (2), superior mesenteric artery (1)	Liver laceration from primary port (1)	Focal ischemic bowel (1), bowel injury and pelvic abscess (1)	
Simon et al. [7]			Renal artery (1)	Splenic injury (4)		
Parsons et al. [18]			Renal vein (1)		Small bowel obstruction (2), fascial dehis. (1), urine leak (1)	
Berger et al. [20]**	Deep vein thrombosis (1)		Renal vein avulsion (1)		Retroperitoneal bleed (1), wound infection (1)	Deep vein thrombosis (1), pleural effusion (1)

**Study patients in citation [8] are subset of [20].

Retroperitoneal

The retroperitoneal approach was described by Gaur in 1992 and popularized by Gill et al. [3, 4]. The patient is positioned in full flank and secured to the operating table. Pressure points are all padded and the table is flexed and the kidney rest raised. The initial incision is made just below the tip of the 12th rib. S-retractors bluntly dissect down to the thoracolumbar fascia which is traversed to gain retroperitoneal access. At this point a dilator balloon is inserted into the retroperitoneal space and inflated with up to 800 cc of air, a technique originally described by Gaur employing a surgical glove inflated in the retroperitoneum [3, 4]. Gill et al. describe laparoscopic examination from within the transparent dissecting balloon to confirm adequate retroperitoneal exposure [3]. Subsequently, the balloon is decompressed and removed and the camera port is introduced employing a fascial retention balloon. This balloon is inflated with up to 30 cc of air and a foam cuff is cinched down on the abdominal wall to create an airtight seal. The shallow nature of the balloon's extent into the operative space facilitates visualization in this smaller operative area. The procedure continues with the placement of two working ports. A port is placed just below the 12th rib extraperitoneally, just lateral to the border of the erector spinae muscle. A 12-mm port is then placed anteriorly three finger breadths cephalad to the iliac crest between the mid- and anterior axillary lines [3]. Others have described alternate placement of these two working ports with the 5-mm port placed anteriorly and the 12-mm port placed at the posterior axillary line [5].

The retroperitoneal dissection confers the advantage of prompt access to the renal hilum. Meticulous dissection through the areolar tissue defines the renal artery pulsations. Once identified, the artery is mobilized, clipped, and divided. The renal vein is then stapled with an Endo-GIA employing vascular staples. The adrenal dissection is performed by working cephalad directly along the great vessel with the anterior aspect of the specimen being freed from the overlying peritoneum. The lower pole of the kidney is freed with ligation and division of the ureter. The specimen is then placed in an impermeable laparoscopic sac that is introduced through a large port. To extract the bagged specimen, the port site incision is either enlarged or the specimen is removed through a small Gibson incision. After confirming hemostasis laparoscopically at reduced pneumoretroperitoneum, ports are removed with fascial reapproximation for port sites greater than 10 mm [3].

Management of the Distal Ureter for Nephroureterectomy

There are a variety of techniques which have been described to manage the bladder cuff excision with laparoscopic nephroureterectomy. No single method has been shown to be superior. Here, as is the case in all of laparoscopic oncology, the goal is to replicate the oncologic principles of the open procedure. Many investigators address the bladder cuff differently depending upon the location of the urothelial tumor. In cases of tumors of the proximal ureter or renal pelvis, the renal dissection begins similarly to radical nephrectomy with early clip ligation without division of the ureter. This laparoscopic dissection follows the transurethral endoscopic preparation of the distal ureter during which the bladder wall is incised to perivesical fat [6]. At our center, topical mitomycin C is employed intravesically during the laparoscopic dissection to help prevent potential implantation of tumor cells from the upper urinary tract. After renal mobilization and ureteral ligation the dissection then continues down into the pelvis to the bladder wall. The ureter is mobilized down to the bladder wall where it has already been freed transurethrally, and the entire specimen is bagged and removed intact in a laparoscopic bag [6]. Distal ureteral tumors by nature of their location may be more likely to seed the bladder or the retroperitoneum during endoscopic dissection. To this end, many authors perform open resection of the distal ureter via a Gibson incision, mobilizing laparoscopically only to the middle third [6, 7].

Gill et al. described a novel technique of distal ureteral management [8]. Under direct cystoscopic visualization, two 2-mm needlescopic ports are inserted suprapubically into the bladder. Through the ipsilateral port to the involved ureteral orifice an endoloop tie is placed into the bladder. Cystoscopically, an open-ended ureteral catheter is placed traversing the endoloop tie and intubating the ureter. Through the other suprapubic port the ureteral orifice of interest is grasped and placed on traction. Using a needlepoint probe on the transurethral resectoscope, the bladder cuff is then developed. Suprapubic traction of the ureteral orifice allows the cystoscopic resection to free periureteral attachments proximal to the orifice. Once the bladder cuff is developed, the endoloop is then cinched to prevent urine and tumor spillage [8]. The patient is then repositioned for a retroperitoneal radical nephrectomy as previously described [3]. Gil et al. also describe two modifications to their technique of kidney resection for nephroureterectomy. First, the balloon dissector used to create the original retroperitoneal working space is advanced caudally to visualize the ureter and mobilize it off of the psoas muscle to create a greater pelvic working space. Additionally, one of the initial steps in the renal dissection is to clip ligate the more proximal ureter to help prevent distension of the distal ureter minimizing spillage [8].

Another laparoscopic technique, known as "the pluck technique," has also been described for nephroureterectomy with only flexible cystoscopy being performed first. A bugbee electrode is used via the flexible endoscope to cauterize the ureteral orifice and the intramural ureter. During the laparoscopic dissection, rostral traction is placed on the ureter everting it, revealing the cauterized intramural ureter. This defines the extent of the laparoscopic dissection and a vascular Endo-GIA stapler is used to ligate, divide, and seal the specimen at the bladder level [9]. This technique has the highest rate of local recurrence of all of the techniques described as the entire distal ureteral urothelium may not be removed. There is also the theoretical risk of intravesical staples becoming a nidus for future stone formation.

Many of the techniques of bladder cuff management do not include repair of the cystotomy, depending rather upon extended post-operative catheter drainage to heal the defect. Some surgeons obtain a cystogram prior to catheter removal. In Shalhav et al.'s series of LNU in which the bladder cuff was stapled laparoscopically, a single patient developed a clinically significant staple line leak related to post-operative hematuria. This particular patient had a history of external beam radiation for prostate cancer and had significant radiation cystitis causing clot retention interfering with effective catheter drainage [10].

In their report comparing 42 LNUs to 35 open nephroureterectomies (ONUs), Gil et al. reported a single incidence of significant extravesical extravasation occurring. The complication, which occurred in the first patient in the series, was managed with fluid drainage via the specimen extraction site [8].

Review of Complications

Introduction

Any discussion of complications of urologic laparoscopy would be incomplete without consideration given to how we tend to report our complications. In short, there is great variation within the urologic literature. Donat examined this in a 2007 report that reviewed 109 urologic oncology studies, including 36 minimally invasive series. The studies were subjected to 10 established criteria for surgical complication reporting set forth as part of the National Surgical Quality Improvement Program (NSQIP) [11, 12]. Twenty-nine of the thirty-six studies that did report complication severity used "major" and "minor" as their grading system. Perhaps most telling about methods of reporting, within these 29 studies there were 26 different definitions of "major" noted [11]. Such variation makes it difficult to compare complication rates fairly from one study to another.

Generally speaking, complication rates as well as the incidence of severe complications seem to decrease as laparoscopic surgeons progress through their learning curve. As described in detail in Table 3, multiple large series have demonstrated, for example, decreasing rates of conversion to open surgery with increasing surgical experience [7, 13–17]. That being said, with increasing surgical skill more complicated procedures are being attempted such as laparoscopic management of very large tumors and those involving renal vein thrombus. As an example, in a series by Parsons et al., the complication rate remained constant during the 5-year study period. According to the authors, this reflected the experience of new surgeons progressing through the laparoscopic learning curve, as well as the continuous evolution of laparoscopic application and techniques [18].

To address the increasing complexity of laparoscopic urology and the difficulties of comparing one series to another, Guillonneau et al. proposed a scoring

Table 3 Laparoscopic learning curve

Study	
Gill et al. [13]	34 complications in series, 71% in first 20 cases
Rassweiler et al. [15]	200 cases total; conversion and reintervention rate for first 50 and last 50: 28 and 4%, respectively
Rassweiler et al. [14]	Majority of technical complications during first 20 cases of each surgeon
Fahlenkamp et al. [16]	2,400 patients; complication rate in first 100 patients and remainder of series: 13.3 and 3.6%, respectively
Soulie et al. [17]	Complication rate in first 100, then subsequent 50 patients: 9 and 4%, respectively. In 350 patient series, 3 open conversions occurred in first 120 patients
Simon et al. [7]	227 LNs in 2 years: first- and second-year complication rate, 8.3 and 2.5%, respectively

system. This European scoring system (ESS) classifies laparoscopic procedures as extremely difficult, very difficult, difficult, moderate, or easy. The very difficult and difficult groups include prostatectomy, radical nephrectomy, and nephroureterectomy, amongst others. Nephrectomy for benign disease was categorized as moderately difficult [19].

Throughout our discussion we will refer to the studies and specific complications in Tables 1 and 2, respectively. Many of these series were not dedicated exclusively to LRN and LNU, but also included nephrectomy for benign disease as in Gill et al. or included multiple other urologic laparoscopic procedures, as in Parsons et al. [13, 18]. Not all of these series stratified their complications by the particular operation, but as much as possible this presentation focuses on those encountered during nephrectomy and nephroureterectomy for malignant disease. The complication rates and conversion rates that can be found in Table 1 refer to the total number of LRNs and LNUs as the denominator. Similarly, the specific complications named in Table 2 occurred during laparoscopic nephrectomy for malignant disease.

Intra-operative Complications

Prolonged Operative Time

A multi-institutional study published in 1995 by Gil et al. took an early look at complications of laparoscopic nephrectomy examining cases at five institutions in the early 1990s [13]. Most of these nephrectomies were performed for benign kidney disease. In these early days of urologic laparoscopy for malignant disease, operative times were longer and complications reflected this. After 8 h radical nephrectomies, three patients had the following complications: post-op myocardial infarction, a brachial plexus palsy, and a lateral thigh compartment syndrome [13]. These positioning related injuries can be minimized by padding all pressure points appropriately and by placing an axillary roll.

Additionally, a number of patients experienced acute congestive heart failure after lengthy laparoscopic procedures. The transient oliguria associated with pneumoperitoneum as well as the substantially smaller insensible fluid losses as compared to open abdominal surgery may not have been readily recognized as they are today. In Rassweiler et al., several patients were converted to an open surgical approach due to hypercarbia, again a function of increased operative time [14]. Operative times have no doubt decreased substantially, but deep venous thrombosis (DVT) still does occur as in Berger et al. [20]. Placement of prophylactic sequential compression stockings prior to the induction of anesthesia can be employed in almost all settings.

Port Site Injuries: Placement and Closure

Laparoscopic port placement injury rates have been estimated at 3 in 1,000 to 5 in 10,000 [21]. A 2001 study examined claims related to entry injuries reported to the Physicians Insurers Association of America over a 20-year period and entry injuries reported to the US FDA over a 3-year period. A total of 506 patients had primary access injuries with 65 deaths. Bowel injury or retroperitoneal vascular injury comprised 76% of all injuries occurring in primary port establishment. Half of the small bowel injuries were unrecognized in the first 24 h, an independent predictor of mortality [21]. Although few if any of these procedures were urologic, bowel and large vascular injuries at the time of port placement constitute the greatest concern. As such, in this review, the major vascular and bowel or visceral injuries that occurred at the time of laparoscopic port placement will be described in the respective sections.

While not occurring during surgery for malignant kidney disease, Gill et al. [13] described a direct trocar injury to a hydronephrotic kidney and a pneumothorax secondary to transpleural placement of a secondary port. Two trocar site hernias, one related to the dilating balloon used during retroperitoneal space development for subsequent nephrectomy, were reported in this multi-center study. The balloon inadvertently straddled the fascia and was inflated in this location. The nephrectomy was completed but the patient presented post-operatively with a port site hernia requiring open repair with mesh [13]. In Soulie et al., two patients required delayed laparotomy following laparoscopic pelvic node dissection. Both were ultimately found to have incarcerated hernias through 10 mm port sites whose fascia was not reapproximated [17]. These, as well as other experiences, now encourage fascial closure of port sites 10 mm or greater in size.

In addition to fascial closure of ports, the extraction of a large radical nephrectomy specimen necessitates a careful closure at the chosen site. Groups in the past have used specimen morcellation or fractionation with subsequent extraction via an impermeable sac in order to obviate the need to significantly extend a laparoscopic incision [2, 22]. Varkarakis et al. showed no significant difference in clinical outcomes between patients who underwent morcellation or intact specimen extraction other than cosmesis at the incision site [23]. Hospitalization time and post-operative analgesic requirement were not affected by the smaller incision through which a morcellated specimen could be removed [23]. So, although the evidence questioning the oncologic safety of specimen morcellation is largely based on case reports, this practice has been largely abandoned due to the concern that employing it may increase the risk of port site metastases [22, 23].

There may, however, be a difference in the incidence of incisional hernias at the specimen extraction site based on a 2009 study from Bird et al. [24]. All four of the patients who developed incisional hernias in this study did so at the paramedian location, two of whom had significantly elevated BMI. Based on the association of elevated BMI with paramedian incisional hernia, these authors changed their treatment algorithm to the use of a lower quadrant incision for specimen extraction in obese patients. The study group treated this way did not develop any incisional hernias [24]. These findings should be considered in the context of others authors' findings who have shown similar rates of major and minor complications when comparing obese and non-obese patients undergoing laparoscopic renal surgery [25]. It is our practice to extract nephrectomy specimens through a Gibson incision after retroperitoneal nephrectomy regardless of BMI. The retroperitoneal space is extended laparoscopically at the end of the procedure to reveal the anterior abdominal wall in the lower quadrant. If the specimen to be extracted is too large, a peritonotomy is performed to accommodate its size.

Illustrating the importance of vigilance during these multi-step procedures, Vallancien et al. described a patient who, at the conclusion of the case, experienced a skin burn from the hot saline used to clean the laparoscopes [26]. Siqueira et al. reported an inferior epigastric injury resulting in an abdominal wall and scrotal hematoma sustained during insertion of a secondary 5-mm port. The injury resolved with conservative management [27].

Vascular Injury

In 1998 the German Urologic Association (GUA) reviewed their experience with laparoscopic nephrectomy, the majority of which were performed for benign disease. Although this study did not specify which complications were specific to the cancer operations, half of their 46 open conversions were emergent, the majority of which were for inability to control bleeding [14]. Several years later, Parsons et al. cited 13 (1.5%) emergent conversions to open surgery overall, 12 of which were for vascular injury [18]. Although laparoscopic experience has broadened, it remains that the majority of emergent open conversions come in the face of uncontrollable hemorrhage.

In radical nephrectomy, the source of this bleeding usually relates to the renal hilar dissection and difficult arterial or venous control. Of significant import to laparoscopic nephrectomy for malignant disease is control of the neovascularity associated with renal cell carcinoma. These multiple and friable vessels can lead to significant bleeding and in our experience are best controlled with bipolar cautery. At our institution the LigaSure vessel-sealing device (Valleylab, Boulder, CO) has been particularly useful in controlling these vessels.

Superior Mesenteric Artery (SMA) Injury

Since 1973 there have been 12 reported cases of superior mesenteric artery (SMA) injuries during left nephrectomy, one also involving the celiac artery [28]. Gill et al. reported a single case of SMA ligation which required an open repair with a Gore-Tex graft [13]. The distance between the left renal artery and the SMA is on average 1 cm. In difficult cases, the left gonadal vein has been used as a guide to the left renal hilum [28]. Overdissection of the left renal hilum or adrenal gland medially can risk inadvertent injury to the SMA. When using an endovascular surgical stapler on the left renal vein, for example, circumferential visualization is important to help ensure that the stapler tips do not "pass point," an error that can result in SMA injury.

Illustrating how devastating an SMA injury can be was the report of a death following this complication by Siqueira et al. [27] The patient was being treated for a left upper pole tumor and had significant atherosclerotic disease. The SMA, thought to be a calcified lymph node, was divided. When brisk bleeding was noted during subsequent dissection, conversion to laparotomy occurred. During the exploration, an SMA injury was confirmed and a tube graft was employed as treatment. Nonetheless, the patient ultimately died after a protracted intensive care unit stay [27].

Adrenal Vascular Injury

The adrenal dissection, classically a component of radical nephrectomy, deserves specific mention as well. The adrenal arteries are controlled in standard fashion, typically employing a combination of locking and non-locking clips as well as bipolar cautery. The adrenal venous drainage is variable and excessive traction can cause venous avulsion leading to brisk bleeding. Clips are employed for venous hemostasis routinely. Ono et al. described brisk adrenal bleeding that was able to be controlled laparoscopically, while Shalhav et al. cited a case of adrenal hemorrhage that ultimately led to re-exploration [2, 10]. This was one of the two major laparoscopic complications in this study, a study that compared LNU to open nephroureterectomy. The patient received 13 units of blood prior to a re-exploration that defined bleeding from the inferior adrenal edge [10].

Variability in Renal Hilar Vascular Anatomy

As previously mentioned, in almost all cases of laparoscopic nephrectomy the most crucial step is arterial and venous control of the renal hilum. The anatomy can be variable and the proximity to the great vessels requires meticulous dissection. A Japanese cadaver study from the National Defense Medical College found a right- and a left-sided incidence of 2.4 and 1.8%, respectively, of renal arteries originating below the origin of the inferior mesenteric artery. Additionally, they found multiple renal veins to be a common occurrence [29]. As an example of the consequences of this variability, one of the two emergent open conversions in Siqueira et al. was due to hemorrhage from an unidentified right lower pole artery during LRN [27]. In the LNU group in this same series, a similar injury occurred during right lower pole dissection, but was able to be controlled laparoscopically [27].

Three phase-contrast imaging with a multidetector CT angiogram (MDCTA) pre-operatively is a commonly employed modality for elucidating the hilar vasculature in preparing for laparoscopic renal surgery, in general. Schlunt et al. showed 100% sensitivity, specificity, and accuracy for renal artery, renal vein, and ureter identification when a radiologist and operating urologist both reviewed the study [30]. Of course, pre-operative imaging cannot always accurately predict intra-operative findings. In Simon et al., there were four elective conversions to open surgery for higher staged tumors than initially predicted based on pre-operative imaging. In one LRN case, a very large appearing renal vein prompted open conversion at which point tumor thrombus in the vena cava was noted. In a different LNU case, dense hilar desmoplastic reaction limited the laparoscopic dissection and open conversion took place [7].

In Ono et al., one case required open conversion and this was secondary to uncontrollable left renal artery bleeding [2]. Attention to the hilum must be paid even during specimen removal. In Gill et al.'s [3] retroperitoneal LRN series, one patient required emergent conversion to an open procedure when brisk bleeding was noted following specimen extraction. At the time of exploratory laparotomy, severe hemorrhage was noted from the renal artery stump and the authors believed that clips had become dislodged during the specimen entrapment and extraction process [3].

Renal vein hemorrhage, more so than renal artery bleeding, can be particularly difficult to control laparoscopically. Berger et al., who expanded upon the Cleveland Clinic experience with LNU from Gill et al. [8], noted two emergent conversions for vascular injury, both due to excessive renal vein bleeding. One of these occurred at the earliest point of hilar dissection, namely the balloon dissection of the retroperitoneal space during primary port placement. During balloon dissection the renal vein was avulsed and emergent conversion ensued [20].

Bleeding can also arise directly from the vena cava at the level of the hilum or from associated venous tributaries due to vessel perforation with laparoscopic instruments or clips. Soulie et al. cited a single major complication in their LRN subset requiring open conversion, a caval injury that occurred during right hilar dissection [17].

Methods of Hemostasis at the Renal Hilum

Fueled by anecdotal reports of surgical clip failures resulting in donor death during living donor nephrectomy, the safety of the different methods used for hilar hemostasis came into question. This issue is relevant to laparoscopic nephrectomy for malignancy as well [31]. These reports which involved clip failure on the donor renal artery stump prompted Friedman et al.'s [31] study based on surveys distributed to hundreds of transplant surgeons. The surveys sought detailed recall of surgical techniques used to control the renal hilum, in particular, the details of any failures of vascular control. The authors concluded that non-locking metal clips should not be applied as the sole means of control of the renal artery and that locking clips do not offer a safety advantage [31]. Based on this report, Teleflex Medical issued a warning in 2006 that non-absorbable polymer ligating (NPL) locking clips were contraindicated for the control of the renal artery during laparoscopic donor nephrectomy [32].

The previous study as well as others led to Hsi et al.'s report based on data from the Food and Drug Administration Manufacturer and User Facility Device Experience database (MAUDE). They retrospectively reviewed 15 years of data reported to this agency regarding failures of hemostatic devices used to control the renal hilum [32]. Reported failures were broken down into those involving endovascular surgical staplers, non-locking titanium clips, and locking non-absorbable polymer ligating clips. No definitive conclusions could be reached on which was the safest hemostatic method because the overall denominator of use of each instrument was unknown, but different mechanisms of common failures were elucidated.

Among the 223 endovascular surgical stapler failures, 177 involved the Endopath (Ethicon Endo-Surgery, Cincinnati, Ohio) and 44 involved the gastrointestinal anastomosis (GIA), both of which stapled and cut in a single step [32]. In contrast, only two reports of endovascular surgical stapler failure involved the thoracoabdominal (TA) stapler (US Surgical, Norwalk, CT) which stapled and cut in separate steps [32]. The technique that we employ on the renal vein at our institution permits direct inspection of the staple line prior to vessel transection by using a non-bladed Endo-GIA (see Figs. 1 and 2). Stapler failure associated with severe hemorrhage and "locking up" of the stapling device following deployment has been reported. Subsequently, the involved surgeons

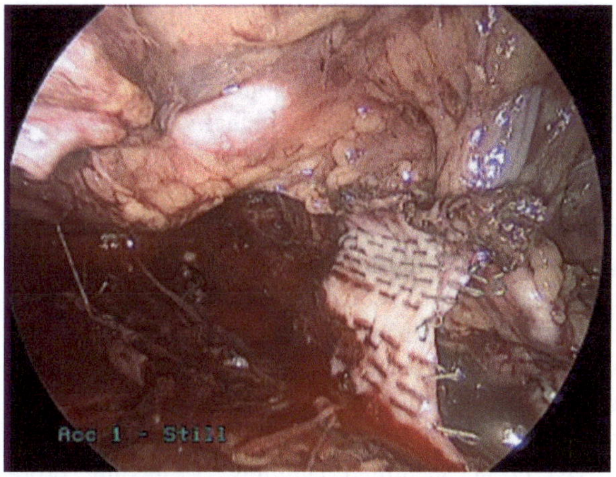

Fig. 1 Inspecting the renal vein prior to transection after placement of two rows of staple lines

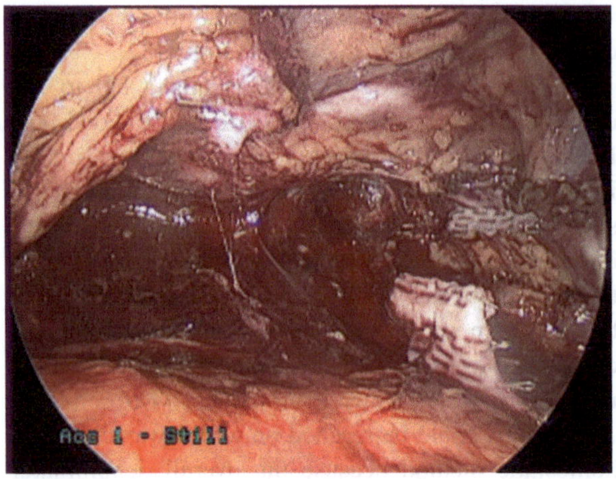

Fig. 2 The stapled and transected renal vein

had difficulty obtaining proximal hemostasis and hemorrhage occurred from forceful removal of the locked device.

The interruption of automatic staple lines because of misplacement over previously placed clips was noted in this study as well as elsewhere in the literature. In Siquiera et al., a study from Indianapolis of 213 laparoscopic nephrectomies, 84 were performed for living donor transplants. There were three endovascular stapler or clip complications described in the donor group, two venous and one arterial. Both venous ligation failures resulted in emergent open conversion, while the arterial injury was successfully controlled laparoscopically [27]. In one of the venous failures, an Endo-GIA stapler misfired during the ligation of a renal vein when a portion of the stapling device engaged over a clip on the adrenal vein. The overlapping portion of the staple line was incomplete but the automatic stapler blade fired nonetheless, resulting in hemorrhage from the proximal renal vein stump [27]. A similar injury was described by Simon et al. in which an Endo-GIA stapler across the renal artery engaged partially over a metal clip on a nearby lumbar vein. The automatic stapler blade transected the artery although the staple line was incomplete [7]. Subsequently, these authors avoid clip placement and prefer the Endo-GIA stapler when dividing peri-hilar vessels, as staple lines can be placed across other staple lines, but not over clips [7].

Hsi et al. identified jamming or feeding problems with non-locking titanium clip devices as well as several instances of clips slipping off of vessels. Additionally, these titanium clips can close in a scissor-like fashion, either rendering a portion of the closure non-hemostatic or, worse, tearing through the vessel with the tip of the scissored clip [32].

In the study by Hsi et al. 18 locking non-absorbable polymer ligating (NPL) clip malfunctions were reported to the FDA, with severe complications and 3 deaths noted [32]. Ten situations in which the clips had become displaced either during the initial surgery or upon re-exploration were noted. Siqueira et al. reported on an NPL clip that had been used to secure the adrenal vein stump that was subsequently dislodged during the arterial dissection [27]. To prevent migration, a 1–2-mm cuff of tissue can be left adjacent to the clip [27]. We agree with Hsi et al. in that thorough dissection is important prior to placement of these locking clips to prevent extraneous tissue from getting caught in the locking mechanism. Visualization of the tip of the locking clip is important as well so as to not force the tip through the vessel wall.

Regarding the portion of vessel left distal to a locking clip, we employ a similar method of renal artery control to the one described by Simforoosh et al. for laparoscopic donor nephrectomy [33]. In this study, 241 patients who underwent laparoscopic donor nephrectomy during an 18-month period had their renal artery and vein controlled with the following technique: a locking non-absorbable polymer ligating (NPL) clip placed on the renal artery near the aorta with a non-locking titanium clip placed a few millimeters distal. The renal vein was controlled with two parallel NPL clips. These authors reported no bleeding complications, clip migration, or slippage [33]. At our institution we place a locking NPL clip on the renal artery with non-locking clips placed distally (see Figs. 3 and 4). As mentioned before, the renal vein is secured with an unbladed Endo-GIA stapler (Fig. 1).

Bowel and Visceral Injury

Introduction

Bowel and solid organ injuries sustained during laparoscopic nephrectomy are also serious complications. These complications may present more insidiously than vascular injury often leading to operative or non-operative intervention rather than emergent conversion to open surgery. When we counsel our patients on

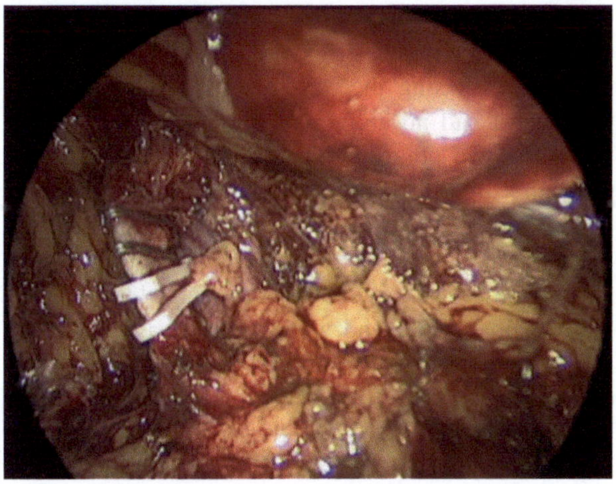

Fig. 3 Retroperitoneal view of renal artery with two locking clips and two non-locking metal clips distally

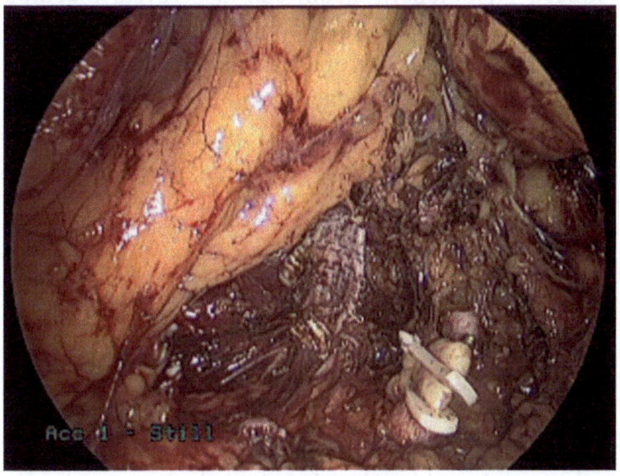

Fig. 4 Renal artery stump with non-locking metal clip distal to locking clips (*foreground*). View of renal vein with Endo-GIA staple line (*background*)

the risk of injury to adjacent structures, it is to these that we refer: on the right side, the ascending colon, liver, duodenum, and diaphragm and on the left, the descending colon, pancreas, and spleen.

Perforated Viscus

Bishoff et al. retrospectively reviewed 915 laparoscopic urologic procedures and identified 10 bowel injuries, including 4 perforations and 6 abrasions, only one of which occurred during laparoscopic radical nephrectomy. However, the presentation and treatment of these injuries is instructive. Of the four perforations, none were recognized intra-operatively, which speaks to the insidious nature of their presentation [34]. Of note, the perforation that occurred during LRN was treated with a percutaneous drain and an enterocutaneous fistula developed [34]. Interestingly, Fahlenkamp et al. reported that over 50% of their bowel injuries were associated with monopolar cautery, none of which were recognized intra-operatively [16].

Stressed in Bishoff's report was the seemingly unusual presentation of the occult perforations and subsequent intra-abdominal abscess. Single port site pain, abdominal distention, diarrhea, and leucopenia were all typical and abscess presented in the absence of fever, peritonitis, nausea, vomiting, or leukocytosis. An acute phase reaction distinct in character from what is experienced during open surgery may account for the signs and symptoms that are different from what would be expected in the setting of similar complications after open surgery [34].

Bowel injuries can occur during port placement, during laparoscopic dissection, as well as during port closure. Gill et al. described an enterocutaneous fistula that arose from a small bowel injury sustained during fascial closure of a port site at the conclusion of a simple nephrectomy. The patient was treated with total parenteral nutrition and bowel rest and the fistula closed spontaneously [13].

We routinely employ a mechanical and antibiotic bowel prep. An empty colon facilitates retraction and exposure; however, sequela of colonic injuries can still arise. Siqueira et al. described a patient who 4 days after a seemingly uneventful LNU presented with lower abdominal pain and was found to have a pelvic abscess on CT exam. The patient was noted on exploration to have a perforated colonic diverticulum probably sustained during dissection along the thin diverticular wall. The injury was treated with a diverting colostomy [27].

Bowel injuries are not always the result of perforation. In Vallencien et al., a patient experienced post-operative bowel obstruction caused by ischemic colonic stenosis, which was effectively managed conservatively [26]. A similar injury was described in Siqueira et al. when after a seemingly uncomplicated left LRN, the patient developed melena. The ensuing workup led to a colonoscopy which found a semi-circumferential ischemic lesion at the splenic flexure. The issue was managed and resolved with conservative measures and was thought to reflect compromise of mesenteric vessels and the marginal vessels at the colonic reflection [27].

Injury to Adjacent Structures

The liver and its relationship with the upper pole of the right kidney posteriorly, where the triangular ligament needs to be incised for mobilization, renders it susceptible to complication. We report on no dissection-related liver injuries but do note a liver injury sustained during primary port insertion, described by Siqueira et al. This injury was repaired laparoscopically by packing with oxidized cellulose and then managed conservatively without the need for reintervention [27].

During the transperitoneal approach to the kidney the duodenum must be mobilized medially, or kocherized, to gain access to the vena cava and renal hilum. Neovascularity to the duodenum from a kidney involved with malignancy can complicate this maneuver. When employing a retroperitoneal approach, overdissection of the hilum medially can potentially violate the duodenum as well. In Ono et al., a single patient sustained a dissection-related duodenal injury that was treated with an open duodenojejunostomy [2]. A more unusual duodenal injury sustained by a patient who had undergone an LNU was described by Fahlenkamp et al. The injury, ultimately noted as duodenal artery bleeding, led to retroperitoneal hemorrhage and death, one of two mortalities in this 2,407 patient review. The authors believed that the hemorrhage may have started due to excessive mesenteric traction [16].

During left nephrectomy, in addition to the descending colon, the spleen and tail of the pancreas are the adjacent organs of interest as both of these structures are in close proximity to the renal hilum. If the pancreas is violated, a surgical drain should be placed. Pancreatic fistula can arise after pancreatic injury as was reported by Rassweiler et al. following a simple nephrectomy [14].

Several splenic injuries have been reported during left LRN and LNU, with treatments ranging from splenectomy to laparoscopic repair with subsequent conservative management, as in the examples seen in Gill et al. and Ono et al., respectively [13, 2]. Simon et al. performed transperitoneal nephrectomy with primary access using the Veress needle providing that the patient had no abdominal surgical history. There were no solid organ or bowel injuries during access using this algorithm, but four splenic injuries occurred during laparoscopic dissection [7]. Two of the four splenic injuries cited in this study required staged open splenectomy. The other two were managed laparoscopically with fibrillar and argon beam coagulation and healed without operative reintervention. These authors concluded that careful dissection of the splenocolic and splenorenal ligaments during left laparoscopic nephrectomy could facilitate safe dissection of the upper pole by allowing the spleen to fall medially and retract superiorly [7]. Direct laparoscopic visualization of the spleen at the conclusion of surgery under reduced pneumoperitoneum can also reveal bleeding masked by elevated intra-abdominal pressures [7]. It is important to remember that post-splenectomy patients require the Pneumovax vaccine.

Post-operative Complications

Specific post-operative complications can be found in Table 2. Several of the injuries listed as post-operative are inseparable from the surgical manipulation that led to them such as the ischemic colonic lesions previously described by Vallencien et al. and Siqueira et al. [26, 27]. Similarly, the urine leaks reported by Shalhav et al. and Parsons et al. were related to the bladder cuff closure during nephroureterectomy [10, 18]. The former complication, which was associated with gross hematuria, was described in the bladder cuff management section.

As is the case with most abdominal surgery, return to normal bowel activity can be delayed, and ileus or bowel obstruction was reported in multiple series (Table 2). However, Parsons et al. reported two small bowel obstructions that ultimately required exploratory laparotomy. In one instance, severe paralytic ileus led to fascial and wound dehiscence and in another, mechanical obstruction arose from herniation through a mesenteric defect [18].

Complications Affecting Oncologic Outcome

In general, dissection during surgery for transitional cell carcinoma (TCC) is more difficult than that for renal cell carcinoma (RCC) of comparable size. In addition to the desmoplastic reaction often associated with TCC that can increase the difficulty of the dissection, port site recurrence has been reported more frequently with TCC and recurrence at the endoscopically resected bladder site is an issue only with nephroureterectomy [35]. This was the case in Arango et al. which reported massive tumor recurrence at the transurethral resection (TUR) site occurring 7 months after LNU for a renal pelvic and calyceal tumor [36].

Tsvian and Sidi reviewed nine reported cases in the urologic literature of port site recurrence. Interestingly, among the five nephrectomies resulting in port site metastases, only two were for TCC and three were for RCC. Importantly, five of the six patients with follow-up reported were not alive at 1 year [22]. Their review included a number of recommendations to minimize the risk of port site recurrence, some of which are routinely employed in oncologic laparoscopy, such as the use of an impermeable specimen extraction sac [22]. A number of cases of port site recurrences have occurred when impermeable extraction sacs either were not used or tore during extraction as in Otani et al.'s report of a tuberculous kidney that harbored an occult TCC [37].

General recommendations to minimize tumor seeding include maintaining trocar fixation, avoiding specimen morcellation, avoiding laparoscopy in the setting of ascites, and minimizing air leakage around the trocars. The latter addresses the so-called chimney effect, the theory, based on a rat model, that peri-trocar air leakage potentiates tumor cell accumulation at the port site [22]. Regarding specimen morcellation, a Brazilian series of 32 LRNs for RCC cited in Tsvian and Sidi's review had 2 port site metastases and subsequently abandoned the practice of specimen morcellation [22]. Additionally, in Castilho et al.'s case report of a port site recurrence 5 months after LRN, both specimen morcellation and the intra-operative recognition of ascites were implicated as risk factors [38]. Despite careful oncologic technique, there are disease-specific factors such as high tumor grade, field effect associated with TCC, and the presence of carcinoma in situ (CIS) that can contribute to the development of port site or TUR site recurrence.

Conclusions

Experience with laparoscopic nephrectomy for malignant disease has evolved significantly since it was first described nearly two decades ago. Despite this vast experience, serious complications exist even in current series. Awareness of the pitfalls that can befall the surgeon and attention to meticulous surgical technique throughout the procedure can serve to limit complications in the future.

References

1. Clayman RV, Kavoussi LR, Soper NJ, et al. Laparoscopic nephrectomy: initial case report. J Urol. 1991; 146:278.
2. Ono Y, Kinukawa T, Hattori R, et al. Laparoscopic radical nephrectomy for renal cell carcinoma: a five-year experience. Urology. 1999;53:280–6.
3. Gill IS, Schweizer D, Hobart MG, et al. Retroperitoneal laparoscopic radical nephrectomy: the Cleveland Clinic experience. J Urol. 2000;163:1665.
4. Gaur, DD. Laparoscopic operative retroperitoneoscopy: use of a new device. J Urol. 1992;148:1137.
5. Pyo P, Chen A, Grasso M. Retroperitoneal laparoscopic partial nephrectomy: surgical experience and outcomes. J Urol. 2008;180:1279.
6. Bariol SV, Stewart GD, McNeill SA, Tolley DA. Oncological control following laparoscopic nephroureterectomy: 7-year outcome. J Urol. 2004;172:1805.
7. Simon SD, Castle EP, Ferrigni RG, et al. Complications of laparoscopic nephrectomy: the Mayo Clinic experience. J Urol. 2004;171:1447.
8. Gill IS, Sung GT, Hobart MG, et al. Laparoscopic radical nephroureterctomy for upper tract transitional cell carcinoma: the Cleveland Clinic experience. J Urol. 2000;164:1513.
9. Sagalowsky AI, Jarrett TW. Management of urothelial tumors of the renal pelvis and ureter. In: Wein AJ, et al., editors. Campbell's urology. 9th ed. Philadelphia: W.B. Sanders Company; 2007. pp. 1653–85.
10. Shalhav AL, Dunn MD, Portis AJ, et al. Laparoscopic nephroureterectomy for upper tract transitional cell cancer: the Washington University experience. J Urol. 2000;163:1100.
11. Donat SM. Standards for surgical complication reporting in urologic oncology: time for a change. Urology. 2007;69:221.

12. Martin RCG, Brennan MF, Jacques DP. Quality of complication reporting in the surgical literature. Ann Surg. 2002;235(6):803.
13. Gill IS, Kavoussi LR, Clayman RV, et al. Complications of laparoscopic nephrectomy in 185 patients: a multi-institutional review. J Urol. 1995;154:479.
14. Rassweiler J, Fornara P, Weber M, et al. Laparoscopic nephrectomy: the experience of the laparoscopy working group of the German Urologic Association. J Urol. 1998;160:18.
15. Rassweiler J, Seemann O, Henkel T, Alken, P. Retroperitoneoscopy – experience with the first 200 patients. J Urol. 1997;157:143.
16. Fahlenkamp D, Rassweiler J, Fornara P, et al. Complications of laparoscopic procedures in urology: experience with 2407 procedures at 4 German centers. J Urol. 1999;162:765.
17. Soulie M, Seguin P, Richeux, L, et al. Urologic complications of laparoscopic surgery: experience with 350 procedures at a single center. J Urol. 2001;165:1960.
18. Parsons JK, Varkarakis I, Rha KH, et al. Complications of Abdominal urologic laparoscopy: longitudinal five-year analysis. Urology. 2004;63:27–32.
19. Guillonneau B, Abbou, CC, Doublet JD, et al. Proposal for a European Scoring System for laparoscopic operations in urology. Eur Urol. 2001;40:2.
20. Berger A, Haber G-P, Kamoi K, et al. Laparoscopic radical nephroureterctomy for upper tract transitional cell carcinoma: oncological outcomes at 7 years. J Urol. 2008;180:849.
21. Chandler JG, Corson SL, Way LW. Three spectra of laparoscopic entry access injuries. J Am Coll Surg. 2001; 192:478.
22. Tsvian A, Sidi AA. Port site metastases in urological laparoscopic surgery. J Urol. 2003;169:1213.
23. Varkarakis I, Rha K, Hernandez F, et al. Laparoscopic specimen extraction: morcellation. BJU Int. 2005;95 Suppl:27.
24. Bird VG, Au JK, Sandman Y, et al. Comparison of different extraction sites used during laparoscopic radical nephrectomy. J Urol. 2009;181:1565.
25. Anast JW, Stoller ML, Meng MV, et al. Differences in complications and outcomes for obese patients undergoing laparoscopic radical, partial, or simple nephrectomy. J Urol. 2004;172:2287.
26. Vallancien G, Cathelineau X, Baumert H, et al. Complications of transperitoneal laparoscopic surgery in urology: review of 1,311 procedures at a single center. J Urol. 2002;168:23.
27. Siqueira TM, Kuo RL, Gardner TA, et al. Major complications in 213 laparoscopic nephrectomy cases: the Indianapolis experience. J Urol. 2002;168:1361.
28. Nevoux P, Zini L, Villers A, et al. Celiac axis and superior mesenteric artery: danger zone for left nephrectomy. J Endourol. 2008;22(11):1.
29. Kaneko N, Kobayashi Y, Okada Y. Anatomic variations of the renal vessels pertinent to transperitoneal vascular control in the management of trauma. Surgery. 2008;143:616.
30. Schlunt LB, Harper JD, Broome DR, et al. Improved detection of renal vascular anatomy using multidetector CT angiography: is 100% detection possible? J Endourol. 2007;21:12.
31. Friedman AL, Peters TG, Jones KW, et al. Fatal and nonfatal hemorrhagic complications of living kidney donation. Ann Surg. 2006;243:126.
32. Hsi RS, Saint-Elie DT, Zimmerman GJ, Baldwin DD. Mechanisms of hemostatic failure during laparoscopic nephrectomy: review of food and drug administration database. Urology. 2007;70(5):888.
33. Simforoosh N, Aminsharifi A, Zand S, Javaherforooshzadeh A. How to improve the safety of polymer clips for vascular control during laparoscopic donor nephrectomy. J Endourol. 2007;21(11):1319.
34. Bishoff JT, Allaf ME, Kirkels W, et al. Laparoscopic bowel injury: incidence and clinical presentation. J Urol. 1999;161:887.
35. Ahmed I, Shaikh NA, Kapadia CR. Track recurrence of renal pelvic transitional cell carcinoma after laparoscopic nephrectomy. BJU. 1998;81:319.
36. Arango O, Bielsa O, Carles J, Gelabert-Mas A. Massive tumor implantation in the endoscopic resected area in modified nephroureterectomy. J Urol. 1997;157:1839.
37. Otani M, Shinichiro I, Tsuji Y. Port site metastasis after laparoscopic nephrectomy: unsuspected transitional cell carcinoma within a tuberculous atrophic kidney. J Urol. 1999;162:286.
38. Castilho LN, Fugita OEH, Mitre AI, Arap S. Port site tumor recurrences of renal cell carcinoma after videolaparoscopic radical nephrectomy. J Urol. 2001;165: 519.

Complications of Laparoscopic Donor Nephrectomy

Alexei Wedmid and Michael A. Palese

Keywords Donor Nephrectomy · Laparoscopy · Complications

Laparoscopic Donor Nephrectomy: An Introduction

The first laparoscopic nephrectomy was performed in 1990 [1] involving a right kidney with renal oncocytoma, opening the door for the first laparoscopic donor nephrectomy 5 years later by Ratner et al. [2].

Early experience with laparoscopic donor nephrectomies had concerns of graft dysfunction, ureteral complications, and loss of right-sided donor kidneys when compared to open donor nephrectomies [3]. Large review studies and meta-analysis of 73 studies involving 6,594 patients comparing open versus laparoscopic donor nephrectomies have since shown equivalent outcomes for the grafts when examining graft function, rejection rate, urologic complications, and patient and graft survival [3–6]. Laparoscopic donor nephrectomy did have longer operating time and warm ischemia time, but this did not translate into higher rates of delayed graft function or loss of graft [5, 6]. Complication rates were similar in number, with laparoscopic donor nephrectomy patients having more gastrointestinal complications (bowel injury, bowel obstruction, internal hernia, and pancreatitis) and open donors having more pulmonary complications (atelectasis, pneumothorax, pulmonary congestion, and hypoxia) and thrombotic complications (deep vein thrombosis, thrombophlebitis, and pulmonary embolism) [5].

Moreover, numerous studies have shown many advantages with laparoscopic over open donor nephrectomy, with donors benefiting from less pain and analgesic requirements, a 1.58-day shorter hospital stay (95% CI 1.87–1.28, $p < 0.001$), and return to work 2.38 weeks earlier (95% CI 3.19–1.57, $p < 0.001$) [6]. In fact, retrospective quality-of-life questionnaires confirm improved bodily pain and physical and emotional role functioning with laparoscopy over open donor nephrectomy at all time points postoperatively, extending to beyond a month after kidney donation [7].

It has become clear that laparoscopic donor nephrectomy is a safe and effective technique for procuring kidney grafts for donation, and due to its advantages in quality of life for the donor, it has spurred an increase in living kidney donation. Since 2001, the number of living persons donating kidneys has exceeded that of cadaveric donors, although a higher number of cadaveric kidneys still exist as both units are harvested [4]. Currently in 2008, living donors account for 41% of all kidney transplants in the United States, with living donors preferred due to superior graft function and patient survival outcomes [8].

In any discussion of complications of donor nephrectomies, it must be stressed that these donors are uniquely healthy individuals, with no benefit to themselves, and therefore any complications are especially drastic. Donors must realize that their act of beneficence is not without risk, and informed consent should be obtained far in advance, allowing ample time for

M.A. Palese (✉)
Department of Urology, Mount Sinai Medical Center, New York, NY, USA
e-mail: michael.palese@mountsinai.org

R. Ghavamian (ed.), *Complications of Laparoscopic and Robotic Urologic Surgery*,
DOI 10.1007/978-1-60761-676-4_11, © Springer Science+Business Media, LLC 2010

the donor to fully understand the details of surgery and risks involved, including possible open conversion, renal failure, and death. While rare, a survey of all United Network for Organ Sharing (UNOS)-listed transplantation programs found donor mortality for both laparoscopic and open organ retrieval to be 0.03% [9]. Furthermore, unique to transplant surgery, we must scrutinize all intraoperative and postoperative techniques to reduce complications in not one but two patients: the donor and the recipient.

Prevention of complications is essential and preoperative evaluation is the first critical step in this process. It is recommended that each transplant center organize a transplant committee to discuss all cases of live organ donation, with evaluation including medical and psychological testing [4]. Preoperative imaging must accurately define vascular anatomy and potential anomalies for donor kidney selection. When comparing multidetector CT angiogram (CTA) to intraoperative surgical findings, the sensitivity, specificity, and accuracy of predicting supernumerary arteries' (including early branches within 1 cm from the aorta) arterial branching were 89, 100, and 97%, respectively, when read by a radiologist alone, rising to 100, 100, 100%, respectively, with a combined preoperative reading with the operating surgeon [10]. CTA is also more accurate than magnetic resonance angiography (MRA), with sensitivities of 100% (vs. 97%) for major vessels, as well as better detection of accessory renal veins and higher resolutions for left lumbar (95% vs. 47%) and left gonadal veins (71% vs. 46%) [11].

Three-dimensional reconstruction is a key component of this committee approach to preoperative CTA imaging, improving surgical approach, preventing intraoperative hemorrhage via a missed accessory or polar vessel, and improving postoperative vascular graft function. Preoperative knowledge of the 21.5% likelihood of multiple arteries and 4.5% likelihood of venous anomalies [12] may even alter kidney selection. While the left kidney is generally preferred for its longer renal vein length, imaging may alter donor kidney selection based on supernumerary vessels or incidental renal masses. Early hesitance to donate the right kidney due to intraoperative difficulties with a short, thin right renal vein leading to presumed graft failure and high thrombosis rates have now been overcome, with a large multi-institutional study showing 98% graft success and no major complications for right laparoscopic donor nephrectomies [13]. Similarly, multiple arteries are associated with a trend in longer warm ischemia time due to multiple vessels, but without any change in blood loss, hospital stay, 1-year graft survival, or overall complications [12].

If differences exist between kidneys, the better kidney should be left in the donor, in order to reduce potential long-term medical complications. Current trends, as measured by a survey of 32 programs, performing approximately 40% of laparoscopic living donors in the United States show that 77% perform right laparoscopic donor nephrectomy either with pure laparoscopic or hand-assisted techniques, yet it still accounts for less than 20% of all donor nephrectomies [14].

Case Description

Patients are positioned in flexed, lateral decubitus with careful padding and arm support. Initial access is obtained using a Veress needle or Hasson technique, and intra-abdominal pneumoperitoneum is limited to 12–15 mmHg. For left-sided nephrectomies, we typically use 3–4 trocars; in right-sided nephrectomies, pure laparoscopy is performed in many centers, although we prefer a hand-assisted technique with three additional trocars.

Dissection begins by opening the lateral peritoneal reflection from the upper sigmoid to splenic flexure and dividing the attachments of the colon, spleen, and pancreatic tail. On the right, we divide the triangular ligament to help retract the liver. For pure laparoscopy, the lateral attachments are left in place to prevent rotation of the kidney and maintain access to the hilum. The gonadal vein is identified and traced superiorly to the left renal vein. The left gonadal, left adrenal, and lumbar veins are isolated and then divided with clips and laparoscopic scissors to obtain maximal vessel length on the renal vein and artery. The ureter is identified lateral to the gonadal vein and an Endo-TA stapler is used to divide the ureteral packet at the level of the iliac vessels. Posterolateral exposure of the kidney is obtained and the harmonic scalpel is used to dissect the adrenal gland off the kidney allowing full mobilization of the kidney on the hilum.

When using standard laparoscopy, a 6-cm Pfannenstiel extraction incision is made and a 15-mm trocar with endobag is introduced under direct vision. Once the recipient team is ready, the kidney and transected ureter are placed in the endobag, and the renal artery and vein are separately divided with vascular staplers. The endobag is carefully closed, delivered, immersed in ice slush, and transferred to the recipient team. Hemostasis is verified and any mesocolic defects closed. The trocar sites are closed under vision, the Pfannenstiel incision or hand-access port is closed in two layers, and local anesthesia is given prior to repositioning the patient supine for extubation.

Postoperatively, the patient receives a clear liquid diet, which is advanced as rapidly as tolerated. Patients receive ketorolac postoperatively, which is converted to oral pain control postoperative day #1. The Foley catheter is removed on postoperative day #1, ambulation encouraged, with usual discharge at 24–48 h postoperatively.

Overall Complication Rates of Laparoscopic Donor Nephrectomy

Laparoscopic donor nephrectomy, like any laparoscopic procedure, bears all the risks of laparoscopy and anesthesia, including injuries related to the entry techniques and trocars, and complications of pneumoperitoneum such as gas embolus and difficulty with cardiopulmonary reserve. These general complications of laparoscopy will not be addressed specifically in this chapter.

Preoperatively, kidney donors are especially healthy surgical patients who have typically undergone extensive screening. Donors include 56% female patients ranging in age from 18 to 74 years, with an overall mean age of 34.9 years, and 24% with multiple arteries whose left kidney is typically donated (Table 1). When performed well, the laparoscopic kidney donor can quickly recover from surgery and its inherent risks.

Early experience led many to believe that a body mass index (BMI) above 30 kg/m^2 resulted in a higher complication rate, but more recent studies have shown that obese donors have no increase in blood loss, serum creatinine, or major complications [14, 22], although their operative time is 30–40 min longer and hospital stay is longer [14, 16]. This allows for a larger potential donor pool, and although 69% of transplant institutions use BMI in the screening process there is no consensus with a BMI cutoff value [14]. While surgical complications may not be affected by BMI, obesity is linked to hypertension and diabetes, and the long-term significance of BMI on medical complications in the donor has not yet been fully assessed.

In the two decades since the first laparoscopic donor nephrectomy, the surgical technique and postoperative management have been refined to a mean operative time of 3–3.5 h, estimated blood loss (EBL) of 148 ml (range 69–344), warm ischemia time (WIT) of 3.3 min (range 2.2–4.9), and hospital stay of 2.43 days (range 1.1–3.3) in large, retrospective studies (Table 2). Over time, the trocars became smaller and the number of trocars decreased, with the extraction site incision remaining a constant 6.6 ± 1 cm, with extraction site moving from umbilical to suprapubic [16].

The largest study, following 738 patients at Maryland [16], reported an average hospital stay of 2.68 days, with postoperative management consisting of clear liquids beginning at 26.5 h and regular diet at 46.8 h. Bowel function returned with bowel sounds at 32.1 h, flatus at 48.1 h, and bowel movements at 63.5 h after surgery. The UCLA group [23] advocates preoperative bowel rest, beginning with clears 2 days before surgery and a mechanical bowel prep the day prior, combined with ketorolac for postoperative pain relief in an effort to shorten mean hospital stay to 1.1 days and hasten bowel function. No readmissions were reported with 97% of patients tolerating clears, passing flatus, and ambulating on postoperative day #1.

Total complication rates in the large published studies range from 4.0 to 31.6% (Table 3), with major complications rates between 1.6 and 7.6% and minor rates between 2.3 and 25.6% depending on the extent of complications included. A modification of the Clavien classification system of complications used for cholecystectomy has been proposed by Kocak et al. [20]. Grade 1 includes minor complications or events that if left alone would have spontaneous resolution or needed simple bedside procedure and compromises 40–62% of total complications [20, 22]. Grade 2–4 are degrees of major complications, with grade 2 describing potentially life-threatening events that usually require intervention but do not result in ongoing disability, grade 3 resulting in residual or lasting disability, and grade 4 resulting in renal failure in the donor or death due to any complication. The learning curve is most noticeable in these major complication

Table 1 Donor characteristics

Study (year)	Patient (*n*)	Mean age (years)	Mean BMI	Gender (% female)	Left kidney (%)	Mean no. of arteries
Maryland (2000) [15]	320	38.7	n/a	57.5	97.5	n/a
Maryland (2004) [16]	738[a]	40.2	27.7	56.9	96	1.3
Cleveland Clinic (2004) [17]	107[b]	40.9	26.1	57	99[b] [79.7%]	n/a
Hopkins (2004) [18]	381	n/a	n/a	n/a	95	n/a
Northwestern (2004) [19]	500	38	28	55	99	1.23
Northwestern (2006) [20]	600[a]	n/a	n/a	n/a	n/a	n/a
UCSF (2005) [21]	530	40.4	26.1	58	84	1.17
Indiana (2007) [22]	253	39.3	26.1	n/a	93.7	n/a
UCLA (2007) [23, 24]	300	36.7	28.3	55.7	99	1.22
Mt Sinai, NY (2007) [25]	500	40.3	27.3	56.2	86.2	n/a

[a]The Maryland 2004 and Northwestern 2006 studies were extended studies of their earlier results, include those patients in their data, and reveal improvements in surgical technique and the learning curve
[b]Cleveland Clinic study included 36 retroperitoneal cases, which were not counted in the numbers and results. These included all but one of the right donor nephrectomies so that actual rate of left nephrectomy was 79.7%

Table 2 Operative outcomes

Study (year)	Patient (*n*)	OR time (min)	EBL (ml)	WIT (s)	Hospital stay (days)
Maryland (2000) [15]	320	214.5 ± 49	146.7 ± 163.2	148.1 ± 68.2	2.75
Maryland (2004) [16]	738[a]	202.1	128 ± 194	169 ± 91	2.7
Cleveland Clinic (2004) [17]	107[b]	220.5	166.2	240.2	2.57
Hopkins (2004) [18]	381	252.9 ± 55.7	344 ± 690	294 ± 204	3.3 ± 4.5
Northwestern (2004) [19]	500	n/a	142.4	157.2 ± 30	1.7
Northwestern (2006) [20]	600[a]	n/a	69 ± 116	n/a	1.5 ± 0.6
UCSF (2005) [21]	530	196 ± 43	n/a	n/a	3.2 ± 1.0
Indiana (2007) [22]	253	199 ± 50	115 ± 285	132 ± 63	2.8 ± 0.9
UCLA (2007) [23, 24]	300	180 ± 55	80 ± 50	240 ± 120	1.1
Mt Sinai, NY (2007) [25]	500	208.2 ± 55.6	197 ± 223	207 ± 91.6	2.3±0.8

[a]The Maryland 2004 and Northwestern 2006 studies were extended studies of their earlier results, include those patients in their data, and reveal improvements in surgical technique and the learning curve
[b]Cleveland Clinic study included 36 retroperitoneal cases, which were not counted in the numbers and results

Table 3 Complication rates

Study (year)	Patient (*n*)	Conversion rate (%)	Intraoperative complication rate (%)	Total complication rate (%)	Major (intraop and post-op) (%)	Minor (%)	Delayed graft function (%)
Maryland (2000) [15]	320	1.6	11.2	31.6	5.9	25.6	2
Maryland (2004) [16]	738[a]	1.6	8.8	27.2	4.2	23.0	2.6
Cleveland Clinic (2004) [17]	107[b]	0	3.7	n/a	n/a	n/a	n/a
Hopkins (2004) [18]	381	2.1	2.6	16.5	7.6	8.9	4.5
Northwestern (2004) [19]	500	1.8	2.8	6.2	2.6	3.6	0.2
Northwestern (2006) [20]	600[a]	1.83	3.2	7.2	4.3	2.8	n/a
UCSF (2005) [21]	530	0.2	1.3	6.4	3.0	3.4	n/a
Indiana (2007) [22]	253	1.2	2.8	10.3	4.0	6.4	4.4
UCLA (2007) [24]	300	1.0	0.6	4.0	1.6	2.3	n/a
Mt Sinai, NY (2007) [25]	500	1.6	5.8	15.6	7.0	8.6	3.0

[a]The Maryland 2004 and Northwestern 2006 studies were extended studies of their earlier results, include those patients in their data, and reveal improvements in surgical technique and the learning curve
[b]Cleveland Clinic study included 36 retroperitoneal cases, which were not counted in the numbers and results

rates, decreasing from 20% in the first 50 cases to 6% in the 200th–250th cases [16].

The Kocak classification scheme for laparoscopic donor nephrectomy further divides grade 2 into grades 2a where treatment is limited to drug or medical management only, grade 2b when additional therapeutic intervention is required, or grade 2c for open conversion of a laparoscopic case. Grade 2c injuries range from 0 to 2.1% (Table 3) with a mean conversion rate of 1.3%. When specified 75–83% were emergent due to vascular bleeding [16, 18]. Other elective causes of open conversion include obesity and failure to progress, small bowel distension and small working space, or intraperitoneal adhesions. Conversion rates are typically higher in the first 100 cases of the series at 6%, lowering to 0.75–1.2% afterward [19, 20]. A similarly statistically significant decline in total donor complication (p=0.03), allograft loss (p=0.001), rate of vascular thrombosis with experience (p=0.01), and rate of ureteral complications (p=0.05) occurs with surgical experience [18].

When complications are separated by time of occurrence, intraoperative complication rates of 0.6–11.2% and postoperative rates of 3.4–20.4% (Table 3). Intraoperative complications consist of bleeding in 93.1% of cases [25], with a meta-analysis of 73 studies [26] showing 1.2% device failure, 0.9% vascular injury, 1.7% venous bleeding, 1.2% arterial bleeding, 1.3% splenic injury, 1.5% conversion to open, and 0.6% transfusion rates. A learning curve is seen with 86.2% of total intraoperative complications occurring in the first 150 cases, compared to 10.3% in the subsequent 150 cases (p=0.003) [25].

Postoperative complications are diverse and include atrial fibrillation, pancreatitis, small bowel obstruction, respiratory distress syndrome, pneumonia, atelectasis, acute pulmonary edema, retroperitoneal hematoma, chylous ascites, urinary retention, epididymitis, UTI, fever, ileus, wound infection, hernias related or unrelated to extraction site, thigh numbness, and arm thrombophlebitis [15, 16, 19]. Reoperation rates of 1.8% have been reported [18].

Graft or recipient complications comprise the final group of surgical complications. Direct injuries to the donated kidney may require pre-transplant repair and include injury of the renal vein or arterial branches, parenchymal lacerations, or perinephric hematoma [16]. Delayed graft function (DGF), defined as the need for dialysis within 1 week of transplant, develops in 0.2–4.5% of recipients (Table 3) and is associated with increased risk of rejection and decreased graft survival [27]. Finally, slow graft recovery, defined as serum creatinine 3.0% mg or greater for 1 week after transplant, may ensue in 11.2–13.3% of recipients [16, 22].

Comparing Alternative Laparoscopic Surgical Techniques

Hand-Assisted Laparoscopic Nephrectomy

Like the laparoscopic donor nephrectomy, the hand-assisted laparoscopic procedure has been shown to be safe and effective, with similar graft survival and decreased perioperative morbidity compared to the traditional open procedure [28]. Proponents of the hand-assisted technique advocate that the hand port leads to decreased warm ischemia time and easier extraction through the already established gel port. A small study [29] of 48 patients confirmed the hand-assisted technique to be up to 50 min faster with a 1.3 min difference in warm ischemia time, which is likely insignificant and had no relevance on postoperative recipient creatinine levels. Other comparative studies [9, 30] have shown the length of surgery to be more dependent on surgical experience than due to the hand-assisted technique.

Total rates of complications were similar between the two techniques at 10.3% vs. 11.1% in a meta-analysis of 73 studies [26], with the pure laparoscopy having statistically significant increase of 3% in more major complications such as splenic injuries and the hand-assisted technique having an equally significant increase in minor complications such as wound infections. The hand-assisted incision is approximately 1–2 cm longer (varying by surgeon hand size) and in most studies has been associated with increased hernias and postoperative ileus with delay to oral intake, likely due to bowel manipulation and fascial stretching [5, 29, 31]. Furthermore, the hand-assisted technique limits the extraction site to one that is usable by surgical reach, at the cost of patient's preference and cosmesis.

In a comparison study [31], the laparoscopic arm had 7.5% open conversions compared to 1.7% in the hand-assisted group, although, once again, this may be due to a learning curve as the majority of conversions were due to failure to progress rather than bleeding complications. Larger studies, including a Northwestern study following their 8-year experience [32], have shown no difference in graft function between the two approaches, with no significant difference for conversion rates, intraoperative or postoperative complications, including incisional morbidity, postoperative ileus, and delayed graft function. Consequently, the decision to use one technique over the other should be left to surgeon's comfort and experience.

Retroperitoneoscopic Donor Nephrectomy

In a small study of 134 donors, retroperitoneoscopic donor nephrectomy has been shown to have similar perioperative times and complication rates as open donor nephrectomy, with no difference in graft function [33]. The theoretical benefits include reduced bowel injury and intraperitoneal complications, decreased risk of herniation, and possibly decreased operative times, once the surgeon learns to operate in the small operative field [34]. However, this technique remains confined to few centers due to smaller working space, difficult landmarks, and topography, as well as likely steeper learning curve than transperitoneal laparoscopy [33].

Earlier experience at the Cleveland Clinic [17] advocated its use on right kidneys to obviate technical difficulties with the right transperitoneal approach and the shorter renal vein, but most centers seem to have bypassed this technique, with further familiarity in transperitoneal right kidney surgery and later series disproving the earlier high rates of vascular complications for right transperitoneal donor nephrectomy.

Robotic-Assisted Laparoscopic Donor Nephrectomy

Robotic-assisted laparoscopic donor nephrectomy has also been described as a variation of laparoscopic donor nephrectomy, for surgeons where pure laparoscopic nephrectomy may not be technically feasible [35, 36]. A study of 38 robotic-assisted cases [35] using three robotic ports and one assistant port reported minimal blood loss, mean operative time of 181 ± 31.72 min, and warm ischemia time of 5.84 ± 1.97 min, while a larger study of 273 patients using robotic hand-assisted donor nephrectomy [36] had similar results with blood loss of 82 ml (range 10–1,500) and mean warm ischemia time of 98 s (range 50–200).

Laparoendoscopic Single-Port Surgery for Donor Nephrectomy

Laparoendoscopic single-site surgery has been proposed for donor nephrectomy to further reduce postoperative pain and incisions (possibly via the umbilicus), thus overall more appealing to potential donors. Its use is still experimental, with instruments for single-port surgery in their infancy and few centers with surgeons knowledgeable in its technique. A recent paper by Gill et al. described their series of four patients with median operating time of 3.3 h (range 3–5 h), minimal blood loss between 50 and 200 ml, and warm ischemia time of 6.2 min (range 4.5–8 min) [37]. Kidney retrieval is the most arduous step [38], with increased retrieval time and warm ischemia. Current evidence is encouraging but will require multicenter, randomized studies to assess its overall feasibility and safety.

Donor Surgical Complications: Unique Surgical Complications in Laparoscopic Donor Nephrectomy and Their Prevention During the Procedure

Positioning and Surgical Entry

Careful patient positioning during the surgery is the first key step in prevention of postoperative complications, associated with the flexed lateral decubutis position, and careful padding of all pressure points is vital in preventing postoperative parasthesias, nerve injuries, and muscle breakdown.

Pulmonary Edema

Unilateral pulmonary edema of the dependent lung has been reported in case reports, likely due to the prolonged lateral decubitus positioning and high intraoperative fluid requirements. In both cases described [39], intravenous fluid volume was nearly 8 L of crystalloid with urine output only 1.5–2.75 L and operating time was greater than 5 h. Diagnosis was confirmed with chest X-ray, and pulmonary edema resolved with oxygen, postoperative fluid restriction, and lasix diuresis in the recovery room.

Deep Venous Thromboembolism (DVT)

A study of 105 laparoscopic donors [40] looking specifically at DVTs with pre- and postoperative ultrasonographies confirmed a 2.3% risk of small, asymptomatic DVTs, even with the use of low molecular weight enoxaparin the night before surgery and intraoperative compression stockings. Donors are considered at low risk for DVT. Compression stocking or serial venous compression boots placed before induction of anesthesia, combined with early ambulation, are warranted. Due to the potential morbidity of DVT and pulmonary embolism, few centers continue to use preoperative anticoagulation, with the secondary risk of intraoperative bleeding.

Rhabdomyolysis

Multiple case reports [41–44] have described renal failure secondary to rhabdomyolysis, with an incidence of about 0.7% [42]. It is described as acute renal failure secondary to myoglobinuria, with an abrupt, sustained change in serum creatinine of >50% over baseline, due to underlying renal vasoconstriction, intraluminal myoglobin cast formation, and direct cytotoxicity from hemoglobin breakdown products. Rhabdomyolysis typically presents with myalgia and pigmenturia, beginning 4 h after surgery. Risk factors for patients at greatest risk include operations greater than 4 h, male sex, high muscle mass, and high BMI [41, 42]. Diagnosis is made by urinalysis with considerable blood on dipstick, but few red blood cells on microscopy. Associated laboratory findings include elevated creatinine phosphokinase (CPK), hyperphosphatemia, hyperkalemia, hypocalcemia, hyperuricemia, and metabolic acidosis. Treatment requires careful monitoring of renal function, with judicious use of alkanization and diuretics. Temporary dialysis is sometimes required. CPK usually peaks on postoperative days 1 and 2 and serum creatinine peak on day 8, but renal function may require up to 2–3 weeks for return to base level [41, 43]. Prevention is crucial, and in addition to adequate padding and expeditious surgery in those patients at high risk, the surgeon should consider not using the kidney bridge, or dropping it early, immediately after visualization of the hilum [43].

Trocar Injuries

Multiple techniques exist for initial access to begin pneumoperitoneum and laparoscopy. When the hand-assisted technique is used, the open Hasson technique is best, with a 0.06% incidence of bowel injuries [45]. However, for pure laparoscopy, the Hasson technique often results in gas leak and other access methods are quicker. Veress needle placement to establish pneumoperitoneum with subsequent optical access is used by many to reduce injuries related to trocar placement and involves fascial and muscle spreading with blunt-tipped trocars, visualizing the layers to facilitate safe insertion. With this technique a 0–0.31% injury rate has been reported in urologic laparoscopic procedures including donor nephrectomies [45, 46], with 50% of the bowel and mesenteric injuries occurring in patients with prior abdominal injuries. Injuries to epigastric vessels were also seen, requiring open ligation. Furthermore, no hernias were noted, even with fascial non-closure of all ports [46].

Renal Mobilization

As with any renal surgery, most intraoperative complications occur when the surgeon has difficulty in the careful dissection of nearby structures while mobilizing the kidney in efforts to expose the hilum.

General Anatomic Considerations

Donor nephrectomy is performed in an adrenal-sparing fashion, and a harmonic scalpel is used to maintain hemostasis while dissecting the adrenal gland off the superior renal pole. When encountered, small inadvertent injuries to the adrenal gland can be cauterized or oversewn, while large injuries may require ipsilateral adrenalectomy. The right adrenal vein is easiest to injure during this dissection, due to its short length and direct insertion into the vena cava.

Further dissection of the superior and posterior aspects of the kidney can create accidental pleural injuries resulting in pneumothorax. This is usually seen as a billowing of the diaphragm into the operative field and, when suspected, should be tested by placing irrigation near the diaphragm and asking the anesthesiologist to hyperexpand the lung to check for air bubbles. When identified, small tears can be repaired with 4-0 chromic suture. Pneumoperitoneum is temporarily reduced, a small Robinson catheter is used to evacuate air from the pneumothorax, and the final hole is closed around the Robinson catheter with a purse-string stitch as the anesthesiologist hyperexpands the lung and the Robinson removed.

Colonic injuries are also common, usually during mobilization off the anterior surface of the kidney. Mesenteric defects in the mesocolon must be avoided, and when identified they must be repaired to prevent internal herniation of small bowel through the defect. If mesenteric injury is severe enough that vascular injury is suspected, the surgeon must evaluate bowel viability for possible bowel resection. A major postoperative problem is bowel function, where ileus may prolong hospitalization and cause readmission. In fact, donors report that normal bowel function does not return for 7–10 days [16]. Narcotics and bed rest prolong slow bowel function, and some prolonged ileus may be due to unrecognized pancreatitis. Furthermore, a high level of suspicion must be reserved for internal hernia and small bowel obstruction through a mesenteric defect. Internal hernia may be differentiated from ileus based on extent of clinical presentation and confirmed with abdominal imaging. Small bowel obstruction typically presents 5–10 days after surgery and requires reoperation. With careful intraoperative vigilance, rates of intestinal hernia are 0.47% [47].

Unique to Left Kidney

Splenic injury is the second most common intraoperative injury in left laparoscopic donor nephrectomy, after vascular/hilar bleeding, with a 1.3% incidence [26]. It is usually encountered during initial exposure or kidney retraction before the splenorenal ligament has been fully divided. Mild-to-moderate splenic tears can be managed by splenorrhaphy, with assistance of hemostatic agents such as BioGlue, Surgicel, FloSeal, and fibrin sealant [48]. Splenectomy is the preferred option for extensive splenic injury, significant blood loss, hemodynamic instability, or ongoing coagulopathy. When splenectomy is performed, it is recommended that the patient is vaccinated for encapsulated organisms such as pneumococcous with the Pneumovax injection.

Injury to the pancreatic tail may also be encountered as it drapes over the renal hilum and medial aspect of the kidney. If lacerated, careful inspection must rule out injury to the pancreatic duct. If only the parenchyma is injured, it should be repaired with simple closure using *non*-absorbable suture, as the pancreatic enzymes will degrade absorbable sutures too quickly, with closed suction drainage of the area. Diet should be advanced slowly postoperatively, as mild pancreatitis and resultant ileus may ensue.

Unique to Right Kidney

Liver injury is the most common inadvertent injury during right laparoscopic donor nephrectomy, most commonly when dissecting the superior pole of the kidney or retracting the liver, especially when this instrument is not visualized by the camera. This can be avoiding by using a self-retaining tooth grasper to elevate the liver, inserted via a 5 mm trocar just below the xiphoid process and clamped to the diaphragm or the sidewall [13]. Hemostasis of the liver can usually be achieved with fulguration or packing of Surgicel, but horizontal mattress suture repair may be required for deeper injuries.

The second portion of the duodenum may be encountered by dissecting the medial aspect of the right kidney to identify the hilum. If injured, the duodenum must be closed in two layers to invert the repair. Postoperatively, nasogastric tube suction must be continued until return of normal gastrointestinal function.

Vascular Dissection and Hilar Control

Dissecting the renal vessels to obtain hilar control and vascular ligation is the portion of the laparoscopic donor nephrectomy with the greatest inherent risk, with total bleeding complication rates of up to 5% [26] and accounting for 75–83% of open conversions [16, 18, 49]. Multiple techniques exist to divide the vessels, in efforts to maximize vessel length, avoid donor bleeding, and secure the vessel stump, in an expeditious fashion, in order to minimize warm ischemia time.

Dissection and Ligation of Tributary Vessels

Obtaining maximal vessel length requires ligation of tributary veins, particularly the gonadal, adrenal, and lumbar veins. Conventional laparoscopic techniques have used clips and scissors to safely divide these veins, with judicious clip use advised to not interfere with stapler deployment and later division of the renal vein. Multiple centers have described "clipless" techniques, using the LigaSure bipolar coagulation for coaptation of vessels 3–7 mm in diameter by fusing collagen in the vessel walls to create a permanent seal [50–53]. Early studies [52] have shown the LigaSure to significantly reduce operating time (164 vs. 68 min) and blood loss (485 vs. 100 ml) by reducing sutures and number of instrument exchanges. However, in a porcine model [54], the LigaSure was deemed inferior to current clip and staple technology, as it was less reliable and required more time for vessel occlusion.

Renal Artery and Vein Division

Due to their larger caliber, bipolar energy is not an option for the renal artery and vein. Traditionally, most transplant centers have used clips to control the renal artery stump. Early experience using non-locking, 10-mm titanium clips resulted in nonsufficient vessel occlusion, requiring three titanium clips placed 2.5 mm apart on the vessel stump to obtain equal security as traditional 2-0 and 0-silk ligatures used in open nephrectomy [55] and hence limiting final vessel length. Most transplant surgeons thus used 10-mm non-absorbable polymer locking clips (Hem-o-lok clips) introduced in 1999 for the artery, typically two clips on the arterial stump and leaving the graft unclipped [4]. Bleeding typically occurs during clip placement, when the vessel has not been fully dissected circumferentially so that additional tissue prevents clip closure, or if tributary vessels are not caught and torn causing accidental bleeding [56]. In vitro studies in a porcine model [57] demonstrate the necessity to apply the Hem-o-lok at 90° to the vessel surface, with a 1 mm cuff between the clip and the vessel division to prevent burst pressure leakage or slippage. Moreover, while most centers use a stapler device on the renal vein due to its larger diameter, some centers worry about known stapler malfunction, as well as its increased cost when compared to clips [56, 58]. Some have successfully used locking clips on the renal vein, facilitating the placement of two clips by gently grasping and pulling the vein with a laparoscopic Babcock to reduce its diameter once the renal artery has been taken. In this series, there were no bleeding complications and no increase in warm ischemia time compared to stapler use when used on donor nephrectomies [58].

In April 2006, the manufacturer of Hem-o-lok clips issued a product safety warning, stating that they were contraindicated in laparoscopic donor nephrectomy for ligating the renal artery, due to nine cases of severe hemorrhage [4]. The US Food and Drug Administration (FDA) did not issue a statement, but most surgeons have switched to other forms of ligation for legal concerns. In fact, in the two cases of arterial hemorrhage resulting in donor death, both used multiple *non-locking* clips [49, 59]. Another two donors have resulted in renal failure, due to severe arterial hemorrhage, cardiac arrest, and contralateral renal failure, but again multiple *non-locking* clips were used [49]. However, in a review of the FDA database for medical devices, there were 27 total problems listed with Hem-o-lok clips, 13 of them being in urologic laparoscopy [59]. Of those 13 incidents, bleeding was the resultant problem in eight cases, with two resultant deaths, making the nephrectomy the only operation in which deaths have resulted [57, 59]. No differentiation was made between instrument failure and user error, but legal concerns exist for the continued use of clip use for control of the renal artery. A 2008 retrospective review [59] by nine institutions performing 1,695 laparoscopic nephrectomies (including 486 donors) attempted to show the safety of the Hem-o-lok clip with no incident dislodgement or failures, either intraoperatively or postoperatively, for up to 6 months after surgery.

Vascular staplers are the current alternative and have traditionally been used on the renal vein due to its diameter. The literature reports up to a 1.7% rate of overall endovascular gastrointestinal anastomosis (Endo-GIA) stapler malfunction [58], although when excluding cases of user error, primary stapler malfunction is rare at 0.3%, typically caused by interposition of clips on tributary vessels or improper usage [60]. Although rare, this failure can cause serious bleeding, often requiring open conversion to retrieve the graft and obtain hemostasis, with resultant increased morbidity to the donor and warm ischemia time for the graft. Most commonly, the Endo-GIA stapler is used, by placing six rows of overlapping staples and cutting in the middle, leaving three rows of staples on each side. The disadvantage of the Endo-GIA is an approximately 1 cm loss of vessel length and the necessity of removal of a row of staples prior to donor kidney perfusion [4]. Others advocate the use of the Endo-TA, which is a non-articulating, non-cutting stapler. If able to be positioned, it gains an extra 5 mm–1 cm in length [4, 51, 61] as it does not leave a lateral row of staples that must be trimmed, with no change in operative time or warm ischemia time [61]. The Endo-TA stapler also allows the surgeon to confirm complete ligation, using a partial cut of the vessel with scissors to confirm absence of back-bleeding, followed by completion of the cut [13]. This technique may be most useful on right-sided nephrectomies when efforts to maximize right renal vein length may cause a deficit of staples at the point where the stapler was firmly pushed against the lower edge of the vein, causing back-bleeding from the vena cava.

En bloc stapling has also been proposed by some centers, with the benefit of decreased need for hilar dissection and its potential bleeding. In a study of 163 patients [62], blood loss and open conversion trended non-significantly lower in en bloc ligation group, compared to individual stapling of the artery and vein. This technique has been hampered by the theoretical risk of arterial venous fistula (AVF), which may lead to diastolic hypertension, abdominal bruits, flank pain, and congestive heart failures. In non-donor studies, incidence of AVF has been associated with infection, inflammation, transfixation sutures, inadequate ligation, recurrent renal neoplasms, and uncontrolled bleeding. A series of 90 patients with en bloc ligation have shown no evidence of AVF at mean 34 months follow-up [62]. However, prior case reports report AVF formation up to 15 years later, and consequently, en bloc stapling should be reserved for urgent/emergent bleeding, as theoretical risk of AVF in the long term cannot be disproven.

Lymphatic Injury and Chylous Ascites

In efforts to maximize vessel length for easier graft implantation and reduced rate of graft thrombosis, extensive perihilar dissection may cause lymphatic injury and leakage. Chylous ascites as a consequence has been described in 0.5% of donors in one study [20] when interruption of major retroperitoneal lymphatic channels causes lymphoperitoneal fistula formation. Meticulous dissection with a bipolar instrument, such as the LigaSure, or clipping of lymphatic tissue is effective in sealing lymphatic tissues and preventing this complication [53, 63]. Case reports of chylous ascites [63–65] had donors present with ascitic fluid, containing a high triglyceride count when tapped, approximately 1–2 weeks postoperatively. Conservative treatment consists of a medium-chain triglyceride diet with low-fat and high-protein content, repeated paracentesis as needed, and diuretics. Second-line treatment involves total parenteral nutrition and a somatostatin analogue, with a resolution rate of 50–60% in 8–12 weeks with these conservative, medical treatments in the lymphadenectomy literature [65]. Due to the healthier nature of donors, more suitable for reintervention, one review [65] recommends surgical intervention if no resolution after 4 weeks, or if a well-visualized lymphatic fistula is seen on bipedal lymphangioram, thereby allowing small fistula to heal, while avoiding long prolonged course of conservative management for larger high-output fistula.

Secondary Sensory Complications of Vascular Dissection

Ipsilateral orchalgia or epididymitis has been reported especially in left donor nephrectomies where the gonadal vein is always ligated. A retrospective review of 145 left-sided male donors showed 9.6% incidence of ipsilateral orchalgia [66] with individual ligation of the gonadal vessels, periureteral tissue, and ureteral over the iliac artery using either surgical clips or a vascular stapler. Donors typically present on postoperative day 5, with 50% complete resolution with NSAIDs and empiric antibiotics at an average of 6.3 ± 7.2 months. Of note, no female donors from this center developed ipsilateral pelvic pain, and there were no significant differences in non-orchalgic donors with respective to operative time, blood loss, or ureteral length. A smaller study of 64 patients [67], using bipolar electrocautery, rather than clips to ligate tributary veins had 21% with ipsilateral testicular pain, including 3.4% with gonadal vein preservation. All pain resolved at a median 34 days after surgery. Larger, retrospective reviews quote rates of 1.04–1.6% orchalgia [18, 25].

The cause is unknown, but likely due to interruption in the innervation of the spermatic plexus [66] or interruption of lymphatic drainage of the testis [67]. Medical treatment with analgesics, NSAIDs, and antidepressants is advocated, with inguinal orchiectomy reserved for unrelenting medical failures and marking the most successful treatment with 73% pain relief [66].

Medial thigh cutaneous parasthesia, or even pelvic pain, has been reported secondary to entrapment of the genitofemoral nerve [66]. This typically occurs when dissecting and ligating the distal ureter and can be reduced by limiting dissection lateral to the gonadal vein when ligating the distal ureter to avoid inadvertent inclusion of the genitofemoral nerve as it exits the psoas muscle.

Injuries During Graft Extraction

Once the donor kidney has been fully dissected and the hilar vessels ligated, the goal is to extract the kidney as expeditiously as possible, for delivery to the ice slush for reperfusion by the recipient surgical team.

Bladder Perforation

Unless a hand port has been used, the kidney is extracted via a Pfannenstiel incision with blunt dissection through the peritoneum. Two reports of bladder perforations have been published [68], both with history of prior tubal ligation, and identified postoperatively with wound infection or urine leak. We recommend careful incision of the fascia and peritoneum before the hilum is ligated, with pneumoperitoneum present and the surgical assistant watching the incision with the laparoscope to ensure no injury occurs. If bladder injury is identified, the bladder should be oversewn in two layers and a Foley catheter is kept postoperatively for 1 week, or until a cystogram confirms no leakage.

Graft Injury

The donor kidney itself is sometimes extracted using an endoextraction bag via this Pfannenstiel incision. Early experiences had endobag breakage or difficult entrapment in 1.6–7% of cases [15, 69], resulting in extraction difficulty and prolonged warm ischemia time. The usual causes are failure to completely dissect the posterior attachments or upper pole of the kidney, or insufficient length of the extraction site [70]. The endoextraction bag has also directly caused kidney injury during extraction, ranging from superficial lacerations [69] to inadvertent decapsulation and grade IV laceration [71], when the kidney is caught between the firm ring of the endobag device and the peritoneal edge.

Techniques preventing graft injury during extraction include placing the kidney in the endoextraction bag and suspending the kidney in it to check for freedom from all attachments, prior to hilar vessel transection, at which point the kidney is quickly withdrawn into the bag [15]. Others insert the endoextraction bag after the colon is medially dropped, using it as a blunt retractor for the colon for assistance in exposing the renal hilum [18]. Caution should be used with this technique not to harm the bag's integrity, as well as confirming that the distal end of the metal ring does not cause injury or abrasion to the spleen or surrounding bowel. With either technique, the laparoscope can be used for direct visualization of the bag during extraction to observe potential issues and maintain proper orientation.

An alternative to the endoextraction bag altogether mimics the hand-assisted technique, while allowing a low, cosmetic incision [72]. An assistant's hand is placed through a small Pfannenstiel incision allowing maintenance of pneumoperitoneum, while at the same time allowing the assistant's hand to confirm that all attachments have been fully dissected before the hilum is divided with the kidney in hand, which is then used to extract the kidney.

Recipient Complications: Differences in Recipient Graft Function as a Result of Surgical Technique

The benefit of the recipient graft must always be another concern for the surgeon performing the laparoscopic donor nephrectomy, with all possible interventions made to maximize graft function, so long as they do not compromise the donor. Nationally, vascular thrombosis, primary non-function, and technical problems account for 0–15% loss of living donor grafts in the immediate postoperative period, compared historically to 0–8% for open donors [22, 34, 73], with 1-year graft survival rates of 93–100% and 1-year recipient survival rates of 97–100% [34]. Delayed graft function (DGF) develops in 0.2–4.5% of live donor recipients (Table 3) and is ultimately associated with increased risk of rejection and decreased graft survival [27].

Despite significant advantages for the donor, early critics worried that the laparoscopic donor nephrectomy may be associated with short-term impaired graft function. This impetus began after early reports of the laparoscopic experience reported higher incidence of delayed graft function, despite equivalent 2-year patient and graft survival [74]. More recent evidence looking at factors affecting recipient functional outcomes include donor screening criteria (female donors into male recipients and highly HLA mismatched kidneys), but no variables related to the laparoscopic procedure itself were statistically significant (prolonged pneumoperitoneum, warm ischemia time, renal artery length, or use of right kidney) [27].

Warm Ischemia Time (WIT)

The laparoscopic approach is linked to longer warm ischemia times, as to date there are no methods of cooling the donor kidney intraoperatively. A study of 469 living donors confirmed that warm ischemia is a dominant risk factor for poor early graft function, defined as delayed or slow graft function after living kidney donation (OR 1.05 per minute of WIT), and predisposes to acute rejection but not overall functional graft survival [75]. Other studies have contradicted this, with WIT not affecting early or long-term graft function at any postoperative time point, as measured by recipient serum creatinine [16, 70].

In the open nephrectomy setting, warm ischemia time of 30 min was shown to be the maximal period of arterial occlusion tolerated before permanent damage was sustained [76], and 60 min of warm ischemia has caused proximal convoluted tubule necrosis in rat studies [77].

Recent studies have also shown no significant difference in WIT between right and left laparoscopic nephrectomies, although WIT is related to difficulties with extraction and learning curve [70]. However, the critical length of WIT remains uncertain, with various reports in animal models and human donor series. It is likely that the small differences caused by the seconds of WIT encountered in laparoscopic donor nephrectomy are negligible. Nonetheless, warm ischemia time should be minimized by planning and practicing safe extraction techniques of the donor kidney.

Effects of Pneumoperitoneum on the Graft

Carbon dioxide pneumoperitoneum decreases stroke volume and cardiac output, with a compensatory increase in mean arterial pressure and systemic vascular resistance at 20 mmHg, but not at 12 mmHg [78]. Prolonged pressures >15 mmHg have also been associated with decreased renal blood flow and oliguria, but its theoretical risk on the graft has not translated into deleterious effect in graft function in multiple animal studies looking at clinical and histologic end points [79–81].

Nonetheless, most surgeons aim to keep pneumoperitoneum at minimal possible working pressures and advocate aggressive fluid hydration (> 10 ml/kg/h) to counter the negative effects of pneumoperitoneum. Others encourage increased renal perfusion with mannitol and/or dopamine hydrochloride administration [73]. These have indeed been shown to produce superior urine production and equivalent graft function compared to open donor nephrectomy [82], although studies have shown dopamine alone to be ineffective in improving renal vein blood flow or oliguria [79].

Recently this dogma of aggressive fluid hydration has been challenged and shown to have no statistical difference in short- or long-term graft function, acute rejection, or postoperative donor complications when compared to conservative goal-directed intraoperative hydration to replete perioperative dehydration and maintain physiological parameters [74]. Some studies have indicated that volume loading after establishment of pneumoperitoneum is too late to counterbalance the collapsed venal system and that the timing of fluids to be more important than the total fluid amount. Overnight prehydration and colloid bolus prior to anesthesia prevented stroke volume decrease during repositioning to the lateral position and improved creatinine clearance for about 48 h duration over controls [83, 84]. In summary, if adequate hydration is the goal, it is important to rehydrate and increase intravascular volume prior to positioning in lateral decubitus position, without overloading the patient and causing pulmonary edema [39], ileus, or wound healing complications.

Ureteral Strictures and Complications

With the early learning curve of the laparoscopic donor nephrectomy, the incidence of ureteral complications was significantly higher than open donor nephrectomy (2–11% vs. 0–6.3%), attributable to the extensive dissection close to the ureteral wall [5, 85]. It is believed that ureteral stenosis or necrosis occurs within 6 months of transplantation [86], due to impaired vascularity from the ureter from aggressive ureteral dissection.

Ureteral stricture is thought to be primarily due to impaired vascularity of the ureter, possibly as a result of harvest technique, although allograft rejection and reimplantation technique also contribute to distal ureteral ischemia. Current rates of ureteral complications are 2–6.3% [16, 18, 86] with 88% of complications occurring within the first 6 months of transplantation, and only 1 presented after 1 year [16]. In a review of donors between 1994 and 2002 [87], 12% of kidneys harvested via laparoscopic nephrectomy required percutaneous nephrostomy drainage, usually within 37 days of transplant for obstruction or fluid collection, and 4.1% eventually required ureteral reconstruction. Stricture rates were independent of warm ischemia time, operating time, and serum creatinine.

Obviously, a large component of the ureteral stricture rate is dependent on the reimplantation technique and possibly stent usage. The surgeon performing the donor nephrectomy can only provide the best possible scaffold to work with by refining ureteral dissection technique. Some reports have suggested the importance of preservation of the gonadal vein with the specimen. The rationale parallels the open nephrectomy, where the ureter is transected en bloc with the gonadal vein at the level of the iliac vessels, avoiding dissection between the ureter and the gonadal vein. An alternative gonadal-sparing technique [18] recommends blunt dissection with minimal electrocautery medial to the gonadal vein, keeping the distal gonadal vein and the mesoureter along the entire length of the ureter down to the pelvic inlet and transecting the gonadal vein at the level of the renal vein. With this modification the ureteral complication rate was decreased from 10.5 to 5.2% [18].

Non-preservation of the gonadal vein simplifies the donor dissection by giving better access to lumbar vein and allowing easier elevation of the ureter. A review of 300 patients who underwent donor nephrectomy via this technique with mean 2-year follow-up [86] proved its safety with no incidence of ureteral strictures in their series. Dissection must preserve hilar fat and periureteral tissue for blood supply, should use bipolar electrocautery when needed for minimal energy dispersion, as well as preserve any lower pole vessels encountered and the "golden triangle" between the gonadal vein stump, renal hilum, and lower pole of the kidney where the superior blood supply to the renal artery supplying the upper ureter exists [85, 86].

Donor Medical Complications

Long-Term Complications of Renal Loss and Donor Safety

Beyond surgical complications, as surgeons operating on a healthy donor, we must always keep in mind the potential medical complications we are inflicting by leaving the donor with a single healthy kidney to withstand hyperfiltration injury, hypertension, and the medical problems they will encounter in their later life. Critics have argued that the recipient's benefit in quality and quantity of life when receiving a kidney from a living donor, compared to a cadaveric kidney, may not outweigh the difference between health and disease for the donor who develops renal complications as a consequence of donation, with overall net societal disutility of the procedure [8].

Due to a lack of long-term donor follow-up, we currently rely on short-term reports from single institutions [5]. These single institution reports are flawed as they usually use head-to-head comparisons with surgeons more experienced in the older open technique and report complications that are part of the learning curve rather than the technique [5]. They also typically neglect long-term medical complications.

At least eight perioperative deaths, from unspecified causes, have been recorded after laparoscopic donor nephrectomy [5]. One report from 2005 stated that 56 of the 50,000 previous kidney donors in the United States had ultimately been listed for transplants themselves, while another 2005 report stated that 104 Americans on the current transplant list had been previous live donors [8].

A retrospective study of 736 patients with mean time of 3 ± 3.2 years since donation [88] showed that serum creatinine, systolic and diastolic blood pressure, and urinary protein all increased significantly from preoperative values. Creatinine clearance fell to 87% of preoperative values, with 6.7% falling to creatinine clearance levels less than 60 ml/ min. One donor developed end-stage renal disease. About 24.3% developed proteinuria exceeding 150 mg/24 h and 10.3% developed hypertension, requiring treatment with an ACE inhibitor. Donors who were overweight (27.8%) and obese (11.5%) postoperatively had higher incidence of diabetes and hypertension. Another study of 162 donors with mean 8-year follow-up [89] found normal residual kidney function and an incidence of non-insulin-dependent diabetes (1.2%) and hypertension (8.7%) in older patients, but this was not statistically different from the general population. A consensus is still lacking on long-term donor outcomes, as a mandatory registry combining experience with complications and long-term outcomes would provide [5]. Currently, UNOS continues to discuss creating such a national donor registry to investigate the long-term surgical and medical complications of kidney donation.

References

1. Clayman RV, Kavoussi LR, Soper NJ, et al. Laparoscopic nephrectomy: initial case report. J Urol. 1991;146:278–82.
2. Ratner LE, Ciseck LJ, Moore RG, et al. Laparoscopic live donor nephrectomy. Transplantation. 1995;60:1047–9.
3. Ratner LE, Montgomery RA, Kavoussi LR. Laparoscopic live donor nephrectomy. A review of the first 5 years. Urol Clin North Am. 2001;28:709–19.
4. Duchene DA, Winfield HN. Laparoscopic donor nephrectomy. Urol Clin North Am. 2008;35:415–24, viii.
5. Shokeir AA. Open versus laparoscopic live donor nephrectomy: a focus on the safety of donors and the need for a donor registry. J Urol. 2007;178:1860–6.
6. Nanidis TG, Antcliffe D, Kokkinos C, et al. Laparoscopic versus open live donor nephrectomy in renal transplantation: a meta-analysis. Ann Surg. 2008;247:58–70.
7. Perry KT, Freedland SJ, Hu JC, et al. Quality of life, pain and return to normal activities following laparoscopic donor nephrectomy versus open mini-incision donor nephrectomy. J Urol. 2003;169:2018–2021.
8. Glannon W. Underestimating the risk in living kidney donation. J Med Ethics. 2008;34:127–8.
9. Giessing M, Turk I, Roigas J, et al. Laparoscopy for living donor nephrectomy – particularities of the currently applied techniques. Transpl Int. 2005;18:1019–27.
10. Schlunt LB, Harper JD, Broome DR, et al. Improved detection of renal vascular anatomy using multidetector CT angiography: Is 100% detection possible? J Endourol. 2007;21:12–7.
11. Bhatti AA, Chugtai A, Haslam P, et al. Prospective study comparing three-dimensional computed tomography and magnetic resonance imaging for evaluating the renal vascular anatomy in potential living renal donors. BJU Int. 2005;96:1105–8.
12. Hsu TH, Su LM, Ratner LE, et al. Impact of renal artery multiplicity on outcomes of renal donors and recipients in laparoscopic donor nephrectomy. Urology 61: 323–327, 2003.
13. Buell JF, Edye M, Johnson M, et al. Are concerns over right laparoscopic donor nephrectomy unwarranted? Ann Surg. 2001;233:645–51.
14. Wright AD, Will TA, Holt DR, et al. Laparoscopic living donor nephrectomy: a look at current trends and practice patterns at major transplant centers across the United States. J Urol. 2008;179:1488–92.
15. Jacobs SC, Cho E, Dunkin BJ, et al. Laparoscopic live donor nephrectomy: the University of Maryland 3-year experience. J Urol. 2000;164:1494–9.
16. Jacobs SC, Cho E, Foster C, et al. Laparoscopic donor nephrectomy: the University of Maryland 6-year experience. J Urol. 2004;171:47–51.

17. Ng CS, Abreu SC, Abou El-Fettouh HI, et al. Right retroperitoneal versus left transperitoneal laparoscopic live donor nephrectomy. Urology. 2004;63:857–61.
18. Su LM, Ratner LE, Montgomery RA, et al. Laparoscopic live donor nephrectomy: trends in donor and recipient morbidity following 381 consecutive cases. Ann Surg. 2004;240:358–63.
19. Leventhal JR, Kocak B, Salvalaggio PR, et al. Laparoscopic donor nephrectomy 1997 to 2003: lessons learned with 500 cases at a single institution. Surgery. 2004;136:881–90.
20. Kocak B, Koffron AJ, Baker TB, et al. Proposed classification of complications after live donor nephrectomy. Urology. 2006;67:927–31.
21. Melcher ML, Carter JT, Posselt A, et al. More than 500 consecutive laparoscopic donor nephrectomies without conversion or repeated surgery. Arch Surg. 2005;140:835–9; discussion 839–40.
22. Sundaram CP, Martin GL, Guise A, et al. Complications after a 5-year experience with laparoscopic donor nephrectomy: the Indiana University experience. Surg Endosc. 2007; 21:724–8.
23. Breda A, Bui MH, Liao JC, et al. Association of bowel rest and ketorolac analgesia with short hospital stay after laparoscopic donor nephrectomy. Urology. 2007;69: 828–31.
24. Breda A, Veale J, Liao J, et al. Complications of laparoscopic living donor nephrectomy and their management: the UCLA experience. Urology. 2007;69:49–52.
25. Chin EH, Hazzan D, Herron DM, et al. Laparoscopic donor nephrectomy: intraoperative safety, immediate morbidity, and delayed complications with 500 cases. Surg Endosc. 2007;21:521–6.
26. Pareek G, Hedican SP, Gee JR, et al. Meta-analysis of the complications of laparoscopic renal surgery: comparison of procedures and techniques. J Urol. 2006;175:1208–13.
27. Abreu SC, Goldfarb DA, Derweesh I, et al. Factors related to delayed graft function after laparoscopic live donor nephrectomy. J Urol. 2004;171:52–7.
28. Lee KS, Hong JH, Jeon SS, et al. Comparison of graft survival in live donor nephrectomy: hand-assisted laparoscopic v open procedures. J Endourol. 2007;21:866–71.
29. Ruiz-Deya G, Cheng S, Palmer E, et al. Open donor, laparoscopic donor and hand assisted laparoscopic donor nephrectomy: a comparison of outcomes. J Urol. 2001;166:1270–3; discussion 1273–4.
30. Bargman V, Sundaram CP, Bernie J, et al. Randomized trial of laparoscopic donor nephrectomy with and without hand assistance. J Endourol. 2006;20:717–22.
31. Velidedeoglu E, Williams N, Brayman KL, et al. Comparison of open, laparoscopic, and hand-assisted approaches to live-donor nephrectomy. Transplantation. 2002;74:169–72.
32. Kocak B, Baker TB, Koffron AJ, et al. Laparoscopic living donor nephrectomy: a single-center sequential experience comparing hand-assisted versus standard technique. Urology. 2007;70:1060–3.
33. Bachmann A, Wolff T, Ruszat R, et al. Retroperitoneoscopic donor nephrectomy: a retrospective, non-randomized comparison of early complications, donor and recipient outcome with the standard open approach. Eur Urol. 2005;48:90–6; discussion 96.
34. Tooher RL, Rao MM, Scott DF, et al. A systematic review of laparoscopic live-donor nephrectomy. Transplantation. 2004;78:404–14.
35. Hubert J, Renoult E, Mourey E, et al. Complete robotic-assistance during laparoscopic living donor nephrectomies: an evaluation of 38 procedures at a single site. Int J Urol. 2007;14:986–9.
36. Horgan S, Galvani C, Gorodner MV, et al. Effect of robotic assistance on the "learning curve" for laparoscopic hand-assisted donor nephrectomy. Surg Endosc. 2007;21: 1512–7.
37. Gill IS, Canes D, Aron M, et al. Single port transumbilical (E-NOTES) donor nephrectomy. J Urol. 2008;180:637–41; discussion 641.
38. Desai M. Single-port surgery for donor nephrectomy: a new era in laparoscopic surgery? Nat Clin Pract Urol. 2009;6:1.
39. Morrisroe SN, Wall RT, Lu AD. Unilateral pulmonary edema after laparoscopic donor nephrectomy: report of two cases. J Endourol. 2007;21:760–2.
40. Biglarnia A, Bergqvist D, Johansson M, et al. Venous thromboembolism in live kidney donors – a prospective study. Transplantation. 2008;86:659–61.
41. Rehman J, Boglia J, Chughtai B, et al. High body mass index in muscular patients and flank position are risk factors for rhabdomyolysis: case report after laparoscopic live-donor nephrectomy. J Endourol. 2006;20:646–50.
42. Glassman DT, Merriam WG, Trabulsi EJ, et al. Rhabdomyolysis after laparoscopic nephrectomy. JSLS. 2007;11:432–7.
43. Kuang W, Ng CS, Matin S, et al. Rhabdomyolysis after laparoscopic donor nephrectomy. Urology. 2002;60:911.
44. Kok NF, Ijzermans JN, Schouten O, et al. Laparoscopic donor nephrectomy in obese donors: easier to implement in overweight women? Transpl Int. 2007;20:956–61.
45. Thomas MA, Rha KH, Ong AM, et al. Optical access trocar injuries in urological laparoscopic surgery. J Urol. 2003;170:61–3.
46. Siqueira TM Jr, Paterson RF, Kuo RL, et al. The use of blunt-tipped 12-mm trocars without fascial closure in laparoscopic live donor nephrectomy. JSLS. 2004;8:47–50.
47. Regan JP, Cho ES, Flowers JL. Small bowel obstruction after laparoscopic donor nephrectomy. Surg Endosc. 2003;17:108–10.
48. Biggs G, Hafron J, Feliciano J, et al. Treatment of splenic injury during laparoscopic nephrectomy with BioGlue, a surgical adhesive. Urology. 2005;66:882.
49. Friedman AL, Peters TG, Jones KW, et al. Fatal and nonfatal hemorrhagic complications of living kidney donation. Ann Surg. 2006;243:126–30.
50. Rosenblatt GS, Conlin MJ. Clipless management of the renal vein during hand-assist laparoscopic donor nephrectomy. BMC Urol. 2006;6:23.
51. Sundaram CP, Bargman V, Bernie JE. Methods of vascular control during laparoscopic donor nephrectomy. J Endourol. 2006;20:467–9; discussion 469–70.
52. Leonardo C, Guaglianone S, De Carli P, et al. Laparoscopic nephrectomy using Ligasure system: preliminary experience. J Endourol. 2005;19:976–8.
53. Constant DL, Florman SS, Mendez F, et al. Use of the LigaSure vessel sealing device in laparoscopic living-donor nephrectomy. Transplantation. 2004;78:1661–4.

54. Landman J, Kerbl K, Rehman J, et al. Evaluation of a vessel sealing system, bipolar electrosurgery, harmonic scalpel, titanium clips, endoscopic gastrointestinal anastomosis vascular staples and sutures for arterial and venous ligation in a porcine model. J Urol. 2003;169:697–700.
55. Kerbl K, Chandhoke PS, Clayman RV, et al. Ligation of the renal pedicle during laparoscopic nephrectomy: a comparison of staples, clips, and sutures. J Laparoendosc Surg. 1993;3:9–12.
56. Casale P, Pomara G, Simone M, et al. Hem-o-lok clips to control both the artery and the vein during laparoscopic nephrectomy: personal experience and review of the literature. J Endourol. 2007;21:915–8.
57. Sooriakumaran P, Kommu SS, Cooke J, et al. Evaluation of a commercial vascular clip: risk factors and predictors of failure from in vitro studies. BJU Int. 2009;103:1410–2.
58. Baumert H, Ballaro A, Arroyo C, et al. The use of polymer (Hem-o-lok) clips for management of the renal hilum during laparoscopic nephrectomy. Eur Urol. 2006;49:816–9.
59. Ponsky L, Cherullo E, Moinzadeh A, et al. The Hem-o-lok clip is safe for laparoscopic nephrectomy: a multi-institutional review. Urology. 2008;71:593–6.
60. Deng DY, Meng MV, Nguyen HT, et al. Laparoscopic linear cutting stapler failure. Urology. 2002;60:415–9; discussion 419–20.
61. Meng MV, Freise CE, Kang SM, et al. Techniques to optimize vascular control during laparoscopic donor nephrectomy. Urology. 2003;61:93–7; discussion 97–8.
62. Kouba E, Smith AM, Derksen JE, et al. Efficacy and safety of en bloc ligation of renal hilum during laparoscopic nephrectomy. Urology. 2007;69:226–9.
63. Sharma A, Heer M, Subramanaym Malladi SV, et al. Chylous ascites after laparoscopic donor nephrectomy. J Endourol. 2005;19:839–40.
64. Shafizadeh SF, Daily PP, Baliga P, et al. Chylous ascites secondary to laparoscopic donor nephrectomy. Urology. 2002;60:345.
65. Caumartin Y, Pouliot F, Sabbagh R, et al. Chylous ascites as a complication of laparoscopic donor nephrectomy. Transpl Int. 2005;18:1378–81.
66. Kim FJ, Pinto P, Su LM, et al. Ipsilateral orchialgia after laparoscopic donor nephrectomy. J Endourol. 2003;17:405–9.
67. Gjertson CK, Sundaram CP. Testicular pain following laparoscopic renal surgery. J Urol. 2008;180:2037–40; discussion 2040–1.
68. Metcalfe PD, Hickey L, Lawen JG. Bladder perforation during laparoscopic donor nephrectomy. Can J Urol. 2004;11:2456–8.
69. Helling TS. Injuries incurred during laparoscopic donor nephrectomy with the endocatch recovery system. Am J Transplant. 2006;6:1088.
70. Soulsby RE, Evans LJ, Rigg KM, et al. Warm ischemic time during laparoscopic live donor nephrectomy: effects on graft function. Transplant Proc. 2005;37:620–2.
71. Mohamed HK, Lin A, Savage SJ, et al. Parenchymal transection of the kidney inflicted by endocatch bag entrapment during a laparoscopic donor nephrectomy. Am J Transplant. 2006;6:232–5.
72. Shalhav AL, Siqueira TM Jr, Gardner TA, et al. Manual specimen retrieval without a pneumoperitoneum preserving device for laparoscopic live donor nephrectomy. J Urol. 2002;168:941–4.
73. Sasaki TM, Finelli F, Bugarin E, et al. Is laparoscopic donor nephrectomy the new criterion standard? Arch Surg. 2000;135:943–7.
74. Bergman S, Feldman LS, Carli F, et al. Intraoperative fluid management in laparoscopic live-donor nephrectomy: challenging the dogma. Surg Endosc. 2004;18:1625–30.
75. Brennan TV, Freise CE, Fuller TF, et al. Early graft function after living donor kidney transplantation predicts rejection but not outcomes. Am J Transplant. 2004;4:971–9.
76. Novick AC: Renal hypothermia: in vivo and ex vivo. Urol Clin North Am. 1983;10:637–44.
77. Jablonski P, Howden B, Leslie E, et al. Recovery of renal function after warm ischemia. I. The effect of chlorpromazine and phenoxybenzamine. Transplantation. 1983;35:535–9.
78. Mertens zur Borg IR, Lim A, Verbrugge SJ, et al. Effect of intraabdominal pressure elevation and positioning on hemodynamic responses during carbon dioxide pneumoperitoneum for laparoscopic donor nephrectomy: a prospective controlled clinical study. Surg Endosc. 2004;18:919–23.
79. McDougall EM, Monk TG, Wolf JS Jr, et al. The effect of prolonged pneumoperitoneum on renal function in an animal model. J Am Coll Surg. 1996;182:317–28.
80. Lind MY, Hazebroek EJ, Bajema IM, et al. Effect of prolonged warm ischemia and pneumoperitoneum on renal function in a rat syngeneic kidney transplantation model. Surg Endosc. 2006;20:1113–8.
81. Iwata T, Gilispie A, Jorns C, et al. Microdialysis monitoring for evaluation of the influence exerted by pneumoperitoneum on the kidney: an experimental study. Surg Endosc. 2008;22:938–42.
82. Bolte SL, Chin LT, Moon TD, et al. Maintaining urine production and early allograft function during laparoscopic donor nephrectomy. Urology. 2006;68:747–50.
83. Mertens zur Borg IR, Kok NF, Lambrou G, et al. Beneficial effects of a new fluid regime on kidney function of donor and recipient during laparoscopic v open donor nephrectomy. J Endourol. 2007;21:1509–15.
84. Mertens zur Borg IR, Di Biase M, Verbrugge S, et al. Comparison of three perioperative fluid regimes for laparoscopic donor nephrectomy: a prospective randomized dose-finding study. Surg Endosc. 2008;22:146–50.
85. Amukele SA, Belletete B, Samadi AA, et al. Urologic complications in renal transplant recipients by donor type. J Endourol. 2006;20:771–5.
86. Breda A, Bui MH, Liao JC, et al. Incidence of ureteral strictures after laparoscopic donor nephrectomy. J Urol. 2006;176:1065–8.
87. Lind MY, Hazebroek EJ, Kirkels WJ, et al. Laparoscopic versus open donor nephrectomy: ureteral complications in recipients. Urology. 2004;63:36–9; discussion 39–40.
88. Rizvi SA, Naqvi SA, Jawad F, et al. Living kidney donor follow-up in a dedicated clinic. Transplantation. 2005;79:1247–51.
89. Sansalone CV, Maione G, Aseni P, et al. Early and late residual renal function and surgical complications in living donors: a 15-year experience at a single institution. Transplant Proc. 2006;38:994–5.

Complications of Laparoscopic Partial Nephrectomy

Ahmed Ghazi, Reinhold Zimmermann, and Gunter Janetschek

Keywords Partial Nephrectomy · Laparoscopy · Hemorrhage · Complications

Introduction

With the widespread use of modern imaging techniques for various unrelated abdominal disorders, a large number of renal masses are found incidentally before producing symptoms. Previously radical nephrectomy (RN) was considered the standard treatment for such tumors [1]. RN is now considered an overtreatment for such cases and is being replaced by nephron-sparing surgery (NSS), which provides similar cancer control [2, 3]. According to the 2007 RCC guidelines of the European Association of Urology, NSS is an established curative approach for the treatment of patients with RCC <4 cm. It can be performed for selected tumors with a maximum diameter of 4–7 cm in centers with experience [4]. Laparoscopic radical nephrectomy (LRN) has become a standard of care within a short period of time. Now, many surgeons are faced with the problem that they are able to offer RN by means of laparoscopy, whereas they revert to open surgery for partial nephrectomy in cases of small renal masses. However, the experience of centers with expertise in laparoscopy shows that laparoscopic partial nephrectomy (LPN) is able to duplicate the fundamental principles of open partial nephrectomy (OPN) [5].

Laparoscopic partial nephrectomy (LPN) for solid renal masses, which was first reported in 1993 by McDougall et al. [6], has become a treatment modality that is increasingly applied by experienced laparoscopic surgeons. Originally LPN was reserved for elective indications, such as small, peripheral, and exophytic tumors, in patients with a normal contralateral kidney. With the maturity of laparoscopic reconstructive techniques, reliable hilar control, and intraoperative ultrasonography, the indications for this procedure have expanded to include both elective and imperative indications for NSS, providing similar functional and oncological outcomes [7, 8]. As this novel technique evolves, information regarding results and potential complications are only now becoming available.

The goal of LPN is to completely remove a renal tumor, obtain effective hemostasis of the tumor bed, and have an appropriate ischemia time, with minimal morbidity to avoid impairment of renal function. However, there are still concerns about the safety of this procedure. There is no doubt that ischemia time of LPN is longer than that of open surgery [3]. Furthermore, in a recent review of the complications of 2775 laparoscopies, LPN was found to be the procedure with the second highest complication rate at 28%, after laparoscopic nephroureterectomy [9]. Nevertheless, the incidence of complications in recent series from centers with expertise ranges from 9 to 33%, which is not significantly different compared to OPN (4.1–38.6%) [3, 10].

To gain a better understanding of the complications associated with a procedure, one must be oriented with the technicalities of such a procedure; we therefore briefly describe our technique of LPN before discussing its various complications.

G. Janetschek (✉)
Department of Urology, Elisabethinen Hospital Linz, Austria
e-mail: guenter.janetschek@elizabethinen.or.at

R. Ghavamian (ed.), *Complications of Laparoscopic and Robotic Urologic Surgery*,
DOI 10.1007/978-1-60761-676-4_12,

Surgical Technique

When we started LPN about 15 years back, it was performed exclusively without hilar control selectively for exophytic tumors not exceeding a diameter of 2 cm. Hemostasis was achieved by bipolar coagulation or argon beam coagulator and additional use of fibrin glue for definitive tissue closure [11]. Since 2001 we use ischemia routinely and have given up using the former technique almost completely, shifting to the resection of larger tumors and, in particular, establishing a completely different concept for LPN [12]. Now it is of great importance to have control of the vessels until the procedure is finished. A preoperative scan with contrast and 3D reconstruction or angio-MRI was used to evaluate tumor location, depth of invasion, proximity to the renal sinus or the hilum, and vascular anatomy. Patient positioning is similar to a classical transperitoneal laparoscopic radical nephrectomy. However, trocar placement varies according to the location of the tumor and the approach (transperitoneal or retroperitoneal) used.

Control of the Vessels

Following mobilization of the colonic flexure, the renal hilum is approached exactly as with radical nephrectomy. The first crucial step in LPN would be dissection and control of the hilum. The renal vein is dissected completely, and the renal artery is left completely undissected within the surrounding connective tissue. Leaving the artery within the surrounding connective tissue a trauma to the intima becomes very unlikely. For induction of ischemia we use a self-made Rummel tourniquet consisting of a 3.5-cm piece of a silicone drainage tube (10 F) and a 18-cm vascular loop folded over once to form a U loop (Fig. 1). The renal vein and the artery with its surrounding connective tissue are looped separately and the tourniquet secured internally by a Hem-o-lok clip (Weck Closure Systems, Research Triangle Park, NC, USA) without inducing ischemia (Figs. 2 and 3).

Tumor Excision

Complete mobilization of the kidney outside the Gerota's fascia is a prerequisite for precise excision of the tumor and reconstruction of the parenchyma. The fat overlying the tumor is widely excised and introduced into an organ bag for later removal. An incision line, which is about 5 mm away from the tumor, is marked with monopolar current. An intraoperative laparoscopic ultrasound probe is a valuable adjunct during this step. Intravenous mannitol (200 ml, 20%) is infused 15 min prior to arterial occlusion. Warm ischemia time is induced by pulling the vascular loop through the silicone tube to entrap the vessels. The tube is then secured under tension with a second Hem-o-lok clip (Fig. 4). Under nearly a bloodless field, tumor excision is done using cold Endo-Scissors. The aim is to achieve a perpendicular incision through the whole layer of the parenchyma. The tumor can be elevated from the tumor bed by placing countertraction with the suction cannula, which also simultaneously aspirates the blood and thereby maintains a clear operative field (Fig. 5). The excised tumor is immediately entrapped within a spring-loaded organ bag left in the abdomen until the end of the procedure.

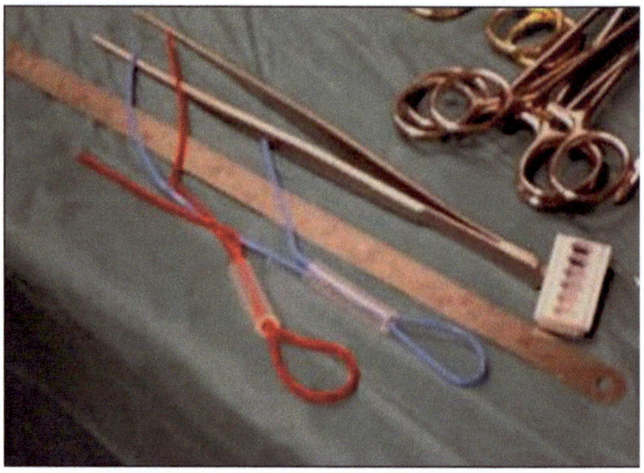

Fig. 1 The self-made Rummel tourniquet for temporary occlusion during laparoscopic partial nephrectomy; the different colors help differentiate the renal artery and vein tourniquets intraoperatively

Reconstruction

Renal repair is started by approximating the interstitial tissue (medulla) using a running 3-0 Vicryl suture with a 26.4-mm 5/8 needle. This suture is secured on both sides with a resorbable Lapra-TY II1 clip

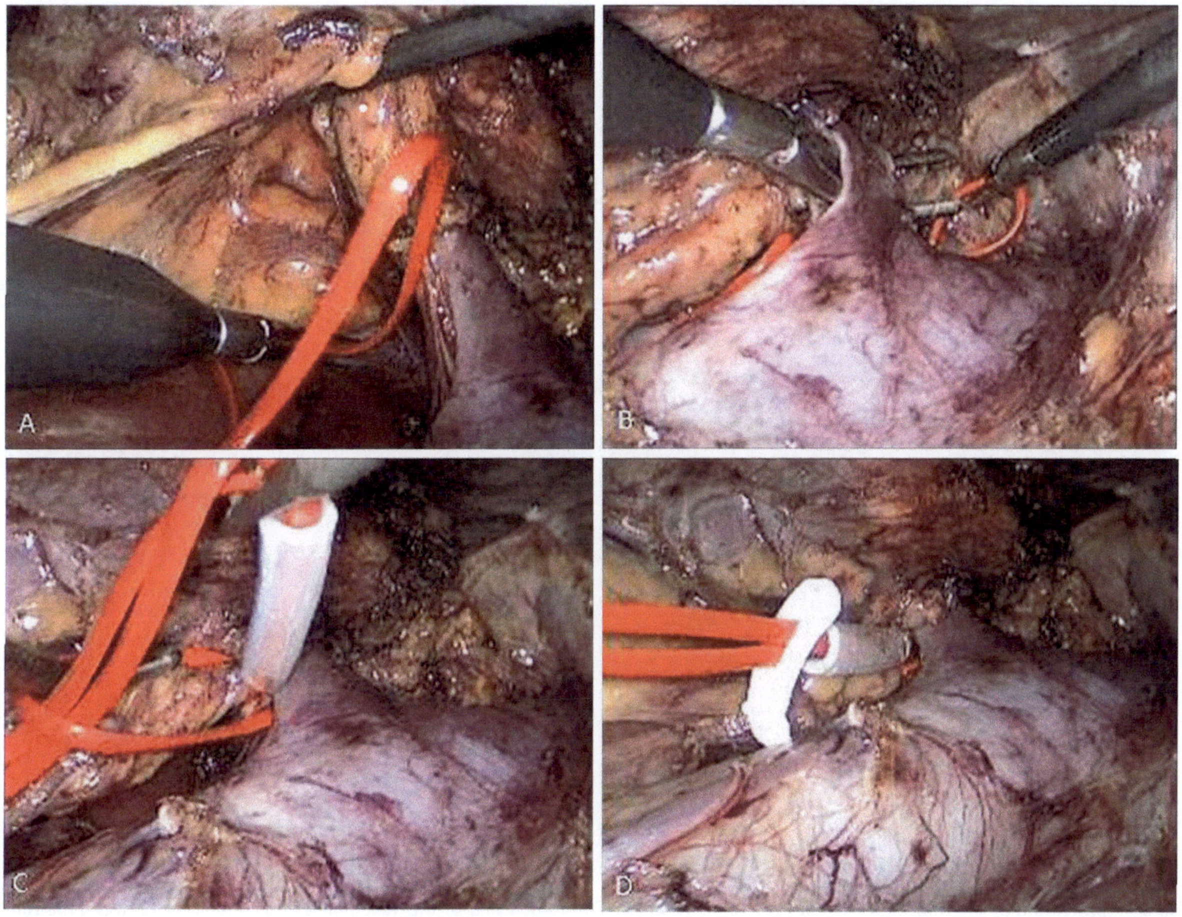

Fig. 2 Application of the tourniquet around the renal artery. (**a**) The folded end of the vascular loop is passed behind both the renal artery and the vein. (**b**) The vascular loop is passed in between the renal artery and the vein. (**c**) Creating a loop around the renal artery. (**d**) Final position of the tourniquet, without induction of ischemia

(Ethicon2, Cincinnati, Ohio, USA) (Fig. 6). This suture achieves closure of the collecting system and the interstitial renal tissue as well as hemostasis. Next, the parenchymal edges are approximated with a second running suture which is applied through the whole thickness of the renal parenchyma, using a Vicryl 1 running suture with an M04 needle. On the terminal end of this suture an XL Hem-o-lok clip is placed. A knot behind it prevents the clip from slipping off. Underneath the suture a bolster of oxidized regenerated cellulose (Tapotamp1) is placed (Fig. 7). This bolster is hemostatic by itself, but also provides hemostasis by pressure on the vessels in the interstitial layer. At each exit point of the parenchyma the suture is tightened and secured by the XL Hem-o-lok clip (Fig. 8). The last stitch is secured by a Lapra-Ty clip in addition to the Hem-o-lock clip. On completion of the renal repair, the second Hem-o-lock clip securing the tourniquet under tension is removed using a Harmonic scalpel. This method allows restoration of renal perfusion while maintaining integrity of the tourniquet around the renal artery, if rapid emergency re-occlusion of the vessels is needed. Recently, we have adopted another innovation. Perfusion is reinstituted after the first parenchymal stitch and the repair is then continued. Following repair, fibrin glue (Tissocul Duo Quick1; Baxter) is applied over the suture line for additional security to avoid delayed bleeding. The special applicator also allows injection of the fibrin directly between the approximated parenchymal rims. The remnants of Gerota's fascia are closed and the kidney is pexed to the lateral abdominal

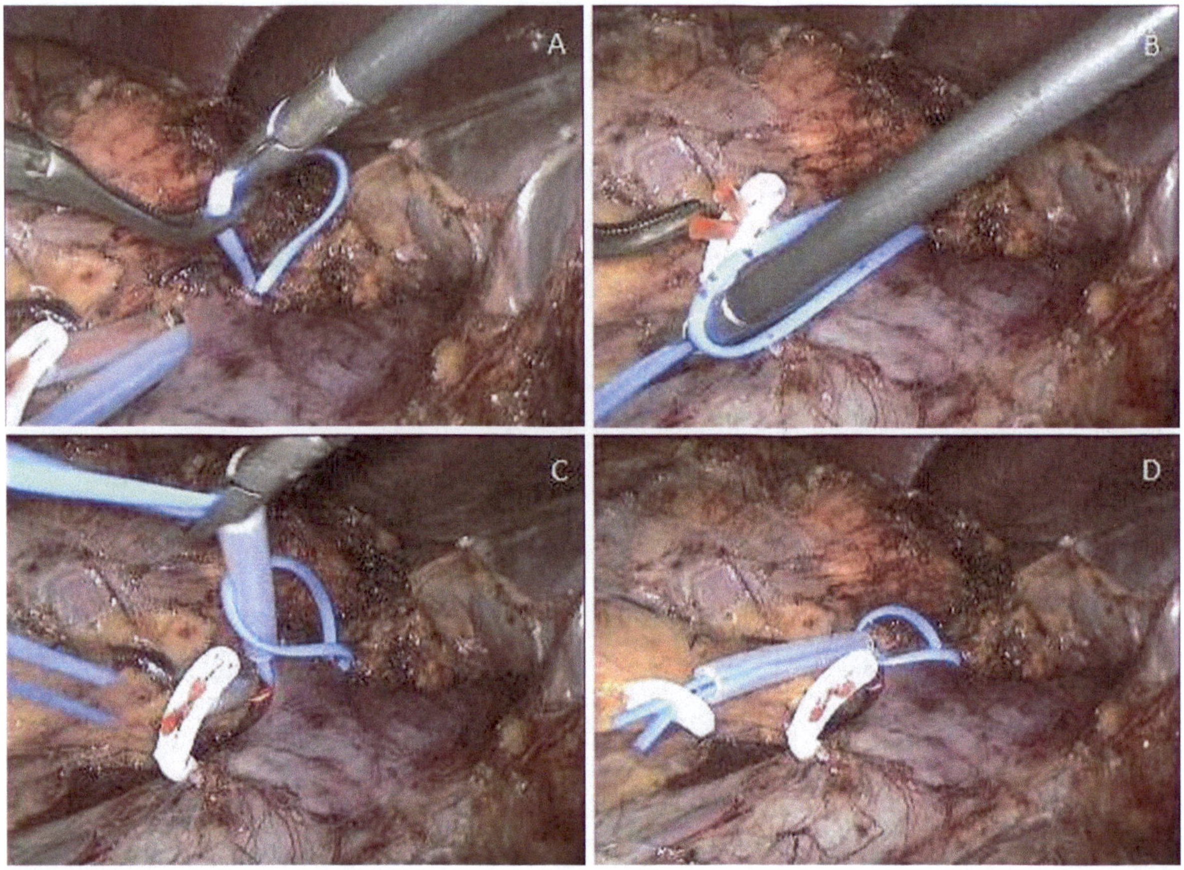

Fig. 3 Application of the tourniquet around the renal vein. (**a**) The folded end of the vascular loop is passed in between the renal artery and the vein. (**b** and **c**) Creating a loop around the renal vein. (**d**) Final position of both tourniquets

wall to avoid torsion. Next, the colon is brought back in its original position and also fixed. A Jackson-Pratt drain is placed routinely. The two specimens are extracted within the organ bags through a 2–3-cm muscle splitting extension of the lower abdominal port site incision.

Follow-Up

Before discharge, ultrasonography of the renal unit is performed routinely. Follow-up at 3 months and then annually thereafter include physical examination and CT or MRI scanning. Renal function was evaluated by determination of serum creatinine and renal scintigraphy with 99mTc-mercaptoacetyltriglycine (99mTc-MAG3).

Complications During LPN

As previously described, LPN is a technically challenging procedure, requiring not only expert laparoscopic skills but also precise intracorporeal suturing to achieve hemostasis and reconstruction of the kidney, within a reasonable ischemic period. Even in expert hands, this procedure has been shown to have a potentially high complication rate [13]. Specifically, bleeding requiring transfusion, urinary leakage, and positive margins are some of the most concerning complications [14]. Also, the need for clamping of the hilum has raised the issue of possible renal injury related to warm ischemia [15, 16]. A complete understanding of these complications is therefore crucial in preventing them.

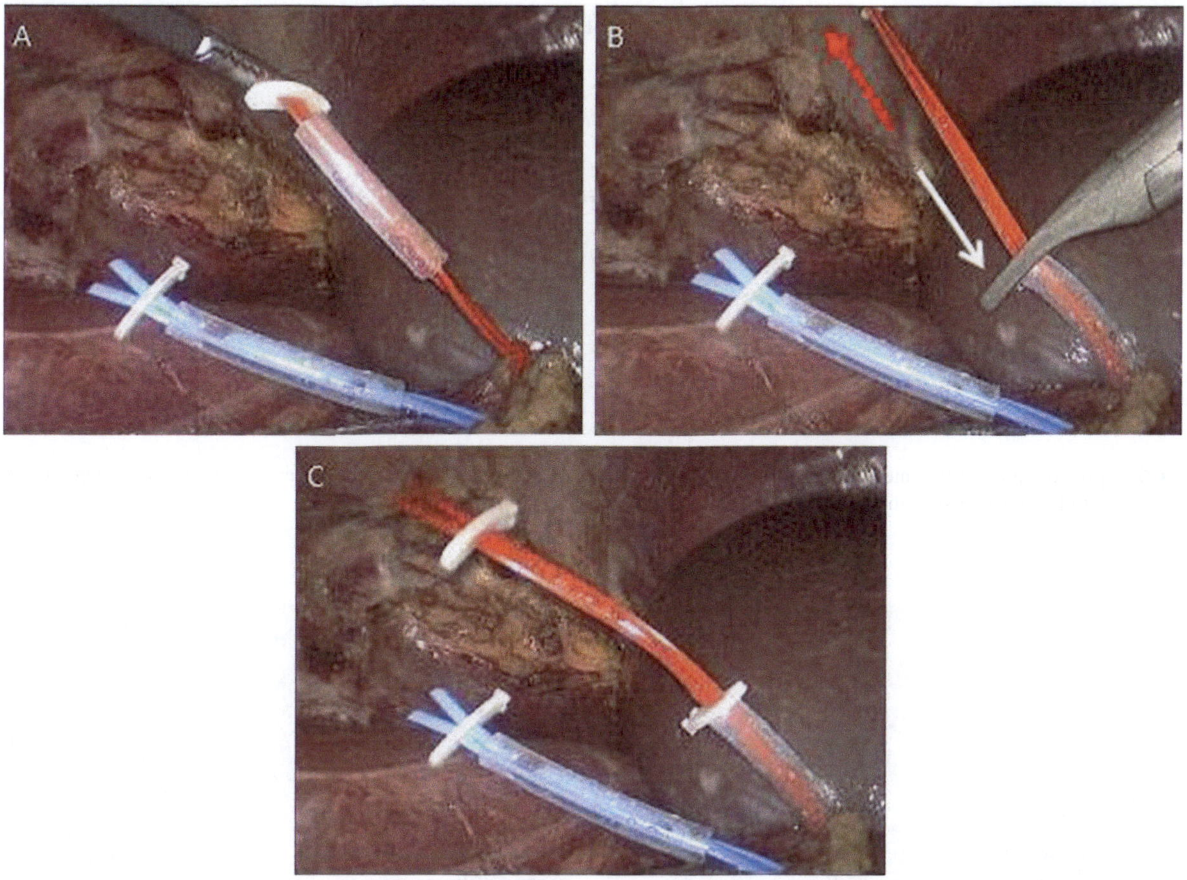

Fig. 4 Induction of ischemia using the Rummel tourniquet. (**a**) The vascular loop is pulled through the silicone tube to entrap the vessels. (**b**) Application of a second Hem-o-lok clip under tension (the *arrows* demonstrate the traction and countertraction forces applied simultaneously to avoid injury to the artery). (**c**) Final position of the tourniquet for vascular occlusion

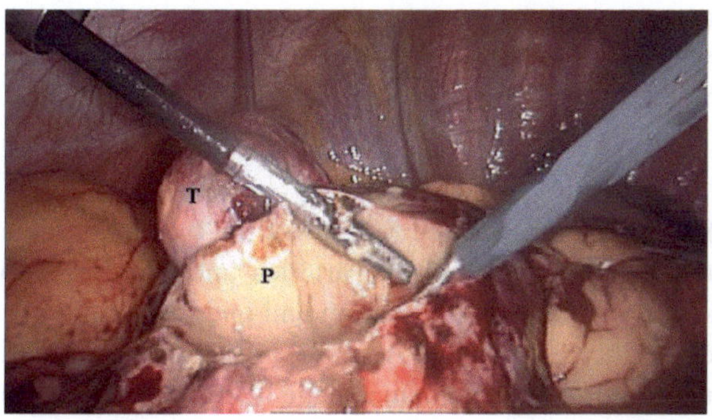

Fig. 5 Excision of the tumor in a relatively bloodless field. T, tumor; P, parenchymal edge

In this context the particular spectrum of complications occurring in LPN is to be described based both on the experiences of a single high-volume laparoscopic center and on the basis of the current literature (Table 1).

Hemorrhage

Hemorrhage from the partial nephrectomy bed is a vital concern intraoperatively and postoperatively. In general, the reported hemorrhage rate fluctuates strongly from 9 to 33% [13, 17–20]. However, it has to be emphasized that not all authors discriminate between intra- and postoperative hemorrhage.

Intraoperative Bleeding

Intraoperative parenchymal hemorrhage can occur during two distinct steps of the operation, each of which has a distinct etiology, that is, (1) during parenchymal

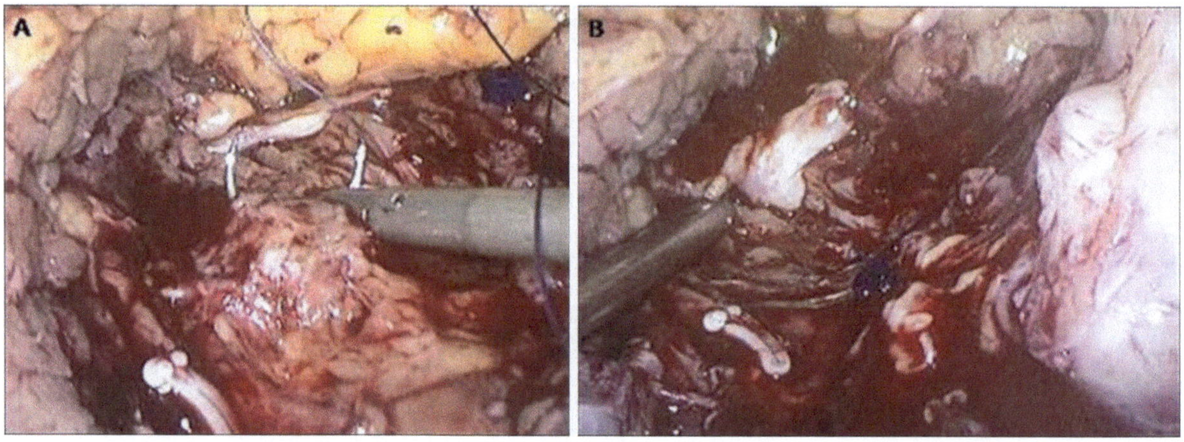

Fig. 6 Approximation of the interstitial tissue (medulla). (**a**) Passage of the needle secured at its end with a PDS locking clip. (**b**) Final view following approximation of the interstitial tissue

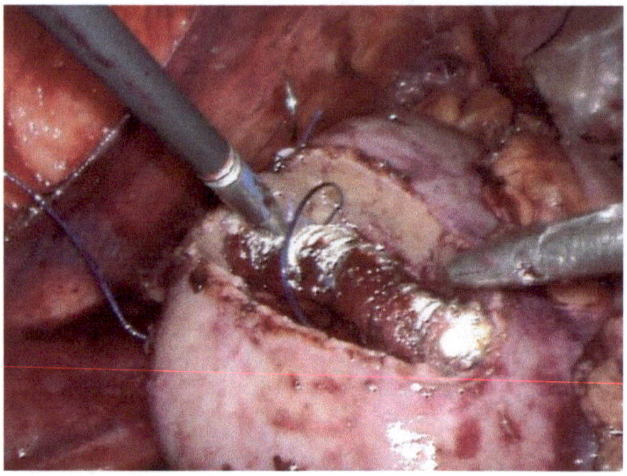

Fig. 7 Renal parenchymal repair using a running suture. The distal end is secured by a non-resorbable clip (Hem-o-lok). Underneath the suture a bolster (Tapotamp) is placed

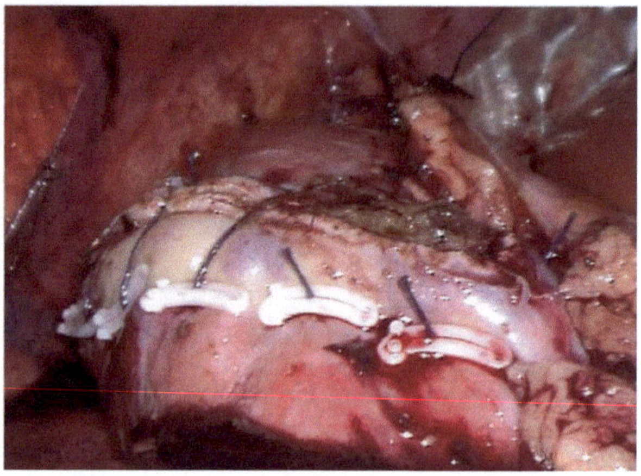

Fig. 8 Renal parenchymal repair is completed. The running suture is tightened and secured by non-resorbable clips (Hem-o-lok)

resection due to inadequate hilar clamping and (2) upon renal revascularization due to inadequate suture repair of the partial nephrectomy bed. Inadequate hilar clamping can occur due to clamp malfunction or a missed renal artery.

The intraoperative blood loss is generally stated to be only minimal to modest. Authors of large series appraise volumes on average between 150 and 250 cc [21]. Overall intraoperative hemorrhage occurred in 3.5% of 200 patients reported by Ramani [13]. However, these 3.5% had a mean blood loss of 1425 cc. In three of seven cases a malfunction of a bulldog clamp was the reason for the bleeding, while two patients had multiple arteries unknown prior to surgery. One open conversion and one LRN had to be done due to bleeding. Abukora [12] informs about a major intraoperative hemorrhage rate of 1.3% (severe) and 2.6% (minor) which was in one case caused by sideslip of a laparoscopic Satinsky clamp and by splenic injury in the second. The malfunction of the Satinsky clamp resulted in conversion to open nephrectomy. However, the rate of transfusion, conversion, and reoperation is overall very low with data ranging from about 2% to not more than 6%.

Table 1 Complications in the largest series of laparoscopic partial nephrectomy [27]

Author	No. of patients	Overall complications (%)	Hemorrhage (%)	Urine leak (%)	Renal failure (%)
Ramani	200	66 (33.0)	20 (10.0)	9 (4.5)	4 (2.0)
Simmons	200	38 (19.0)	11 (5.5)	4 (2.0)	1 (0.5)
Wright	49	7 (14.3)	1 (2.0)	4 (2.1)	0
Venkatesh	123	26 (21.1)	3 (2.4)	13 (10.6)	0
Schiff	66	6 (9.0)	1 (1.5)	2 (3.0)	0
Link	217	27 (12.4)	4 (1.8)	3 (1.4)	3 (1.4)
Bollens	39	12 (30.7)	1 (2.5)	3 (7.7)	0
Abukora	78	23 (29.5)	6 (7.7)	5 (6.4)	0
Porpigilia	90	22 (24.4)	7 (7.8)	4 (4.4)	0
Total	1062	227 (21.4)	54 (5.1)	45 (4.2)	7 (0.7)

Postoperative Bleeding

Acute

Only a minority of authors discriminate between acute, postoperative, and delayed occurrence of hemorrhage. Simmons reports about four postoperative events (2%) resulting exclusively from surgical bleeding and blood loss within a range from 200 to 1000 cc [21]. Two patients had to return to operation room, one was managed laparoscopically and the other by open surgery, both without loss of kidney. Further, five patients developed delayed hemorrhage between postoperative days 7–14. Reasons forming the basis of the bleeding remained unclear in three cases: one patient suffered from a fall with subsequent bleeding and one more was diagnosed with a pseudoaneurysm. One of these patients had to undergo nephrectomy and three were controlled by transfusion only. The patients with pseudoaneurysms were successfully treated by angioembolization [21].

Delayed

In the series by Simmons there were four patients (2%) with postoperative bleeding who became symptomatic at day 1 (0–1) [21]. Their blood loss was on an average 425 cc: one had an open nephrectomy, one was operated laparoscopically, and two were managed solely by transfusion. On the other hand, five patients (2.5%) endured delayed bleeding on average at day 12 (7–16). This led to open surgery in one case, one had angioembolization of a pseudoaneurysm, and three were managed with transfusion. In our series there was only one patient (1.3%) with delayed bleeding who could be managed conservatively (12). Of the complications reported by Ramani [13], four (2%) patients had postoperative bleeding on the second day after surgery (4). Three received transfusion and one was successfully treated with bed rest. In another eight patients (4%), delayed bleeding occurred on an average at day 16 following surgery. Only two (1%) had to undergo open reoperation, while the rest were treated conservatively, including transfusion. In a smaller series describing several modifications of the LPN technique, only one perirenal hematoma occurred (4%) without the requirement of further measures like transfusion or surgical interventions [22]. Link has seen three postoperative bleeds (1.4%) but without providing further details [12].

Management

When a postoperative hemorrhage is diagnosed, the management chosen depends on the severity at presentation [21, 23, 24]. Depending on the presentation, immediate postoperative bleeding may be managed with transfusion and observation or may necessitate reoperation for surgical hemostasis [21, 24]. We recommend an attempt at laparoscopic management if a second-look surgery becomes mandatory. Usually one does not encounter severe hemorrhage with this approach. A vascular injury such as pseudoaneurysm or arteriovenous fistula may cause a sudden onset of bleeding into the collecting system, several days after surgery and following an uneventful postoperative course. Such bleeding is best treated with selective angioembolization [25] (see Chapter 5, p. 54, Fig. 7).

Prevention

The most likely causes of intraoperative hemorrhage were malfunction of the bulldog clamp (3.5%), multiple arteries (1.5%), and Satinsky clamp malfunction (0.5%). The reasons for postoperative and delayed hemorrhage remained unclear in the majority of cases [13]. However, the most likely source of postoperative and delayed hemorrhage would be the partial nephrectomy bed and therefore adequate control of this bed is vital for prevention of bleeding. To obtain the optimal hemostatic effect, the interstitial tissue (medulla) is approximated using a running suture, which not only provides adequate closure of the collecting system but is also considered a fundamental step in hemostasis. The surgeon must be cautious that this suture does not reach too deep into the interstitial tissue to avoid damage of underlying renal vessels. Such a vascular injury may result in arteriovenous fistula or formation of a pseudoaneurysm, which may be potential sources of bleeding. Furthermore, the second running suture for approximation of the parenchyma edges must be applied through the whole thickness of the renal parenchyma and cinched down tightly over the bolsters. This provides compression of the parenchyma incorporated within the suture path as well as approximation of the cut parenchymal edge against the bolster, thereby achieving hemostasis. However, care must be taken that the suture is always pulled in a right angle to the parenchyma, otherwise it may tear through the tissue resulting in an injury which is difficult to repair. In addition, a majority of surgeons perform LPN with the aid of hemostatic agents and/or sealants under a bolster to prevent bleeding and urine leak [24]. These agents include gelatin matrix thrombin tissue sealant (FloSeal; Baxter Healthcare, Deerfield, IL, USA), fibrin glue (Tisseel; Baxter Healthcare, Deerfield, IL, USA), bovine serum albumin-based adhesive (BioGlue; CryoLife, Kennesaw, GA, USA), cyanoacrylate glue (Glubran; General Enterprise Marketing,Viareggio, Lucca, Italy), and oxidized regenerated cellulose (Surgicel; Ethicon, Somerville, NJ, USA). Only when used in conjunction with the primary measurements described will they effectively reduce the incidence of bleeding and urine leakage [2, 12, 14, 17, 26].

Regarding hilar control, different techniques can be utilized, namely the laparoscopic bulldog, Satinsky clamp, and the Rummel tourniquet (5-mm umbilical tape and 10-F silicon tape). The use of the bulldog clamp can be dangerous because it may sideslip during the procedure, an event which was previously discussed. Furthermore, it can be reasonably time consuming to remove the bulldog clamps particularly in the event of a perihilar bleeding which can lead to a prolonged ischemia time. The Satinsky clamp harbors the additional risk of an incomplete occlusion of the vessels mainly in the situation that a small vessel lying in the distal part of the clamp may remain unoccluded. This may result in unforeseen bleeding from the resection area and venous congestion. In this context we have made the decision to use, now in our center, solely the Rummel tourniquet. The tourniquet once placed is safe and reliable (no possibility of slippage), ensures permanent control of the vessels, and can be left in place till the end of the procedure without any disadvantageous effect, allowing rapid reclamping in cases of inadvertent bleeding. In addition, no supplementary trocar is required and several tourniquets could be applied without problems. The only essentially slight restriction is that the use of the tourniquet requires some more dissection of the vascular hilus which may result in a longer operation time. However, this is crucial, and the length of ischemia time is not influenced by this measure at all. Finally, the authors advocate complete bed rest for 24 h postoperatively, followed by 2 weeks of restricted physical activity in an attempt to minimize physical jarring of the freshly operated renal remnant.

Urinary Leakage

In the large majority of patients who develop a urinary fistula, the pelvicalyceal system had been entered intraoperatively requiring suture repair. It can be considered as a typical by-product of NSS and is not specific for LPN at all. The frequency of urinary leakage occurrence varies between 1.5 and 4.5% [3]. Therefore, it has to be considered as the second most frequent complication following LPN.

Ramani [13] reported an overall incidence of urine leakage of 4.5% out of a series of 200 patients, of whom 89% had intraoperative pelvicalyceal entry requiring suture repair . Management involved cystoscopic placement of a double-J stent in eight cases, two of whom also required CT-guided percutaneous drainage. One asymptomatic patient was treated expectantly. Operative re-exploration was not required in any of the patients. In another cohort also involving 200 patients, Simmons and Gill [21] reported urinary leak in four (2%) patients. In all patients, intraoperative calyceal entry was identified by retrograde injection of methylene blue via a ureteric catheter placed preoperatively. Postoperative management was either by stenting of the ureter in three or CT-guided percutaneous drainage in one. The duration of stenting ranged from 2 to 6 months. The authors reported two consecutive cohorts [12, 22] in which 3.8% (3 of 78 patients) and 0% (0 of 25) of patients developed urinary leakage postoperatively; in both cohorts, methylene blue instillation through a ureteric catheter was not used to identify violation of the collecting system and repair was performed by approximating the interstitial tissue (medulla) using a running suture. The leak was managed conservatively in three patients and settled within 2 weeks.

In a large series of LPN, urinary leakage was diagnosed in 3.1% of the laparoscopic cases. The management was in almost 92% conservatively; however, in two cases a nephrectomy had to be done.

Management

The time of first manifestation is of broad variability and ranges from only few days after surgery to several months [13]. Not all patients become symptomatic but many are diagnosed only by chance. The management is predominantly endoscopic by insertion of a stent for usually 1–2 months (range in the literature after LPN 30–90 days) [13]. Percutaneous drainage is required only in exceptional cases because the urinary drainage achieved by the stent is sufficient for closure of the urinary collecting system defect. Rarely, a nephrectomy may be the definitive option when no other treatments have succeeded in resolving the leakage [7].

Prevention

It is well documented in the literature that the depth of the lesion is associated with increased injuries to the collecting system [23, 24, 27, 28]. Although routine preoperative placement of ureteral stent is not a common practice [27], few authors have suggested an intraoperative placement of a single J externalized ureteral stent for retrograde injection of methylene blue to assist with collecting system identification and repair [28]. Recently routine placement was eliminated and used only in select patients when there is a higher likelihood to enter the collecting system (i.e., for endophytic and hilar tumors) [29]. However, with experience, any calyceal entry can be identified without the use of a ureteral catheter [30]. We advocate such an approach and the interstitial suture as described before is very effective for this purpose, keeping our fistula rate as low as 1.5% [12]. The suture within the interstitial layer develops hemostatic effects as well. The use of hemostatic agents and/or sealants during LPN has been reported to decrease the incidence of urine leak as well [17, 24].

Positive Surgical Margins (PSMs)

To achieve acceptance as the standard of care in nephron-sparing surgery the laparoscopic approach must achieve the oncological standards attained by the open approach. Although LPN has many advantages, they must not come at the expense of adequate cancer control. The positive margin rate of 3.5% is comparable to that in open series of partial nephrectomy (0–14.3%) [14, 31–34].

Breda et al. [35] recently performed a survey on LPN. Over 855 cases were collected, and 21 cases (2.4%) were identified with positive margins. The mean tumor size was 2.7 cm. Response to the positive margin was not uniform, with 14 patients undergoing immediate nephrectomy and 7 followed expectantly. Long-term outcomes in these seven patients were not available.

Similarly, Permpongkosol et al. [36] reported 511 LPNs performed by two surgeons and found nine patients (1.8%) with a positive margin during a mean follow-up of 40 months. Comparable to all LPN series, mean tumor size was 2.8 cm. Two patients were treated with completion radical nephrectomy, neither with identifiable tumor in the nephrectomy specimen. One von Hippel Lindau (VHL) patient died of metastatic RCC disease, and the remaining six patients were disease-free at median follow-up of almost 3 years. Because oncologic outcomes of LPN must match the standards of OPN, the recent report of 5-year outcomes by Lane and Gill [37] was a crucial milestone.

In this cohort of 56, only one had a positive surgical margin and this patient remains disease free at greater than 6.5 years follow-up. The vast majority were pT1a, with a mean tumor size of 2.9 cm. Overall and cancer-specific survival rates at 5 years were 86 and 100%, respectively. The authors acknowledge the limitations inherent in their analysis, particularly that 5-year data were applicable to only 37 patients with malignancy.

The authors [12] reported their 10-year experience with LPN in 78 patients, including unclamped LPN in 29 and clamped LPN in 49 (cold ischemia in 24 and warm ischemia in 25 patients). The mean tumor size was 1.97 and 2.2 cm in unclamped and clamped groups, respectively. At a mean follow-up of 24 and 12 months for the clamped and unclamped groups, respectively, there were no recurrences. Frank et al. [38] compared the outcomes of patients with central and peripheral tumors treated with LPN. After LPN the positive margin rate was similar for central and peripheral tumors, leading to the conclusion that the position of the tumor does not predict positive margin outcomes. Furthermore, the mean tumor sizes in previous studies of LPN have been small (2.6–3.3 cm), suggesting a potential effect of tumor size in the attainment of negative surgical margins [7, 14, 29, 31, 39].

Management

Tumor at the surgical margin suggests incomplete cancer removal, potentially increasing the risk of local or distant recurrence. Therefore, the treatment of patients with a positive surgical margin remains a challenge, with controversy persisting over the need for more rigorous follow-up or for immediate adjunctive therapy including repeat partial nephrectomy or completion of nephrectomy. Recent studies addressing the impact of PSM in partial nephrectomy specimens have suggested that a PSM does not necessarily indicate residual disease [14, 35, 40]. Therefore, select patients with a positive surgical margin may be safely offered vigilant monitoring [14, 35, 41]. However, more data are required before this option can be advocated.

Prevention

PSMs during LPN are due to either the inadequate sectioning of the tumor or the presence of multicentric tumors not identified during investigation [42]. Detailed three-dimensional preoperative imaging and intraoperative ultrasound are helpful in this regard. Nevertheless, tumor resection in a bloodless field to maintain visual confirmation of normal parenchyma at the resection bed remains the primary measure in prevention of PSMs. This can only be achieved under ischemic conditions with hilar vascular control. During ischemia normal renal tissue and tumor can be distinguished precisely so that complete resection without violation of the tumor can be continuously monitored. This is of utmost importance during resection of central tumors closely related to the renal vasculature when adequate surgical margins are difficult to achieve. It has also been documented that the absolute width of normal parenchyma excised has no impact on long-term disease progression, provided that the surgical bed is free of residual tumor [31, 43].

Warm Ischemia Time (WIT)

As previously discussed, clamping the renal hilum during LPN is considered a fundamental part of the operation; doing so diminishes blood loss and obtains a "dry" field such that one can perform precise tumor excision, visualize the collecting system, and repair it in case of calyceal entry [44, 45]. Despite the visualization offered by hilar control, warm ischemia remains a concern because prolonged ischemia may adversely affect renal function. There are incomplete data regarding the maximum warm ischemia time (WIT) compatible with preservation of renal function; however, 30 min is historically the generally safe accepted limit, under which full recovery of renal function is expected [46, 47]. The safety of this limit in humans is supported by analysis of a series of LPN after which dimercapto-succinic acid scans performed showed no loss of renal function [45, 48, 49]. Functional recovery appears to occur within hours after 20 min of warm ischemia and days after 30 min, and may take several weeks after 60 min of clamping [47].

Porpiglia et al. [15] performed a prospective study in 18 patients who underwent a LPN with a WIT >30 min. The authors found that the loss of renal function was maximal between 32 and 42 min. The statistical analysis demonstrated that the loss of function evaluated by serum creatinine, GFR, and renal scintigraphy was not influenced by pathologic lesion size, patient age, or presence of comorbidities but was significantly influenced by the duration of warm ischemia ($p < 0.05$). They concluded that kidney damage occurs when warm ischemia is >30 min and that efforts should be made to limit warm ischemia to <30 min. Desai and coworkers [48] recently also evaluated the impact of warm ischemia on renal function in 179 patients after LPN. The authors concluded that pre-existing azotemia and advanced age increased the risk of postoperative kidney dysfunction if the warm ischemia time exceeded 30 min. On the other hand, Bhayani et al. [50] underwent LPN in a total of 118 patients with a normal contralateral kidney. Patients were divided into three groups based on WIT (no renal occlusion, warm ischemia less than 30, and warm ischemia greater than 30 min). Using only serum creatinine levels, they demonstrated that a WIT up to 55 min does not influence long-term renal function after LPN. Thus, during LPN efforts to minimize warm ischemia are important but they should not jeopardize cancer control, hemostasis, or collecting system closure. However, using only serum creatinine levels as an indicator of renal damage in patients with a normal contralateral kidney is meaningless and can be reliable only in cases with solitary kidneys. Gill et al. [51] reported that the postoperative decrease in renal function following LPN in solitary kidneys was impacted by several factors including a WIT of more than 30 min (when comparing 30 min or less vs. more than 30 min of warm ischemia, postoperative serum creatinine increased from the baseline preoperative value by 15% vs. 43%).

Management

According to Rocca Rossetti [52], warm ischemia in open surgery can be classified as follows: (1) <10 min – harmless; (2) up to 30 min – generally reversible lesions; (3) >30 min – risk of irreversible parenchymal lesions increasing rapidly with the ischemic time; and (4) >60 min – irreversible lesions. Therefore, the only actual means of preventing irreversible renal damage is to keep WIT within the acceptable safe limit of 30 min, or even within a more secure and less injurious limit of 20 min.

Prevention

Experts in LPN have shown that ischemia times are longer with the laparoscopic approach as compared to open surgery [5, 12, 44]. Achieving resection of the tumor and closure of the renal parenchyma with hemostasis within 30 min during LPN requires a strong laparoscopic technique. The replacement of knotting by clips not only has the advantage to speed up the procedure but also has the additional advantage that the large surface of the clips allows perfect hemostasis by applying high pressure to the renal parenchyma. This technique is advocated not only by the authors but also by several surgeons [4, 22, 53].

Recently, we have adopted another innovation introduced by Baumert et al. [54]. Perfusion is reinstituted after the first parenchymal stitch and the repair is then continued. We never have experienced severe bleeding by doing so. On the contrary, bleeding spots in the parenchyma mark potential bleeding sources. They indicate where the next suture should be placed so that the risk of delayed hemorrhage is decreased. In our experience, early declamping substantially reduced the WIT by about 10 min [16]. Other authors have also confirmed these findings [55]. Finally, the choice of the transperitoneal approach facilitates complete mobilization of the kidney so that an ideal angle between the needle holder and the incision line of the kidney can always be achieved, which is a prerequisite for precise and fast placement of the suture. In case of a posteriorly located tumor, the kidney is tilted medially for 180° so that the tumor is in an anterior position. Other authors also concur with the use of this approach for LPN [20]. However, we have experience with the retroperitoneal approach as well, which we consider ideal in lower pole posterior tumors, and the suture technique and Rummel tourniquet placement have proven reliable [12].

Despite the aforementioned techniques used to reduce WIT during LPN, there will remain difficult cases where WIT longer than 30 min is expected [29, 53, 56, 57]. In light of this, several techniques of regional hypothermia during LPN have been reported including laparoscopic ice slush cooling, intraureteral cooling, and intravascular hypothermic perfusion [58–60]. Although hypothermia affords cellular protection and allows as much as 3 h of ischemia without permanent renal injury [47], achieving hypothermia during LPN is somewhat cumbersome and therefore reserved for cases when prolonged warm ischemia may adversely affect renal function.

The use of protective measures against ischemia to help reduce the possible hypoxic injuries to the kidney has been the routine practice during partial nephrectomy, regardless of the approach used. The main protective mechanism is adequate hydration prior to the induction of ischemia, which is initiated by the delivery of intravenous mannitol (12.5 g) and/or furosemide (10–20 mg) 5–10 min before vessels are clamped. This promotes diuresis and minimizes the sequelae of renal reperfusion injury caused by the accumulation of free radicals [3]. Therefore, our technique of renal hypothermia by means of arterial perfusion has a twofold mechanism of protection against renal injury. Besides the effect of cooling, toxic radicals are continuously washed out of the kidney, preventing essential damage.

Other Complications

Arterial Injury

Complete dissection and skeletonization of the artery harbors the risk of direct trauma to the arterial wall and its intima during occlusion. As a consequence, obliteration of the arterial lumen may occur. We experienced a case of silent loss of a kidney following an uneventful LPN, which was most probably as a result of this. Henceforth the vein is selectively dissected, looped, and eventually occluded leaving the renal artery completely undissected within the surrounding connective tissue which is separately looped en bloc, minimizing the risk of its injury.

Pseudoaneurysm of Renal Artery

Renal artery pseudoaneursym (RAP) is a rare complication after partial nephrectomy. The patients usually present with macroscopic hematuria and flank pain from 1 day up to 3 weeks following LPN. The diagnosis can be made either by contrast-enhanced CT or by renal angiography which are both conclusive diagnostic imaging methods for RAP. Angiographic selective embolization is a safe and efficacious technique for treatment, and very infrequently it requires nephrectomy due to persistent bleeding. In big series of LPN the frequency of this complication is identified as about 1–2% presenting mostly around 2 weeks after surgery. The authors thoroughly describe the presentation, evaluation, management, and prevention of hemorrhage due to renal artery pseudoaneurysm following LPN [25, 61].

Even more exceptional is the occurrence of an arteriovenous fistula as a complication of LPN. Remaining conscious of the frequency of these conditions, they have nevertheless to be considered in patients with typical clinical presentation.

Urinary Obstruction

Link et al. [19] reported two patients with postoperative ipsilateral ureteropelvic junction (UPJ) obstruction. In one case a dense stricture formed, for which endoscopic incision failed. The second patient subsequently presented with a nonfunctioning, obstructed kidney and underwent nephrectomy. In these two cases, there were right upper pole tumors, suggesting that injury to the UPJ was not a direct result of the tumor resection step of LPN. The etiology of postoperative UPJ obstruction in the setting of LPN remains unclear, but it could include ischemia due to mobilization or reaction to hemostatic agents. A case of UPJ obstruction following LPN was also reported in the series from the Cleveland Clinic in 2003 [14].

The authors also reported a case in which one patient had major urinary leakage through the drain. It was noted that the ureter was inadvertently obstructed by a Hem-o-lok clip applied at the end of a hemostatic suture. This was managed by laparoscopic re-exploration, removal of the clip, and JJ stent insertion [12].

Infection

We also experienced a case of infection following partial nephrectomy for stone disease, which resulted in a perirenal abscess. This was most probably due to the presence and postoperative extravasation of infection-laden urine. Therefore, appropriate antimicrobial coverage must be taken into consideration following partial nephrectomy for similar indications.

Hemorrhagic Congestion

Hemorrhagic congestion is a result of incomplete occlusion of the artery or the presence of a missed accessory artery, while the vein is completely occluded during induction of ischemia. Without outflow, the kidney becomes congested with blood causing irreversible renal damage. This can occur during enbloc clamping with a Statinsky clamp. Therefore, it would be best to avoid individual dissection of the renal artery and vein. This maneuver can cause arterial vasospasm, increase the risk of vascular injury, and increase operating time [18, 24, 53].

Risk Factors for Complications

Porpiglia et al. [10] retrospectively analyzed 90 patients who underwent LPN. Patient age, BMI, tumor size, location and pattern of growth, surgical approach (transperitoneal vs. retroperitoneal), WIT, hemostatic technique, maximum thickness of the margin of resection, and histology were collected and analyzed to identify any risk factors for complications during LPN. On univariate analysis (no multivariate analysis was performed), only tumor growth pattern (cortical vs. corticomedullar) was found to correlate with the occurrence of complications, with a significantly higher rate of complications for corticomedullar lesions ($p = 0.02$).

Simmons and Gill [21] evaluated age, BMI, ASA grade, CCI score, tumor size, laterality and centrality, preoperative serum creatinine, EBL, operative time, and WIT of patients undergoing LPN. They found no correlation on univariate and multivariate analysis between the above variables and complications during LPN. However, in a recent report from Turna et al. [62], prolonged warm ischemia time, increased intraoperative blood loss, and solitary kidney status were found to be independent risk factors on multivariate analysis for the development of postoperative complications after LPN, suggesting that all three factors should be considered when planning an LPN in order to minimize complications.

Conclusion

Laparoscopic NSS has evolved significantly in a decade. The hilar control, reconstruction, hemostasis by suture, and cold ischemia were the major advancements. The procedure still remains challenging with the potential of significant complications, which require considerable expertise in laparoscopic environment. Nevertheless, the technique continues to evolve and with effective, reliable, and safe cold ischemia, it will come into the realms of average urologists in the future.

References

1. Matin SF. Laparoscopic approaches to urologic malignancies. Curr Treat Options Oncol. 2003;4:373.
2. Fergany AF, Hafez KS, Novick AC. Long-term results of nephron sparing surgery for localized renal cell carcinoma: 10-year follow up. J Urol. 2000;163(2):442–5.
3. Porpiglia F, Volpe A, Billia M, Scarpa RM. Laparoscopic versus open partial nephrectomy: analysis of the current literature. Eur Urol. 2008;53:732–43.
4. Ljungberg B, Hanbury DC, Kuczyk MA, et al. Renal cell carcinoma guideline. Eur Urol. 2007;51:1502–10.
5. Gill IS, Desai MM, Kaouk JH, et al. Laparoscopic partial nephrectomy for renal tumor: duplicating open surgical techniques. J Urol. 2002;167:467–9.
6. McDougall EM, Clayman RV, Anderson K. Laparoscopic wedge resection of a renal tumor: initial experience. J Laparoendosc Surg. 1993;3:577.
7. Gill IS, Kavoussi LR, Lane BR, Blute ML, Babineau D, Colombo JR, Frank I, Permpongkosol S, Weight CJ, Kaouk JH, Kattan MW, Novick C. Comparison of 1,800 laparoscopic and open partial nephrectomies for single renal tumors. J Urol. 2007;178:41–6.
8. Marszalek M, et al. Laparoscopic and open partial nephrectomy: a matched-pair comparison of 200 patients. Eur Urol. 2009. doi:10.1016/j.eururo.2009.01.042.
9. Permpongsol S, Link RE, Su LM, et al. Complications of 2775 laparoscopic procedures: 1993 to 2005. J Urol. 2007;177:580–5.
10. Porpiglia F, Volpe A, Billia M, Renard J, Scarpa RM. Assessment of risk factors for complications of laparoscopic partial nephrectomy. Eur Urol. 2008;53:590–6.
11. Janetschek G, Jeschke K, Peschel R, Strohmeyer D, Henning K, Bartsch G. Laparoscopic surgery for stage 1 renal cell carcinoma: radical nephrectomy and wedge resection. Eur Urol. 2000;38:131–8.
12. Abukora F, Nambirajan T, Albqami N, Leeb K, Jeschke S, Gschwendtner M, Janetschek G. Laparoscopic nephron sparing surgery: evolution in a decade. Eur Urol. 2005;47:488–93.

13. Ramani AP, Desai MM, Steinberg AP, et al. Complications of laparoscopic partial nephrectomy in 200 cases. J Urol. 2005;173:42–7.
14. Gill IS, Matin SF, Desai MM, et al. Comparative analysis of laparoscopic versus open partial nephrectomy for renal tumors in 200 patients. J Urol. 2003;170:64–8.
15. Porpiglia F, Renard J, Billia M, et al. Is renal warm ischemia over 30 minutes during laparoscopic partial nephrectomy possible? One-year results of a prospective study. Eur Urol. 2007;52:1170–8.
16. Janetschek G. Laparoscopic partial nephrectomy for RCC: how can we avoid ischemic damage of the renal parenchyma? Eur Urol. 2007;52:1303–5.
17. Gill IS, Ramani AP, Spaliviero M, Xu M, Finelli A, Kaouk JH, Desai MM. Improved haemostasis during laparoscopic partial nephrectomy using gelatine matrix thrombin sealant. Urology. 2002;65:463–6.
18. Orvieto MA, Chien GW, Tolhurst SR, Rapp DE, Steinberg GD, Mikhail AA, Brendler CB, Shalhav AR. Simplifying laparoscopic partial nephrectomy: technical considerations for reproducible outcomes. Urology. 2005;66:976–80.
19. Link RE, Bhayani SB, Allaf ME, Varkarakis I, Inagaki T, Rogers C. Exploring the learning curve, pathological outcomes and perioperative morbidity of laparoscopic partial nephrectomy performed for renal mess. J Urol. 2005;173:1690–4.
20. Wright JL, Porter JR. Laparoscopic partial nephrectomy: comparison of transperitoneal and retroperitoneal approaches. J Urol. 2005;174:841–5.
21. Simmons MN, Gill IS. Decreased complications of contemporary laparoscopic partial nephrectomy: use of a standardized reporting system. J Urol. 2007;177:2067–73.
22. Häcker A, Albadour A, Jauker W, Ziegerhofer J, Albquami N, Jeschke S, Leeb K, Janetschek G. Nephron-sparing surgery for renal tumours: acceleration and facilitation of the laparoscopic technique. Eur Urol. 2007;51:358–65.
23. Nadu A, Mor Y, Laufer M, et al. Laparoscopic partial nephrectomy: single center experience with 140 patients evolution of the surgical technique and its impact on patient outcomes. J Urol. 2007;178:435–9.
24. Breda A, Stepanian SV, Lam JS, et al. Use of haemostatic agents and glues during laparoscopic partial nephrectomy: a multi-institutional survey from the United States and Europe of 1,347 cases. Eur Urol. 2007;52:798–803.
25. Singh D, Gill IS. Renal artery pseudoaneurysm following laparoscopic partial nephrectomy. J Urol. 2005;174(6):2256–9.
26. Weld KJ, Venkatesh R, Huang J, Landman J. Evolution of surgical technique and patient outcomes for laparoscopic partial nephrectomy. Urology. 2006;67:506–7.
27. Zimmermann R, Janetschek G. Complications of laparoscopic partial nephrectomy. World J Urol. 2008;26:127–33.
28. Meeks JJ, Zhao LC, Navai N, Perry KT Jr., Nadler RB, Smith ND. Risk factors and management of urine leaks after partial nephrectomy. J Urol. (In press).
29. Venkatesh R, Weld K, Ames CD, et al. Laparoscopic partial nephrectomy for renal masses: effect of tumor location. Urology. 2006;67:1169–74.
30. Bove P, Bhayani SB, Rha KH, Allaf ME, Jarrett TW, Kavoussi LR. Necessity of ureteral catheter during laparoscopic partial nephrectomy. J Urol. 2004;172:458–60.
31. Sutherland SE, Resnick MI, Maclennan GT, Goldman HB. Does the size of the surgical margin in partial nephrectomy for renal cell cancer really matter? J Urol. 2002;167:61.
32. Thrasher JB, Robertson JE, Paulson DF. Expanding indications for conservative renal surgery in renal cell carcinoma. Urology. 1994;43:160.
33. Gerard C, Ballereau C, Leroy X, Lemaitre L, Villers A, Biserte J. Long-term oncological results after conservative surgery for unifocal renal cancer. Prog Urol. 2003;13:14.
34. Licht MR, Novick AC, Goormastic M. Nephron sparing surgery in incidental versus suspected renal cell carcinoma. J Urol. 1994;152:39.
35. Breda A, Stepanian SV, Liao J, et al. Positive margins in laparoscopic partial nephrectomy in 855 cases: a multi institutional survey from the United States and Europe. J Urol. 2007;178:47–50.
36. Permpongkosol S, Bagga HS, Romero FR, Sroka M, Jarrett TW, Kavoussi LR. Laparoscopic versus open partial nephrectomy for the treatment of pathological T1N0M0 renal cell carcinoma: a 5-year survival rate. J Urol. 2006;176:1984–8.
37. Lane BR, Gill IS. 5-year outcomes of laparoscopic partial nephrectomy. J Urol. 2007;177:70–4.
38. Frank I, Colombo JR Jr, Rubinstein M, Desai M, Kaouk J, Gill IS. Laparoscopic partial nephrectomy for centrally located renal tumors. J Urol. 2006;175:849–52.
39. Porpiglia F, Fiori C, Terrone C, Bollito E, Fontana D, Scarpa RM. Assessment of surgical margins in renal cell carcinoma after nephron sparing: a comparative study: laparoscopy vs. open surgery. J Urol. 2005;173:1098–101.
40. Permpongkosol S, Colombo JR Jr, Gill IS, Kavoussi LR. Positive surgical parenchymal margin after laparoscopic partial nephrectomy for renal cell carcinoma: oncological outcomes. J Urol. 2006;176:2401.
41. Yossepowitch O, Thompson RH, Leibovich BC, et al. Positive surgical margins at partial nephrectomy: predictors and oncological outcomes. J Urol. 2008;179:2158–63.
42. Campbell SC, Novick AC. Surgical technique and morbidity of elective partial nephrectomy. Semin Urol Oncol. 1995;13:281.
43 Castilla EA, Liou LS, Abrahams NA, et al. Prognostic importance of resection margin width after nephron-sparing surgery for renal cell carcinoma. Urology. 2002;60:993–7.
44. Guillonneau B, Bermudez H, Gholami S, et al. Laparoscopic partial nephrectomy for renal tumor: single center experience comparing clamping and no clamping techniques of the renal vasculature. J Urol. 2003;169:483–6.
45. Nadu A, Kitrey N, Mor Y, Golomb J, Ramon J. Laparoscopic partial nephrectomy: is it advantageous and safe to clamp the renal artery? Urology. 2005;66: 279–82.
46. Marberger M. Renal ischaemia: not a problem in laparoscopic partial nephrectomy? BJU Int. 2006;99:3–8.
47. Novick AC. Renal hypothermia: in vivo and ex vivo. Urol Clin North Am. 1983;10:637–44.
48. Desai MM, Gill IS, Ramani AP, et al. The impact of warm ischaemia on renal function after laparoscopic partial nephrectomy. BJU Int. 2005;95:377–83.
49. Shekarriz B, Shah G, Upadhyay J. Impact of temporary hilar clamping during laparoscopic partial nephrectomy on

postoperative renal function: a prospective study. J Urol. 2004;172:54–7.
50. Bhayani SB, Rha KH, Pinto PA, et al. Laparoscopic partial nephrectomy: effect of warm ischemia on serum creatinine. J Urol. 2004;172:1264–6.
51. Gill IS, Colombo Jr JR, Moinzadeh A, Finelli A, Ukimura O, Tucker K, et al. Laparoscopic partial nephrectomy in solitary kidney. J Urol. 2006;175:454–8.
52. Rocca Rosetti S. Impact of acute ischemia on human kidney. In: Margerger M, Dreikorn K, editors. Renal preservation. Baltimore: Williams & Wilkins; 1983. pp. 21–37.
53. Haber GP, Gill IS. Laparoscopic partial nephrectomy: contemporary technique and outcomes. Eur Urol. 2006;49:660.
54. Baumert H, Ballaro A, Shah N, Mansouri D, Zafar N, Molinié V, Neal D. Reducing warm ischemia time during laparoscopic partial nephrectomy: a prospective comparison of two renal closure techniques. Eur Urol. 2007;52(4):1164–9.
55. Nguyen MM, Gill IS. Halving ischemia time during laparoscopic partial nephrectomy. J Urol. 2008;179:627–32; discussion 32.
56. Frank I, Columbo JR Jr, Rubinstein M, et al. Laparoscopic partial nephrectomy for centrally located renal tumors. J Urol. 2006;175:849–52.
57. Lattouf J-B, Beri A, Oswald D, Grull M, Leeb K, Janetschek G. Laparoscopic partial nephrectomy for hilar tumors: technique and results. Eur Urol. 2008;54:409–18.
58. Gill IS, Abreu SC, Desai MM, Steinberg AP, Ramani AP, Ng C, et al. Laparoscopic ice slush renal hypothermia for partial nephrectomy: the initial experience. J Urol. 2003;170: 52.
59. Janetschek G, Abdelmaksoud A, Bagheri F, Al-Zahrani H, Leeb K, Gschwendtner M. Laparoscopic partial nephrectomy in cold ischemia: renal artery perfusion. J Urol. 2004;171:68.
60. Landman J, Venkatesh R, Lee D, Vanlangendonck R, Morissey K, Andriole GL, et al. Renal hypothermia achieved by retrograde endoscopic cold saline perfusion: technique and initial clinical application. Urology. 2003;61:1023.
61. Cohenpour M, Strauss S, Gottlieb P, Peer A, Rimon U, Stav K, Gayer G. Pseudoaneursym of the renal artery following partial nephrectomy: imaging findings and coil embolization. Clin Radiol. 2007;62(11):1104–9.
62. Turna B, Frota R, Kamoi K, et al. Risk factor analysis of postoperative complications in laparoscopic partial nephrectomy. J Urol. 2008;179:1289–94; discussion 1294–5.

Complications of Robotic Partial Nephrectomy

Matthew Sand, Elias Hyams, and Michael Stifelman

Keywords Partial nephrectomy · Kidney cancer · Complications · Robotic surgery

Introduction

Partial nephrectomy has emerged as the standard of care for the treatment of small renal tumors. Laparoscopic partial nephrectomy (LPN) has been performed for over 15 years and has demonstrated satisfactory oncologic outcomes, decreased patient morbidity, and shorter recovery time compared to open surgery [1–3]. Robotic-assisted laparoscopic partial nephrectomy (RALPN) is an emerging technique that shares the minimally invasive advantages of LPN and may provide technical advantages specific to robotic systems (e.g., improved visualization and dexterity during reconstruction) [4, 5]. Furthermore, early literature on RALPN has demonstrated possible advantages in terms of warm ischemia time (WIT) and blood loss compared with laparoscopy [4, 5].

As the experience with RALPN is early, the incidence and the risk of complications are not well documented; however, they seem to parallel those of LPN in the initial series. Importantly, as the primary surgeon is at the console during robotic surgery, prevention of intra-operative complications is even more crucial, though this can be mitigated by the presence of a skilled side surgeon. This chapter reviews the epidemiology, prevention, diagnosis, and treatment of both intra- and post-operative complications associated with RALPN.

Technique

Pre-operatively, all patients are consented for RALPN with the possibility of radical nephrectomy or open surgery. All patients receive a bowel prep the day prior to surgery including one bottle of magnesium citrate in the afternoon, 1–2 fleets enemas the night prior, and a clear liquid diet the day prior. Golytely is preferred to magnesium citrate in patients with renal insufficiency. The patient is brought to the operating room and given general anesthesia. Sequential compression devices are applied to both lower extremities, and the patient is dosed with prophylactic intravenous antibiotics. The patient is placed in a modified semi-flank position with all pressure points carefully padded. The patient is shaved, prepped, and draped in standard sterile fashion. An initial Hasson® balloon port is placed superior to the umbilicus under direct vision. This may be placed further laterally toward the side of interest depending on patient's body habitus (obese patients should have trocars placed further laterally). The abdomen is insufflated and the robotic ports are placed either with a three- or four-arm configuration based on surgeon preference. When using a standard system, we utilize a V-type configuration and triangulate the ports depending on whether the tumor is in the upper, the mid, or the lower pole. Working ports of 5 and 10 mm are placed medial to the camera port (inferiorly and superiorly, respectively) at the level of the robotic ports (Fig. 1). With the newer S system we

M. Stifelman (✉)
Department of Urology, New York University Medical Center, New York, NY, USA
e-mail: michael.stifelman@nyumc.org

R. Ghavamian (ed.), *Complications of Laparoscopic and Robotic Urologic Surgery*,
DOI 10.1007/978-1-60761-676-4_13,

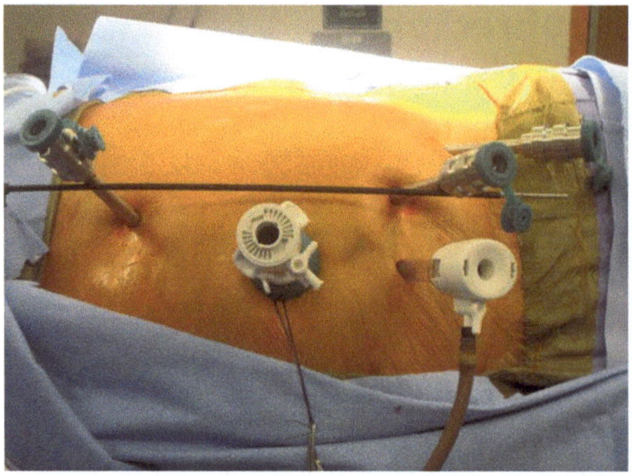

Fig. 1 Positioning of robotic ports

use the same configuration for all tumor locations and decide on fourth arm based on patient's body habitus. The fourth-arm port is placed inferiorly and laterally to the camera, near the side wall. The Jackson-Pratt drain will eventually be placed through this port site. The assistant 10-mm port is placed between the camera and inferior robotic ports. To gain initial exposure of the kidney, hilum, ureter, and tumor, we use the monopolar hot shears in the right robotic arm and PK forceps in the left arm. For right-sided tumors, the right colon is reflected medially, the liver is retracted superiorly, and the duodenum is kocherized. Landmarks identified include adrenal gland superiorly, inferior vena cava medially, and gonadal vein inferiorly. On the left side, lateral attachments to the spleen are divided and the spleen, pancreas, and colon are reflected medially. Landmarks identified include the adrenal superiorly, aorta medially, and gonadal vein inferiorly. Next the ureter is isolated, and the lower pole packet is retracted anteriorly. All posterior attachments to the kidney are dissected with blunt and sharp techniques to the upper pole and the kidney is placed on traction anteriorly allowing the hilum to be placed on stretch. The renal artery and the vein are dissected out individually. The assistant or the fourth arm provides traction on the kidney, while the console surgeon has two hands free to perform the dissection. A laparoscopic Doppler probe (VTI, Nashua, NH) is used to aid in the identification of both the main and accessory renal veins and arteries. The assistant's second port is used for suction and retraction. Perirenal fat is removed from the area of interest without violating the overlying Gerota's fascia. The goal is to obtain complete exposure of the capsule surrounding the tumor with adequate margins to enable complete resection and visualization of tumor-free tissue at the margins. A laparoscopic ultrasound probe is used to characterize the tumor in three dimensions to guide tumor excision. The anticipated excision line is scored on the capsule with cautery prior to clamping of the renal artery.

Prior to clamping, the back table is checked to ensure that all necessary instruments are available. The Surgicel® bolster is placed in the abdomen off to the side so that it is ready for reconstruction after tumor removal. Mannitol (12.5 g) is administered intravenously prior to arterial clamping. The primary surgeon and the side surgeon at this time discuss the plan for tumor resection and reconstruction. Typically the renal artery is clamped without clamping of the renal vein. Both renal artery and vein may be clamped together if there is concern for back-bleeding or the tumor is involving the renal hilar vessels, fat, or pelvis. The tumor is excised with a robotic cold shears. The left-hand or assistant grasper is used to maintain optimal positioning of the kidney to allow for tumor resection. The assistant uses the suction to aspirate any blood that may be obscuring the deep tumor margin and to give gentle countertraction on the normal parenchyma during excision. Tumor is grossly inspected and placed to the side or in an entrapment bag. With the tumor excised, robotic needle drivers are used to oversew the collecting system entry if present or obvious open vessels with a running or a figure-of-eight 2-0 Vicryl suture. A TissueLink® device is then used to cauterize the cortex of the resection bed. Surgicel® bolster is placed in the defect and interrupted 2-0 Vicryl sutures with Weck clips at the end are placed through the capsule across the defect. A Weck clip is placed on the contralateral side of the stitch and cinched down until dimpling is noted in the capsule. A Lapra-Ty® is then placed to ensure that it does not slip [6]. The arterial clamp is removed typically after the bolster is placed and capsular re-approximation is complete but may be removed before bolster placement to ensure that specific vessels are oversewn and to reduce warm ischemia time.

Importantly, a laparoscopic Doppler probe is used pre- and post-clamping to confirm the effectiveness of clamping by assessing flow in the parenchyma adjacent to the tumor. If there is persistent arterial signal after clamping of the renal artery, an accessory renal artery is sought and clamped. After clamp removal, perfusion of the parenchyma is rechecked with the Doppler probe. A second dose of 12.5 g mannitol is given after clamp removal. The abdomen is thoroughly inspected for bleeding with insufflation pressure decreased to 5 mmHg and mean arterial pressure increased to >90 mmHg. Bleeding is also evaluated after Valsalva maneuver by the anesthesiologist. The kidney is typically placed back into normal anatomic position and pexed with clips or a running suture. A single JP drain is placed near the resection bed in a dependent position and left to straight drainage. All the ports are removed under direct vision.

Robotic Versus Laparoscopic Partial Nephrectomy

We believe, after completing over 150 standard laparoscopic procedures followed by 100 robotic procedures, that robotics offers significant benefits. Increased dexterity and range of motion have clear advantages in tumor resection and renorrhaphy. Excising a tumor may require alterations in the angle of resection that may be facilitated by robotic techniques. Improved magnification may enable improved recognition of the tumor's gross margin. After tumor excision, oversewing large vessels and collecting system injury within the defect requires intracorporeal suturing, for which robotics has the greatest advantage. There is greater precision and dexterity with robotic suturing as well as improved visualization within the defect. This advantage also applies to renorrhaphy as sutures are placed across the defect over a bolster. While skilled laparoscopists may be very successful with laparoscopic suturing and needle handling, robotics provides an indisputable advantage for most surgeons. Even for skilled laparoscopists, tumors that are difficult to access (e.g., posterior) or more complex (e.g., near the hilum) may be facilitated with the precision and improved range of motion of robotic tools.

Disadvantages of robotic partial nephrectomy are important to recognize. The significant learning curve must be overcome as the surgeon adapts to a new surgical environment and increased surgical magnification. Due to the higher magnification, it is more difficult to pan out the camera to achieve a global surgical view and more difficult to change the camera and instrument configuration in comparison to standard laparoscopy. Therefore, one must rely on strict identification of surgical landmarks to help overcome these challenges. Additionally, there is an increased reliance on the side surgeon, especially when a three-arm approach is utilized. Due to the primary surgeon's location at the robotic console, the assistant surgeon must be responsible for providing traction, exposure, suction, irrigation, clamping, and passing of instruments, needles, and adjunct hemostatic agents. However, this dependence of the side surgeon may be somewhat overcome with the four-arm approach, in which the assistant utilizes only one port and is relegated to suction, clamping, and passage of needles. We have observed with experience using the four-arm approach that the side surgeons' role may be minimized so that a senior surgeon is not required. Finally, robotics adds complexity to the setup and preparation of the operating room in comparison to traditional laparoscopy. However, with OR training and repetition, this too can be minimized as our time to incision is no different with robotic versus laparoscopic procedures.

Literature Review

RALPN has been performed for over 5 years with recent publication of multiple case series [4, 5, 7–14]. Authors describe subjective benefits including improved dexterity during exposure of complex tumors and renal reconstruction [4, 5, 12]. There is variable data in terms of objective differences between robotics and laparoscopy. The largest study of RALPN reported benefits of this technique in terms of warm ischemia time and estimated blood loss [5]. Decreases in WIT, operative time, and hospital stay were also observed in the robotic cohort in another smaller retrospective comparison [4]. There have been no reported differences between RALPN and LPN in terms of intra- or post-operative complications in any series [4, 5, 7–14]. Table 1 provides a summary of all series of RALPN published to date, while Table 2 lists the rates and types of complications reported. Despite our experience, definitive evaluation of RALPN in terms of outcomes and complications will require larger, prospective studies comparing the standard of care.

Table 1 Summary of contemporary RALPN series

	Study (reference to literature review)									
Variable	Wang	Caruso	Aron	Michli	Deane	Gettman	Kaul	Ho	Rogers	Benway
No. of cases	40	10	12	20	11	13	10	20	11	129
Mean tumor size (cm)	2.5	1.95	2.4	2.7	3.1	3.5	2.3	3.5	3.8	2.9
Side R/L	17/23	NR	7/5	10/10	4/7	7/6	6/4	9/11	5/6	NR
Mean OR time	140	279	242	142	228.7	215	155	82.8	202	189
Mean EBL (ml)	136	240	329	263	115	170	92	189	220	155
Mean WIT (min)	19	26.4	23	28.1	32.1	22	21	21.7	28.9	19.7
Mean LOS (days)	2.5	2.6	4.7	2.8	2	4.3	3.5	4.8	2.6	2.4
Length of f/u (avg. mos)	NR	NR	7.4	NR	16	2–11	15	NR	NR	NR
Intra-operative complications	0	2	1	1	0	0	0	0	0	0
Post-operative complications	8	1	3	2	1	1	2	0	2	11

Table 2 Summary of types of complications of RALPN

	Study (reference to literature review)									
	Wang (40 pts)	Caruso (10 pts)	Aron (12 pts)	Michli (20 pts)	Deane (11 pts)	Gettman (13 pts)	Kaul (10 pts)	Ho (20 pts)	Rogers (11 pts)	Benway (129 pts)
Overall complication rate (%)	20	30	33	15	18	8	20	0	18	8.5
Bleeding	3	2	0	0	1	0	1	0	0	4
Urine leak	1	0	0	0	0	0	1	0	2	3
GI (ileus)	0	0	1	0	0	1	0	0	0	1 (C. diff)
Medical	4	0	2 (PE, CHF)	1 (PE)	0	0	0	0	0	2 (MI, PE)
Other	0	1 (retention)	1 (robotic camera malfunction)	2 (postoperative abscess, lost needle requiring ex-lap)	0	0	0	0	0	1 (rectus hematoma)

Intra-operative Complications

To date, 10 RALPN series have been published with a combined sample size of 264 patients [4, 5, 7–14]. Among these patients, only four intra-operative complications have been reported (1.5%). Two cases of intra-operative hemorrhage occurred requiring conversion to open surgery [7]. One hemorrhage occurred after unclamping of the hilum and the other occurred due to venous back-bleeding from an unclamped renal vein [7]. One robotic camera malfunction occurred requiring conversion to traditional laparoscopy [8]. Finally, one series reported loss of a free needle in the patient as it was being removed without direct vision through a port. Open conversion was required to locate and remove this needle [9].

There have been several comparisons of robotic and laparoscopic partial nephrectomy in the literature; however, these series have been retrospective and most have been relatively small. The most recent and largest comparison to date (129 RALPNs versus 118 LPNs) demonstrated no statistically significant difference in complication rates [5]. Specifically, no intra-operative complications were noted in the RALPN series with only one reported in the LPN series (adrenal injury requiring adrenalectomy) [5]. Three other smaller studies comparing RALPN to LPN have been published. The Washington University group compared 40 RALPNs to 62 LPNs and observed statistically significant reductions in WIT, operative time, and length of hospital stay in the robotic cohort without any difference in complication rate [4]. Two other smaller studies showed no significant differences in peri-operative variables or complication rates between the two procedures [8, 10].

Post-operative Complications

Post-operative complications in published series of RALPN are summarized in Table 2 [4, 5, 7–14]. Thirty-one post-operative complications were reported in 264 cases in the literature (11.7%). Nine post-operative hemorrhagic complications (3.5%), seven urine leaks (2.7%), three gastrointestinal complications (two cases of ileus and 1 case of *Clostridium difficile* colitis), and nine medical complications (pulmonary embolism, congestive heart failure, and myocardial infarction) have been reported. Additionally, one post-operative abscess was reported adjacent to the tumor resection bed which failed intravenous antibiotic therapy and eventually required nephrectomy [9]. Only one case each of post-operative urinary retention and rectus hematoma (managed expectantly) has been reported.

The rates of specific post-operative complications appear comparable between RALPN and LPN. For instance, rate of urinoma and post-operative hemorrhage after LPN was 4.5 and 6%, respectively, in the Cleveland Clinic series focusing specifically on complications of LPN [15]. A 123-patient LPN series from Washington University in St. Louis reported 26 overall complications (21%), specifically 3 hemorrhagic complications (2.4%), 13 urine leaks (10.6%), and 10 medical complications (8%) [16]. Another large study of 217 patients from Johns Hopkins reported 4 hemorrhagic complications (1.8%), 3 urine leaks (1.4%), 3 wound infections (1.4%), 2 cases of post-operative renal failure (0.9%), and 15 medical complications (6.9%) [17].

Thus the safety of RALPN appears clear. As there is likely selection bias in the early experience with RALPN, it is important that definitive comparisons with LPN in terms of outcomes and specific complications be drawn from prospective and ideally randomized studies.

Diagnosis of Complications

Maintaining a high index of suspicion and a consistent diagnostic protocol is important to enable early detection of complications of RALPN. This section will focus on strategies to diagnose the most common complications described above. Strategies for treatment are reviewed in the subsequent sections.

Urine Leak

Urine leak is the most commonly reported complication of RALPN. Pre-operatively, careful review of imaging may suggest tumor proximity to the collecting system, which might necessitate entry into a calyx. Importantly, entry into the collecting system may be necessary to obtain a negative deep margin and should not be viewed as problematic per se. Intra-operatively, various techniques have been described to facilitate recognition of collecting system entry. Close inspection of the resection bed may reveal gross evidence of collecting system entry. In more subtle cases, authors have described retrograde placement of a 5-Fr open-ended ureteral catheter at the beginning of the case to allow for injection of methylene blue to identify leak intra-operatively and/or the integrity of collecting system repair [18]. Additionally, indigo carmine can be given intravenously for the same effect. A long spinal needle can be used to inject methylene blue directly into the renal pelvis as well. We do not routinely perform these maneuvers as gross inspection is typically sufficient. No data has been published to show that these techniques result in lower incidence of urine leaks; however, they may be useful tools.

To allow for complete decompression of the urinary tract and maximize healing of the collecting system, we leave a 20-Fr Foley catheter in place for 48 h on a routine basis. Additionally, a Jackson-Pratt drain is left near the resection bed in a dependent position and placed to bulb suction. Maximal drainage of the urinary tract is critical for prevention of urine leakage. Our standard protocol is to remove the Foley catheter on post-operative day 2 and observe the JP drain for increased output. The JP fluid is sent for creatinine level 4–6 h later and if it is consistent with serum creatinine, it is removed. If there is evidence of leakage (i.e., continued high output and elevated JP creatinine level), the drain is left in place and managed as described below.

Anytime a leak is suspected, we recommend obtaining a CT urogram with delayed images (Fig. 2). The

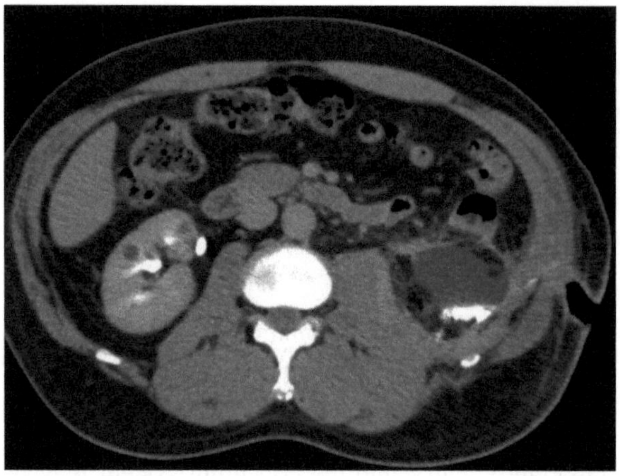

Fig. 2 CT urogram demonstrating urinoma inferior to kidney after lower pole RALP. Contrast enhancement within urinoma occurred during delayed phase of CT indicating communication between collecting system and fluid collection

goal of this study is to determine if there is collection that needs to be drained, where the current drain sits in relation to the area of leak, and to rule out ureteral obstruction. Management of urine leak is described below in detail.

Hemorrhage

Hemorrhage can occur at any point during the case, from hilar dissection through tumor resection and clamp removal, as well as post-operatively in immediate or delayed form. Intra-operative hemorrhage can be prevented by meticulous dissection and avoidance of the use of monopolar cautery near large vessels. A laparoscopic Doppler probe can be used to identify hilar vessels and improve recognition of vital structures during dissection. A skilled side surgeon is helpful in appropriately manipulating tissues and minimizing risk of iatrogenic injury.

Post-operative bleeding can occur in immediate or delayed form. Immediate post-operative bleeding most often results from inadequate closure of the renal defect or unrecognized surgical bleeding from another source. This can typically be prevented by careful inspection of the renal bed and renal hilum at the end of the case. Decreasing insufflation pressure to 5 mmHg as well as ensuring that the mean arterial pressure is at least 90 mmHg during inspection can reveal more subtle yet significant bleeding. Significant immediate post-operative hemorrhage is usually readily identified clinically by hemodynamic instability as well as a decreasing hematocrit. A baseline hematocrit should be obtained post-operatively and compared to a delayed hematocrit at 4 h post-operatively. Observation of these patients in a monitored setting is also mandatory.

Delayed hemorrhage can occur at any interval post-operatively and is usually attributable to pseudoaneurysm, arteriovenous (AV) fistula, or arteriocalyceal fistula. Communication of pseudoaneurysm or AV fistula with the collecting system will result in gross hematuria that can be severe. The typical pathogenesis of this complication involves undetectable injury to the wall of a segmental branch of the renal artery. An incomplete disruption of the arterial wall can result in pseudoaneurysm or AV fistula formation as the wall attempts to heal. Significant bleeding occurs when the defective vessel fistulizes with a portion of the collecting system resulting in significant hematuria and hemorrhage. Hematuria is the most common presentation of delayed hemorrhage after RALPN and any degree of hematuria should be carefully evaluated.

If there is mild gross hematuria, a CT or an MR angiogram is the initial study of choice. These modalities will identify the vascular complications described above [19]. Renal ultrasonography with Doppler flow study may also be useful [19]. If gross hematuria is substantial (i.e., requires clot evacuation and decreasing hematocrit is noted), patients should be taken directly for renal angiography with potential embolization by interventional radiology (Figs. 3 and 4). As there is a high likelihood of vascular fistula to the urinary tract in this setting, proceeding directly to angiography with a therapeutic option will decrease the overall intravenous contrast load, decrease radiation exposure for a patient, and avoid any potential delay in treatment. It is important to have a low index of suspicion with post-operative hematuria as rapid diagnosis and treatment of vascular complications is critical to avoid serious morbidity and even mortality.

Bowel Injury

Bowel injury during RALPN can be classified as either recognized or unrecognized during the procedure.

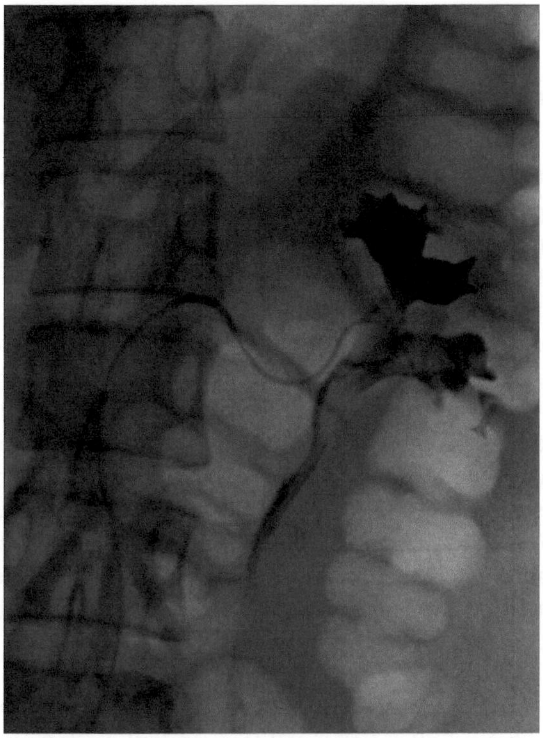

Fig. 3 Renal angiogram demonstrating third-order inferior branch of renal artery with abnormal fistulous connection with adjacent lower pole calyx. Note the filling of renal collecting system with contrast during angiographic phase consistent with arteriocalyceal fistula

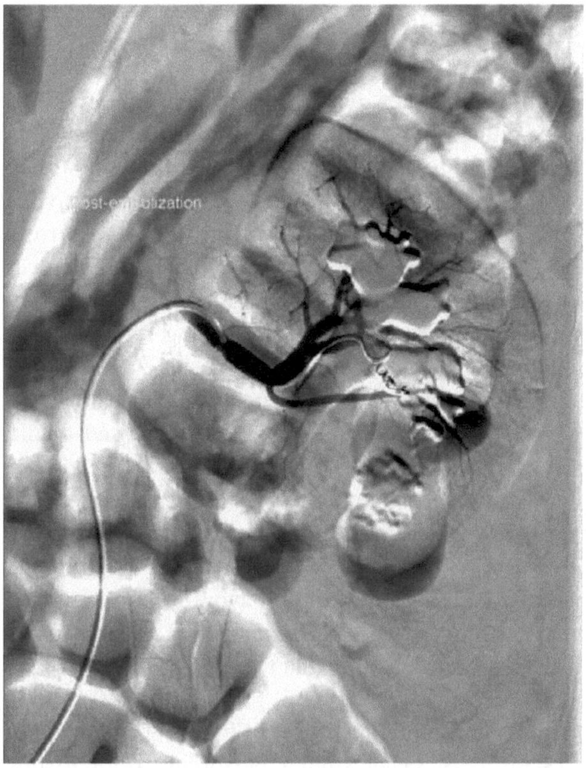

Fig. 4 Renal angiogram of same kidney after superselective arterial embolization. Note coils in position preventing contrast from perfusing the affected segment of the kidney

High index of suspicion for this complication allows for intra-operative recognition and prevention of more significant later morbidity. Incidence of laparoscopic bowel injury during urologic surgery was reported in a large meta-analysis to be 0.13% (266/205,969 cases), of which 69% were unrecognized at the time of surgery [20]. Bowel injury can occur during laparoscopic port placement or removal/closure or may occur as a result of thermal injury during the procedure. The degree of bowel injury varies from superficial abrasions to small enterotomies to frank perforation. Diagnostic evaluation of unrecognized bowel injuries usually begins when the patient begins to exhibit characteristic signs and symptoms, including single trocar site pain, abdominal distention, nausea/vomiting, fever, and leukopenia or leukocytosis [20]. Immediate surgical exploration and repair are indicated if suspicion of bowel injury is high, while CT scan with oral and IV contrast will usually identify the injury or associated abscess if the patient is stable and the clinical picture is less clear.

Rhabdomyolysis

Similar to other surgical procedures performed in the lateral decubitus position, rhabdomyolysis may occur due to compression at pressure points related to positioning. Male sex, high body mass index, prolonged operative times, and the lateral decubitus position are all risk factors for developing rhabdomyolysis during laparoscopic procedures [21]. Diagnostic consideration for rhabdomyolysis typically occurs when the patient reports discrete musculoskeletal pain nearly immediately upon recovering from anesthesia. Serum creatinine phosphokinase and creatinine should be trended to follow the clinical course. Imaging studies are not typically necessary but if performed may show a hematoma within the affected muscle. Rarely, compartment syndrome may occur requiring fasciotomy; gluteal compartment syndrome requiring operative intervention has been reported during urologic laparoscopy [21].

Renal Insufficiency

Renal insufficiency due to nephron loss is significantly reduced with partial versus radical nephrectomy. Nonetheless, warm ischemia while on clamp may result in transient renal insufficiency post-operatively. Renal ischemia can result in acute tubular necrosis (ATN) demonstrated by elevated serum creatinine over several days. Renal vascular occlusion is typically necessary to minimize hemorrhage during resection and repair and to allow for satisfactory visualization. Small exophytic tumors may be resected off-clamp; however, the hilum should always be completely exposed should clamping be required. Significant debate is seen in the literature regarding maximum WIT to minimize renal functional impairment. One recent study reports minimizing WIT to under 40 min as ideal to minimize risk of ATN and to potentially avoid more permanent renal insufficiency [22]. The incidence of renal functional impairment was found to be more than two-fold higher in cases with a WIT greater than 40 min in patients with a pre-operative GFR of >60 ml/min per 1.73 m^2 [22]. Other studies performed prior to this more recent study demonstrated stable post-operative renal function with WIT up to 50 min [23–27]. An additional study reports that nadir glomerular filtration rate (GFR) is most affected by WIT greater than 20 min, with each additional minute over 20 min resulting in significantly reduced nadir GFRs [28]. Overall, it is clear that minimizing ischemia time is helpful for maximizing outcomes for renal function, but reducing ischemia time must be weighed against imperatives of cancer control (e.g., visualization during resection) and potentially the amount of blood loss. Patient factors profoundly influence how much renal ischemia is "safe," as patients with preexisting renal insufficiency, risk factors for nephropathy, or solitary kidney will have less renal reserve [28].

As renal insufficiency commonly occurs after RALPN, close monitoring of urine output and serum creatinine post-operatively is routine. If renal function further deteriorates or persists post-operatively, there should be a low threshold for obtaining nephrology consultation. A renal ultrasound may be performed to ensure that there is no postrenal etiology including clot obstruction, though this will likely be more apparent clinically (e.g., flank pain). Additionally, intraperitoneal urine leak may cause an increase in serum creatinine secondary to peritoneal absorption.

Treatment/Prevention of Complications

Urine Leak

Prevention of urine leak by effective intra-operative repair of collecting system defects is of critical importance in partial nephrectomy. Although robotic systems make suture reconstruction technically easier than conventional laparoscopy, multiple synthetic compounds have been developed to augment creation of a watertight seal in collecting system closure. Seven synthetic agents were compared in a porcine model of laparoscopic partial nephrectomy to determine each agent's effectiveness in sealing collecting system defects [29]. The result of this study showed no clear advantage for one synthetic agent but the best results were observed using a combination of a sutured surgical bolster and Floseal®, which best mimics the techniques used in open repair [29].

Urine leaks vary in severity and thus the treatment strategy varies accordingly. JP drain fluid creatinine is assessed after Foley catheter removal as described above. If there is elevated JP creatinine, the drain is left in place and output is monitored. If there is continued elevation of the creatinine level after 1 week, a CT urogram should be performed to assess for urine leak (seen particularly on delayed images) and to rule out urinoma. If there is evidence of leakage with or without urinoma, the drain should be left in place to continue bulb suction. If urine leakage does not resolve after 1 week, imaging should be repeated to rule out accumulating fluid collection. If there is persistent leak without urinoma, the drain should be converted to straight drainage. If leakage does not resolve with straight drainage, the drain should be gradually devanced over several weeks to allow for fistulization and gradual sealing of the collecting system. If there is high output drainage that is persistent, retrograde placement of a ureteral stent or placement of a percutaneous nephrostomy tube away from the site of surgery should be considered. Distal obstruction (e.g., secondary to blood clot) should be ruled out with CT urogram or other urography.

If there is urinoma, the position of the JP drain should be studied to determine proximity to the fluid collection. If the drain has been removed or is out of position, percutaneous drainage should be performed. If the drain is noted on the resection bed, it should be repositioned so that it is not preventing sealing of the site of leak. Serial imaging should be performed to confirm improvement and resolution of the urinoma.

Almost all urinary leakage will resolve with maximal drainage of the urinary tract. Foley catheters should be left in place or replaced in patients with known or suspected high voiding pressure, or if a ureteral stent is placed to prevent reflux. High post-voiding residuals or high voiding pressures due to outlet obstruction may promote or worsen the severity of urine leaks in patients with concomitant ureteral reflux, and careful monitoring of these issues may prevent or minimize leaks [18]. Re-exploration and repair of the collecting system versus nephrectomy are rarely indicated but have been performed in this setting [18].

Hemorrhage

Intra-operative bleeding is commonly encountered and can typically be addressed in minimally invasive fashion. Venous bleeding from smaller vessels typically resolves by increasing the insufflation pressure and holding direct pressure. Hemostatic agents like Floseal® can be used as well. The combination of pressure, hemostatic agents, and patience is usually successful for addressing most venous bleeding. Injury to a larger vein (e.g., inferior vena cava) may require direct repair with prolene suture. Robotic systems, given finer motion and improved dexterity, may facilitate vascular reconstruction when necessary. Arterial bleeding will not typically resolve with pressure and/or hemostatic agents and requires control of smaller vessels and repair of larger vessels. The threshold to convert to open for control of vasculature depends on surgeon's experience and comfort addressing these injuries in prompt fashion.

Bleeding can also occur intra-operatively after removal of the arterial clamp. This is desired to an extent because it allows for identification of specific vessels that require oversewing. Prior to releasing the clamp, we recommend oversewing exposed vessels and/or collecting system injury in figure-of-eight or running fashion with Vicryl suture. Also we recommend the use of the TissueLink® device to seal the parenchyma to prevent bleeding off-clamp. After specific areas of bleeding are oversewn, we use a Surgicel bolster in the defect secured with parenchymal sutures that are compressive over the bolster. The sutures are tensioned using Weck clips and Lapra-Ty's as described in the literature [6]. Prior to completing the procedure, the insufflation pressure should be decreased to 5 mmHg and mean arterial pressure should be at least 90 mmHg to ensure that there is no significant bleeding. If significant bleeding is noted and does not resolve with pressure and/or additional hemostatic agents, it may be necessary to take down the reconstruction and address a specific area of bleeding.

Treatment strategies for hemorrhage associated with RALPN depend on whether the bleeding is immediate or delayed. Immediate post-operative hemorrhage can be managed conservatively initially with close monitoring of vital signs, serial CBCs, and transfusions as indicated. Hemodynamic instability or inadequate response to conservative strategies necessitates operative re-exploration.

As mentioned above, delayed hemorrhage is typically due to pseudoaneurysm or AV fistula formation with resultant fistulization to the collecting system. During RALPN, specific strategies can be employed to minimize the risk of arterial wall injury. Precise closure of the resection bed with the avoidance of deep passes with large needles may decrease the likelihood of this complication [4]. If significant gross hematuria is noted or there has been diagnosis of pseudoaneurysm/AV fistula on abdominal imaging, percutaneous angiography with superselective embolization is typically effective and, if performed initially, functions as both a diagnostic and a therapeutic modality [19] (Fig. 4). It is critical to aggressively diagnose and treat these vascular complications to avoid further patient morbidity. If angioembolization fails to control the bleeding, re-exploration to achieve hemostasis is indicated. Nephrectomy can be performed as a last resort option if the bleeding is not controllable by the other described measures.

Bowel Injury

Bowel injuries recognized during RALPN require intra-operative repair. The degree of injury determines the type of repair, with specifics of the types of repair being outside of the scope of this chapter. If a serosal injury (e.g., abrasion) is noted, this should be oversewed immediately. If a small laceration is noted, this can be repaired in two layers, but a larger laceration may require bowel resection and necessitates general surgery involvement. There should be a low threshold to consult general surgery intra-operatively for both practical and legal purposes. If a more extensive injury or contamination is noted, bowel diversion may be necessary.

Unrecognized bowel injuries are overwhelmingly repaired by laparotomy with a small subset of patients managed conservatively with total parenteral nutrition [20]. Small bowel injuries are more likely to be treated conservatively as enteric contents are typically sterile in the small bowel [20]. Early recognition of bowel injury is critical as rapid progression to sepsis and cardiovascular collapse can occur with delay in treatment.

Rhabdomyolysis

The treatment for rhabdomyolysis depends on the severity of the course. There is no absolute cutoff with regard to the level of creatinine phosphokinase (CK) that is used to define clinical rhabdomyolysis. Many clinicians use five times the upper limit of normal (1000 IU/L), but typically much higher levels of CK are necessary to cause clinical concern. Rhabdomyolysis can be complicated by acute renal failure (occurring in 4–33% of patients), compartment syndrome, cardiac dysrhythmias via electrolyte abnormalities, and disseminated intravascular coagulopathy; thus if patients exhibit clinical findings consistent with rhabdomyolysis, careful screening of these associated complications is imperative [30]. Management includes intravenous fluid hydration with the initiation of sodium bicarbonate therapy for urine alkalinization in order to prevent myoglobin deposition in the glomeruli and progressive nephropathy [30]. If compartment syndrome occurs, fasciotomy may be necessary [21].

Renal Insufficiency

As mentioned previously, minimization of renal ischemia is critical in decreasing the risk of post-operative renal insufficiency as well as longer term renal dysfunction. A recent large multi-institutional series comparing robotic to conventional laparoscopic PN showed significantly shorter WIT in the robotic cohort, 19.7 versus 28.4 min (p <0.001) [5]. Further investigation comparing robotics to conventional laparoscopy will have to be performed to determine if this shorter WIT results in superior long-term post-operative renal functional outcomes as could be inferred. In addition to minimizing WIT, studies have suggested that clamping of the renal artery alone provides sufficient control of bleeding during resection while allowing for some venous backflow perfusion to limit total renal ischemia during resection [28]. Recently described techniques of early unclamping of the renal hilum after running an initial suture along the resection bed with complete hemostasis and closure being obtained off-clamp have also been shown to decrease ischemia and resultant nephropathy [31].

Adequate renal perfusion pre- and post-clamping also minimizes the degree of ischemia–reperfusion injury to the kidney. As patients are NPO for 8–12 h pre-operatively, sufficient fluid resuscitation should be given at the beginning of the case to return patients to a normovolemic fluid status. Intra-operatively, administration of mannitol (12.5 g IV) before and after arterial clamping has been shown to decrease the risk of ATN associated with renal ischemia. The proposed mechanisms of action of mannitol include acting as a free radical scavenger, decreasing intracellular edema, decreasing intra-renal vascular resistance, increasing blood flow and GFR of superficial nephrons, and promoting osmotic diuresis [32]. Additionally, administration of furosemide after unclamping of the renal hilum promotes osmotic diuresis and may reduce the risk of ischemic nephropathy [32].

Conclusion

RALPN is a safe and effective approach to the treatment of small renal tumors. Studies have demonstrated a similar profile of potential complications compared to LPN. Robotic systems clearly provide subjective benefits to the surgeon in terms of dexterity, visualization, and ergonomics, and may ultimately decrease the risk of certain complications particularly for more complex tumors and among surgeons not already skilled in traditional laparoscopy. Key principles to minimize the risk of complications include maximal drainage of the urinary tract to decrease risk of and effectively treat urine leakage, prompt diagnosis and treatment vascular complications with a low threshold for angioembolization, and minimization of warm ischemia time to prevent renal dysfunction. Future studies of RALPN will further delineate its benefits and provide more information regarding its comparability with LPN.

References

1. Porpiglia F, Volpe A, Billia M, Scarpa RM. Laparoscopic versus open partial nephrectomy: analysis of the current literature. Eur Urol. 2008;53(4):732–42.
2. Romero FR, Rais-Bahrami S, et al. Laparoscopic partial nephrectomy in obese and non-obese patients: comparison with open surgery. Urology. 2008 May;71(5):806–9.
3. Gong EM, Orvieto MA, et al. Comparison of laparoscopic and open partial nephrectomy in clinical T1a renal tumors. J Endourol. 2008;22(5):953–7.
4. Wang AJ, Bhayani SB. Robotic partial nephrectomy versus laparoscopic partial nephrectomy for renal cell carcinoma: single-surgeon analysis of >100 consecutive procedures. Urology. 2009 Feb;73(2):306–10.
5. Benway BN, Bhayani SB, Rogers CG, et al. Robot assisted partial nephrectomy versus laparoscopic partial nephrectomy for renal tumors: a multi-institutional analysis of perioperative outcomes. J Urol. 2009;182(3):866–72.
6. Benway BM, Wang AJ, Cabello JM, Bhayani SB. Robotic partial nephrectomy with sliding-clip renorrhaphy: technique and outcomes. Eur Urol. 2009;55(3):592–9.
7. Caruso RP, Phillips CK, Kau E, Taneja ST, Stifelman MS. Robot assisted laparoscopic partial nephrectomy: initial experience. J Urol. 2006;176:36–9.
8. Aron M, Koenig P, et al. Robotic and laparoscopic partial nephrectomy: a matched-pair comparison from a high-volume centre. BJU Int. 2008;102:86–92.
9. Michli EE, Parra RO. Robotic-assisted laparoscopic partial nephrectomy: initial clinical experience. Urology. 2009 Feb;73(2):302–5.
10. Dean LA, Lee HJ, et al. Robotic versus standard laparoscopic partial/wedge nephrectomy: a comparison of intraoperative and perioperative results from a single institution. J Endourol. 2008;22(5):947–52.
11. Gettman MT, Blute ML, et al. Robotic-assisted laparoscopic partial nephrectomy: technique and initial clinical experience with DaVinci robotic system. Urology. 2004;64:914–8.
12. Kaul S, Laungani R, et al. DaVinci-assisted robotic partial nephrectomy: technique and results at a mean of 15 months of follow-up. Eur Urol. 2007 Jan;51(1):186–91.
13. Ho H, Schwentner C, et al. Robotic-assisted laparoscopic partial nephrectomy: surgical technique and clinical outcomes at 1 year. BJU Int. 2009;103(5):663–8.
14. Rogers CG, Metwalli A, et al. Robotic partial nephrectomy for renal hilar tumors: a multi-institutional analysis. J Urol. 2008;180:2353–6.
15. Ramani AP, Desai MM, et al. Complications of laparoscopic partial nephrectomy in 200 cases. J Urol. 2005;173:42–7.
16. Venkatesh R, Weld K, Ames CD, et al. Laparoscopic partial nephrectomy for renal masses: effect of tumor location. Urology. 2006;67:1169–74.
17. Link RE, Bhayani SB, Allaf ME, et al. Exploring the learning curve, pathological outcomes and perioperative morbidity of laparoscopic partial nephrectomy performed for renal mass. J Urol. 2005;173:1690–4.
18. Meeks JJ, Zhao LC, et al. Risk factors and management of urine leaks after partial nephrectomy. J Urol. 2008;180:2375–8.
19. Cohenpour M, Strauss S, et al. Pseudoaneurysm of the renal artery following partial nephrectomy: imaging findings and coil embolization. Clin Radiol. 2007;62:1104–9.
20. Bishoff JT, Allaf ME, et al. Laparoscopic bowel injury: incidence and clinical presentation. J Urol. 1999;161:887–90.
21. Glassman DT, Merriam WG. Rhabdomyolysis after laparoscopic nephrectomy. J Soc Laparoendosc Surg. 2007;11:432–7.
22. Mufarrij PW, Shah OD, Berger AD, Stifelman MD. Robotic reconstruction of the upper urinary tract. J Urol. 2007;178(5):2002–5.
23. Godoy G, Ramanathan V, Kanofsky JA, O'malley RL, Taureen BU, Taneja SS, Stifelman MD. Effect of warm ischemia time during laparoscopic partial nephrectomy on early post-operative glomerular filtration rate. J Urol. 2009;181(6):2438–43.
24. Bhayani SB, Rha KH, Pinto PA, Ong AM, Allaf ME, Trock BJ, et al. Laparoscopic partial nephrectomy: effect of warm ischemia on serum creatinine. J Urol. 2004;172:1264.
25. Desai MM, Gill IS, Ramani AP, Spaliviero M, Rybicki L, Kaouk JH. The impact of warm ischaemia on renal function after laparoscopic partial nephrectomy. BJU Int. 2005;95:377.
26. Lane BR, Gill IS. 5-Year outcomes of laparoscopic partial nephrectomy. J Urol. 2007;177:70.
27. Saranchuk JW, Touijer AK, Hakimian P, Snyder ME, Russo P. Partial nephrectomy for patients with a solitary kidney: the Memorial Sloan-Kettering experience. BJU Int. 2004;94:1323.
28. Lane BR, Babineau DC, et al. Factors predicting renal functional outcome after partial nephrectomy. J Urol. 2008;180:2363–9.
29. Johnston WK, Kelel KM, et al. Acute integrity of closure for partial nephrectomy: comparison of 7 agents in a hypertensive porcine model. J Urol. 2006;175(6):2307–11.
30. Reisiger KE, Landman J, et al. Laparoscopic surgery and the risk of rhabdomyolysis: diagnosis and treatment. Urology. 2005;66:29–35.
31. Baumert H, Ballaro A, Shah N, et al. Reducing warm ischemia time during laparoscopic partial nephrectomy: a prospective comparison of two renal closure techniques. Eur Urol. 2007;52(4):1164–9.
32. Nosowsky EE, Kaufman JJ. The protective action of mannitol in renal artery occlusion. J Urol. 1963;89:295–9.

Complications of Laparoscopic Retroperitoneal Lymph Node Dissection

Mohamed A. Atalla, Eboni J. Woodard, and Louis R. Kavoussi

Keywords Testicular cancer · Laparoscopy · Complications · Lymph nodes

Patients with stage I nonseminomatous germ cell tumors (NSGCT) have several treatment options, including surveillance, chemotherapy, and retroperitoneal lymph node dissection (RPLND) [1]. The primary, and often only, site of metastasis in NSGCT is the retroperitoneal lymph nodes. Fifteen to forty percent of patients are clinically understaged, despite improvement in radiographic techniques. Open RPLND is the standard of care for staging and treatment. With advances in surgical technique, perioperative morbidity and mortality have been minimized, but up to 70% of patients undergoing RPLND receive no therapeutic benefit [2]. This outcome makes the minimally invasive approach a sensible option.

Laparoscopic RPLND first emerged as a diagnostic and staging tool. With advances in imaging technology, the development of automated suturing devices, the advent of hemostatic agents, and the increasing skill level of surgeons, laparoscopic RPLND has evolved into a therapeutic operation that upholds all the necessary oncological principles that open surgery provides [3]. Nevertheless, laparoscopic RPLND is a technically challenging procedure that should be reserved for experienced laparoscopic surgeons who are also comfortable performing open RPLND and applying advanced vascular skills as necessary.

The indications for RPLND in low-stage NSCGT are clinical stage I or IIA, negative serum tumor markers, and the absence of comorbidities that would preclude safe surgery. More recently, laparoscopic RPLND has also been offered to patients with residual masses following primary chemotherapy. In the hands of an experienced laparoscopic surgeon, the benefits of laparoscopic RPLND include shorter convalescence, more favorable cosmetic results, less postoperative pain and morbidity, and reduced operative blood loss and length of hospital stay [4].

Postchemotherapy laparoscopic RPLND is more technically demanding, due to the resulting desmoplastic reaction, and should be performed in centers with experience in primary laparoscopic RPLND. Permpongkosol [5] reported on 16 consecutive patients who underwent postchemotherapy laparoscopic RPLND by a single surgeon, with 14 dissections successfully completed. Seven patients (43.8%) developed complications and two (12.5%) required open conversion. All intraoperative complications were vascular injuries. Underscoring the importance of surgeon's experience, all operative complications occurred during the first half of the series. Retrograde ejaculation is several fold more common in postchemotherapy than in primary laparoscopic RPLND [6]. No perioperative mortality has been reported with either procedure.

Procedure

Laparoscopic RPLND is performed in the supine position, with the arms padded and secured to the patient's side. The abdomen is insufflated with a Veress needle.

M.A. Atalla (✉)
Smith Institute for Urology, 450 Lakeville Road, New Hyde Park, NY 11042, USA
e-mail: atalla@att.net

R. Ghavamian (ed.), *Complications of Laparoscopic and Robotic Urologic Surgery*,
DOI 10.1007/978-1-60761-676-4_14, © Springer Science+Business Media, LLC 2010

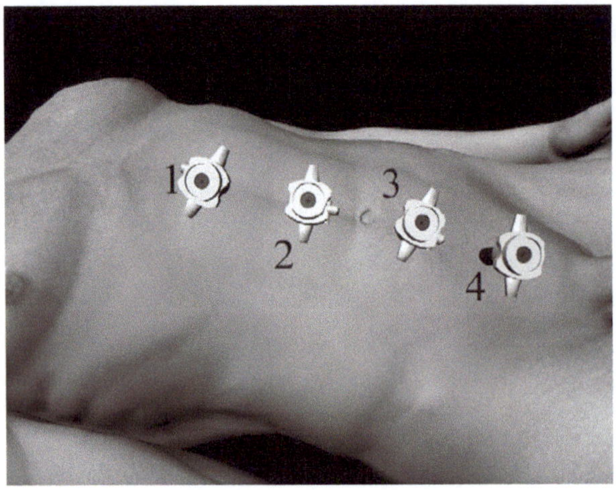

Fig. 1 Port placement for laparoscopic RPLND

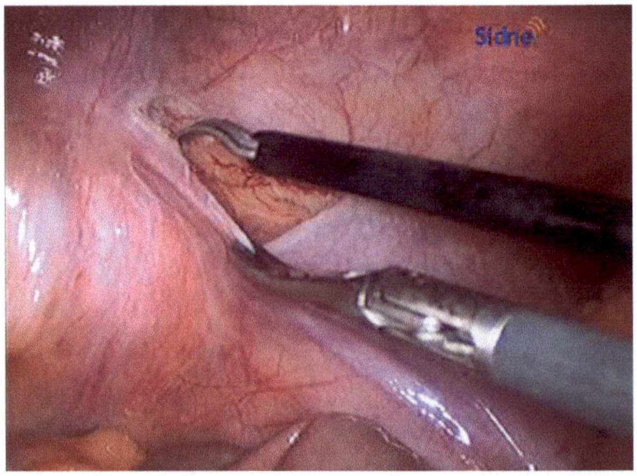

Fig. 2 Dissection of the spermatic cord at the internal inguinal ring

Four 12-mm trocars are placed in the midline, equally spaced beginning 2 cm inferior to the xiphoid process and extending to the symphysis pubis (Fig. 1).

Reflection of the colon is carried out differently, depending on the side being approached. On the left side, the white line of Toldt is incised from the level of the spleen to the iliac vessels. The splenocolic and colorenal ligaments are divided for added mobility. On the right side, the peritoneum is incised superior to the hepatic flexure and medially to Winslow's foramen. The Kocher maneuver is performed in the second portion of the duodenum to expose the inferior vena cava (IVC).

When incising the posterior peritoneum, dissection is avoided lateral to Gerota's fascia to prevent the kidney from falling into the operative field. The use of electrocautery near the bowel is avoided to prevent inadvertent thermal injury. During colon mobilization, any mesenteric holes should be repaired immediately. If not, these defects can be a source of bleeding and lead to the formation of internal hernias postoperatively.

The spermatic cord is first dissected (Fig. 2). The camera is placed in the second lowest port and a retractor is placed in the subxyphoid port. The cord is identified at the internal ring and dissected toward the IVC on the right and the renal vein on the left. Placement of a lateral trocar at the level of the umbilicus in the midaxillary line may facilitate the dissection. The roof of the internal ring may be opened, but care must be taken to avoid injury to the inferior epigastric vessels. Clips should be placed on the cord to prevent bleeding if the cord is inadvertently avulsed. The dissection is extended distally until the orchiectomy suture is encountered.

The cord is traced proximally to identify the IVC (right), the left renal vein (left), and the aorta. The cord is adherent to the lower pole of Gerota's fascia and dissection with ligation is needed to free the cord in this area. It is important to identify the ureter early to avoid inadvertent injury. Once the cord is dissected, the camera is shifted to the second uppermost port. A paddle retractor is placed in the lowermost port. The renal vessels are next identified and clips are used generously to ligate lymphatics and prevent a postoperative lymphocele. On the right side, the lymphatic tissue is split from the surface of the IVC and bluntly dissected both medially and laterally. Care should be taken during the insertion of the clipped gonadal vein to avoid bleeding. On the left side, the left renal vein is traced to the IVC, and the tissue is rolled medially off the IVC to help create the interaortocaval package.

The anterior tissue is rolled to lead to the posterior dissection. Lumbar vessels and lymphatics should be meticulously clipped. The sympathetic chain is distinguished from prominent lymphatic channels: the former should be left intact. Lower pole renal vessels should be anticipated. The interaortocaval lymphatic tissue is excised with great caution to avoid major vascular injury. When the dissection follows the surface of the aorta, care must be taken to avoid avulsing the gonadal arteries or injuring the inferior mesenteric artery. In some instances, however, it may be necessary to divide the inferior mesenteric artery. The retrocaval and retroaortic nodes are the last to be dissected. With the great vessels retracted anteriorly, the nodal packet is teased off the undersurface of the great vessels in a "split-and-roll" technique (Fig. 3).

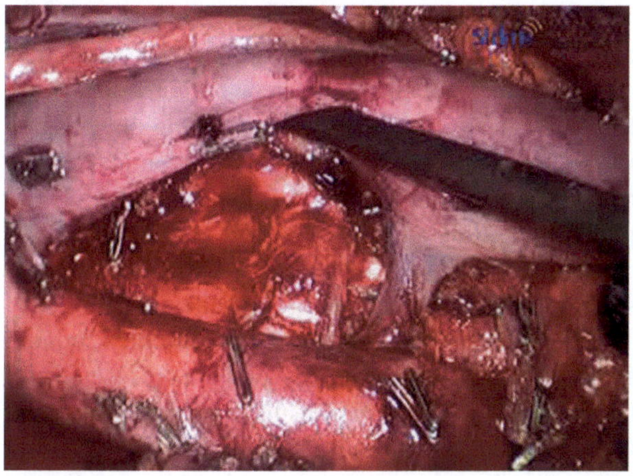

Fig. 3 Retrocaval dissection completed

At the conclusion of the dissection, the abdomen is carefully inspected for bleeding or injury to the surrounding viscera. All trocars are removed under direct vision, and the port sites are closed with a wound closure device.

Postoperatively, patients can be managed on a standard patient care unit. The Foley catheter is usually removed on postoperative day 1. Diet can be advanced on postoperative day 1, as bowel function usually returns within 24 h. Early ambulation is encouraged. Patients are usually ready for discharge on postoperative day 2.

Postchemotherapy laparoscopic RPLND presents special challenges when compared to primary laparoscopic RPLND [5]. To be considered for such a procedure, patients with stage II or III disease should have negative tumor markers and have demonstrated a response to prior therapy, as evidenced by a decrease in the size of the initial mass. Because of the difficulties and morbidities involved, some reports have recommended limiting laparoscopic RPLND for residual tumors less than 5 cm in size [7]. Desmoplastic tissue changes following chemotherapy may make standard templates difficult to follow (Fig. 4). Nevertheless, a bilateral RPLND is performed in addition to removing the residual tumor mass. Fine bipolar grasping forceps can be helpful and hemostatic agents may be used.

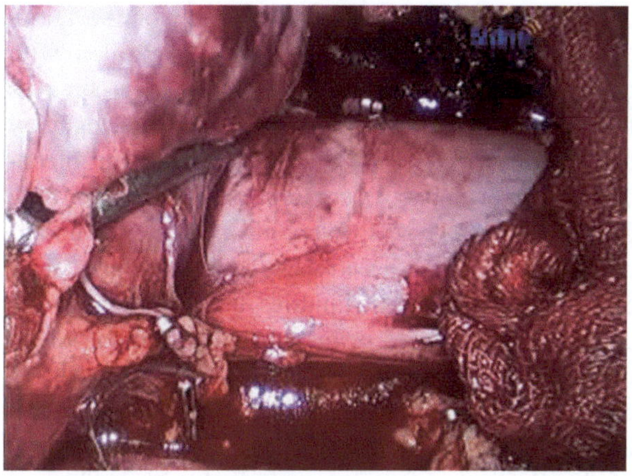

Fig. 4 Dissection of a precaval residual mass following chemotherapy for testis cancer

Complications

Initial series of laparoscopic RPLND reported complication rates between 5.6 and 46.7%. Later reports indicated a decrease in the complication rate to 9.4–25.7% [8]. Open conversion rates were higher in early series (5.8–13.3%) but diminished as larger series with greater experience emerged (1.1–5.4%). This likely reflects improved proficiency with laparoscopic handling of intraoperative complications.

Complications can be grouped into intraoperative, early postoperative, and delayed postoperative. Intraoperative complications include injury to major vessels and other organs. In the early postoperative period, complications include bowel complications, pulmonary embolism, and lymphoceles. Delayed complications include ejaculatory disorders and ureteral strictures.

Bleeding and Vascular Injury

Intraoperative bleeding is the most frequent complication of laparoscopic RPLND [6]. Troublesome bleeding can occur from lumbar, gonadal, or mesenteric vessels, as well as from vasa vasorum of the aorta. Most bleeding of this type can be controlled with electrocautery, clips, and hemostatic agents such as fibrin glue or Surgicel. Intracorporeal suturing may be required for persistent bleeding. Significant bleeding can occur due to laceration of renal or lower pole accessory renal vessels. Every effort should be undertaken to repair injuries to these vessels without their division. IVC or aortic injuries usually occur while controlling tributaries or branches. If a lumbar vessel retracts into the psoas muscle, uncontrolled bleeding can be managed with indirect pressure or a figure-of-eight stitch placed deep in the muscle. Lacerations of the IVC can often be controlled with prolonged direct pressure and, if necessary, hemostatic agents. It is important not to re-explore these lacerations after hemostasis is achieved, as the forming clot may be inadvertently dislodged. Laceration of the aorta can be managed initially with direct pressure, but usually require intracorporeal suturing or open conversion. An Endostitch with a LapraTy at the end can accelerate suturing.

Significant intraoperative bleeding is also the leading cause for open conversion in laparoscopic RPLND (5.1–11.8%) [8, 9]. Improvement in laparoscopic equipments and techniques and development of effective hemostatic agents and clips have allowed versatility in the management of significant vascular injuries with a less frequent need for open conversion. Major vascular injuries may require more complex maneuvers such as vascular clamping and intracorporeal suturing. If such maneuvers are not successful, it is best to make a controlled open conversion for appropriate control of hemorrhage.

Organ Injury

Bowel injury is rarely reported (1–2%), but potentially catastrophic, particularly if unrecognized. Injuries that are directly visualized intraoperatively are best managed immediately. Intestinal abrasions and sharp injuries can result during the course of dissection or intestinal mobilization. These injuries can be repaired primarily using silk suture. Bowel perforation or significant thermal injuries result during dissection or during trocar and instrument introduction. Such injuries usually require excision and often necessitate segmental resection with primary anastomosis. Repairs are followed by copious irrigation when soiling has occurred.

Injuries that are not recognized intraoperatively pose a more significant clinical challenge [10]. The clinical picture is distinctly different from that of bowel injuries following laparotomy. Subtle signs are masked by postoperative pain, analgesics, and postoperative antibiotics. Delayed recognition is often heralded by port site pain, diarrhea, abdominal distention, low-grade fevers, and leukopenia. While diagnosis is mostly clinical, contrast-enhanced abdominal CT is often helpful in confirmation. When the index of suspicion is high enough, immediate repair with abscess drainage is indicated. This can be initiated and occasionally accomplished laparoscopically.

The ureters can also be inadvertently injured sharply, using thermal energy or by excessive skeletonization and devascularization. Care in dissection is the main preventive technique. Intraoperative recognition of sharp ureteral injury should be followed by primary repair over an indwelling stent and external drainage. Thermal ureteral injury should be treated with excision and reimplantation (with or without psoas hitch and bladder flaps), with primary uretero-ureterostomy reserved to proximal injuries only. Postchemotherapy RPLND patients may benefit from preoperative ureteral catheter placement if the residual mass intimately involves one of the ureters. Unrecognized ureteral injuries will usually present late with low-grade fevers, vague abdominal pain, and abdominal distention due to the resultant ileus. Serum creatinine may be elevated, while hyponatremia and hyperkalemia may also be observed. The diagnosis is confirmed with CT urography. Injuries that are recognized postoperatively may be managed by retrograde pyelography and stent placement. If this fails, a percutaneous nephrostomy should be placed, followed by a delayed repair. In all instances, intraperitoneal urinary collections should also be percutaneously drained.

In the upper abdomen, the pancreas, gallbladder, spleen, and liver can rarely be injured. Intraoperative pancreatic injury should be repaired promptly, and a wide caliber drain should be placed. Persistent pancreatic leaks may require bowel rest, parenteral rest, and octreotide to help reduce exocrine secretions. Injury to the gallbladder may require cholecystectomy. Splenic and liver injuries can usually be conservatively treated with argon beam coagulation and hemostatic agents.

Organ injury can also result from vascular injury. Irreparable renal vascular injury may necessitate nephrectomy. Accessory renal vascular injury should not lead to nephrectomy. These vessels are often injured when their course is anomalous or during the interaortocaval, retroaortic, or retrocaval dissections. Inferior mesenteric artery or vein injury should not have deleterious effect. Superior mesenteric artery injury, on the other hand, is detrimental and requires open reconstruction and possible bowel resection if infarction results.

Ejaculatory Dysfunction

Operative template modification has allowed preservation of antegrade ejaculation in most patients [11]. Sympathetic chain injury can result in ejaculatory dysfunction in 0–4.8% of cases, similar to open RPLND [6]. This is best avoided by careful dissection of lymphatics posterior to the IVC and distinction from sympathetic chain fibers, which they can closely resemble. Due to the risk of ejaculatory dysfunction, patients should be encouraged to undergo preoperative sperm banking.

Chylous Ascites

Chylous ascites (1.2–6.6%) and lymphoceles (3.4–13.2%) are delayed postoperative complications [9, 12]. They can be avoided by liberal clipping of lymphatic channels during dissection. Preoperatively, to reduce the risk of lymphatic complications, patients are started on a low-fat diet 1–2 weeks before surgery, which they continue up to 2 weeks postoperatively.

Patients with chylous ascites typically present with abdominal distention and the sensation of abdominal fullness. Other nonspecific symptoms include abdominal pain, nausea, vomiting, and dyspnea, owing to the ascites restricting the movement of the diaphragm. Rarely, chylous ascites may present as milky drainage from the incision or excessive prolonged drainage from surgical drains. Most patients will present within 1 month. Laboratory studies can aid in the diagnosis of chylous ascites. Findings may include hypoalbuminemia, lymphocytopenia, anemia, hyperuricemia, elevated LFTs, hyponatremia, normal cholesterol, and triglyceride levels.

The diagnosis of chylous ascites is made by paracentesis and the analysis of the ascitic fluid. Chylous ascites fluid is white or milky in appearance with an elevated triglyceride level (110–8100 mg/dl), total fat content of 4–40 g/L, and specific gravity greater than that of serum (1.010–1.054). The leukocyte count is usually elevated (232–2560 cells/mm^3), but cultures should be sterile. Cholesterol level is usually low and amylase and glucose levels are normal. Protein content varies from 1.4 to 6.4 g/dL, with a mean of 3.7 g/dL, depending on dietary intake and serum proteins.

Imaging of the abdomen and lymphatic system has a role in both diagnosis and management of chylous ascites. An abdominal CT scan can demonstrate ascites. However, the presence of ascites on CT is not specific, as it is difficult to distinguish simple ascites from chylous ascites. Lymphangiography traditionally has been the standard modality for evaluating chylous ascites, but lymphoscintigraphy provides a noninvasive and more physiologic alternative.

Treatment is aimed at decreasing the flow of lymph in the mesenteric lymphatic glands, consequently limiting the leakage of lymph into the peritoneum. Patients can often be managed conservatively with therapeutic paracentesis (repeated drainage may be necessary), total parental nutrition, and/or a low-fat, medium-chain triglyceride diet. Salt restriction and diuretics may also be of benefit. The use of octreotide, a somatostatin analog, has been shown to speed up the resolution of chylous ascites. Octreotide is beneficial when given early in the course of treatment, typically at a dose of 100 μg administered subcutaneously three times per day. Refractory chylous ascites may require surgical intervention, including re-exploration to identify the site of leakage followed by placement of a surgical clip or a suture (Fig. 5). Peritoneovenous shunting is an alternative therapeutic option for patients who are poor surgical candidates.

Lymphocele formation is another complication that may require intervention. Simple lymphoceles can be managed with CT-guided drainage and sclerosis or placement of percutaneous catheters. Loculated lymphoceles can be more difficult to manage and

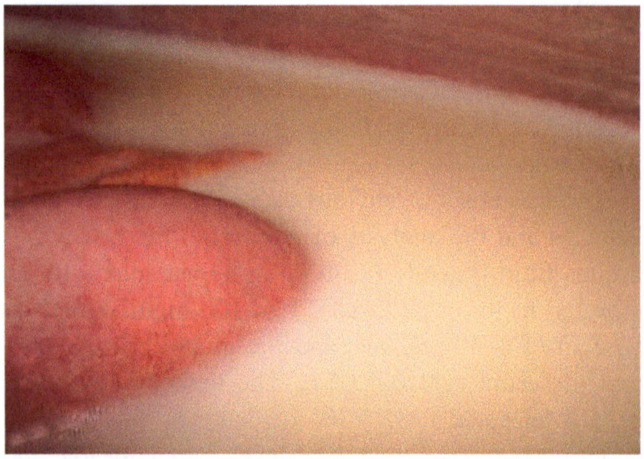

Fig. 5 Chylous ascites

may require multiple drainage catheters, reserving laparoscopic or open marsupialization as a last resort [13].

Small Bowel Obstruction

Bowel obstruction can result from fascial hernial defects stemming from improper closure of port sites. Internal hernias can also result in bowel obstruction if mesenteric defects caused during dissection are not appropriately closed. These defects should be closed with absorbable sutures or clips.

Conclusions

Laparoscopic RPLND is a challenging procedure that requires advanced laparoscopic skills to duplicate the oncological efficacy of open RPLND. It is critical to recognize potential difficulties and complications and take appropriate steps to minimize these risks before they result in an adverse event. It is equally important to recognize any vascular or organ injury intraoperatively, as delayed recognition of such injuries is typically more morbid. Each of these complications is more likely to result in postchemotherapy laparoscopic RPLND. As a result, open conversion is more frequent in the postchemotherapy patient. Finally, complications will occur, but having a high level of suspicion for both common and unusual events allows the surgeon to minimize the most catastrophic sequelae.

References

1. Bosl GJ, Bajorin DF, Sheinfeld J. Cancer of the testis. In: DeVita VT, Hellman S, Rosenberg SA, editors. Cancer, principles & practice of oncology. 7th ed. Philadelphia, PA: Lippincott Williams & Wilkins; 2005. pp. 1269–93.
2. Lashley DB, Lowe BA. A rational approach to managing stage I nonseminomatous germ cell cancer. Urol Clin North Am. 1998;25:405.
3. Allaf ME, Bhayani SB, Link RE, et al. Laparoscopic retroperitoneal lymph node dissection: duplication of open technique. Urology. 2005;65:575.
4. Janetschek G, Hobisch A, Peschel R, et al. Laparoscopic retroperitoneal lymph node dissection for clinical stage I nonseminomatous testicular carcinoma: long-term outcome. J Urol. 2000;163:1793.
5. Permpongkosol S, Lima GC, Warlick CA, et al. Postchemotherapy laparoscopic retroperitoneal lymph node dissection: evaluation of complications. Urology. 2007;69:361.
6. Kenney PA, Tuerk IA. Complications of laparoscopic retroperitoneal lymph node dissection in testicular cancer. World J Urol. 2008;26:561.
7. Janetschek G, Hobisch A, Hittmair A, et al. Laparoscopic retroperitoneal lymphadenectomy after chemotherapy for stage IIB nonseminomatous testicular carcinoma. J Urol. 1999;161:477.
8. Rassweiler JJ, Scheitlin W, Heidenreich A, et al. Laparoscopic retroperitoneal lymph node dissection: does it still have a role in the management of clinical stage I nonseminomatous testis cancer? A European perspective. Eur Urol. 2008;54:1004.
9. Neyer M, Peschel R, Akkad T, et al. Long-term results of laparoscopic retroperitoneal lymph-node dissection for clinical stage I nonseminomatous germ-cell testicular cancer. J Endourol. 2007;21:180.
10. Bishoff JT, Allaf ME, Kirkels W, et al. Laparoscopic bowel injury: incidence and clinical presentation. J Urol. 1999;161:887.
11. Donohue JP, Thornhill JA, Foster RS, et al. Retroperitoneal lymphadenectomy for clinical stage A testis cancer (1965 to 1989): modifications of technique and impact on ejaculation. J Urol. 1993;149:237.
12. Link RE, Amin N, Kavoussi LR. Chylous ascites following retroperitoneal lymphadenectomy for testes cancer. Nat Clin Pract Urol. 2006;3:226.
13. Varga Z, Hegele A, Olbert P, et al. Laparoscopic peritoneal drainage of symptomatic lymphoceles after pelvic lymph node dissection using methylene blue instillation. Urol Int. 2006;76:335.

Complications of Laparoscopic and Robotic Pyeloplasty

Elias Hyams and Michael Stifelman

Keywords Pyeloplasty · Complication · Urinary leakage · Robotic · Obstruction

Introduction

In the last decade, treatment of ureteropelvic junction (UPJ) obstruction has increasingly shifted from open to minimally invasive surgery. In particular, laparoscopic pyeloplasty (LP) has evolved into the standard of care for definitive management of this disease based on comparable mid- to long-term outcomes and decreased morbidity compared to open surgery [1–3]. The dissemination of LP in the community has been limited by the technical difficulty of intracorporeal suturing; thus LP has been performed primarily at advanced laparoscopic centers. Recently robotic techniques have been introduced to minimally invasive pyeloplasty with the goal of facilitating intracorporeal suturing. Series of robotic-assisted laparoscopic pyeloplasty (RALP) and limited comparisons with LP have demonstrated equivalent outcomes with clear subjective benefits compared to laparoscopy. Both procedures have been uniformly shown to be safe with low complication rates; reported complications have been both general to urologic laparoscopy (e.g., vascular or bowel injury) and specific to upper tract reconstruction (e.g., urinary leak, stent migration). The purpose of this chapter is to review literature regarding intra- and postoperative complications of minimally invasive pyeloplasty and to discuss the diagnosis, treatment, and prevention of these complications.

Description of Procedure

The technique of robotic-assisted laparoscopic dismembered pyeloplasty is reviewed. Cases are typically performed transperitoneally, though retroperitoneal RALP can be considered if there has been significant prior abdominal surgery in the relevant upper quadrant. The patient is placed in a modified semilateral position with all pressure points carefully padded and sequential compression devices applied to both lower extremities. Prophylactic antibiotics are administered prior to incision. Three robotic trocars are typically placed in a V configuration with an accessory 5-mm trocar in the suprapubic crease. For right-sided repairs, an additional 5-mm subxiphoid accessory trocar is placed to facilitate liver retraction. The proximal ureter and the renal pelvis are dissected and crossing vessels if present are carefully identified and isolated (Fig. 1). A diamond-shaped incision is made at the UPJ with robotic Potts scissors (Intuitive Surgical, Sunnyvale, CA, USA). The redundant UPJ tissue is used as a handle to manipulate the proximal ureter. The proximal ureter is spatulated laterally and the excess renal pelvis is excised. If renal calculi are present, a flexible nephroscope is introduced through one of the ports and used to inspect the calices after the obstructed UPJ has been transected. Stones are removed using a stone basket through the nephroscope or using robotic

M. Stifelman (✉)
Department of Urology, New York University School of Medicine, New York, NY, USA
e-mail: michael.stifelman@nyumc.org

R. Ghavamian (ed.), *Complications of Laparoscopic and Robotic Urologic Surgery*,
DOI 10.1007/978-1-60761-676-4_15,

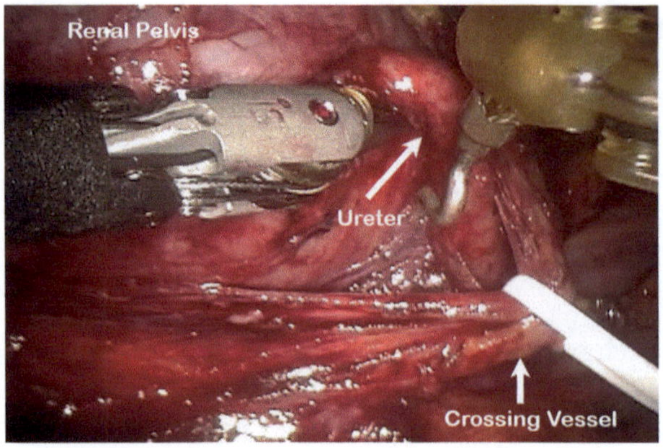

Fig. 1 Crossing vessel isolated in vessel loop with exposure of renal pelvis and ureter

graspers. Stent placement may be performed retrograde or anterograde, though the authors prefer anterograde placement because it does not require bladder access intraoperatively. After placement of the posterior stitches, the stent is placed in an anterograde fashion. A 4-0 polyglactin suture on an RB-1 needle is used to perform a running anastomosis (Fig. 2). A self-suction Jackson-Pratt drain is placed near the anastomosis, exiting through the most inferior robotic port site. A Foley catheter is left in place postoperatively. If there are no complications, the Foley catheter and surgical drain are removed before hospital discharge (typically postoperative day 2). A KUB X-ray is obtained in the recovery room to confirm positioning of the ureteral stent. The ureteral stent is removed 4–6 weeks postoperatively. Patients are imaged approximately 3 months postoperatively with diuretic renal scan or intravenous pyelography to assess the drainage of the repaired system.

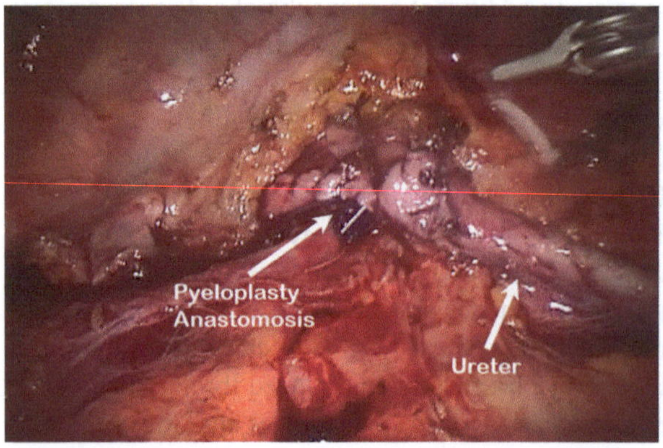

Fig. 2 Completion of anastomosis using robotic techniques

Review of Literature

The first report of LP was published in 1993 by Schuessler et al. [4]. Since then it has become the standard of care at centers where advanced laparoscopy is performed based on both comparable outcomes and decreased morbidity compared to open surgery [5]. LP has been shown to be safe and effective for both primary and secondary UPJ obstruction and using trans- and retroperitoneal approaches [6, 7]. Types of laparoscopic reconstruction have included Anderson–Hynes dismembered pyeloplasty (typically with crossing vessels or a redundant renal pelvis), Y–V plasty (typically with no crossing vessels or a high insertion), and others [8]. Robotic assistance was first reported by Sung in 1999 and numerous series have demonstrated equivalence or superiority of this technique, particularly regarding facilitated intracorporeal suturing [9, 10]. In robotic pyeloplasty series, there have been negligible intraoperative complications [9–16].

Series of LP have demonstrated a low intraoperative complication rate [6, 8, 17]. In one series of 147 patients having transperitoneal LP, there were two cases of bowel injury including a serosal injury to the small bowel and an inadvertently clipped colonic diverticulum [8]. Both injuries were repaired laparoscopically during the same surgery. There were no intraoperative complications in one large series of patients having extraperitoneal LP [18]. Other large series of LP have demonstrated no intraoperative complications [19, 20]. In the largest multi-institutional series to date of RALP, one minor intraoperative complication (splenic laceration) was noted among 140 patients; this was successfully managed with pressure and topical hemostatic agents [16].

A meta-analysis of complications of LP found that the intraoperative complication rate ranged from 2 to 2.3% [17]. This study stratified intraoperative complications using the Satava classification [21]. Grade 1 incidents (no consequences for the patient) included inadvertent transection of a lower pole artery, loss of a needle in the retroperitoneum, and hypercapnia.

Grade 2 incidents (recognized and repaired intraoperatively) included cutting or migration of a ureteral stent, colonic injury, and inability to dissect the UPJ or to approximate the ureter and the renal pelvis. Finally, grade 3 incidents (requiring postoperative reintervention) included a colonic injury and massive bleeding from a port site.

Both pure laparoscopic and robotic techniques have been used safely to perform secondary pyeloplasty after endopyelotomy and primary pyeloplasty [5, 6, 11, 22]. One intraoperative complication occurred in a series of 36 patients having laparoscopic transperitoneal repair of secondary UPJ obstruction; this patient had bleeding requiring conversion to open surgery [6]. No intraoperative complications were noted in 23 patients having secondary robotic pyeloplasty in a large multi-institutional study of RALP [16]. Minimally invasive pyeloplasty has also been safely performed in patients with upper urinary tract anomalies [11, 23].

The rate of conversion from laparoscopic to open pyeloplasty has been reported to be up to 1.6% [7]. Rassweiler et al. [24] reported a single conversion in their large series of retroperitoneal LP based on significant anastomotic tension and the requirement for open dissection and fixation of the kidney during suturing. The risk of conversion is higher during the early portion of the learning curve for LP and decreases significantly as experience improves [7]. Mufarrij et al. [16] reported no open conversions in a series of 140 patients having RALP. Two procedures of 29 were converted to open in another series of RALP; both conversions occurred in patients undergoing secondary pyeloplasty after failed endopyelotomy [25]. Facilitated intracorporeal suturing with robotic techniques may limit the rate of conversion based on failure to progress, particularly early in a surgeon's laparoscopic experience.

Risk of significant bleeding from laparoscopic or robotic pyeloplasty is low. Soulie et al. reported 2 of 61 patients developing hematoma in the lumbar fossa following LP, while Rassweiler et al. reported 5 cases of postoperative hematoma in 143 patients undergoing LP [24, 26].

See Tables 1 and 2 for summaries of postoperative complications from major series of laparoscopic and robotic pyeloplasty. Importantly, these studies do not use standardized definitions of what constitutes a "complication"; thus they may not be directly comparable. Minor and major complications are often grouped together in determining the total complication rate in these studies.

The postoperative complication rate for LP has been reported to be from 2 to 22% [24, 27, 28]. A meta-analysis of LP series revealed an 8% postoperative complication rate including hematoma, urinoma, pyelonephritis, bowel serosal injury, transient ileus, thrombophlebitis, and ureteropelvic junction (UPJ) anastomotic stricture [29]. Another meta-analysis of complications of LP reported a postoperative complication rate of 12.9–15.8% in large series [17]. Increasing experience with LP within series has revealed decreasing rates of postoperative complications [27]. Extraperitoneal LP has had published complication rates up to 13% [26].

Postoperative complication rates for RALP have also been low. In the largest series to date, 7.1% major and 2.9% minor complication rates were reported [16]. The most common major complication in this series (7 of 10) was stent migration, with no difference between the use of retrograde and anterograde techniques for stent placement. The authors mention now erring on the side of longer stent placement and relying on reflux of methylene blue dye through the proximal end of the stent to confirm anterograde placement. One patient in this series had gluteal necrosis with a BMI of 42 during a 5-h procedure, requiring subsequent fasciotomy. The authors mention that their operative times have decreased and that they do not flex the table during surgery for obese patients to allow for more even distribution of weight. Additionally, one patient in this series developed an obstructing blood clot in the renal pelvis necessitating percutaneous nephrostomy tube placement that was left in place until stent removal. The authors mention that irrigation of the renal pelvis prior to closure can help to minimize likelihood of this complication. Lastly, one patient had worsening hydronephrosis and pyelonephritis postoperatively requiring stent exchange.

In another series of 92 patients having RALP, 3 patients (3%) had early complications requiring reintervention [9]. One patient required stent exchange and percutaneous nephrostomy tube placement for clot-related obstruction of the renal pelvis and colic with urine extravasation; one patient bled into the collecting system 2 days postoperatively and despite conservative treatment required open secondary pyeloplasty; and one patient with excessive urine extravasation after

Table 1 Postoperative complications of laparoscopic pyeloplasty

Series	No. of cases	Approach	Postoperative complication rate (%)	Postoperative complications
Symons [39]	118	Trans	10.2 (12)	Infection (4), anastomotic leak (5), hematoma (1), hematuria (2)
Rassweiler [17]	189	Retro	7.9 (15)	Hematoma (6), urine extravasation (4), stent obstruction (2), severe UTI (2), pulmonary embolism (1)
Moon [40]	170	167 retro and 3 trans	7 (12)	Colon injury requiring right hemicolectomy POD 6; re-exploration for port site bleeding 12 h postoperatively; MI; perinephric urinoma treated conservatively; heavy hematuria; port-site infection; uncomplicated UTI; unexplained postoperative fever/rigor; ipsilateral renal pelvic stones (3)
Romero [41]	188	Trans	6.4 (12)	Urinary leak (5), stent migration (2), ureteral obstruction (2), bleeding (1), bilateral pleural effusion (1), seroma (1)
Inagaki [8]	147	Trans	7.5 (11)	Laparoscopic repositioning of drainage tube for urinary leakage (2); retroperitoneal hematoma; diagnostic laparoscopy (negative) for suspected bowel injury; blood transfusion (2); CHF; superficial antecubital thrombophlebitis; transient ileus; persistent urinoma
Davenport [42]	83	66 trans and 17 retro	14.4 (12)	Urine leak after Foley catheter removal (6), acute urinary retention (2), persistent drain site leak (1), asthma exacerbation from NSAID use (1), DVT (1), perirectal bleed (1)
Zhang [2]	50	Retro	4 (2)	Prolonged duration of retroperitoneal drain for urine leak (2)
Mandhani [19]	92	Trans	18.4	Paralytic ileus (6), blood transfusion, prolonged drain output (6), pyelonephritis, meatoplasty, SWL, ureteroscopy for stent migration, percutaneous stenting, repair of port site hernia
Eden [7]	124	Retro	4.1 (5)	Myocardial infarction 6 h postoperatively; bleeding from a subcostal artery lacerated during port insertion requiring return to OR 10 h postoperatively; superficial port site infection; renal calculus formation (2)
Hemal [43]	24	12 trans and 12 retro	12.5 (3)	Prolonged ileus (3) (all transperitoneal)
Sundaram [6]	36	Trans (all secondary)	22.2 (8)	Anastomotic leakage at postoperative cystogram POD 2 (4) (three managed with continued Foley catheter and retroperitoneal drain, one required PCN); UTI, pneumonia; atelectasis; fever; bilateral upper extremity weakness thought related to patient positioning; renal calculus formation at 2 months
Klingler [44]	40	Trans	17.5 (7)	Anastomotic stricture; reoperation (2) (nephrectomy in one patient for recurrent stricture/urosepsis/deteriorated renal function, open ureterocalicostomy in one patient for ischemic anastomosis/recurrent stricture); renal pelvic clot retention (2) requiring PCN in one patient; urinoma; urosepsis from recurrent UTI (2) requiring PCN in one patient
Jarrett [45]	100	Trans	11 (11)	Urinary ascites secondary to drain migration requiring laparoscopic exploration and drain repositioning (2); retroperitoneal bleeding requiring PCN; blood transfusion (3); CHF; pneumonia; superficial antecubital thrombophlebitis; transient ileus; persistent urinoma requiring percutaneous drainage
Turk [20]	49	Trans	2 (1)	Anastomotic leakage POD 1 requiring laparoscopic repair
Soulie [26]	55	Retro	12.7 (7)	Hematoma (3), urinoma, severe pyelonephritis, anastomotic stricture (2) requiring open pyeloplasty at 3 weeks and delayed balloon incision at 13 months

Table 2 Postoperative complications of robotic-assisted laparoscopic pyeloplasty

Series	No. of procedures	Postoperative complication rate	Postoperative complications
Mufarrij [16]	140	7.1 (10) (major) and 2.9 (4) (minor)	*Major*: stent migration (7), clot obstruction, gluteal compartment syndrome requiring fasciotomy, pyelonephritis/obstruction; *minor*: febrile UTI, urine leak (2), splenic laceration (intraoperative)
Yanke [25]	29	6.9 (2)	Readmission for flank pain (no intervention), pyelonephritis
Schwentner [9]	92	3.3 (3)	Bleeding into renal pelvis/colic with urine extravasation requiring stent exchange and PCN; bleeding into collecting system 2 days postoperatively initially managed conservatively, then requiring open pyeloplasty 3 months later; insufficient closure of resected renal pelvis and excessive urine extravasation requiring transperitoneal exploration and primary closure of renal pelvis
Chammas [46]	100	3 (3)	Pyelonephritis (3)
Weise [12]	31	6.5 (2)	Afebrile UTI, urine leak with ileus treated non-operatively
Palese [11]	35	11.4 (4)	UTI requiring oral antibiotics; pyelonephritis requiring IV antibiotics (2); gluteal compartment syndrome
Patel [15]	50	2 (1)	Renal colic after stent removal at 21 days requiring restenting (retrograde pyelogram showed widely patent anastomosis)
Bernie [13]	7	28.6	Febrile UTI requiring IV antibiotics, gross hematuria from bleeding at anastomotic site requiring readmission, and conservative treatment
Gettman [10]	9	11 (1)	Urinary leakage requiring open exploration and repair of incompletely closed renal pelvis

inadequate closure of the renal pelvis required open repair of the renal pelvis. This last patient had prior treatment of UPJ obstruction, but the exact treatment is not mentioned. Two other patients in this series had prior pyeloplasty, and nine had prior endopyelotomy or ureteroscopy, none of whom had significant complications. In one series of 31 patients with RALP, there were 1 non-febrile UTI and 1 urine leak with ileus that was treated non-operatively [12].

Urine leakage occurs in up to 2.3% of patients having LP and can occur despite meticulous suturing and ureteral stent placement [8, 28]. Soulie et al. reported 2 of 61 patients developing postoperative urinoma [26]. Rassweiler et al. reported urinary extravasation in 2 of 143 patients after LP [17]. Secondary pyeloplasty and congenital abnormalities may be risk factors for urinary leak [10].

Success rates for both laparoscopic and robotic pyeloplasty are high and early restricturing is uncommon [9, 30]. Mufarrij et al. reported that 3 of 140 patients required treatment of recurrent stricture after robotic pyeloplasty, two requiring endopyelotomy and one requiring repeat pyeloplasty [16]. The authors attributed these failures most likely to ischemia and/or technical factors.

Operative Planning

Comprehensive preoperative planning may minimize the risk of complications related to minimally invasive pyeloplasty. First, the upper urinary tract anatomy must be delineated in terms of anatomic variation and the disease process. Planning should include CT or MR angiography to assess for crossing vessels and delineate hilar anatomy. CT and MR urography can be used to characterize the lesion of interest, i.e., the length and location of stricture. Diuretic renal scans are useful to assess relative renal function and degree of obstruction. Patients should have mechanical bowel prep prior to reconstructive urologic surgery to increase working space and improve exposure. If a secondary repair is being performed or if there has been prior abdominal surgery, bowel adhesions may be present and bowel decompression may facilitate exposure and visualization and decrease risk of injury.

The decision to perform minimally invasive versus open pyeloplasty depends primarily on surgeon's preference and experience. Regarding the use of pure laparoscopy versus robotic assistance, there is little data to suggest that one approach is superior to the other. Limited comparisons have yielded conflicting data and have not included long-term follow-up [13, 14, 31, 32]. Robotic techniques are likely to have greatest advantage for surgeons without considerable laparoscopic suturing experience. Ultimately surgeons should select the technique with which they are most familiar.

Selection of transperitoneal versus retroperitoneal approaches for pyeloplasty also depends primarily on surgeon's preference. Both approaches have been shown to be safe and effective for upper tract surgery [26]. Retroperitoneal access may be safer in patients with extensive prior abdominal surgery, though disadvantages include limited working space and a potentially steeper learning curve [33].

Prevention of Complications

General principles of peri-operative care apply to patients having minimally invasive pyeloplasty including the use of bilateral sequential compression boots, prophylactic antibiotics, and generous padding to all pressure points.

Laparoscopic suturing is the most challenging aspect of LP. Technical complications of suturing (e.g., stricture, urinary extravasation) may be minimized by meticulous technique, but patient factors (e.g., chronic steroid use, secondary repair) may influence whether these complications occur. Technologies like Lapra-Ty clips (Ethicon Endosurgery, Piscataway, NJ, USA) may be used to minimize tissue trauma during suturing [34]. Also robotic assistance has decreased the learning curve for anastomotic suturing and may reduce complications related to the suture line early in a surgeon's experience.

Creating a tension-free anastomosis is critical to decrease the risk of complications related to ureteral ischemia and suture line breakdown. Too much ureter or pelvis may be inadvertently removed leading to difficulty in creating a tension-free suture line. Redundant renal pelvis should not be removed until the anastomosis is complete. Creating a relaxed suture line may be particularly difficult during secondary repair because of a small renal pelvis or an ischemic tissue. Intraoperative techniques for safely creating more length include nephropexy, reverse psoas hitch (tacking the pelvis to the psoas muscle), and creating a "handle" in the renal pelvis to decrease the manipulation of healthy tissue (Fig. 3a, b). Traction sutures can also be placed in the ureter or the pelvis to decrease the risk of ischemia from tissue manipulation. Risk of urinary leakage may be reduced by control of suture tension during collecting system closure, e.g., with Lapra-Ty's [34]. Also if there is excess fibrosis around the ureter, particularly during secondary pyeloplasty, this should be removed prior to creation of the anastomosis to avoid incorporating this tissue into the repair.

Inadvertent injury to major vessels can be minimized with good operative planning including CT or MR angiography to identify crossing vessels

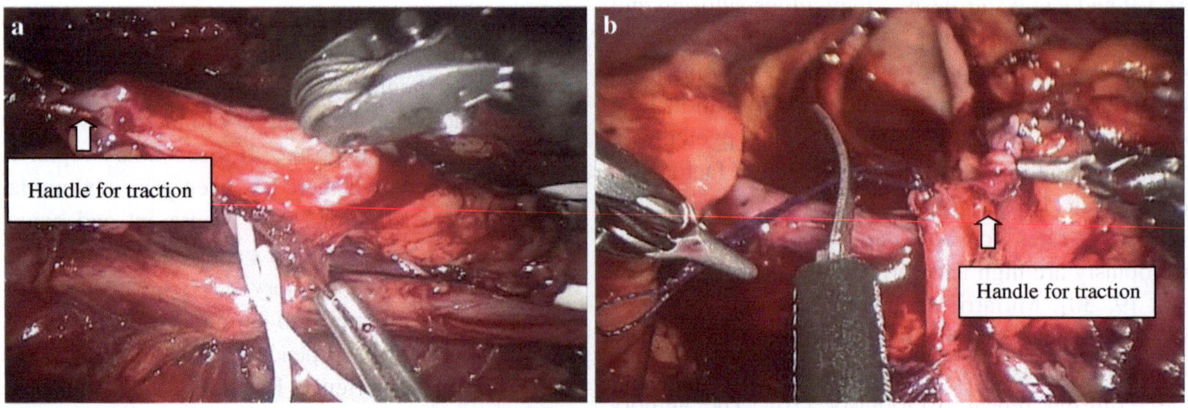

Fig. 3 (**a**) Robotic grasper using handle of nonviable tissue to facilitate spatulation of ureter with Potts scissors. (**b**) Robotic grasper using handle of tissue that will not be used in the anastomosis to enable positioning of proximal and distal tissues during suturing

and/or anomalous vascular anatomy. However, as these modalities are not completely reliable, a laparoscopic Doppler probe (VTI, Nashua, NH, USA) can be used to improve the detection of aberrant vessels and potentially decrease the risk of vascular injury [35] (Fig. 4).

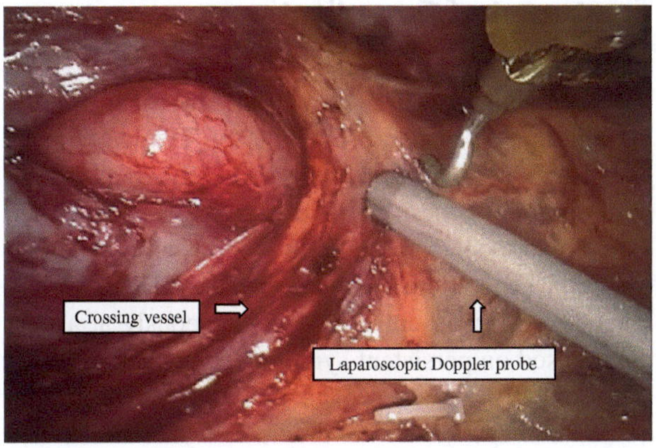

Fig. 4 Laparoscopic Doppler probe confirming flow in crossing vessel

Ureteral stent placement is important to minimize the risk of urinary leakage. Complications of stent placement include submucosal tunneling and incomplete advancement into the bladder or the kidney, depending on the direction of placement. Retrograde stenting requires a second surgeon to place the stent cystoscopically, while the laparoscopic surgeon confirms placement in the renal pelvis. If anterograde placement is performed, the bladder can be filled with 300 cc of methylene blue, and refluxed dye confirms correct distal positioning of the stent. Confirmation by flexible cystoscopy can also be employed to confirm antegrade placement and corrective measures taken at the time of surgery. There is initial evidence that stentless LP in patients having primary repairs is safe; however, this data is preliminary [36].

We leave a percutaneous drain near the anastomosis for at least 2 days to minimize the risk of urinoma formation while healing occurs and to aid in the detection of urinary leak. A Foley catheter is also left in place for at least 2 days postoperatively. On postoperative day 2, the Foley catheter is removed and the drain output is observed to ensure that there is no increased drainage. Approximately 4–6 h after Foley removal, the drain fluid is sent for creatinine level. If the fluid creatinine level is equal to serum, then the drain is removed. If there is evidence of urine leak, patients are managed as described below.

Diagnosis of Complications

Postoperative complications comprise the majority of complications from laparoscopic or robotic surgery [26]. Also, intraoperative injuries may not be recognized until the postoperative period. Symptoms that cannot be explained by physical exam or routine studies should prompt further evaluation. Computed tomography is the study of choice in most patients with unexplained pain, fever, leukocytosis, or decreasing hematocrit following urologic laparoscopy [37].

Bleeding is rare after minimally invasive pyeloplasty. A retroperitoneal bleeding may manifest with a decreasing hematocrit and/or hemodynamic instability. If there is no hemodynamic instability, CT scan is the preferred modality for diagnosis of a retroperitoneal bleeding as well as postoperative hematoma [37]. Delayed bleeding can occur as well; in one series, a patient required hospitalization for retroperitoneal bleeding 1 month after LP [8].

Urinoma is another important complication following minimally invasive pyeloplasty. Urinoma may be indicated by flank or abdominal pain, fever, or elevated liver function tests on the right side [37]. In the early postoperative period, leakage can be detected by persistently elevated drain output and can be confirmed by checking drain fluid creatinine. If there is suspicion for urine leak or urinoma formation, CT with intravenous contrast and delayed images is the diagnostic modality of choice (Fig. 5). There should be a low threshold to perform abdominal imaging to rule out urinoma and/or distal obstruction in the setting of high drain output, significant pain especially associated with leg flexion, and/or elevated drain fluid creatinine.

If a patient presents with ipsilateral flank pain prior to stent removal, imaging should be performed (e.g., KUB) to ensure that the stent is in proper position. Postoperatively, patients should have a KUB in the recovery room to ensure good positioning (Fig. 6). Renal sonogram can be performed for flank pain to ensure that there is no acute obstruction, e.g., secondary to clot, though this may be difficult to ascertain if there is a chronically dilated renal pelvis, and thus we prefer computed tomography.

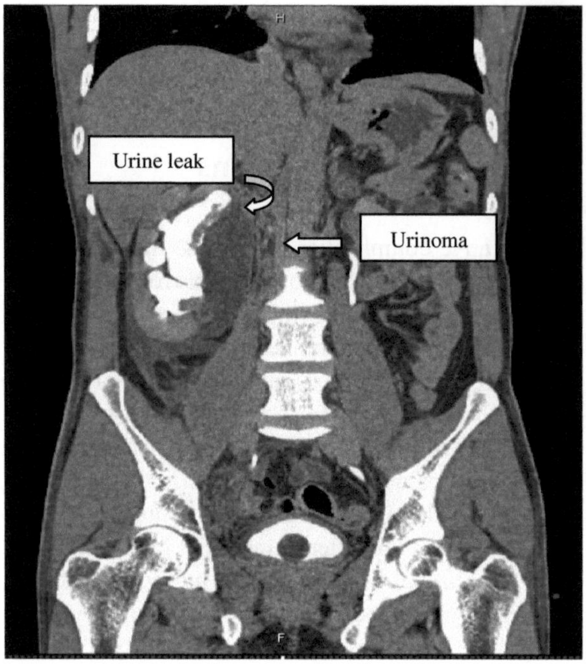

Fig. 5 CT urogram demonstrating small leak at the right superior renal pelvis closure site

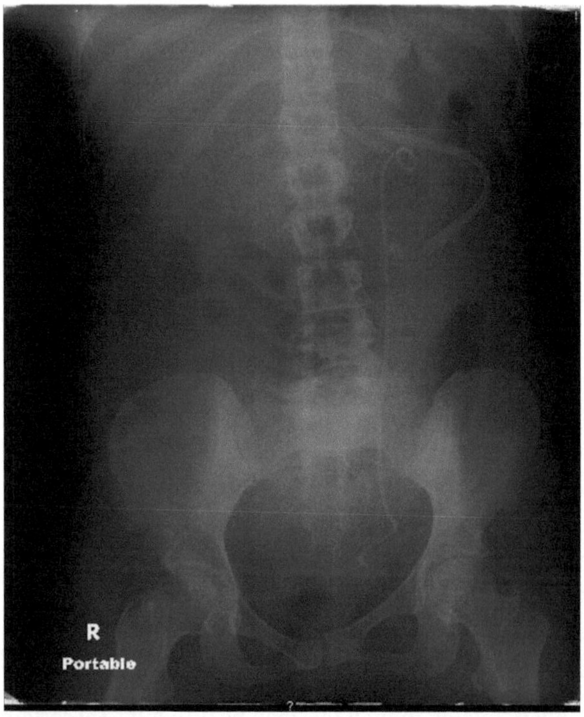

Fig. 6 KUB demonstrating left ureteral stent out of position following robotic pyeloplasty. Distal loop of stent is in the distal ureter rather than the bladder

Stents are typically removed 4–6 weeks after repair and the anastomosis evaluated at 6–8 weeks by renal scan or intravenous pyelogram (IVP). Depending on the timing of restricturing, this process may be considered a treatment failure or a complication.

Treatment of Complications

Bleeding or hematoma formation can occur following minimally invasive pyeloplasty. Hematoma can generally be managed conservatively by following serial hematocrits and transfusing as necessary. Hemodynamic instability or precipitous drop in hematocrit may necessitate urgent reoperation. There may be a need to drain a hematoma percutaneously at a later point based on persistent symptoms or infection [26].

Essentially any urine leak will resolve with adequate drainage (external drain, Foley catheter, and ureteral stent). When a urine leak is suspected by persistent high output or symptoms, fluid creatinine should be assessed and abdominal imaging should be performed to rule out urinoma and to confirm stent and drain positioning. When urinoma is present, we should ensure that the drain is in proper position within the collection. If not, a second drain is placed under CT guidance. We should also confirm that the ureteral stent has not migrated into the ureter and does not require ureteroscopic adjustment. If urinoma is noted after stent removal, the stent should be replaced or a nephroureteral stent should be placed. If there is no Foley catheter, it should be replaced to maximize drainage. In treating urinoma, we leave the drain on suction for 1 week and then obtain repeat imaging. If there is resolution of urinoma but still high output/evidence of urinary leakage, the suction is removed and the drain is left to straight drainage. If high output/evidence of leakage persists, drains are gradually advanced out. The Foley catheter is left in place until the leak has resolved. We utilize similar principles in managing urine leak post-partial nephrectomy.

There are generally no significant sequelae from urinary leakage but periureteral scarring can occur. Repeat laparoscopy to suture an insufficiently closed site is rarely necessary but has been reported [20]. Reactive pleural effusions can occur from urinary leakage abutting the diaphragm; these may require drainage if symptoms develop or there is consideration of infection.

Stent obstruction or migration can occur after minimally invasive pyeloplasty. If stent obstruction has occurred, the stent should be changed or percutaneous nephrostomy tube placement with or without anterograde stenting should be performed. Stent migration can also occur requiring repositioning via ureteroscopy or removal depending on timing relative to surgery [19]. If stent migration below the anastomosis is identified late, stenosis may require reoperation [26].

Acute obstruction after stent removal may require repeat stenting or nephrostomy tube placement depending on symptoms, presence of infection, and serum creatinine [27, 38]. If early restricturing occurs, the next step is to characterize the stricture with drainage imaging (e.g., IVP, CT urogram). Short annular strictures can be initially treated with endourologic techniques such as balloon dilation or endopyelotomy. However, secondary pyeloplasty may ultimately be required if these interventions fail or longer strictures are present, and alternative techniques like ureterocalicostomy may be necessary depending on patient anatomy (e.g., insufficient renal pelvis for anastomosis) [26].

Conclusions

Minimally invasive pyeloplasty has become the standard of care for definitive management of UPJ obstruction. Inexperience with laparoscopic suturing has been the main obstacle to widespread performance of minimally invasive repairs. Advantages of robotic systems (i.e., facilitated intracorporeal suturing) may enable more urologists to safely and effectively perform this procedure. Fundamental tenets of minimally invasive pyeloplasty hold true for both laparoscopic and robotic procedures: careful tissue handling to minimize risk of ischemia and maximizing drainage of the upper tract postoperatively. Vigilant postoperative care can ensure early detection and effective treatment of complications should they occur.

References

1. Klingler HC, Remzi M, Janetschek G, et al. Comparison of open versus laparoscopic pyeloplasty techniques in treatment of uretero-pelvic junction obstruction. Eur Urol. 2003;44(3):340–5.
2. Zhang X, Li HZ, Ma X, Zheng T, Lang B, Zhang J, Fu B, Xu K, Guo XL. Retrospective comparison of retroperitoneal laparoscopic versus open dismembered pyeloplasty for ureteropelvic junction obstruction. J Urol. 2006;176(3):1077–80.
3. Calvert RC, Morsy MM, Zelhof B, Rhodes M, Burgess NA. Comparison of laparoscopic and open pyeloplasty in 100 patients with pelvi-ureteric junction obstruction. Surg Endosc. 2008;22(2):411–4.
4. Schuessler WW, Grune MT, Tecuanahuey LV, et al. Laparoscopic dismembered pyeloplasty. J Urol. 1993;150:1795.
5. Vakarakis IM, Bhayani SB, Allaf ME, et al. Management of secondary ureteropelvic junction obstruction after failed primary laparoscopic pyeloplasty. J Urol. 2004;172: 180–2.
6. Sundaram CP, Gruss RL, Rehman J, et al. Laparoscopic pyeloplasty for secondary ureteropelvic junction obstruction. J Urol. 2003;169:2037–40.
7. Eden C, Gianduzzo T, Chang C, et al. Extraperitoneal laparoscopic pyeloplasty for primary and secondary ureteropelvic junction obstruction. J Urol. 2004;172: 2308–11.
8. Inagaki T, Rha KH, Ong AM, et al. Laparoscopic pyeloplasty: current status. BJU Int. 2005;92(Suppl 2):102–5.
9. Schwentner C, Pelzer A, Neururer R, et al. Robotic Anderson-Hynes pyeloplasty: 5-year experience of one center. BJU Int. 2007;100(4):880–5.
10. Gettman MT, Peschel R, Neururer R, et al. A comparison of laparoscopic pyeloplasty performed with the da Vinci robotic system versus standard laparoscopic techniques: initial clinical results. Eur Urol. 2002;42(5):453–7.
11. Palese MA, Stifelman MD, Munver R. Robot-assisted laparoscopic dismembered pyeloplasty: a combined experience. J Endourol. 2005;19(3):382–6.
12. Weise ES, Winfield HN. Robotic computer-assisted pyeloplasty versus conventional laparoscopic pyeloplasty. J Endourol. 2006;20(10):813–9.
13. Bernie JE, Venkatesh R, Brown J, et al. Comparison of laparoscopic pyeloplasty with and without robotic assistance. JSLS. 2005;9:258–61.
14. Link RE, Bhayani SB, Kavoussi LR. A prospective comparison of robotic and laparoscopic pyeloplasty. Ann Surg. 2006;243(4):486–91.
15. Patel V, et al. Robotic-assisted laparoscopic dismembered pyeloplasty. Urology. 2005;66(1):45–9.
16. Mufarrij PW, Woods M, Shah OD, et al. Robotic dismembered pyeloplasty: a 6-year, multi-institutional experience. J Urol. 2008;180(4):1391–6.
17. Rassweiler JJ, Teber D, Frede T. Complications of laparoscopic pyeloplasty. World J Urol. 2008;26:539–47.
18. Soulie M, Salomon L, Seguin P, et al. Multi-institutional study of complications in 1085 laparoscopic urologic procedures. Urology. 2001;58:899–903.
19. Mandhani A, Kumar D, Kumar A, et al. Safety profile and complications of transperitoneal laparoscopic pyeloplasty: a critical analysis. J Endourol. 2005;19(7): 797–802.
20. Turk IA, Davis JW, Winkelman B, et al. Laparoscopic dismembered pyeloplasty – the method of choice in the presence of an enlarged renal pelvis and crossing vessels. Eur Urol. 2002;42(3):268–75.

21. Satava RM. Identification and reduction of surgical error using simulation. Minim Invasive Ther Allied Technol. 2005;14:257–61.
22. Shapiro EY, Cho JS, Srinivasan A, et al. Long-term follow-up for salvage laparoscopic pyeloplasty after failed open pyeloplasty. Urology. 2009;73:115–8.
23. Bove P, Ong AM, Rha KH, et al. Laparoscopic management of ureteropelvic junction obstruction in patients with upper urinary tract anomalies. J Urol. 2004;171:77–9.
24. Rassweiler JJ, Subotic S, Feist-Schwenk M, et al. Minimally invasive treatment of ureteropelvic junction obstruction: long-term experience with an algorithm for laser endopyelotomy and laparoscopic retroperitoneal pyeloplasty. J Urol. 2007;1777:1000–5.
25. Yanke BV, Lallas CD, Pagnani C, Bagley DH. Robot-assisted laparoscopic pyeloplasty: technical considerations and outcomes. J Endourol. 2008;22(6):1291–95.
26. Soulie M, Salomon L, Patard JJ, et al. Extra-peritoneal laparoscopic pyeloplasty: a multi-center study of 55 procedures. J Urol. 2001;16:48–50.
27. Iwamura M, Soh S, Irie A, et al. Laparoscopic pyeloplasty for ureteropelvic junction obstruction: outcome of initial 12 procedures. Int J Urol. 2004;11:449–55.
28. Permpongkosol S, Link RE, Su L, et al. Complications of 2,775 urological laparoscopic procedures: 1993 to 2005. J Urol. 2007;177:580–5.
29. Kaouk JH, Gill IS. Laparoscopic reconstructive urology. J Urol. 2003;170:1070–8.
30. El-Shazly MA, Moon DA, Eden CG. Laparoscopic pyeloplasty: status and review of literature. J Endourol. 2007;21(7):673–8.
31. Peschel R, Neururer R, Bartsch G, Gettman MT. Robotic pyeloplasty: technique and results. Urol Clin North Am. 2004;31(4):737–41.
32. Winfield HN. Management of adult ureteropelvic junction obstruction – is it time for a new gold standard? J Urol, 2006;176(3):866–7.
33. Viterbo R, Greenberg RE, Al-Saleem T, et al. Prior abdominal surgery and radiation do not complicate the retroperitoneoscopic approach to the kidney or adrenal gland. J Urol. 2005;174:446–50.
34. Shalhav AL, Orvieto MA, Chien GW, et al. Minimizing knot tying during reconstructive laparoscopic urology. Urology. 2006;68:508–13.
35. Hyams ES, Kanofsky JA, Stifelman MD. Laparoscopic Doppler technology: applications in laparoscopic pyeloplasty and radical and partial nephrectomy. Urology. 2008;71(5):952–6.
36. Shalhav AL, Mikhail AA, Orvieto MA, et al. Adult stentless laparoscopic pyeloplasty. JSLS. 2007;11(1):8–13.
37. Cadeddu JA, Regan F, Kavoussi LR, et al. The role of computerized tomography in the evaluation of complications after laparoscopic urological surgery. J Urol. 1997;158:1349–52.
38. Parsons JK, Varkarakis I, Rha KH, et al. Complications of abdominal urologic laparoscopy: longitudinal five-year analysis. Urology. 2004;63:27–32.
39. Symons SJ, Bhirud PS, Jain V, Shetty AS, Desai MR. Laparoscopic pyeloplasty: our new gold standard. J Endourol. 2009;23(3). Epub ahead of print.
40. Moon DA, El-Shazly MA, Chang CM, et al. Laparoscopic pyeloplasty: evolution of a new gold standard. Urology. 2006;67(5):932–6.
41. Romero FR, Wagner AA, Trapp C, Permpongkosol S, Muntener M, Link RE, Kavoussi LR. Transmesenteric laparoscopic pyeloplasty. J Urol. 2006;176:2526–9.
42. Davenport K, Minervini A, Timoney AG, Keeley FX Jr. Our experience with retroperitoneal and transperitoneal laparoscopic pyeloplasty for pelvi-ureteric junction obstruction. Eur Urol. 2005;48(6):973–7.
43. Hemal AK, Goel R, Goel A. Cost-effective laparoscopic pyeloplasty: single center experience. Int J Urol. 2003;10(11):563–8.
44. Klingler HC, Remzi M, Janetschek G, Kratzik C, Marberger MJ. Comparison of open versus laparoscopic pyeloplasty techniques in treatment of uretero-pelvic junction obstruction. Eur Urol. 2003;44(3):340–5.
45. Jarrett TW, Chan DY, Charambura TC, et al. Laparoscopic pyeloplasty: the first 100 cases. J Urol. 2002;167:1253–6.
46. Chammas MF Jr, Hubert J, Patel VR. Robotically assisted laparoscopic pyeloplasty: a transatlantic comparison of techniques and outcomes. BJU Int. 2007;99:1113–7.

Complications of Laparoscopic and Robotic Ureteral Surgery

Ugur Boylu and Raju Thomas

Keywords Robotics · Reimplantation · Ureter · Laparoscopy · Complications

Introduction

Over the past two decades, technological innovations have remarkably improved the delivery of urologic care. The management of ureteral diseases has undergone a tremendous evolution in the range of available options. Various minimally invasive surgical options have become available, for instance, in treating ureteropelvic junction obstruction (UPJO) including antegrade and retrograde endopyelotomy, Acucise^{TM} incisional endopyelotomy, and percutaneous endopyeloplasty. More recently, the introduction of laparoscopic and robotic surgery has opened new doors for diverse application of these techniques in minimally invasive urologic surgery. In particular, laparoscopic pyeloplasty has evolved into the standard of care for UPJO [1, 2]. Recently, robotic-assisted pyeloplasty has been introduced with the distinct advantage of facilitating intracorporeal suturing. Decision regarding the appropriate treatment option for UPJO depends on several factors such as degree of hydronephrosis, function of affected renal unit, presence of kidney stones, length of obstructing segment, presence of crossing vessels, availability of necessary surgical equipment, and above all, surgeon's experience. Utilizing the same principles advocated for the management of the UPJO, laparoscopic and robotic surgery are also being utilized for the treatment of other problems, such as vesicoureteral reflux disease and ureteral strictures. However, every technological advancement introduces new potential complications in addition to already existing ones. Surgeons must be aware of the possible complications associated with the introduction of new equipment and techniques, appropriate prevention of these complications, and finally prompt diagnosis and management of these complications. One cannot overemphasize the importance of surgeons being fully familiar with newly introduced equipment and being aware of potential complications, especially during the learning curve associated with mastering a particular technique.

Operative Techniques

Ureteroureterostomy

The operative techniques for laparoscopic and robotic-assisted ureteroureterostomy and lessons we have learned from laparoscopic and robotic pyeloplasty are similar. Following cystoscopy and placement of an ipsilateral 5-Fr open-ended ureter catheter and a retrograde pyelogram to assess the length of the obstructing strictured segment, the patient is placed in a modified 45° lateral decubitus position. The 5-Fr open-ended catheter is positioned just distal to the obstructing segment and secured to a Foley catheter.

R. Thomas (✉)
Department of Urology, Center for Minimally Invasive & Robotic Surgery, Tulane University School of Medicine, New Orleans, LA, USA
e-mail: rthomas@tulane.edu

R. Ghavamian (ed.), *Complications of Laparoscopic and Robotic Urologic Surgery*,
DOI 10.1007/978-1-60761-676-4_16,

A 12-mm port is usually placed at the umbilicus for the laparoscopic/robotic camera. Two ports are placed 30° cranially and caudally off an axis from the umbilicus to the strictured segment, approximately 8–10 cm from the umbilicus (Fig. 1). The fourth port (used by the bedside surgeon in robotic surgery to assist in dissection, suction, and intracorporeal introduction and removal of sutures/needles) is placed near the midline inferior to the umbilicus. The trocar placements need to be adjusted depending on the size of the patient and location of the stricture, taking into consideration the basic principles of laparoscopic and robotic ergonomics and the need to facilitate suturing the anastomosis. For right-sided procedures, an additional port could be placed in the subxiphoid area for liver retraction, if necessary. Following achievement of pneumoperitoneum, the colon is reflected medially. The ureteral ends are identified, isolated, and adequate proximal and distal ureterolysis is performed. The strictured segment is transected, the ureteral ends are spatulated in opposite directions 180° apart, and all fibrous, strictured, and unhealthy appearing tissues are excised.

The anastomosis of the ureteral ends begins at the posterior aspect using a 4-0 polyglactin suture on RB-1 needle. We suggest using two such sutures starting posteriorly and running them in either direction and culminating anteriorly. A double pigtail stent is passed over a guide wire, preferably in a retrograde fashion into the ureter. Although ureteral stent placement is a subjective matter and based on the surgeon's preference, it is important to note that the placement of a ureteral stent intraoperatively for a ureteral stricture is more challenging than that for laparoscopic or robotic pyeloplasty. Thus, placing a 5-Fr open-ended catheter just distal to the strictured segment is highly recommended. A super-stiff or similar guidewire is passed through the open-ended catheter by the assistant and retrieved by the laparoscopic or robotic surgeon. This guidewire is introduced into the proximal ureteral segment and a stent is loaded onto the guidewire and advanced, under direct vision, into the renal pelvis. This maneuver is performed after completion of the posterior sutures. After visual guidance has secured the stent in place, the anterior portion of the anastomosis is completed. Caution is advised during stent placement so as not to push the stent into the ureteral orifice. Confirmation of the distal curl of the stent in the bladder can be done using a flexible cystoscope. After the anastomosis is satisfactorily completed, periureteral fat is reapproximated over the anastomosis. A closed-suction drain is placed, which is managed as with any similar drain, and the double pigtail stent is left indwelling for approximately 4–6 weeks.

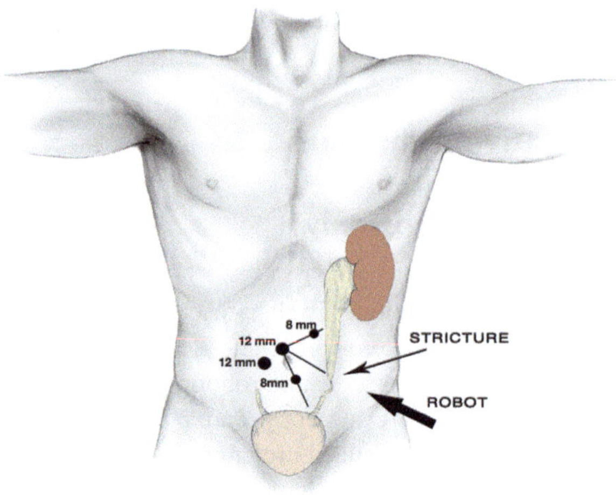

Fig. 1 Port placement for laparoscopic and robotic ureteroureterostomy

A tension-free anastomosis is crucial. Thus, if the ureteroureterostomy appears to be under undue tension, additional procedures should be considered. Additional procedures include further ureterolysis in each direction and tension-decreasing procedures, such as reverse nephropexy [3] (Fig. 2). The perceived advantages of robotic-assisted ureteroureterostomy vs. laparoscopic ureteroureterostomy are improved dexterity, articulation, precision with tissue and needle handling and placement of suture, shorter learning curve for novice surgeons, improved visualization of the operative field, shorter operative times, and equivalent outcomes to open surgery and conventional laparoscopy.

In summary, the principles of laparoscopic and robotic ureteroureterostomy for ureteral stricture disease should mimic those of open surgical technique. These include knowing the exact location and extent of the strictured segment, dissecting and excising the disease segment, spatulating the ends, appropriate stent placement, and producing a tension-free anastomosis.

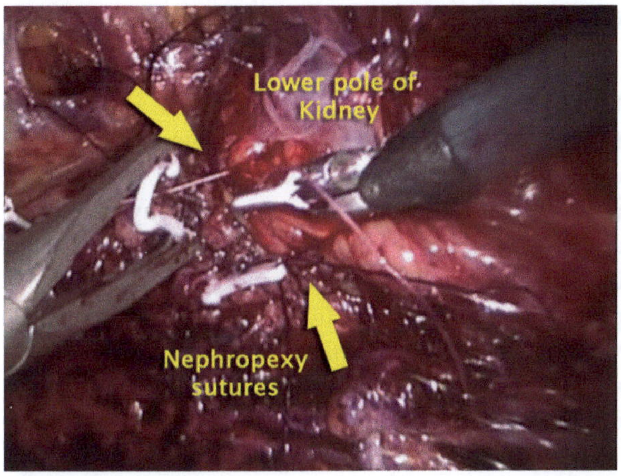

Fig. 2 Reverse nephropexy. *Arrows* indicate the nephropexy sutures with surgical clips

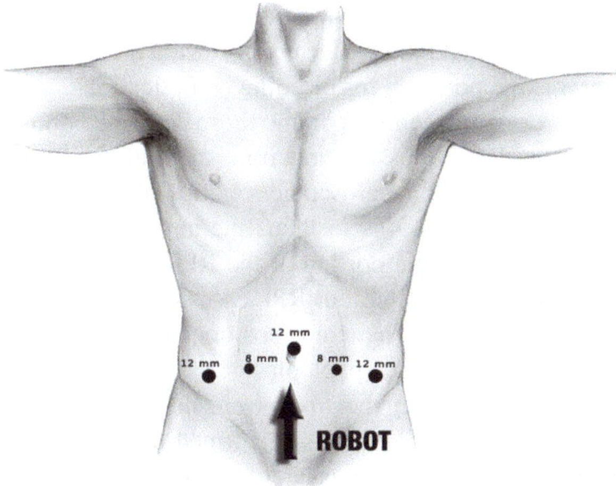

Fig. 3 Port placement for laparoscopic and robotic-assisted ureteral reimplantation

Ureteral Reimplantation

After appropriate preoperative workup to delineate the length of the ureteral stricture, the patient is placed in a lithotomy position. A 5-Fr open-ended ureteral catheter is passed into the affected ureter; however, this is usually impossible due to the stricture. After achieving pneumoperitoneum with the Veress needle, a 12-mm port is placed at the umbilicus and two ports are placed in the midclavicular line approximately 2 fingerbreadths below the level of the umbilicus. Additionally, one port is placed lateral to the abovementioned ports for suction, retraction, and suture delivery (Fig. 3). The line of Toldt is incised and the ipsilateral colon is reflected medially. The ureter is identified at the level of the crossing of the iliac vessels and dissected free just above the level of fibrosis/stricture. The dissection is continued caudally as far as possible. The ureter is transected as distally as possible and spatulated. The bladder is dissected posteriorly and mobilized anteriorly and ipsilaterally. The placement of a double pigtail stent is highly recommended. If possible, a direct ureteroneocystostomy is performed but in cases with longer strictured segment or more proximal strictures, a Boari flap with or without a psoas hitch is utilized [4]. The posterior ureterovesical anastomosis is closed with 4-0 polyglactin sutures. The distal end of the pigtail stent is placed into the bladder and the anterior ureterovesical anastomosis is completed with the same 4/0 polyglactin suture. In select cases, an anti-reflux procedure may be desired. The anastomosis is tested for leakage by bladder irrigation and is then covered with perivesical fat. A closed drain, such as a Jackson-Pratt drain, is placed and the ports are closed. A Foley catheter drains the bladder. The drain, the Foley catheter, and the ureteral stent are managed in a routine manner based on sound urologic principles.

Infrequently Performed Ureteral Procedures

Although reported series have addressed infrequent problems such as the laparoscopic ureteral management of retroperitoneal fibrosis (RPF) [5] and retrocaval ureters [6, 7], such techniques follow the principles of open surgical management and these complex procedures are recommended for urologists with overall significant experience in laparoscopic and robotic techniques.

The key to such advanced laparoscopic and robotic procedures is appropriate preoperative workup and anatomic delineation of the ureteral course through the RPF or around the inferior vena cava (IVC). In the case of RPF, surgical candidates must have a biopsy of the RPF tissue to rule out malignancy. The right ureteral dissection must be performed with utmost caution since the RPF draws the ureter toward the IVC and presents the potential for bleeding complications.

The trocar placements mimic those described above for ureteral strictures and ureteroneocystostomy. Thus, the experienced laparoscopic/robotic surgeon will place the trocars so as to focus the axis of the camera toward the main portion of the RPF or the course of the retrocaval ureter. For RPF cases, a ureteral stent is preplaced and the patient is positioned in a modified flank position (as for a pyeloplasty or ureteral stricture management). After the trocars are in place, careful but meticulous dissection is performed to free up the ureter. Intraoperative biopsies of the RPF tissue may be indicated. After the ureter has been isolated adequately, we recommend intraperitoneal placement of the involved ureter by reapproximating the peritoneal incision behind the ureter and securing the ureter away from the retroperitoneum, as described with open surgical approaches [8]. Caution is advised during this dissection not to strip the ureter or place undue tension or traction on the ureter. Bilateral laparoscopic/robotic management of RPF is possible but requires prolonged operative time since patients have to be repositioned for the other side.

For the rare case of retrocaval ureter, the ureter is carefully dissected off the IVC and reapproximated in the normal anatomic position and stented, as described in section "Ureteroureterostomy" on ureteral strictures.

Literature Review: Complications of Laparoscopic and Robotic Ureteral Surgery

The critical step in avoiding complications is to be aware of potential problems and to be prepared to identify and promptly manage any adverse events. Toward this goal, it is essential to have adequate preoperative workup to delineate the location and the extent of the pathology of the ureter needing reconstructive intervention. The status of the surrounding tissues and adjacent organs is a necessity to minimize any potential complications. To be fully cognizant of the task at hand, we recommend preoperative workup, including CT scans, renal functional studies, and retrograde pyelograms.

Complications of Ureteral Reimplantation

Ureteral reimplantation in adults is essentially performed for distal ureteral pathologies resulting in ureteral stricture. In 1992, Nezhat et al. [9] reported the first laparoscopic ureteroneocystostomy. The operation is particularly challenging and requires a high degree of laparoscopic skill. Therefore, it is not widely performed by urologists. In 2003, Yohannes et al. [10] were the first to describe their experience with robotic-assisted ureteral reimplantation for ureteral stricture disease.

Complications of laparoscopic and robotic-assisted ureteral implantation are summarized in Table 1. Unlike the pyeloplasty series, both laparoscopic and robotic ureteral reimplantation series are limited in the number of case series published. Therefore, it is difficult to define the associated complications and their morbidity. The complication rates in published series ranged from 5.6 to 33% [11–15]. Although the complication rates were higher in earlier smaller series, recent published data containing more than 10 patients reported complication rates ranging from 5.6 to 13.3% [13, 16, 17]. Recently, Seideman et al. [16] published the largest series of laparoscopic ureteral reimplantation with 45 patients. Intraoperative complications included two ureterotomies performed in areas of normal ureter in patients with retroperitoneal fibrosis. Postoperative complications included colitis, ileus, and respiratory distress in one patient and small bowel obstruction in another patient, which resolved with nasogastric suction and bowel rest. Additionally, urinary leak was treated with conservative management in three patients. Simmons et al. reported one patient who underwent a Boari flap procedure and developed a postoperative urinoma, verified on computed tomography [17]. This patient was treated with bladder catheter decompression and the urinoma resolved after 2 weeks. Rassweiler et al. [15] performed 10 laparoscopic ureteral reimplantations and reported two complications in this series. Two patients suffered from prolonged ileus for 4 days, whereas the authors reported more serious complications (two intra-abdominal bleeding and hematoma with urinary leakage, and one anastomotic stricture with urinary leakage) in their open ureteral reimplantation group. In a series of eight patients with laparoscopic ureteroneocystostomy, Castillo et al. reported one pulmonary

Table 1 Complications in laparoscopic and robotic-assisted ureteral reimplantation series

Series	Year	Number of patients	Technique	Conversion to open	Number of complications (%)	Complications
Fugita [12]	2001	3	L	0	1 (33%)	Colitis
Nezhat [14]	2004	6	L	0	2 (33%)	Stent discomfort, leg pain
Castillo [11]	2005	8	L	0	2 (25%)	Urinary leak, pulmonary embolism
Rassweiler [15]	2006	10	L	0	2 (20%)	Ileus
Simmons [17]	2007	12	L	0	1 (8.3)	Urinary leak
Ogan [18]	2008	6	L	1 (16.7%)	0	–
Modi [13]	2008	18	L	1 (5.6%)	1 (5.6%)	Bradycardia, arrhythmia
Symons [34]	2009	6	L	0	0	–
Seideman [16]	2009	45	L	0	6 (13.3%)	Ureterotomy, colitis, ileus, respiratory distress, small bowel obstruction, urinary leak
Mufarrij [20]	2007	4	R	0	0	–
Laungani [19]	2008	3	R	0	0	–
Patil [4]	2008	12	R	0	0	–
Williams [21]	2009	8	R	0	0	–

L, laparoscopic; R, robotic assisted

embolism in a patient with prostate cancer who had undergone perineal prostatectomy and one uroperitoneum in a patient with a medical history of cervical carcinoma, hysterectomy, and radiotherapy [11]. In the latter patient, exploratory laparoscopy revealed a small opening in the bladder closure, which was repaired with intracorporeal suturing. In another study with 18 cases of laparoscopic ureteral reimplantation, Modi et al. [13] reported one (5.6%) intraoperative bradycardia and arrhythmia due to hypercarbia and pneumoperitoneum. The procedure was terminated and following the stabilization of the patient after 48 h, open ureteroneocystostomy was performed. Additionally, one open conversion (16.7%) was reported by Ogan et al. [18] in a series of six patients with laparoscopic ureteral reimplantation.

Complications of robotic-assisted ureteral reimplantation are unclear (Table 1). There are four series of robotic-assisted ureteral reimplantation with smaller number of patients (range 3–12) [4, 19–21]. There were no intraoperative and postoperative complications or conversion to open ureteroneocystostomy in these studies. In summary, although the number of series and the number of patients in each series are small, the reason for fewer complications might be due to facilitated suturing, three-dimensional visualization, and improved articulation of robotic systems.

Complications of Ureteroureterostomy and Other Ureteral Surgery

Laparoscopic ureteroureterostomy was introduced by Nezhat et al. in 1992 [9]. In their study involving eight laparoscopic ureteroureterostomy patients, seven were found to have patent anastomosis with a follow-up of 2–6 months [22]. One patient had mild ureteral stricture, which resolved with transvesical ureteral dilatation. Polascik and Chen [7] reported management of a retrocaval ureter case with laparoscopic ureteroureterostomy. Ameda et al. [6] reported two ureteroureterostomies without any intra- or postoperative complications. Recently, Mufarrij et al. [20] reported two robotic-assisted ureteroureterostomies without any major or minor complications. Thiel et al. [23] published a robotic-assisted ureteroureterostomy case report. The overall clinical experience in laparoscopic and robotic-assisted ureteroureterostomy is, however, limited.

Though principles of pyeloplasty mimic ureteroureterostomy, there are certain differences that need to be highlighted. One of the most challenging aspects of ureteroureterostomy is the need for tension-free anastomosis. This principle is less of a concern with pyeloplasty since the patulous renal pelvis is more forgiving and amenable to a tension-free anastomosis. Thus, the surgeon should be aware of the need to perform adequate proximal and distal ureterolysis in an effort to make the ureteroureterostomy anastomosis as tension free as possible. More importantly, additional procedures such as a reverse nephropexy may be indicated to achieve this goal and should be clearly indicated in the surgical consent form. Patient selection for this technique is crucial since the inability to perform a tension-free anastomosis may require additional procedures, which may not be laparoscopically or robotically feasible in a given patient.

Placement of an indwelling ureteral stent during ureteroureterostomy is also challenging since the two ends of the ureter need stabilization for appropriate stenting. One consideration is retrograde placement of an open-ended ureteral catheter up to the strictured segment. This catheter can then be introduced into the proximally dissected ureteral segment and a guide wire is subsequently placed through the open-ended ureteral catheter for stent placement.

Prevention and Management of Complications

Preoperative Preparation and Planning

Detailed preoperative preparation could minimize the risk of complications related to ureteral surgery. As mentioned earlier, comprehensive imaging will help to delineate the anatomy and therefore the surgical approach for reconstruction. In patients with ureteral strictures, RPF, and such ureteral pathology, a CT scan should be performed to assess the retroperitoneum for any associated pathology, such as tumors, which can cause secondary strictures. Additionally, the CT scan assesses the status of the renal parenchyma and degree of hydronephrosis. We would also recommend a MAG-3 renal scan to assess the individual renal functional status. CT and MR urography can be used to assess the length and location of the strictured segment. For ureteral strictures, an open-ended ureteral catheter should be passed beyond the stricture if the stricture is not completely obstructing the ureter. This maneuver will facilitate intraoperative identification of the ureter amidst the strictured and fibrosed tissue. This will add to the tactile feedback while dissecting through the fibrous tissue. Retrograde and antegrade imaging can be used to identify the length and the location of the ureteral stricture or fistulae. Depending on the size and the location of the stricture, a direct ureteroneocystostomy or a Boari flap, etc. can be performed [8] (Table 2).

The decision to perform a laparoscopic, an open, or a robotic-assisted surgical procedure depends on patient selection, available instruments, and, most importantly, the surgeon's experience. Publications comparing laparoscopic and robotic-assisted pyeloplasty are unable to demonstrate the superiority of any one technique [24, 25]. In a recent meta-analysis, robotic-assisted and laparoscopic pyeloplasty appeared to be equivalent with regard to postoperative leaks, hospital readmission, success rates, and operative time [26]. As far as ureteroneocystostomy is concerned, because of limited available data comparing robotic-assisted vs. laparoscopic ureteral reimplantation, the selection of the appropriate technique depends primarily on surgeon's preference and experience. Robotic techniques have the advantage of improved perception of depth and facilitated suturing compared to pure laparoscopic techniques. This advantage has directly led to easier and wider dissemination of the robotic techniques for urologic reconstruction and has also directly increased the proliferation and accessibility of this minimally invasive technique for a greater number of patients.

Table 2 Recommended ureteral reconstructive surgical techniques based on ureteral defect lengths [8]

Technique	Ureteral defect length (cm)
Ureteroureterostomy	2–3
Ureteroneocystostomy	4–5
Psoas hitch	6–10
Boari flap	12–15
Reverse nephropexy	5–8

In the literature, transperitoneal and retroperitoneal approaches have been shown to be similarly effective and safe for laparoscopic pyeloplasty [27]. The decision between a transperitoneal and an extraperitoneal approach depends on available equipment and surgeon's experience.

Complications Specific to Laparoscopic and Robotic Urologic Reconstructive Procedures

Bleeding

Caution should be exercised when dissecting in close proximity to major blood vessels. The renal collecting system is close to the aorta, renal vessels, inferior vena cava (IVC), iliac vessels and is thus vulnerable to trauma while dissecting through and around strictured ureteral segment. This is especially true in secondary strictures and in RPF, especially on the right side when it can be closely adherent to the IVC. Significant bleeding, though relatively rare, may need open surgical intervention.

Urinary Extravasation

Some degree of urinary extravasation is to be expected since the anastomosis takes time to become watertight. Management is outlined below. However, prudent management of drains and Foley catheter can greatly minimize such events.

Tension at Anastomosis

Any tension at the anastomotic site is a harbinger of future problems such as the recurrence of the stricture and is a source of significant frustrations during the operative procedure. Section "Management of Complications" outlines management strategies.

Stent Migration (Proximal or Distal)

Prompt diagnosis and management can save a lot of grief for the patient and the urologist alike. Stent-associated problems are more common than is appreciated. Strict adherence to sound stenting and troubleshooting, as described earlier in this chapter, can minimize postoperative stent-related complications.

Recurrence of Primary Pathology

Meticulous attention to surgical detail and being cognizant of the above-mentioned potential adverse events would positively impact success rates. Recurrence of ureteral strictures is multifactorial. Causes range from inadequate excision of the diseased ureteral segment to vascular supply problems to tension at the anastomotic sites, hence the importance of management details from the preoperative diagnostic stage to the intraoperative details, so as to achieve optimum results.

Diagnosis of Complications

Even though the published rates of complications for ureteroureterostomy and ureteroneocystostomy are quite low, any unusual symptom/s should prompt further evaluation. In urologic laparoscopy, since abdominal findings are known to be subtle and atypical, a CT scan is indicated in patients with significant clinical findings in whom routine examination and tests are not diagnostic [28]. Postoperative bleeding, bowel injury, urinary leak/urinoma, or renal obstruction can reliably be identified with CT.

Urinoma is one of the most common and potentially severe complications of the urinary tract surgery. It may present fever and flank or abdominal pain. Peritonitis may develop due to urinary ascites. Urinary leakage is the initiator of fistulas. Persistent high-volume drainage through the drain site in early postoperative phase should be suspected as being secondary to urinary extravasation. High creatinine levels in the drain fluid can confirm urinary leakage. A CT scan with contrast and delayed images will differentiate a generalized urinary leak from an organized urinoma (Fig. 4). Premature removal of a drain can lead to urinoma formation.

Although significant bleeding rarely occurs after minimally invasive procedures, such as ureteroureterostomy and ureteroneocystostomy, vital signs

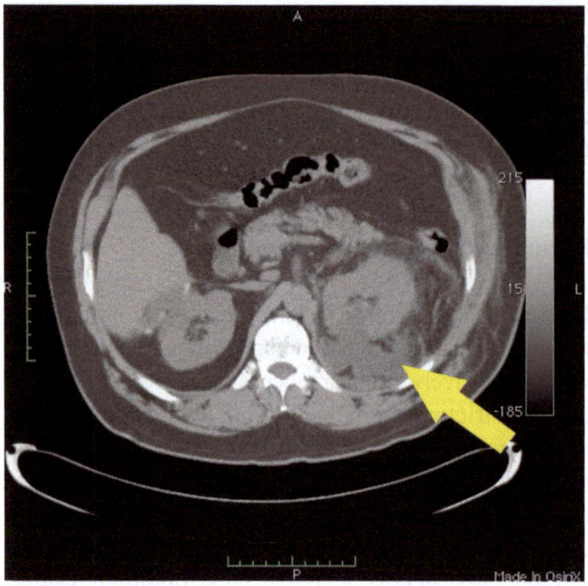

Fig. 4 A urinoma on the left side demonstrated in CT scan

and serial hematocrits should be monitored carefully in the early postoperative period. A decrease in blood pressure and hematocrit may be a sign of bleeding. Additionally, clot formation in the ureter secondary to bleeding may result in secondary obstruction and insufficient drainage of the renal unit, thereby causing urinary extravasation.

In patients with flank pain or discomfort, a KUB should be performed to ensure proper stent position. A migrated stent can result in obstruction of the renal pelvis and urine leakage. Any malpositioned stent should be repositioned immediately using basic endourologic techniques. Renal ultrasound may be convenient to evaluate the obstruction and blood clots in renal pelvis; however, CT scanning is diagnostic for clotted hematoma in the renal pelvis. Such an event needs close monitoring and the need for a percutaneous nephrostomy tube depends on patient's symptoms and urinary leakage.

Management of Complications

Bleeding

Intraoperative bleeding should be relatively easy to diagnose and treat. Treatment options include use of hemostatic agents, judicious electrocautery use, appropriate use of suturing skills and techniques, and surgical clips. Prompt open surgical intervention may be needed if laparoscopic and robotic techniques are inadequate. Other methods such as temporarily increasing the pressure of the pneumoperitoneum may be helpful in achieving hemostasis when used with the abovementioned techniques.

In patients with delayed signs of bleeding, such as decreasing hematocrit and symptoms of hemodynamic shock, urgent reoperation may be needed. Port site bleeding is not uncommon for laparoscopy and should be checked first [29]. If hemodynamic stability exists, hematomas should be handled conservatively and drained later only if infection or persistent symptoms arise.

Urinary Extravasation

Resolution of any urinary leak is dependent on appropriate management of the drain, the Foley catheter, and the ureteral stent. In cases with persistent high drain output, fluid creatinine should be assessed, since the drain is usually intraperitoneal. CT scan with contrast should be performed to evaluate for any extravasation, check the drain position, and rule out urinoma. To confirm proper stent position, a simple KUB should suffice. If urinoma is diagnosed after the removal of the stent, which may be secondary to inadequate healing, the stent should be replaced and the cause of urinoma investigated. If the Foley catheter is removed, it should be replaced to promote a low-pressure urinary drainage system. In treating an urinoma, use of a suction drain is preferable to a non-suction drain. If there is persistence of urinary leakage, especially in the early postoperative period, drains are gradually removed away from the anastomosis site to promote healing. The Foley catheter is left in place until the leak has resolved. These principles are similar to those described in managing urine leak following partial nephrectomy [30].

Tension at Anastomosis

All urologic reconstructive procedures should be performed in a tension-free manner. Tension at the anastomosis is a potential complication that should be noticed and managed intraoperatively. This principle of reconstructive urologic surgery is of paramount importance. Because of the absence of haptic feedback with laparoscopic and robotic procedures, the tension at the anastomosis should be carefully visualized. Every effort should be made to promote the tension-free anastomosis; failure to do so markedly increases the risk of secondary recurrence. In cases with longer segment of stricture, additional reconstructive techniques may be required (Table 2). Appropriate preoperative counseling to inform the patient of possible additional intraoperative measures that may be needed, as well as the patient's consent, is critical.

Stent Migration

Stent migration is one of the most common complications of the ureteral surgery [31, 32]. It can occur after pyeloplasty, ureteroureterostomy, and ureteroneocystostomy. If the ureteral stent is obstructed, the stent should be changed with a percutaneous access either in an antegrade fashion or in a retrograde fashion. If the stent has migrated proximally or distally, early diagnosis and repositioning is required. Flank pain, abdominal symptoms, or increased urinary output through the drain site should alert one to the possibility of a malpositioned ureteral stent. Prompt correlation of patients' symptoms with objective findings, such as hydronephrosis, is recommended so as not to delay diagnosis of a correctable problem. The consequences of late identification of stent migration are urinary leak, urinoma, and secondary stenosis [29, 33].

Recurrence of Primary Ureteral Stricture

The success rates of minimally invasive reconstructive urologic procedures are close to those of open surgical equivalents if the basic principles of managing ureteral strictures are applied. Thus, if the ureteral pathology is not treated appropriately, the success rate will be less than optimal. Secondary strictures are always more difficult to manage due to the challenges in dissection at the site of the resulting fibrosis and adhesions. Secondary treatment choices are dependent on the length and the location of the stricture. Short annular strictures can be initially treated endoscopically. Nevertheless, reoperation (repeat laparoscopic, robotic-assisted, or open surgical intervention) may be required if endopyelotomy/endoureterotomy or balloon dilation fails or if longer strictures have resulted. To provide a tension-free anastomosis, different reconstructive surgical techniques may be utilized based on the length of the stricture. The recommended management strategy to treat ureteral strictures based on stricture length is summarized in Table 2 [8].

Conclusion

Laparoscopic and robotic-assisted ureteroureterostomy and ureteral reimplantation appears to be an effective and feasible alternative in today's wide range of surgical options for management of ureteral strictures and other ureteral pathologies. Available data are limited in defining the complications and associated morbidity in some of the infrequently encountered procedures such as ureteral stenosis secondary to retroperitoneal fibrosis. Another problem is the unavailability of standardized complication classifications. Nevertheless, the basic principles and techniques of ureteral surgery can ultimately be applied to laparoscopic and robotic ureteral surgery with the advantages of minimally invasive surgery such as less morbidity, faster convalescence, and better cosmesis. The importance of being aware of these complications and above all being well trained on newer technology such as the robot will go a long way in decreasing complications and thereby morbidity and mortality in our patients.

References

1. Klingler HC, Remzi M, Janetschek G, Kratzik C, Marberger MJ. Comparison of open versus laparoscopic pyeloplasty techniques in treatment of uretero-pelvic junction obstruction. Eur Urol. 2003;44:340–5.
2. Zhang X, Li HZ, Ma X, Zheng T, Lang B, Zhang J, Fu B, Xu K, Guo XL. Retrospective comparison of retroperitoneal laparoscopic versus open dismembered pyeloplasty for ureteropelvic junction obstruction. J Urol. 2006;176:1077–80.
3. Boylu U, Lee BR, Thomas R. Robotic-assisted laparoscopic pyeloplasty and nephropexy for ureteropelvic junction obstruction and nephroptosis. J Laparoendosc Adv Surg Tech A. 2009;19(3):379–82.
4. Patil NN, Mottrie A, Sundaram B, Patel VR. Robotic-assisted laparoscopic ureteral reimplantation with psoas

hitch: a multi-institutional, multinational evaluation. Urology. 2008;72:47–50; discussion 50.
5. Kavoussi LR, Clayman RV, Brunt LM, Soper NJ. Laparoscopic ureterolysis. J Urol. 1992;147:426–9.
6. Ameda K, Kakizaki H, Harabayashi T, Watarai Y, Nonomura K, Koyanagi T. Laparoscopic ureteroureterostomy for retrocaval ureter. Int J Urol. 2001;8:71–4.
7. Polascik TJ, Chen RN. Laparoscopic ureteroureterostomy for retrocaval ureter. J Urol. 1998;160:121–2.
8. Hsu TH, Streem SB, Nakada SY. Management of upper urinary tract obstruction. In: Wein AJ, editors. Campbell-Walsh urology, vol. 2. Philadelphia: Saunders Elsevier; 2007.
9. Nezhat C, Nezhat F, Green B. Laparoscopic treatment of obstructed ureter due to endometriosis by resection and ureteroureterostomy: a case report. J Urol. 1992;148: 865–8.
10. Yohannes P, Chiou RK, Pelinkovic D. Rapid communication: pure robot-assisted laparoscopic ureteral reimplantation for ureteral stricture disease: case report. J Endourol. 2003;17:891–3.
11. Castillo OA, Litvak JP, Kerkebe M, Olivares R, Urena RD. Early experience with the laparoscopic Boari flap at a single institution. J Urol. 2005;173:862–5.
12. Fugita OE, Dinlenc C, Kavoussi L. The laparoscopic Boari flap. J Urol. 2001;166:51–3.
13. Modi P, Gupta R, Rizvi SJ. Laparoscopic ureteroneocystostomy and psoas hitch for post-hysterectomy ureterovaginal fistula. J Urol. 2008;180:615–7.
14. Nezhat CH, Malik S, Nezhat F, Nezhat C. Laparoscopic ureteroneocystostomy and vesicopsoas hitch for infiltrative endometriosis. JSLS. 2004;8:3–7.
15. Rassweiler JJ, Gözen AS, Erdogru T, Sugiono M, Teber D. Ureteral reimplantation for management of ureteral strictures: a retrospective comparison of laparoscopic and open techniques. Eur Urol. 2007;51:512–22; discussion 522–3.
16. Seideman CA, Huckabay C, Smith KD, Permpongkosol S, Nadjafi-Semnani M, Lee BR, Richstone L, Kavoussi LR. Laparoscopic ureteral reimplantation: technique and outcomes. J Urol. 2009;181:1742–6.
17. Simmons MN, Gill IS, Fergany AF, Kaouk JH, Desai MM. Laparoscopic ureteral reconstruction for benign stricture disease. Urology. 2007;69:280–4.
18. Ogan K, Abbott JT, Wilmot C, Pattaras JG. Laparoscopic ureteral reimplant for distal ureteral strictures. JSLS. 2008;12:13–7.
19. Laungani R, Patil N, Krane LS, Hemal AK, Raja S, Bhandari M, Menon M. Robotic-assisted ureterovaginal fistula repair: report of efficacy and feasibility. J Laparoendosc Adv Surg Tech A. 2008;18: 731–4.
20. Mufarrij PW, Shah OD, Berger AD, Stifelman MD. Robotic reconstruction of the upper urinary tract. J Urol. 2007;178:2002–5.
21. Williams SK, Leveillee RJ. Expanding the horizons: robot-assisted reconstructive surgery of the distal ureter. J Endourol. 2009;23:457–61.
22. Nezhat CH, Nezhat F, Seidman D, Nezhat C. Laparoscopic ureteroureterostomy: a prospective follow-up of 9 patients. Prim Care Update Ob Gyns. 1998;5:200.
23. Thiel DD, Badger WJ, Winfield HN. Robot-assisted laparoscopic excision and ureteroureterostomy for congenital midureteral stricture. J Endourol. 2008;22:2667–9.
24. Bernie JE, Venkatesh R, Brown J, Gardner TA, Sundaram CP. Comparison of laparoscopic pyeloplasty with and without robotic assistance. JSLS. 2005;9:258–61.
25. Link RE, Bhayani SB, Kavoussi LR. A prospective comparison of robotic and laparoscopic pyeloplasty. Ann Surg. 2006;243:486–91.
26. Braga LH, Pace K, Demaria J, Lorenzo AJ. Systematic review and meta-analysis of robotic-assisted versus conventional laparoscopic pyeloplasty for patients with ureteropelvic junction obstruction: effect on operative time, length of hospital stay, postoperative complications, and success rate. Eur Urol. 2009 [Epub ahead of print].
27. Soulie M, Salomon L, Patard JJ, Mouly P, Manunta A, Antiphon P, Lobel B, Abbou CC, Plante P. Extraperitoneal laparoscopic pyeloplasty: a multicenter study of 55 procedures. J Urol. 2001;166:48–50.
28. Cadeddu JA, Regan F, Kavoussi LR, Moore RG. The role of computerized tomography in the evaluation of complications after laparoscopic urological surgery. J Urol. 1997;158:1349–52.
29. Rassweiler JJ, Teber D, Frede T. Complications of laparoscopic pyeloplasty. World J Urol. 2008;26:539–47.
30. Urena R, Mendez F, Woods M, Thomas R, Davis R. Laparoscopic partial nephrectomy of solid renal masses without hilar clamping using a monopolar radio frequency device. J Urol. 2004;171:1054–6.
31. Mandhani A, Kumar D, Kumar A, Kapoor R, Dubey D, Srivastava A, Bhandari M. Safety profile and complications of transperitoneal laparoscopic pyeloplasty: a critical analysis. J Endourol. 2005;19:797–802.
32. Romero FR, Wagner AA, Trapp C, Permpongkosol S, Muntener M, Link RE, Kavoussi LR. Transmesenteric laparoscopic pyeloplasty. J Urol. 2006;176:2526–9.
33. Mufarrij PW, Woods M, Shah OD, Palese MA, Berger AD, Thomas R, Stifelman MD. Robotic dismembered pyeloplasty: a 6-year, multi-institutional experience. J Urol. 2008;180:1391–6.
34. Symons S, Kurien A, Desai M. Laparoscopic ureteral reimplantation: a single center experience and literature review. J Endourol. 2009;23:269–74.

Complications of Robotic Prostatectomy

Akshay Bhandari and Mani Menon

Keywords Robotic · Prostatectomy · Prostate · Cancer · Potency · Continence

Introduction

Robotic prostatectomy has now become the most common surgical procedure for the treatment of prostate cancer in the United States. In 2008, over 70,000 robotic prostatectomies were performed worldwide (Intuitive Surgical). While there are no randomized trials that compare outcomes of open and laparoscopic prostatectomy, it is commonly assumed that minimally invasive surgery is associated with less morbidity and complications than is open surgery. Some of it could be related to the increased blood loss seen with radical retropubic prostatectomy and the indirect effects on homeostasis. The complication rates of radical retropubic prostatectomy reported from centers of excellence are low and range from 6 to 10% [1, 2]. However, data from the analysis of population-based registries suggest a complication rate of around 30% of which 20% are medical and 10% surgical [3, 4]. A recent population-based analysis comparing minimally invasive and retropubic radical prostatectomy during 2003–2005 concluded that men undergoing minimally invasive prostatectomy when compared to retropubic radical prostatectomy experienced significantly fewer 30-day complications, blood transfusions, anastomotic strictures, and shorter length of stay [5].

We started our robotic prostatectomy program in 2001 and have performed over 4,200 robotic prostatectomies as of this writing. Over this time period, our technique has undergone several modifications [6–10]. In the past we have published our complication rates for over 1,200 patients [11–13]. Although there have been some recent reports of complications from robotic prostatectomy, the overall literature addressing the complications of robotic prostatectomy is sparse. We currently hold the largest series of robotic prostatectomy and have therefore drawn heavily upon our own experience in preparing this chapter.

Technique of Vattikuti Institute Prostatectomy (VIP)

The VIP technique has undergone several modifications over the years [6–8, 10, 14]. In contrast to the Montsouris technique [15], we approach the bladder neck initially (antegrade approach). Earlier on in our experience, we switched to a running urethrovesical anastomosis using a double-armed suture. In addition we have abandoned bulk ligation of dorsal venous complex in favor of precise suturing of individual veins after urethral transection. We have also described the lateral prostatic fascia nerve-sparing technique (Veil of Aphrodite) [7]. Other modifications include endopelvic fascia sparing, extended pelvic lymphadenectomy to include hypogastric group of nodes, two-layer anastomosis [16], and, most recently, catheterless urethrovesical anastomosis [8].

A. Bhandari (✉)
Vattikuti Urology Institute, Henry Ford Health System, 2799 W. Grand Blvd., Detroit, MI, 48202, USA
e-mail: abhanda1@hfhs.org

R. Ghavamian (ed.), *Complications of Laparoscopic and Robotic Urologic Surgery*,
DOI 10.1007/978-1-60761-676-4_17, © Springer Science+Business Media, LLC 2010

Patient Selection

We do not have set exclusion criteria. Any patient who is a candidate for radical retropubic prostatectomy is considered a candidate for VIP. Relative contraindications for this procedure are the same as those for laparoscopy. These include advanced obstructive lung disease, abnormalities of cardiac output, and significant prior abdominal surgeries. Having said that, 30% of the patients who presented to us for robotic prostatectomy had a history of prior abdominal or inguinal surgery.

Patient Positioning and Port Placement

Patient is placed in lithotomy position with the help of stirrups. Pressure points are carefully padded with foam pads. Patient is secured to the table with heavy tape and the table in then moved to a steep Trendelenburg position. Pneumoperitoneum is then established using a Veress needle. Ports are placed under direct vision. The abdomen is transilluminated in a dark room to outline abdominal vessels during port placement. We use a standard six-port technique.

Developing of the Extraperitoneal Space

Using a 30° angled-up lens, a transverse peritoneal incision is made extending from one medial umbilical ligament to the other. The incision is extended in an inverted U to the level of the vasa on either side. The space of Retzius is entered through the areolar tissue anterior to the bladder.

Lymph Node Dissection

The extent of the lymph node dissection earlier on in our experience included the external iliac and the obturator group of lymph nodes. However, we now routinely include the internal iliac group of nodes, overlying the hypogastric vein. This dissection is typically carried out caudal to the origin of the obliterated umbilical artery so as to avoid injury to the ureter.

Bladder Neck Transection and Posterior Dissection

We approach the bladder neck directly without opening the endopelvic fascia or ligating the dorsal vein complex. The Foley balloon is deflated while keeping it in the bladder and the anterior bladder wall is grasped in the midline by the assistant and lifted directly toward the ceiling. This simple maneuver aids in clearly identifying the bladder neck. A 1-cm incision is made in the anterior bladder neck in the midline to expose the Foley catheter. The left-sided assistant then grasps the tip of the Foley catheter with firm anterior traction, thus exposing the posterior bladder neck, which is then incised.

The posterior bladder neck is then dissected away from the prostate and the fascial layer anterior to the vasa and seminal vesicles is incised, thus exposing the vasa and seminal vesicles. The vasa are then dissected and transected and the distal end is held by the left assistant, whereas the proximal end is held by the right assistant to provide the necessary exposure and counter-traction. The artery to the seminal vesicles is then controlled using clips or fine coagulation and the seminal vesicles are dissected away. This exposes the Denonvilliers' fascia, which is carefully incised and a plane developed between the prostate and the perirectal fat. This dissection is carried down to the apex of the prostate and laterally to the pedicles of the prostate.

Next, the seminal vesicle is retracted superomedially by the contralateral assistant and the pedicle is placed on traction. The pedicles are controlled by either clipping or coagulating the vessels individually by bipolar coagulation.

Nerve Sparing

For standard nerve sparing, the major neurovascular bundles that run posterolaterally are preserved in the usual fashion. Minimal bipolar coagulation or no cautery is used for this step. If a more extensive nerve sparing is planned, the prostatic fascia is incised anteriorly to create the "Veil of Aphrodite" that has also been described as "high anterior release" [17] or "curtain dissection" [18] by others. For this, the avascular plane between the prostatic fascia and the prostate is entered deep into the venous sinuses of the Santorini plexus.

Apical Dissection and Urethral Transection

Prior to performing apical dissection, we ensure that the Foley catheter is within the prostatic urethra. With the assistant firmly retracting the prostate toward the patients' head, the dorsal venous complex is transected without its bulk ligation. It is important not to skeletonize the urethra as minimal manipulation hastens the return of continence. The urethra is transected using a cold scissor about 5 mm distal to the prostatic notch and the free specimen is placed in an endobag.

The dorsal venous complex is then controlled with a running 2-0 braided polyglactin suture on a 17-mm tapered needle. Pneumoperitoneum is lowered and perineal pressure is applied by the assistant to ensure good control of the dorsal venous complex as increased abdominal pressure may falsely mask any open venous sinuses.

Urethrovesical Anastomosis

In our hands, urinary continence rate 30 days after prostatectomy is 90% with a single-layer, continuous-suture mucosa-to-mucosa anastomosis. This is perhaps the result of three factors: not opening up endopelvic fascia, not dissecting the dorsal vein complex to place a controlling suture, and guillotine amputation of the urethra. In a randomized control study [16], we did not see improvement in continence with reconstruction of the periurethral tissues. This is in contrast to reports from surgeons who open up the endopelvic fascia and ligate the dorsal vein, prior to transecting the bladder neck. However, we did see a decrease in anastomotic leaks and pelvic hematomas. Because the two-layer anastomosis adds extra strength to the one-layer variant, we have started to perform a two-layer anastomosis routinely. For this too, 3-zero double-armed monofilament sutures are used. The first suture of the outer layer is passed through the Denonvilliers' fascia and then through the posterior rhabdosphincter. After four passes from right to left which creates a posterior plate (Fig. 1a), the suture is then locked and its one end is held gently by an assistant.

Using the other double-armed suture the urethrovesical anastomosis (inner layer) is then performed. The first suture is passed outside-in on the posterior bladder wall at the 4 o'clock position, continuing into the urethra at the corresponding site inside-out. After three passes in the bladder neck and two in the urethra, the bladder is then cinched down to the urethra gently. After a few more throws, the direction of the stitch is then changed such that the passage is now inside-out on the bladder neck and outside-in on

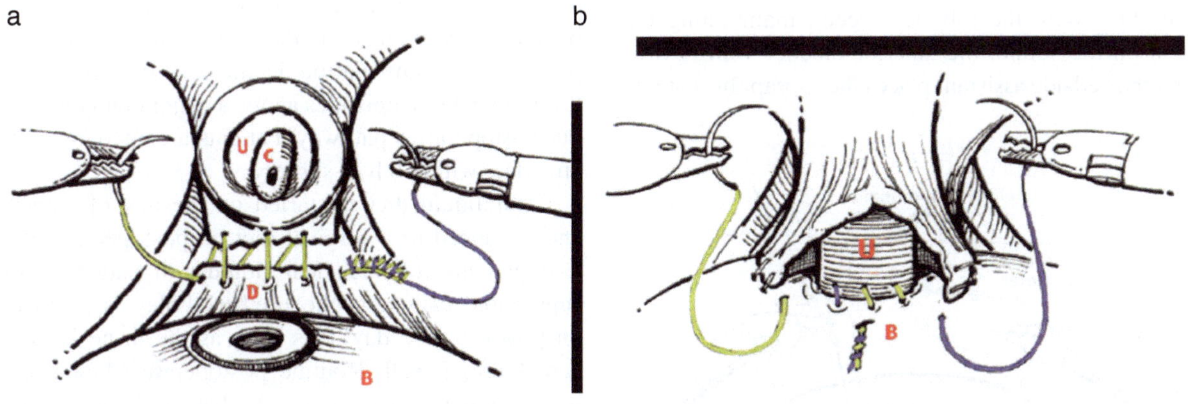

Fig. 1 (**a**) Posterior outer layer approximating the Denonvilliers' fascia and posterior rhabdosphincter. (**b**) After completing the urethrovesical anastomosis (*inner layer*), the anterior puboprostatic tissue is approximated to the midline bladder tissue to complete the anterior pubovesical collar reconstruction. B, bladder; C, Foley catheter; D, Denonvilliers' fascia; U, urethra

the urethra. The suture is then run clockwise to the 11 o'clock position. Next, the other end of the suture is run in a counter-clockwise fashion from the 4 o'clock position to the 11 o'clock position starting inside-out on the bladder and outside-in on the urethra. Both ends of the suture are then tied to each other to complete the inner layer of the anastomosis. A fresh 20-Fr Foley catheter is placed by the assistant and the integrity of the anastomosis tested by instilling 250 cc of saline.

Finally the outer layer is completed by suturing the puboprostatic ligament to the anterior pubovesical collar (Fig. 1b).

Suprapubic Catheter Placement

Under robotic visualization of the anterior abdominal wall, a 14-Fr Rutner (Bard Medical, Covington, GA) suprapubic catheter is percutaneously placed in the midline approximately one-third of the distance from the umbilicus to the pubic symphysis by the bedside assistant. Before placement in the bladder, the bedside assistant inserts a 2-0 nonabsorbable polypropylene suture on a straight needle through the skin and abdominal wall adjacent to the suprapubic catheter. The console surgeon grasps the needle and places a full-thickness horizontal mattress suture through the anterior bladder wall. The needle is then passed back through the anterior abdominal wall approximately 1 cm lateral to the initial needle puncture where it is grasped by the bedside assistant once it is through the skin. With the robotic surgeon maintaining tension on the suture, the anterior bladder wall is lifted and the bedside assistant places the suprapubic catheter

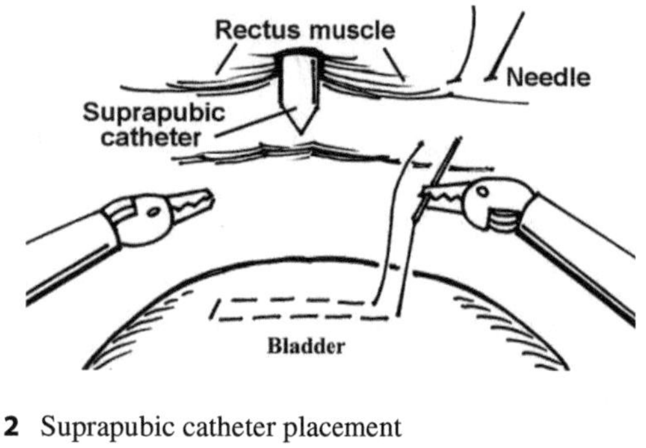

Fig. 2 Suprapubic catheter placement

(Fig. 2). Prompt drainage of irrigation fluid confirms proper placement of the catheter. The catheter balloon is then instilled with 4 cc sterile water. Once the specimen is extracted and pneumoperitoneum is no longer present, the external suture is tied onto the skin with the help of a button, thereby anchoring the anterior bladder wall to the anterior abdominal wall. The Foley catheter is plugged and the suprapubic catheter is connected to gravity drainage.

Specimen Retrieval

A Jackson-Pratt drain is placed only if there is a persistent anastomotic leak. This is passed through the left assistant port in the iliac fossa and secured on the outside with a #3-0 nylon suture. The specimen that is already placed in an endobag is removed by enlarging the umbilical port incision as required. The fascia is closed with interrupted #1 polyester suture and the skin is closed with subcuticular sutures.

Postoperative Care

Patients receive a liter bolus in the recovery room. Intravenous ketorolac and oral acetaminophen with codeine are used for pain control. Antibiotics are only used perioperatively for 24 h. We routinely use 5,000 units of unfractionated subcutaneous heparin every 8 h along with sequential compression devices for thromboembolic prophylaxis in the immediate postoperative period. Early ambulation is the key to minimizing thromboembolic episodes and is a major component of our postoperative pathway. Patients are encouraged to ambulate within 6 h of surgery.

Clear liquid diet is started on the day of surgery and advanced to a surgical diet on postoperative day 1 if patients tolerate clear liquids. In patients with suprapubic catheters, the urethral Foley is removed on postoperative day 1 as long as the urine is clear and draining well. Routine postoperative hematocrit is not drawn. Patients are discharged home with a catheter and follow-up in 7 days for a catheter removal under cystographic control. Patients with a suprapubic catheter are asked to clamp the catheter starting on postoperative day 5 and are asked to record postvoid residual volumes.

Data Collection

We used hospital claims data to analyze complications in all 4,000 patients undergoing VIP at our institute from 2001 to 2008. Data was cross validated with a prospectively collected database. Preoperative and intraoperative patient data were also obtained from our database. Complications are graded into four groups using the original Clavien classification system [19] (Table 1). We also sub-categorized complications broadly into medical and surgical complications. In the following section, we discuss these complications in detail. The numbers in parentheses after each complication represent the complications that we have had in our series of 4,000 patients.

Table 1 Complications in 4,000 patients undergoing Vattikuti Institute prostatectomy (original Clavien classification system [19])

Complications	No. (%)
Clavien grade I	151 (3.8)
Surgical	
Retention	59 (1.5)
CT-guided drainage	34 (0.9)
Ileus	29 (0.7)
Rectal injury	14 (0.4)
Other surgical	2 (<0.1)
Medical	
Neutropenia, arrhythmia, pneumonia	13 (0.3)
Clavien grade II	30 (0.8)
Surgical	
Re-exploration	22 (0.6)
Robotic	10 (0.3)
Open	12 (0.3)
Other surgical	5 (0.1)
Medical	
Respiratory distress	3 (<0.1)
Clavien grade III	17 (0.4)
Surgical	
Bowel injury	6 (0.1)
Recto-urethral fistula	1 (<0.1)
Medical	
Thromboembolic, cardiac	10 (0.3)
Clavien grade IV	1 (<0.1)
Total surgical	172 (4.3)
Total medical	27 (0.7)
Total complications	199 (5)

Complications

Anesthesia-Related Complications (<0.1%)

While some anesthetic complications are common for both minimally invasive surgery and open surgery, others are unique to minimally invasive surgery. Most of these complications are related to insufflation of abdomen with carbon dioxide and the subsequent rise in intraabdominal pressure.

Sinus bradycardia is frequently observed and is attributed to multiple factors including insufflation with carbon dioxide, increased vagal response from stretching of the peritoneal structures, steep Trendelenburg position, and hypercapnia. This is usually managed successfully by promptly administering atropine, desufflating the abdomen, and reversing the Trendelenburg position. If not managed appropriately and in a timely manner, asystolic cardiac arrest may develop. We report one such case where we had to abort a procedure due to asystole. Patient was appropriately resuscitated and underwent an uneventful procedure at a later date after undergoing a thorough cardiac evaluation.

Increased intraabdominal pressure causes an increase in intrathoracic pressure and an increase in both pulmonary and systemic vascular resistance. This causes increased blood pressure and decreased cardiac output, which may be significant in patients with borderline cardiac output at baseline.

Fluid management can be very challenging in these patients due to inability to accurately measure urine output. Overhydration causes increased urine output that can obscure the operative field and make the anastomosis very challenging. Fluid overload in a steep Trendelenburg position can also cause significant facial edema, specifically early in the learning curve when operative times are in excess of 3 h. We typically prefer to limit intravenous fluids to less than 1,000 cc for the entire case till the point of anastomosis. We report one case of severe bronchial edema requiring emergent re-intubation.

We have experienced once case of severe anaphylaxis, presumably from latex in a patient with no known allergies. We also report a case of infiltration of intravenous fluids into subcutaneous tissue leading to significant swelling of the forearm. To prevent this complication, the bedside surgeon should ensure proper functioning of the intravenous line after the arms are tucked to the patient's side and secured, as it can be a challenge to troubleshoot once the patient is draped and the robot is docked.

Corneal abrasions are not an uncommon complication and although not associated with any long-term sequelae in our experience, they can be a cause of significant pain and discomfort in the immediate postoperative period. Most cases are due to lagophthalmos (failure of eyelids to close) that leads to drying of the cornea. We have virtually eliminated this complication by carefully covering the eyes with an eye patch.

Non-vascular Access-Related Complications (0.1%)

Most of the access-related complications are the same for any laparoscopic procedure. These could range from minor bleeding to major vascular or visceral catastrophe. In a large study, Chandler et al. [20] reported that most of the access-related complications occur at the time of initial access and that 75% of these involved puncture to the bowel or retroperitoneal vessels. It cannot be adequately stressed that basic laparoscopic skills are an essential requirement prior to establishing a successful robotic prostatectomy program. At our institution, we use the closed technique of establishing access, wherein a Veress needle is used to puncture the peritoneal cavity blindly followed by insufflation of carbon dioxide. Thereafter, the first trocar is introduced blindly into the peritoneal cavity. The camera is introduced through this trocar and subsequent trocars are placed under vision. Proponents of the open technique described by Hasson [21] consider it to be safer than the closed technique; however, there to our knowledge, there are no studies that have confirmed this claim. Another alternative is to use an optical trocar to enter the abdomen under direct view [22]. In patients with significant abdominal surgeries, we sometimes use a hybrid technique, wherein the Veress needle is used to establish pneumoperitoneum following which a 5-mm optical trocar with a 0° lens is used to enter the abdomen under direct vision. In the end, the surgeon should use the technique he or she is comfortable with.

Subcutaneous Emphysema and Air Embolism (0%)

Subcutaneous emphysema could be caused by improper placement of Veress needle or due to leakage of carbon dioxide around ports when the incisions are too large. Murdock et al. [23] reported that longer operative times and greater number of ports predispose to subcutaneous emphysema. While subcutaneous emphysema mostly involves a limited area and is largely inconsequential, rarely it can track all the way up to the neck and severely compromise oxygenation. Its incidence can be minimized by limiting the incision to the size of the port and also by avoiding multiple passes through the peritoneum while placing ports. Once discovered, it can be managed by placing a purse-string suture around the leaking port and by decreasing the intraabdominal pressure. In our experience, subcutaneous emphysema is an uncommon problem and has not yet been associated with any adverse event.

Carbon dioxide embolism is another rare but lethal complication of laparoscopy. When encountered, it is invariably caused by insufflation through a Veress needle that has punctured a blood vessel or an organ [24, 25]. It is best avoided by simply confirming proper placement of the Veress needle prior to insufflation. This can be done using a syringe half filled with saline. The syringe is first aspirated and then saline is injected and the water column is observed. If blood is aspirated or if the column does not drop freely, the needle should be repositioned. Carbon dioxide embolism results in sudden onset of bradycardia and hypotension. It manifests as an abrupt decline in oxygen saturation and a sudden increase in end-tidal carbon dioxide followed by a rapid decrease. Management is immediate desufflation of peritoneum, turning the patient to a left lateral decubitus while still in Trendelenburg position and hyperventilation with 100% oxygen.

Visceral Injury (0.1%)

Both solid and hollow visceral organs can be potentially injured during insertion of Veress needle or placement of trocars. Bowel injuries can be associated with a significant morbidity as well as mortality. In a large review carried out by van der Voort et al. [26], the incidence of laparoscopy bowel perforation was about

0.4%. Small bowel injuries were most frequent. A trocar or a Veress needle caused most of the bowel injuries (42%). Approximately 70% of laparoscopy-induced bowel injuries were seen in patients with adhesions or previous laparotomy. While 67% of the bowel injuries were recognized within 24 h of surgery, the mortality rate associated with laparoscopy-induced bowel injury was almost 4%.

Of the six bowel injuries recorded in our cohort, four patients had a history of prior abdominal surgery requiring extensive lysis of adhesions. The other two were probably the result of instrument passage. However, approximately 30% of our patients had previous abdominal or inguinal surgery and the overall incidence of iatrogenic bowel injury in this cohort was about 0.2%. Proper patient selection is the key to establishing a successful minimally invasive program and it may be advisable to restrict robotic prostatectomy to patients who have not had prior abdominal surgery, during the learning phase. An extraperitoneal or a perineal approach may be indicated in these patients. We have rarely performed adhesiolysis through a minilaparotomy in some of these patients. The robot is then docked after open port placement and the prostatectomy completed.

Injury to solid organs is uncommon. We report one case of renal hematoma from puncture of a pelvic kidney with a Veress needle. A small renal hematoma was noted, which was observed for sometime intraoperatively. It was stable and we therefore proceeded with the prostatectomy. Barring gross hematuria, there were no adverse sequelae.

Other potential organs that can be injured are the urinary bladder and stomach. Placing a Foley catheter and a oro-gastric tube in all patients, prior to insertion of the Veress needle, may reduce the risk of occurrence of these injuries.

Vascular Complications (<0.1%)

Access Related (<0.1%)

The incidence of access-related vascular injuries reported in the laparoscopic literature is low, ranging from 0.03 to 0.2% [27–29]. Like visceral injuries, majority of access-related vascular injuries are caused by either the first trocar or the Veress needle [30, 31]. In fact, Champault et al. [32] reported that 83% of the serious vascular injuries occur during the placement of the first trocar. The aorta and common iliac vessels are most frequently injured. It is generally recommended that the access phase of laparoscopy be performed with the patient lying level, without any Trendelenburg tilt. Trendelenburg rotates the sacral promontory and brings the aortic bifurcation close to the umbilicus, thus increasing the chances of vascular injury [33]. Also, intraabdominal pressure rather than volume of carbon dioxide insufflated should be used as a guide to determine when to place the primary trocar. We insufflate the abdomen to 20 mmHg for port placement and then decrease the intraabdominal pressure to 15 mmHg. We have thus far encountered one major vascular injury during access, resulting in a contained, non-expanding retroperitoneal hematoma. The procedure was aborted, patient was managed conservatively, and the robotic prostatectomy was completed on a later date.

Injury to accessory abdominal vessels, such as inferior epigastric artery and vein, can occur during secondary port placement. Chandler et al. [20] reported that injury during secondary port placement was to abdominal wall vessels in 35% of the cases and to the aorta or iliac artery in 30% of cases. We recommend port placement under proper transillumination in a dark room to prevent injury to these accessory abdominal vessels. It is also recommended that all ports be removed under direct vision at the conclusion of the procedure and the port sites observed for arterial bleeders. If discovered, cauterizing these bleeders alone is usually insufficient. A figure-of-eight suture should be placed for adequate control.

Access Unrelated (<0.1%)

Majority of vascular injuries in radical prostatectomy occur during pelvic lymphadenectomy [34, 35]. Commonly injured vessels are the external iliac and the obturator. As described in our technique, we routinely perform an extended node dissection to include the internal iliac group of lymph nodes and this puts the hypogastric vein at risk of injury. While we have never experienced any vascular injury as a direct cause of surgical dissection, we have had to explore one patient for bleeding from an accessory obturator artery presumably from an injury caused by a suture needle.

The stereotactic vision and the precision of the robotic instruments along with motion scaling help in preventing inadvertent movements. There is obviously no substitute for a thorough knowledge of vascular anatomy of the pelvis.

Rectal Injury (0.3%)

The reported rate for rectal injury in laparoscopic prostatectomy is 1–3.3% [36–41]. We report an incidence of about 0.3%, Patel et al. [42] reported an incidence of 0.1% in 1,800 patients, and Fischer et al. [43] reported an incidence of 1% in 210 patients undergoing robotic prostatectomy.

In our experience, most of the rectal injuries occurred posterolaterally, close to the apex. The majority of these patients had aggressive apical cancer and were undergoing a planned wide excision. In three instances, cancer had extended into the rectal serosa, and excision of the rectal wall was required to achieve negative margins. In patients with clinical T3 or high-volume Gleason 8 or 9 disease, we administer a mechanical bowel cleansing with polyethylene glycol (GoLYTELY). Rectal injuries are identified intraoperatively and repaired primarily in two layers, an inner mucosal layer and an outer seromuscular layer with a running #3-0 polyglactin suture. Anal dilation is performed in all patients. Patients were kept on a clear liquid diet for 72 h and received broad-spectrum antibiotic coverage postoperatively.

Ten of the eleven patients were discharged home within 72 h with no complications. However, one patient developed a recto-vesical fistula that needed a diverting colostomy followed by delayed repair of fistula. This patient had locally extensive carcinoma, and gross fecal spillage was noted at the time of surgery, because of non-compliance with the bowel prep. In patients with aggressive local disease we now routinely order a complete bowel preparation preoperatively.

Ureteral Injury (<0.1)

This is a rare complication but often missed intraoperatively. It can happen during extended lymphadenectomy and during posterior dissection. We have encountered two ureteral injuries thus far. One of these was presumably during extended pelvic lymphadenectomy during a salvage prostatectomy in a patient with a recurrence after brachytherapy. The other occurred in a patient with prior inguinal hernia repair with mesh which resulted in a distorted anatomy. Both these injuries were missed intraoperatively and required delayed exploration and repair. The first patient underwent a transureteroureterostomy and the other was managed with a psoas hitch combined with a Boari flap. Hu et al. [44] reported one ureteral injury in 322 patients undergoing robotic prostatectomy. Several large open prostatectomy series have also reported a very low incidence of ureteral injury [1, 45].

We also report one case of obstruction of the ureteral orifice during urethrovesical anastomosis. Patient was explored the next day with robotic assistance. The anastomosis was taken down and it was discovered that he had a complete duplication on one side and the ectopic ureteral orifice was incorporated within the anastomosis. While we do not routinely use indigo carmine or methylene blue, some authors have found it helpful to locate the ureteral orifices. The ureteral orifices can be very close to the bladder neck in patients with large median lobes and the urethrovesical anastomosis should be performed using utmost care in these patients. We recommend the use of a small needle such as a 17-mm, half-circle tapered needle for anastomosis.

Postoperative Anemia and Blood Transfusion (1.9%)

Blood loss in minimally invasive prostatectomy is significantly lower than that in open prostatectomy. Available robotic series report a mean blood loss in the range of 100–300 cc and a transfusion rate in the range of 0.3–2% [43, 46–48]. Our mean blood loss is about 140 cc and transfusion rate is 1.9%. Only one patient had required intraoperative blood transfusion in our series.

The lower blood loss associated with robotic prostatectomy could be attributed to pneumoperitoneum and the superior vision and high magnification of the endoscopes. The dorsal vein complex can often be a source of troublesome bleeding. As our technique has evolved, we have abandoned bulk ligation of the dorsal venous complex in favor of precise suturing of individual veins after urethral transection. It is helpful to lower the intraabdominal pressure and apply perineal pressure to identify all bleeding sinuses.

Meticulous hemostasis is also required during dissection of the pedicle and neurovascular bundles. In our experience, patients undergoing a more aggressive nerve sparing such as the "Veil of Aphrodite" experience a higher blood loss as thermal coagulation is used very sparingly. For this, the plane of dissection is between the prostatic capsule and the prostatic fascia which contains several venous sinuses. If these vessels are not carefully controlled, then often result is troublesome pelvic hematomas that can jeopardize the urethrovesical anastomosis.

Patients on anticoagulation with warfarin often pose a unique set of challenges. We analyzed our data on patients with chronic anticoagulation undergoing robotic prostatectomy and found that patients on perioperative bridging therapy with subcutaneous low molecular weight heparin had a significantly higher transfusion rate (23% vs. 2%) than did patients not on perioperative bridging therapy [49]. However, this did not translate into increased complications or readmissions.

In general, patients on anticoagulation or antiplatelet agents, those with bleeding diatheses and large prostate volumes (>100 cc), and those who undergo a very aggressive nerve sparing or wide excision are at a higher risk of developing complications from bleeding postoperatively. A cystogram should be routinely performed in such patients. A sausage-shaped bladder is usually seen in patients who develop a large pelvic hematoma. These patients can sometimes develop a delayed leak. Therefore our practice is to keep a Foley catheter in place for a minimum of 2 weeks in these patients. An organized pelvic hematoma can cause partial or complete disruption of the urethrovesical anastomosis. We have seen this in three patients, who were explored robotically. The anastomosis was completely taken down, clots were evacuated, and anastomosis was re-done.

Management of Acute Postoperative Hemorrhage After Robotic Prostatectomy

Acute postsurgical hemorrhage is a rare but life-threatening complication of radical prostatectomy and in many cases may require re-operation. Acute postoperative hemorrhage is defined as bleeding in the postoperative period requiring blood transfusions to maintain hemodynamic stability or severe bleeding necessitating immediate surgical exploration. We have explored 10 patients thus far for acute postoperative hemorrhage. Of these, seven patients were explored minimally invasively with robotic assistance and the other three underwent open exploration. We were able to identify a clear source of bleeding in six of the seven patients who underwent robotic exploration. Of these, three were in the pelvis and three were rectus sheath hematomas. Overall, the median hospitalization for patients who underwent robotic exploration was 3 days and these patients did better than those that underwent open exploration. Based on our experience, we have developed an algorithm for the management of postoperative hypotension following robotic prostatectomy (Fig. 3).

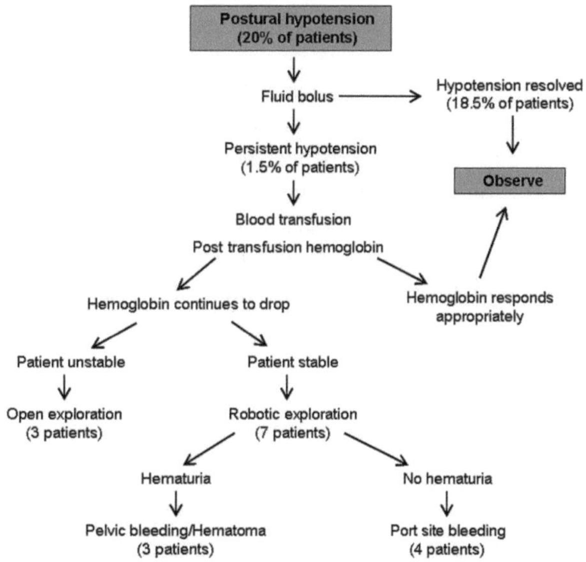

Fig. 3 Algorithm of management of postoperative hypotension following robotic prostatectomy

Urinary Ascites (0.7%)

This is perhaps one of the most disturbing complications in our series. Urinary ascites leads to chemical peritonitis and resulting ileus. While this complication is not life threatening and resolves with percutaneous drainage, these patients usually present with severe abdominal pain and distension, closely mimicking acute abdomen from bowel injury. The differentiation between a urinary leak and a bowel injury is critical, as the management is vastly different. Patients with urinary ascites usually have an elevated serum creatinine secondary to urinary absorption and cystographic evidence of a urinary leak. While cystographic leaks are common with open approach, they seldom cause symptoms as they are extraperitoneal. A CT cystogram should be obtained emergently in these patients and any fluid collection should be drained percutaneously under CT or ultrasound guidance. Patients with urinary peritonitis appear desperately ill but recover dramatically with drainage. If the patient does not improve immediately, he should be re-imaged and if needed re-drained. On the contrary, patients with unrecognized bowel injury are desperately ill and will not recover unless the injury is repaired. Figure 4 shows our algorithm of managing patients with unexplained postoperative pain that lasts >48 h.

Nine of the 26 patients (35%), who presented with urinary ascites, also required blood transfusions and had large pelvic hematomas on imaging. Pelvic hematomas tend to organize and distract the anastomosis. Thus some of these patients may have a normal initial cystogram and then may present later with a delayed leak on repeat cystogram.

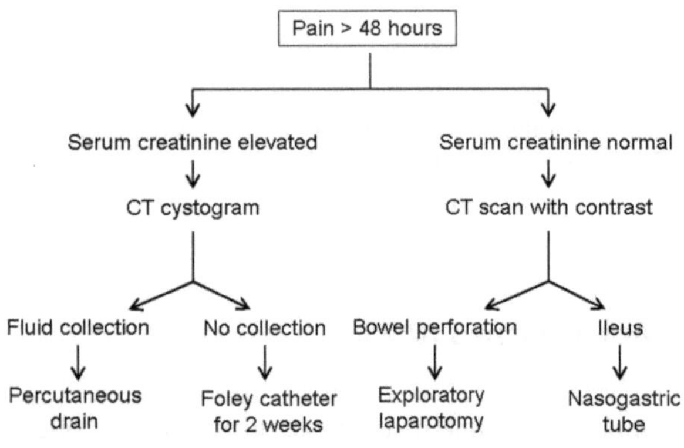

Fig. 4 Algorithm of managing patients with unexplained postoperative pain lasting >48 h following robotic prostatectomy

We adopted the two-layer anastomosis in an attempt to improve early continence but found no improvement in our hands [16]. However, we continue to perform a two-layer anastomosis as we have observed a lower incidence of cystographic leaks in these patients. We attribute this difference to better hemostasis, and therefore fewer pelvic hematomas. Whether this will ultimately decrease the incidence of urinary ascites requiring CT-guided drainage is yet to be seen.

Postoperative Ileus (0.7%)

Certain patients present with typical postoperative ileus that is unrelated to urinary ascites. Etiologies include bleeding or peritoneal irritation from carbon dioxide. The patients are best managed with bowel rest and sometime may require placement of a nasogastric tube until bowel function returns.

Bowel Complications (0.2%)

These include bowel injuries unrelated to access, incisional and port site hernias, and incarcerated hernias. Bowel can be injured during instrument passage by the bedside assistants. We report two such cases in our series. We also report three cases of incisional hernia. At the end of the procedure we extract the specimen through a vertical midline or a paramedian incision. The fascia is then closed with interrupted #1 polyester suture. Using meticulous technique and taking adequate fascial bites, wound dehiscence can be minimized; however, one patient was on chronic steroids and had very weak fascia. His closure broke down twice and he ultimately required definitive closure with a dermal graft. The other two were not associated with any identifiable risk factors and were probably purely technical.

Port site hernias are a rare occurrence after laparoscopy. It is felt that port site hernia in adults is usually confined to port sizes >10 mm. We use dilating trocars as these are associated with a lower incidence of bleeding as well as port site hernias [50]. Two 12-mm ports are used. One port is placed periumbilically and the second one is placed in the right anterior to mid-axillary line, slightly above the iliac crest. While the periumbilical port site is extended for specimen extraction and its fascia then closed, we do not routinely close fascia on the other 12-mm port site, given its location. We have encountered two port site hernias thus far and both of these were at the 8-mm robotic trocar sites.

Up to 5% of our patients have an incidental inguinal hernia that is discovered during robotic prostatectomy. Early in our experience we were not very compulsive in repairing these hernias. However, we have had two patients who presented with incarcerated inguinal hernia within a week of their robotic prostatectomy. Because of this, we have now changed our practice and are more aggressive in repairing these inguinal hernias with a simple plug and a mesh. This can be done relatively easily with the robot and it only adds 5 min to the operating time. Other robotic series have reported a 0.6–1% incidence of incisional/incarcerated hernias [43, 46].

Early recognition of bowel complications is particularly important as patients with laparoscopic bowel injuries or hernias will present with atypical signs and symptoms. Bishoff et al. [51] reported their experience with laparoscopic bowel injuries and found that majority of injuries (69%) were unrecognized intraoperatively. They also observed that interestingly majority of these patients initially presented with leukopenia rather than leukocytosis. A high index of suspicion is needed to diagnose this entity as patients may rapidly deteriorate due to overwhelming sepsis.

Lymphocele (0.2%)

This is a rare complication in our series, perhaps because of the intraperitoneal approach. While only eight patients presented with symptomatic lymphocele requiring percutaneous drainage, the incidence of asymptomatic lymphoceles is probably greater. In general, extended lymph node dissection and an extraperitoneal approach are associated with a higher incidence of lymphocele formation. Incidence of lymphocele causing deep venous thrombosis is also higher with extraperitoneal approach. Feicke et al. [52] reported a 5% incidence of symptomatic lymphocele in 99 patients undergoing extended pelvic lymphadenectomy during robotic prostatectomy. We occasionally observe lower extremity lymphedema in patients undergoing pelvic lymphadenectomy; however, it is a transient occurrence and usually resolves within 4–6 weeks.

Urinary Retention (1.5%)

Early in our experience, we were removing Foley catheters at 1–4 days postoperatively and experienced a high incidence of urinary retention (4.7%). While the anastomosis is watertight, there is significant edema at the urethrovesical anastomosis for the first few days. Since then, we have modified our pathway and now leave catheters in for an average of 7 days. With this, we have noticed a significant decrease in urinary retention to 0.9%. Patel et al. [42] report a retention rate of 0.4% in 1,800 patients.

When patients present with urinary retention, a well-lubricated Coudé tip catheter is passed gently into the bladder. In certain cases, an assistant could place a gloved finger in the rectum to support the urethrovesical anastomosis. If there is any suspicion about proper placement of the catheter, we recommend obtaining a limited cystogram to confirm location of the catheter. A flexible cystoscopy followed by passage of a guidewire may be used only as a second resort.

Medical Complications (0.5%)

In a population-based analysis comparing minimally invasive radical prostatectomy with radical retropubic prostatectomy, Hu et al. [5] reported that incidence of cardiac (1% vs. 1.7%), respiratory (2.5% vs. 4.6%), and other medical complications (4.8% vs. 5.6%) was significantly lower for minimally invasive prostatectomy. Our results confirm these findings. Fourteen patients in our series had a major medical complication such as deep venous thrombosis or pulmonary embolism (seven patients), stroke (one patient), myocardial infarction (three patients), and respiratory complication (three patients). There were six minor medical complications. Other robotic prostatectomy series also report a similar low incidence of medical complications [42].

We attribute this low incidence of medical complications to several factors:

1. The average time to ambulation is significantly less in patients undergoing minimally invasive prostatectomy than in those undergoing open prostatectomy. In fact, majority of our patients are ambulating within 6 h of their surgery.
2. As previously described, due to the transperitoneal nature of our technique, the incidence of significant lymphoceles and thus deep venous thrombosis and pulmonary embolism is very low.
3. The minimal blood loss associated with minimally invasive prostatectomy leads to less fluid electrolyte imbalance and therefore a low incidence of other medical complications such as cardiac arrhythmias.
4. Short operative times.

We have experienced one death, presumably from a massive myocardial infarction on postoperative day 21.

Delayed Complications

The incidence of bladder neck contracture after robotic prostatectomy is low and is in the range of 0.1–1% [42, 43, 48]. The two most common delayed complications of radical prostatectomy are urinary incontinence and impotence. We have published outcomes of over 2,500 patients undergoing Vattikuti Institute prostatectomy [6, 10].

Continence

About 23.7% of the patients reported having complete continence (zero pads) immediately after catheter removal, 50% of the patients reported continence within 4 weeks, and 90% of the patients reported continence at 3 months. At 12 months follow-up, 84% of the patients had total urinary control and 8% used a liner for security reasons or for occasional stress incontinence. About 95.2% of the patients were socially dry ($\leq$1 pad per day) at 12 months and <1% of the patients were completely incontinent. Other robotic series have confirmed similar results [47, 48, 53]. While the overall continence rates at 12 months are comparable to those of open radical prostatectomy [54, 55], the median time to continence appears to be shorter for robotic prostatectomy. While there have been some recent reports of improvement in early continence by restoring Denonvilliers' fascia [56–58], we found no such improvement in early continence rates in a randomized trial [16]. In our experience, early continence rates were high without fascial reconstruction (see Section "Urethrovesical Anastomosis").

Potency

Potency rates were best in patients undergoing bilateral extended nerve sparing ("Veil of Aphrodite"). We used the sexual health inventory for men (SHIM) questionnaire to measure sexual function. In patients with no preoperative erectile dysfunction (defined as SHIM score >21) undergoing bilateral veil nerve sparing, intercourse was reported in 93% of the patients; however, only 73% of the patients reported return to baseline. In comparison, in patients with no preoperative erectile dysfunction undergoing bilateral standard nerve sparing, only 68% of the patients reported intercourse and only 39% of the patients reported return to baseline [10]. Other robotic series have reported overall potency of 70–80% at 12 months [48, 53, 59].

Conclusion

Robotic radical prostatectomy is a safe procedure with less blood loss and is associated with a low medical as well as surgical complication rate. Yet, it is still a major procedure with potentially major complications that require prompt diagnosis and management. Persistent pain after 48 h is the harbinger of a potential problem and warrants aggressive investigation. Patients who develop urinary peritonitis after a transperitoneal prostatectomy may present with acute abdomen and should be treated with percutaneous drainage; others should be explored to rule out a bowel injury. Patients with acute postoperative hemorrhage after robotic prostatectomy do well with prompt exploration using robotic or minimally invasive techniques where possible. Like any major procedure, certain complications of robotic prostatectomy can be minimized by proper patient selection and meticulous surgical technique.

References

1. Catalona WJ, Carvalhal GF, Mager DE, et al. Potency, continence and complication rates in 1,870 consecutive radical retropubic prostatectomies. J Urol. 1999;162:433.
2. Lepor H, Nieder AM, Ferrandino MN. Intraoperative and postoperative complications of radical retropubic prostatectomy in a consecutive series of 1,000 cases. J Urol. 2001;166:1729.
3. Alibhai SM, Leach M, Tomlinson G, et al. 30-Day mortality and major complications after radical prostatectomy: influence of age and comorbidity. J Natl Cancer Inst. 2005;97:1525.
4. Bianco FJ Jr, Riedel ER, Begg CB, et al. Variations among high volume surgeons in the rate of complications after radical prostatectomy: further evidence that technique matters. J Urol. 2005;173:2099.
5. Hu JC, Hevelone ND, Ferreira MD, et al. Patterns of care for radical prostatectomy in the United States from 2003 to 2005. J Urol. 2008;180:1969.
6. Badani KK, Kaul S, Menon M. Evolution of robotic radical prostatectomy: assessment after 2766 procedures. Cancer. 2007;110:1951.
7. Kaul S, Bhandari A, Hemal A, et al. Robotic radical prostatectomy with preservation of the prostatic fascia: a feasibility study. Urology. 2005;66:1261.
8. Krane LS, Bhandari M, Peabody JO, Menon M. Impact of percutaneous suprapubic tube drainage on patient discomfort after radical prostatectomy. Eur Urol. 2009; 56:325.
9. Menon M, Hemal AK. Vattikuti Institute prostatectomy: a technique of robotic radical prostatectomy: experience in more than 1000 cases. J Endourol. 2004;18:611.
10. Menon M, Shrivastava A, Kaul S, et al. Vattikuti Institute prostatectomy: contemporary technique and analysis of results. Eur Urol. 2007;51:648.
11. Bhandari A, McIntire L, Kaul SA, et al. Perioperative complications of robotic radical prostatectomy after the learning curve. J Urol. 2005;174:915.
12. Menon M, Bhandari A. Complications of robotic prostatectomy. In: Loughlin KR, editors. Complications of urologic surgery and practice. Diagnosis, prevention, and management. Informa Healthcare, 369; 2007.
13. Tewari A, Srivasatava A, Menon M. A prospective comparison of radical retropubic and robot-assisted prostatectomy: experience in one institution. BJU Int. 2003;92:205.
14. Menon M, Tewari A, Peabody JO, et al. Vattikuti Institute prostatectomy, a technique of robotic radical prostatectomy for management of localized carcinoma of the prostate: experience of over 1100 cases. Urol Clin North Am. 2004;31:701.
15. Guillonneau B, Vallancien G. Laparoscopic radical prostatectomy: the Montsouris technique. J Urol. 2000;163:1643.
16. Menon M, Muhletaler F, Campos M, et al. Assessment of early continence after reconstruction of the periprostatic tissues in patients undergoing computer assisted (robotic) prostatectomy: results of a 2 group parallel randomized controlled trial. J Urol. 2008;180:1018.
17. Nielsen ME, Schaeffer EM, Marschke P, et al. High anterior release of the levator fascia improves sexual function following open radical retropubic prostatectomy. J Urol. 2008;180:2557.
18. Lunacek A, Schwentner C, Fritsch H, et al. Anatomical radical retropubic prostatectomy: 'curtain dissection' of the neurovascular bundle. BJU Int. 2005;95:1226.
19. Clavien PA, Sanabria JR, Strasberg SM. Proposed classification of complications of surgery with examples of utility in cholecystectomy. Surgery. 1992;111:518.
20. Chandler JG, Corson SL, Way LW. Three spectra of laparoscopic entry access injuries. J Am Coll Surg. 2001;192:478.
21. Hasson HM. Open laparoscopy: a report of 150 cases. J Reprod Med. 1974; 12:234.
22. String A, Berber E, Foroutani A, et al. Use of the optical access trocar for safe and rapid entry in various laparoscopic procedures. Surg Endosc. 2001;15:570.
23. Murdock CM, Wolff AJ, Van Geem T. Risk factors for hypercarbia, subcutaneous emphysema, pneumothorax, and pneumomediastinum during laparoscopy. Obstet Gynecol. 2000;95:704.
24. Cobb WS, Fleishman HA, Kercher KW, et al. Gas embolism during laparoscopic cholecystectomy. J Laparoendosc Adv Surg Tech A. 2005;15:387.
25. Scoletta P, Morsiani E, Ferrocci G, et al. Carbon dioxide embolization: is it a complication of laparoscopic cholecystectomy? Minerva Chir. 2003;58:313.
26. van der Voort M, Heijnsdijk EA, Gouma DJ. Bowel injury as a complication of laparoscopy. Br J Surg. 2004;91:1253.
27. Bonjer HJ, Hazebroek EJ, Kazemier G, et al. Open versus closed establishment of pneumoperitoneum in laparoscopic surgery. Br J Surg. 1997;84:599.
28. Hashizume M, Sugimachi K. Needle and trocar injury during laparoscopic surgery in Japan. Surg Endosc. 1997;11:1198.
29. Mac Cordick C, Lecuru F, Rizk E, et al. Morbidity in laparoscopic gynecological surgery: results of a prospective single-center study. Surg Endosc. 1999;13:57.
30. Catarci M, Carlini M, Gentileschi P, et al. Major and minor injuries during the creation of pneumoperitoneum. A multicenter study on 12,919 cases. Surg Endosc. 2001; 15:566.
31. Schafer M, Lauper M, Krahenbuhl L. Trocar and Veress needle injuries during laparoscopy. Surg Endosc. 2001;15:275.
32. Champault G, Cazacu F, Taffinder N. Serious trocar accidents in laparoscopic surgery: a French survey of 103,852 operations. Surg Laparosc Endosc. 1996;6:367.
33. Ahmad G, Duffy JM, Watson AJ. Laparoscopic entry techniques and complications. Int J Gynaecol Obstet. 2007;99:52.
34. Lazzeri M, Benaim G, Turini D, et al. Iatrogenic external iliac artery disruption during open pelvic lymph node dissection: successful repair with hypogastric artery transposition. Scand J Urol Nephrol. 1997;31:205.
35. Safi KC, Teber D, Moazen M, et al. Laparoscopic repair of external iliac-artery transection during laparoscopic radical prostatectomy. J Endourol. 2006;20:237.
36. Bollens R, Vanden Bossche M, Roumeguere T, et al. Extraperitoneal laparoscopic radical prostatectomy. Results after 50 cases. Eur Urol. 2001;40:65.
37. Gill IS, Zippe CD. Laparoscopic radical prostatectomy: technique. Urol Clin North Am. 2001;28:423.

38. Guillonneau B, Vallancien G. Laparoscopic radical prostatectomy: the Montsouris experience. J Urol. 2000;163:418.
39. Hoznek A, Salomon L, Olsson LE, et al. Laparoscopic radical prostatectomy. The Creteil experience. Eur Urol. 2001;40:38.
40. Rassweiler J, Sentker L, Seemann O, et al. Laparoscopic radical prostatectomy with the Heilbronn technique: an analysis of the first 180 cases. J Urol. 2001;166:2101.
41. Turk I, Deger S, Winkelmann B, et al. Laparoscopic radical prostatectomy. Technical aspects and experience with 125 cases. Eur Urol. 2001;40:46.
42. Dangle P, Patil N, Palmer J, Samavedi S, Coughlin G, Patel VR. Operative complications of robotic-assisted radical prostatectomy. Eur Urol. 2008;Suppl 7.
43. Fischer B, Engel N, Fehr JL, et al. Complications of robotic assisted radical prostatectomy. World J Urol. 2008;26:595.
44. Hu JC, Nelson RA, Wilson TG, et al. Perioperative complications of laparoscopic and robotic assisted laparoscopic radical prostatectomy. J Urol. 2006;175:541.
45. Lepor H, Kaci L. Contemporary evaluation of operative parameters and complications related to open radical retropubic prostatectomy. Urology. 2003;62:702.
46. Ahlering TE, Skarecky D, Lee D, et al. Successful transfer of open surgical skills to a laparoscopic environment using a robotic interface: initial experience with laparoscopic radical prostatectomy. J Urol. 2003;170:1738.
47. Patel VR, Thaly R, Shah K. Robotic radical prostatectomy: outcomes of 500 cases. BJU Int. 2007;99:1109.
48. Zorn KC, Gofrit ON, Orvieto MA, et al. Robotic-assisted laparoscopic prostatectomy: functional and pathologic outcomes with interfascial nerve preservation. Eur Urol. 2007;51:755.
49. Krane LS, Laungani R, Satyanarayana R, et al. Robotic-assisted radical prostatectomy in patients receiving chronic anticoagulation therapy: role of perioperative bridging. Urology. 2008;72:1351.
50. Bhoyrul S, Payne J, Steffes B, et al. A randomized prospective study of radially expanding trocars in laparoscopic surgery. J Gastrointest Surg. 2000;4:392.
51. Bishoff JT, Allaf ME, Kirkels W, et al. Laparoscopic bowel injury: incidence and clinical presentation. J Urol. 1999;161:887.
52. Feicke A, Baumgartner M, Talimi S, et al. Robotic-assisted laparoscopic extended pelvic lymph node dissection for prostate cancer: surgical technique and experience with the first 99 cases. Eur Urol. 2008;55:876.
53. Joseph JV, Rosenbaum R, Madeb R, et al. Robotic extraperitoneal radical prostatectomy: an alternative approach. J Urol. 2006;175:945.
54. Graefen M, Walz J, Huland H. Open retropubic nerve-sparing radical prostatectomy. Eur Urol. 2006;49:38.
55. Walsh PC, Marschke P, Ricker D, et al. Patient-reported urinary continence and sexual function after anatomic radical prostatectomy. Urology. 2000;55:58.
56. Nguyen MM, Kamoi K, Stein RJ, et al. Early continence outcomes of posterior musculofascial plate reconstruction during robotic and laparoscopic prostatectomy. BJU Int. 2008;101:1135.
57. Rocco B, Gregori A, Stener S, et al. Posterior reconstruction of the rhabdosphincter allows a rapid recovery of continence after transperitoneal videolaparoscopic radical prostatectomy. Eur Urol. 2007;51:996.
58. Tewari AK, Bigelow K, Rao S, et al. Anatomic restoration technique of continence mechanism and preservation of puboprostatic collar: a novel modification to achieve early urinary continence in men undergoing robotic prostatectomy. Urology. 2007;69:726.
59. Patel VR, Tully AS, Holmes R, et al. Robotic radical prostatectomy in the community setting – the learning curve and beyond: initial 200 cases. J Urol. 2005;174:269.

Methods and Maneuvers for Improving Functional Outcomes During Robotic Radical Prostatectomy

Gerald Y. Tan, Philip J. Dorsey, Jr, and Ashutosh K. Tewari

Keywords Robotic · Prostatectomy · Prostate · Cancer · Potency · Continence · Margins · Anatomy

Introduction

Prostate cancer remains a pressing public health concern worldwide. In 2009, more than 192,000 men were diagnosed with the disease, and more than 27,000 men died from it in the United States alone [1]. The advent of serum prostate-specific antigen (PSA) screening, coupled with a rising incidence of needle biopsies in asymptomatic men, has contributed to prostate cancer becoming the most common cancer in men in the United States [1, 2] and other parts of the world [3]. With increasing evidence of improved long-term survival and progression-free outcomes [4–10], radical prostatectomy has become increasingly popular as the treatment of first choice for organ-confined disease.

Since its inception in 2001, robotic-assisted surgery utilizing the da Vinci® Surgical System (Intuitive Surgical Inc, Sunnyvale, CA) has radically transformed the landscape of oncologic surgery for prostate cancer. Over 55,000 radical prostatectomies were performed with da Vinci® robotic assistance in the United States in 2007 [11], and over 70,000 worldwide in 2008 (source: Intuitive Surgical Inc, Sunnyvale, CA). The benefits of the da Vinci® System over conventional laparoscopy are readily apparent: superior ergonomics, optical magnification of the operative field within direct control of the console surgeon, and enhanced dexterity, precision, and control of operative movements. The patented robotic instruments have additional articulating joints (EndoWrist®; Intuitive Surgical Inc, Sunnyvale, CA) that permit seven degrees of freedom of movement, empowering the minimally invasive surgeon to perform intracorporeal suturing, and dissection intuitively and effortlessly. Its current state-of-the-art version, the da Vinci® S™ HD Surgical System (Intuitive Surgical Inc, Sunnyvale, CA), integrates 3D high-definition vision capability with the existing robotic platform, providing twice the effective viewing resolution with improved clarity and detail of tissue planes. Its digital zoom function reduces interference between endoscope and instruments, while the integrated touchscreen monitor permits telestration for improved proctoring and team communication. In addition, the TilePro™ multi-image stereo viewer enables simultaneous display of multiple video inputs in the surgeon console, integrating display of the patient's ultrasound, CT, and MRI images [12]. For patients, the benefits of smaller incisions, less blood loss and need for transfusions, postoperative pain, and shorter hospitalization stay have proved hugely popular and have been demonstrated in several recent meta-analyses [13, 14].

With advances in both surgical techniques and technologies, patient's expectations following radical prostatectomy have also changed. More men are now being diagnosed with curable prostate cancer at a younger age. For these men, the primary consideration is no longer complete clearance of cancer, which they

A.K. Tewari (✉)
Director, LeFrak Institute of Robotic Surgery, Director, Prostate Cancer Institute, Ronald P. Lynch Professor of Urologic Oncology, James Brady Foundation Department of Urology, Weill Medical College of Cornell University, New York Presbyterian Hospital, 525 East 68th Street, Starr 900, New York, NY 10065, USA
e-mail: ashtewarimd@gmail.com

R. Ghavamian (ed.), *Complications of Laparoscopic and Robotic Urologic Surgery*, DOI 10.1007/978-1-60761-676-4_18, © Springer Science+Business Media, LLC 2010 have come to expect of their surgeons. Instead, patients nowadays are more concerned about the impact of radical prostatectomy on their quality of life, specifically on their continence and sexual function following extirpative surgery, evaluating these outcomes against those reported with radiation and focal therapies such as cryotherapy and high-intensity focused ultrasound in making their final decision on treatment [10]. It is therefore timely for us to review methods and maneuvers that may be adopted by the robotic surgeon to optimize functional outcomes following da Vinci® computer-aided radical prostatectomy.

Optimizing Continence Recovery After Robotic Radical Prostatectomy

Introduction

Next to developing metastatic progression of cancer following surgery, urinary incontinence remains the most feared complication of men undergoing radical prostatectomy [15]. The incidence of postprostatectomy incontinence (PPI) has varied from 2 to 66% in reported series [16]. Urinary incontinence has the most negative effect on patients' quality of life [17], causing psychological distress and social inhibition for fear of public embarrassment for patients. Recurring costs for both chronic conservative treatment of PPI and secondary procedures such as transurethral bulking injection therapy or artificial urinary sphincter implants for refractory PPI place a further onerous burden on health-care systems and individual finances [18].

Anatomy of Male Continence Mechanism

Urinary continence in men required both a compliant bladder and a competent urethral sphincter complex working together in harmony. The male urethral sphincter complex comprises (1) the ring-shaped *internal sphincter* at the bladder neck; (2) the circularly orientated Ω-shaped *urethral rhabdosphincter*, comprising both striated and smooth muscular components; (3) the longitudinally orientated *smooth muscle component of the prostatomembranous urethra*; and (4) connective tissue structures of the pelvis [19, 20] (Fig. 1). Findings from cadaveric anatomic dissections and electron microscopy studies suggest a dual basis for continence control: (1) the striated periurethral muscles provide tonic contraction necessary for passive continence at rest, while (2) rapid muscular contraction of the pelvic floor expedites voluntary interruption of urinary stream or during sudden rises of intrabdominal pressure [21–23].

Anatomic studies by Myers [24] and Steiner [25] also elegantly demonstrated that the urethral rhabdosphincter is suspended and stabilized both anteriorly and posteriorly by its musculofascial investments from the apical prostate to the perineal membrane where the rhabdosphincter inserts into the perineal body, providing all-round stability and suspensory support for the rhabdosphincter. In addition, the urethral rhabdosphincter complex is innervated by both the autonomous nervous system via the pelvic nerve and inferior hypogastric plexus and the somatic system via the pudendal nerve. The inferior hypogastric plexus, situated at the tips of the seminal vesicles, conducts sympathetic impulses from ganglia of T11–L2, as well as parasympathetic innervation from sacral nerve roots S2, S3, and S4 via its intrapelvic branches to the inner urethral smooth muscle and mucosa [26, 27].

Risk Factors for Postprostatectomy Incontinence

Results from numerous studies have identified the following risk factors for postprostatectomy incontinence: (1) patient age more than 70 years [28, 29]; (2) short membranous urethral length on both preoperative and postoperative endorectal magnetic resonance imaging [30–32]; (3) postprostatectomy anastomotic strictures [28, 29, 33]; (4) surgical technique [28]; (5) low institutional and surgeon caseload [34–36]. Other studies report worse continence outcomes in patients where the neurovascular bundles were not preserved [37, 38], in obese patients [28], those with large prostate glands [39–41], and those with previous prostate surgery [28, 42], although the evidence for these latter factors is less robust.

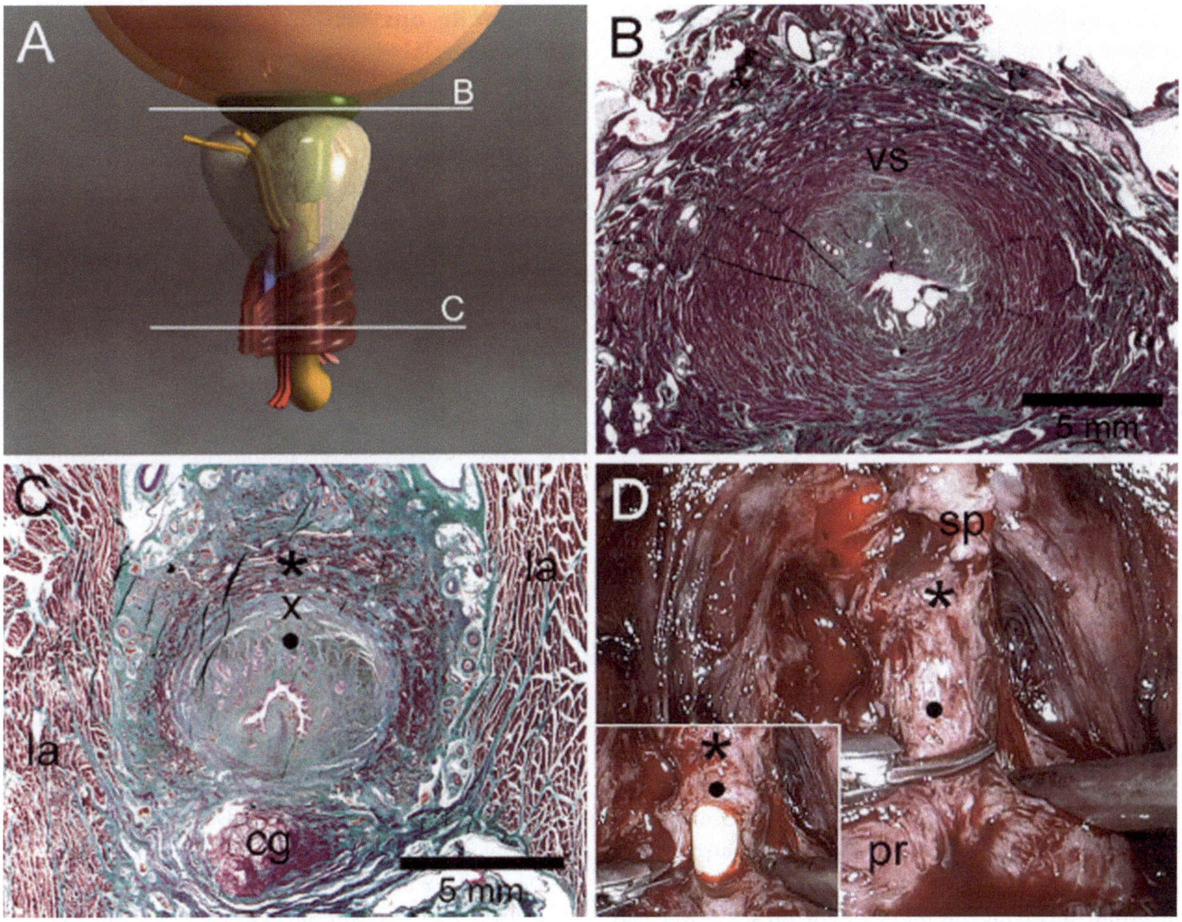

Fig. 1 (**a**) Graphic illustration of the male continence mechanism, posterolateral view. Note the Ω-shaped rhabdosphincter wrapped around the prostatomembranous urethra in *red* and *blue*, and the internal vesical sphincter at the level of the baldder neck in *green*. (**b**) Transverse section of the bladder neck demonstrating the circular-shaped *vesical (internal) sphincter* (vs). (**c**) Transverse section of the *urethral rhabdosphincter* at level of membranous urethra comprising of a smooth muscular part (X) and a striated part (*). The smooth muscular part of the urethra (longitudinal musculature) is evident close to the urethral lumen, as makred by the *dot* (·). Cowpers gland (cg), levator ani (la). (**d**) Intraoperative picture of apical dissection during laparoscopic radical prostatectomy. Santorini plexus (sp), prostate (pr). During apical dissection the Santorini plexus, the urethral sphincter and inner longitudinal smooth muscular layer of the urethra can be freed and dissected in steps. The urethral catheter becomes visible after incision of the inner smooth muscular layer. © Elsevier Inc. – Stolzenburg et al. [19]

Assessment of Postprostatectomy Incontinence

Walsh et al. first defined urinary continence following radical prostatectomy as patients not requiring the use of any pads [43]. This strict definition has been embraced by many investigators, although Eastham [28], Lepor [44], and several others still define postprostatectomy continence as using either none or up to one pad a day in reporting their results.

Initial evaluation of PPI currently includes a review of the patient's medical history and comorbidities, physical examination looking at rectal tone and neurologic function; bladder ultrasonography postmicturition for residual urine; urine analysis to rule out treatable urinary tract infection; a urine diary; an incontinence questionnaire for subjective assessment, e.g., the International Consultation on Incontinence Questionnaire-Short Form (ICIQ-SF); and a standardized 1-h pad test. The ICIQ-SF is currently recommended by the European Association of Urology for its simplicity and ease of use [45, 46]. Failing a trial of lifestyle intervention, bladder training and pelvic floor muscle therapy (with or without pharmacotherapy), further evaluation for refractory PPI with urodynamic studies and urethrocystoscopy is warranted to confirm intrinsic sphincter deficiency.

Surgical Maneuvers for Optimizing Continence Outcomes

Optimizing Preservation of Urethral Rhabdosphincter Length

The membranous urethra and sphincter complex serve as the cornerstone of the continence mechanism. As such, every effort to optimally preserve membranous urethral sphincter length during radical prostatectomy contributes to early return of continence. van Randenborgh et al. [47] reported maximizing functional urethral length by carefully dissecting out the distal intraprostatic urethra. Comparing 403 men who received this technical modification to a control group of 610 patients with standard excision of the urethra, the group receiving urethral length preservation had accelerated return to both early (33% vs. 15%) and final continence (89% vs. 76%) without pads without oncologic compromise of surgical margin postivity. Our group [48] also demonstrated that a preoperative membranous urethral length of less than 14 mm was associated with delayed return to continence in patients undergoing conventional robotic-assisted prostatectomy (25 vs. 12 weeks, $p = 0.037$). However, in patients who underwent reconstruction of anterior support structures, as well as a later group who underwent total anatomic restoration of the periprostatic tissue, this association of shorter MUL with poorer continence recovery was successfully ameliorated by the technical modifications. In this series, the mean time for achieving continence in patients with short vs. longer preoperative MUL was 7.4 vs. 6.2 weeks for anterior reconstruction and 3.6 vs. 2.7 weeks for total anatomic restoration. We describe our technique of total anatomic restoration in a later section.

Posterior Reconstruction of the Denonvilliers' Musculofascial Plate

Caudal retraction of the remnant urethral stump following prostatectomy is a commonly encountered problem, placing tension on the newly fashioned vesicourethral anastomosis. To prevent stump recession, Rocco et al. introduced the concept of posterior reconstruction of Denonvilliers' musculofascial plate (PRDMP) [49–51]. Following excision of the prostate, seminal vesicles, and vasa deferentia, the posterior median fibrous raphe is fixed to the residual Denonvilliers' fascia with two polyglactin 3-0 sutures. The reinforced posterior Denonvilliers' musculofasical plate is then attached to the posterior bladder wall with two sutures applied 1–2 cm cranial to the bladder neck, the new cranial landmark serving as the point for sphincter fixation. The vesicourethral anastomosis is then fashioned with 6–8 polyglactin 3-0o sutures, with the anterior sutures incorporating the puboprostatic ligaments (Fig. 2). In both their series of open retropubic prostatectomies, Francesco Rocco et al. [49, 50] found that continence rates were significantly improved in patients undergoing PRDMP compared to conventional anastomosis construction – 62.4% vs. 14.0% at discharge, 74.0% vs. 30% at 1 month, and 85.2% vs. 46% at 3 months follow-up. Bernardo Rocco et al. [51] reported similar success with the PRDMP technique in their early series of patients undergoing transperitoneal laparoscopic radical prostatectomy, with continence rates of 74.2% vs. 25% at catheter removal and 83.8% vs. 32.3% at 30 days follow-up. Nguyen et al. [52] from the Cleveland Clinic also reported significant improvement with the Rocco technique of posterior musculofascial plate reconstruction in their cohort of patients undergoing laparoscopic or robotic prostatectomy – 34% vs. 3% at 3 days following catheter removal and 56% vs. 17% at 6 weeks follow-up.

Preservation of the Bladder Neck and Internal Sphincter

Recognizing that excision of the bladder neck during radical prostatectomy potentially injures the internal vesical sphincter, several investigators have explored the benefit of careful dissection and preservation of the

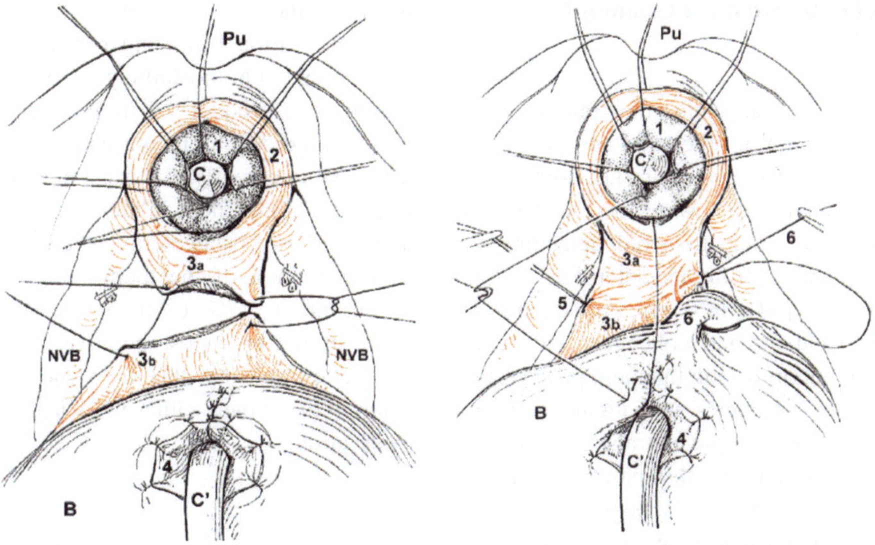

Fig. 2 Posterior reconstruction of urethral rhabdosphincter and Denonvilliers' musculofascial plate. (*Left*) Suturing the rhabdosphincter and median fibrous raphe to the remnant Denonvilliers' fascia. (*Right*) Fixation of the rhabdosphincter and Denonvilliers' fascia to the posterior bladder wall 2 cm superiorly to the bladder neck. Pubis (Pu), Foley catheter in membranous urethra (C), bladder catheter (C'), bladder (B), neurovascular bundle (NVB), membranous urethra (1), anterolateral wall of rhabdosphincter (2), sectioned posterior wall of rhabdosphincter (3a), sectioned Denonvilliers' fascia (3b), bladder neck eversion (4), posterior vesicourethral anastomosis (7). © Elsevier, Inc. – Rocco et al. [50]

bladder neck and prostatic urethra while dissecting free the cancerous prostate gland [53–58]. The majority of these studies have reported earlier return of continence with bladder neck preservation (BNP) without compromise of cancer control, although long-term continence rates were similar. In a systematic review of the literature, Cambio and Evans [59] found that BNP was not associated with margin positivity at the bladder neck, nor local/biochemical recurrence in properly selected patients. In addition, many studies also report a decreased incidence of bladder neck contracture with bladder neck preservation, which may indirectly affect continence outcomes.

Bladder Neck Intussusception

Walsh and Marschke [60] first proposed bladder neck intussusception (BNI) as a means of preventing the bladder neck from opening during vesical filling by using two 2-0 Maxon Lembert buttressing sutures placed lateral and posterior to the reconstructed bladder neck. They demonstrated significantly earlier return of continence at 3 months in the BNI group (82% vs. 54%, $p = 0.0035$), although bladder neck contracture rates were similar in both groups. Wille et al. [61] also reported earlier continence in a prospective randomized non-controlled trial – in their series of 272 men undergoing radical retropubic prostatectomy, continence rates at 3 months follow-up were significantly improved in the BNI group compared to the control group (77% vs. 60%, $p = 0.009$), although final continence status at 12 months was comparable.

Bladder Neck Mucosal Eversion

Everting the bladder neck mucosa before vesicourethral anastomosis construction has been advocated as a means of augmenting tension-free mucosal coaptation and decreasing subsequent contracture formation and prolonged incontinence [62]. However, in a prospective controlled trial involving 100 patients, Srougi et al. reported no significant benefit of bladder neck mucosal eversion on either bladder neck contracture or continence outcome [63].

Preservation of Puboprostatic Ligaments and Arcus Tendineus

Steiner first proposed incising the puboprostatic ligaments just proximal to the prostate apex with dissecting scissors while avoiding the dorsal vein complex, after which there were no further finger dissections in the plane to avoid detaching the urethral rhabdosphincter from its anterolateral ligamentous attachments [64]. In a randomized trial of 100 patients, Stolzenburg and colleagues [65] compared the effect of puboprostatic ligament preservation on early continence outcomes in patients undergoing nerve-sparing laparoscopic extraperitoneal radical prostatectomy. They found that patients receiving PPL preservation had significantly better early continence than their counterparts receiving conventional surgery without compromise of surgical margins (24% vs. 12% at 2 weeks and 76% vs. 48% at 3 months follow-up). Based on our cadaveric studies of the continence mechanism, we have also found significantly earlier continence recovery after robotic-assisted radical prostatectomy with preservation of the puboprostatic ligaments, arcus tendineus, and puboperinealis musculofascial collar [66–68].

Preservation of Neurovascular Bundles and Continence Nerves

Building on their anatomic findings, Hollabaugh and Steiner proposed a continence nerve-sparing "no-touch" approach to retropubic radical prostatectomy with the following modifications: (1) avoiding use of the right-angle clamp below the posterior urethra to develop a plane between the urethra and rectum, which may cause injury to the contralateral intrapelvic branch of the pudendal nerve and the pelvic nerve from the inferior hypogastric plexus as they enter the rhabdosphincter; (2) cutting the posterior rhabdosphincter under direct vision without use of a right-angle clamp or put on traction with an umbilical tape; (3) transecting the rectourethralis muscle at the prostatic apex after releasing the neurovascular bundles; and (4) placing the vesicourethral anastomotic sutures away from the 5 and 7 o'clock positions to avoid snaring the innervations of the external striated urethral sphincter [69]. The role of innervation in continence is also suggested by other findings: John et al. [70] found that trigonal denervation following radical prostatectomy, as assessed by immunostaining of trigonal biopsies for protein gene product 9.5 immunoreactive nerve fiber density, predicted an increased risk of urinary incontinence. More recently, Catarin and colleagues [71] also reported that pudendal-related perineal reflexes appear unaffected by prostatectomy, whereas autonomic afferent denervation of the membranous urethra mucosa was found in 77% of men after prostatectomy, as demonstrated by a postoperative increase in urethra–anal reflex sensory threshold and latency. In their cohort, 92% of men with urinary leakage demonstrated denervation.

Anatomic Restoration Technique During Robotic Radical Prostatectomy

We believe that during conventional anastomosis following radical prostatectomy, the vesicourethral anastomosis and bladder neck become biomechanically unstable at the following sites: (a) tension is exerted on the healing anastomosis from spontaneous urethral stump recession into the pelvic floor; (b) the posteriorly deficient Ω-shaped urethral rhabdosphincter lies unsupported posteriorly, impairing efficient contraction of the sphincter mechanism; (c) the posterior bladder neck lies unsupported in the retrotrigonal fossa created by excision of the seminal vesicles; and (d) the anterior and lateral bladder neck lie unsupported as well (Fig. 3). The overall effect appears to be pelvic descent of the bladder pressing on the unsupported anastomosis. As a result, during micturition the contractile forces generated by the detrusor musculature are directed inferiorly at the anastomosis, causing additional stress on the continence mechanism (Fig. 4).

As such, we have developed the following paradigm of seven key principles for optimizing early continence recovery following radical prostatectomy, which we have described as the anatomic restoration technique (ART): (1) preservation of anterior fibrotendinous support structures, chiefly the arcus tendineus and the puboprostatic ligaments; (2) optimization of functional membranous urethral length; (3) reinforcement of unstable posterior bladder neck in the unsupported retrotrigonal fossa left by excised seminal vesicles; (4) reinforcement of the posteriorly deficient Ω-shaped

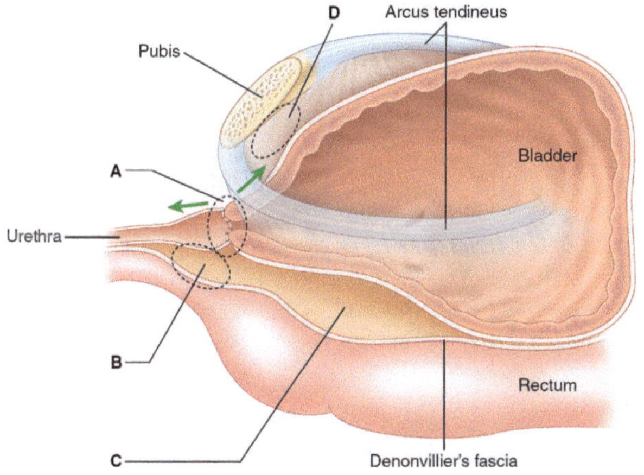

Fig. 3 Points of postulated biomechanical instability associated with the conventional vesicourethral anastomosis (sagittal view): (**a**) tension on the vesicourethral anastomosis from spontaneous urethral stump recession into the pelvic floor; (**b**) the posteriorly deficient Ω-shaped urethral rhabdosphincter lies unsupported posteriorly, impairing efficient contraction of the sphincter mechanism; (**c**) the posterior bladder neck lies unsupported in the retrotrigonal fossa created by excision of the seminal vesicles; (**d**) the anterior and lateral bladder neck lie unsupported as well. © Elsevier Inc. – Tan et al. [72]

urethral sphincter complex for suspensory support; (5) fashioning of a tension-free, stable vesicourethral anastomosis; (6) prevention of urethral stump recession and optimizing mucosal coaptation; (7) alleviation of pelvic descent and downward pressure of the bladder on the anastomosis during micturition (Fig. 5a, b).

The benefits of this approach appear to be threefold. First, it provides circumferential dynamic suspensory support for the urethral sphincter complex, as documented by postoperative cystographic studies (Fig. 6). Second, it avoids pelvic prolapse and downward pressure of the bladder on the healing anastomosis during micturition. Third, tension at the anastomosis is relieved with improved mucosal apposition and coaptation. We recently reported our experience with the anatomic restoration technique (ART) in a cohort of 530 patients [72], wherein we defined continence as zero pad usage. We found that the ART resulted in significantly earlier return of continence (38.6, 82.6, 90.5, and 97.5 % at 1, 6, 12, and 24 weeks follow-up, respectively) and significantly lower incidence of anastomotic strictures and clinically significant leaks compared to men receiving conventional anastomosis.

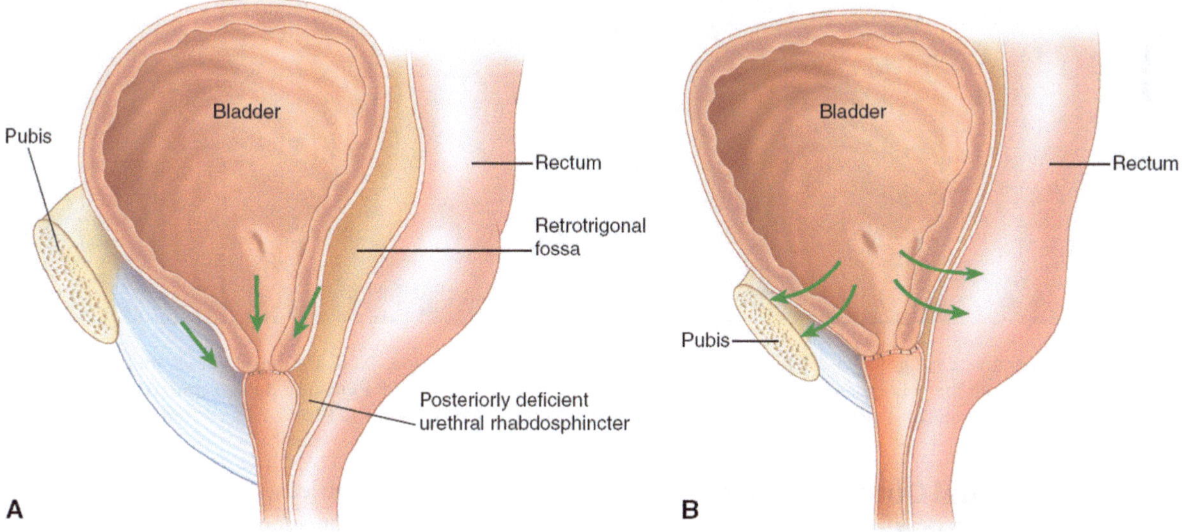

Fig. 4 Biomechanical forces acting on the vesicourethral anastomosis in the *upright* position. (**a**) In the conventional vesicourethral anastomosis, pelvic descent of the bladder presses on the unsupported anastomosis. During micturition, the contractile forces generated by the detrusor musculature are directed inferiorly at the anastomosis (*green arrows*), causing additional stress on the continence mechanism. (**b**) In our technique, the bladder is hitched up anterolaterally by the suspension sutures through the arcus tendineus, ameliorating downward tension on the healing anastomosis. During micturition, the same contractile forces (*green arrows*) are dissipated away from the anastomosis and urethral rhabdosphincter. © Elsevier Inc. – Tan et al. [72]

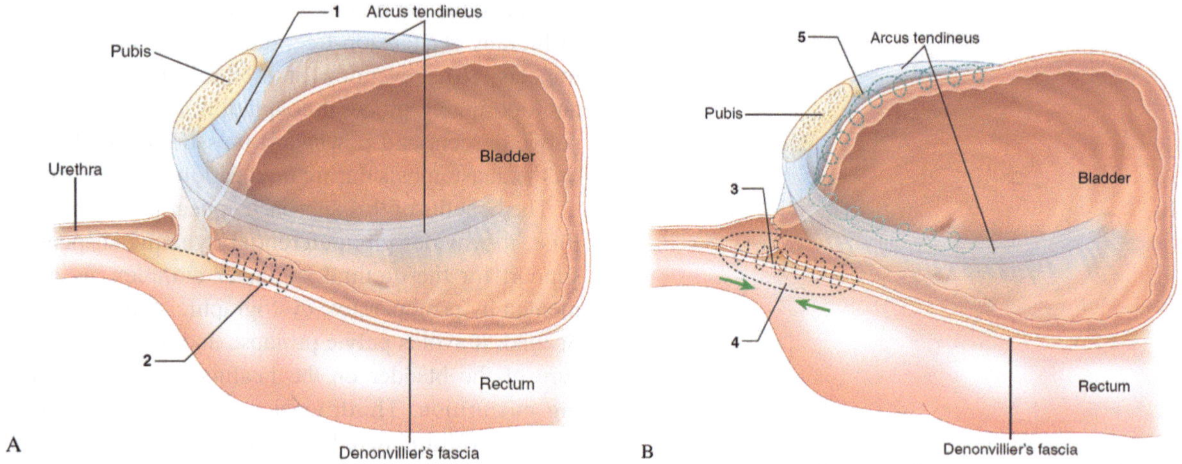

Fig. 5 (**a**) Anatomic restoration of vesicourethral junction: (1) preservation of anterior support structures, i.e., puboprostatic ligaments and arcus tendineus; (2) posterior bladder neck reinforced with 0 Vicryl suture, obliterating retrotrigonal space. (**b**) Anatomic restoration of vesicourethral junction: (3) the posteriorly deficient urethral rhabdosphincter reinforced against Denonvilliers' musculofascial plate; (4) Denonvilliers' musculofascial plate reconstructed, preventing urethral stump recession, relieving tension on the anastomosis, and improving mucosal coaptation at the anastomosis; (5) anterior suspension sutures to the arcus tendineus and puboprostatic ligaments alleviate downward prolapse of the bladder on the anastomosis. © Elsevier Inc. – Tan et al. [72]

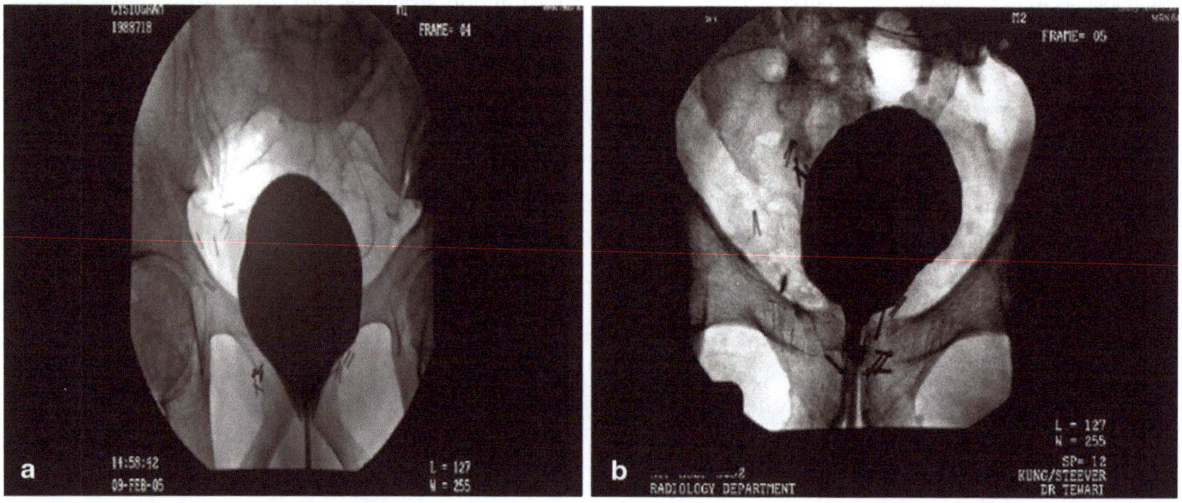

Fig. 6 (**a**) Postoperative cystogram in a patient with conventional anastomosis. Note the pelvic descent of the anastomosis. (**b**) Postoperative cystogram of a patient who underwent total anatomic restoration. Note the anastomosis and bladder neck being well suspended above the pubic ramus as a result of our technical modifications. © Elsevier Inc. – Tan et al. [72]

Optimizing Sexual Outcomes After Robotic Radical Prostatectomy

Introduction

The advent of PSA screening has resulted in a downward stage migration of prostate cancer, with prostate cancer patients being diagnosed at a younger age with early organ-confined disease. Preservation of sexual function has become an increasing priority for these men in considering radical prostatectomy as a treatment option. Despite advances in techniques and surgical technologies, return of erectile function sufficient for sexual intercourse at a year after surgery varies from 15 to 87% in contemporary series of radical prostatectomy [13, 14, 73]. Data from the Prostate Cancer Outcomes Study suggest that sexual dysfunction following radical prostatectomy has a significant impact on the quality of life for men, impacting everyday interactions with women and affecting their own perceptions of their masculinity, particularly in younger men [74, 75].

Risk Factors for Postprostatectomy Erectile Dysfunction

Penile erection is a complex event dependent on vascular and neurogenic factors. Penile tumescence is a direct result of increased arterial blood flow and engorgement of the corpora cavernosum and spongiosum with occlusion of the subtunical venules to retain blood during continued stimulation. The arterial supply of the penis is provided by the internal pudendal arteries, which are the terminal branches of the hypogastic artery. In the flaccid state, penile blood flow is reduced due to tonic contraction of the vascular smooth muscle. During tumescence, however, autonomic nerve-induced relaxation of the vascular and corporal smooth muscle results in rapid arterial filling and engorgement of the cavernosal sinusoids. This is brought about by cholinergic and non-adrenergic non-cholinergic mechanisms involving the release of nitric oxide and other mediators, which cause production of intracellular cyclic GMP and subsequent depletion of intracellular calcium in vascular smooth muscle. The expanding sinusoids within the corpora cavernosa compress the subtunical venules against the tunica albuginea, trapping venous flow to maintain erection [76].

Sexual dysfunction following radical prostatectomy is believed to be multi-factorial. Quinlan and Walsh [77] first reported in 1991 that patient age, clinical and pathologic stage of cancer, and preservation of the neurovascular bundles are significantly associated with recovery of potency after radical prostatectomy. More recent studies by Rabbani [78] and Dubbelman [79] further supported the observations that patient age, their preoperative potency status, and the aggressiveness of nerve sparing were most predictive of potency recovery after surgery. Surgeon's experience and surgical volume [94], intraoperative neurovascular bundle injury, penile ischemia and subsequent fibrosis, and veno-occlusive disease are further variables for successful return of sexual function following surgery [76].

Anatomic Basis of Erectogenic Nerve Preservation

Neurovascular Bundles and Cavernosal Nerves

Much of the progress achieved in the past two decades in improving potency outcomes after radical prostatectomy has been wrought through an improved appreciation of the anatomic basis of the nerves responsible for erection. The autonomic neural system is directly responsible for penile erection. The inferior hypogastric plexus (IHP) is responsible for the mechanisms of erection, ejaculation, and urinary continence. The IHP contains sympathetic and parasympathetic components. The sympathetic fibers arise from the T11 to L2 ganglia, while the parasympathetic fibers originate from the ventral rami of S3 and S4. The IHP is a dense network of neural fibers located within a fibro-fatty, sub-peritoneal plate between the urinary bladder and rectum [80].

In 1982, Walsh and Donker [81] first published their seminal study detailing the anatomy of the nerves supplying the corpora cavernosa in male stillborns. Subsequent cadaveric and intraoperative studies by Walsh and colleagues [82, 83] at the Johns Hopkins Institute further elucidated that the neurovascular bundles (NVB) run posterolateral to the prostate between two layers of lateral pelvic fascia – the prostatic fascia medially and levator fascia laterally (Fig. 7). The NVBs comprise the cavernosal nerves (CN) directly responsible for erectile function, which originate from the most inferior portion of the IHP; the arterial branches from the inferior vescial artery; and venous vessels. The majority of these cavernous nerve fibers, approximately 6 mm wide, then run caudally at the 3 and 9 o'clock position of the membranous urethra beneath the striated sphincter at the prostatic apex (Fig. 8).

Variations of Course of Neurovascular Bundles

More recent studies suggest that the course of the NVBs is more complex than previously described by Walsh. In 2004, Costello and colleagues demonstrated in cadaveric dissections that the NVBs descend posterior to the seminal vesicles, converging at the mid-prostatic level and then diverging on approaching the prostatic apex, being hard to distinguish [84].

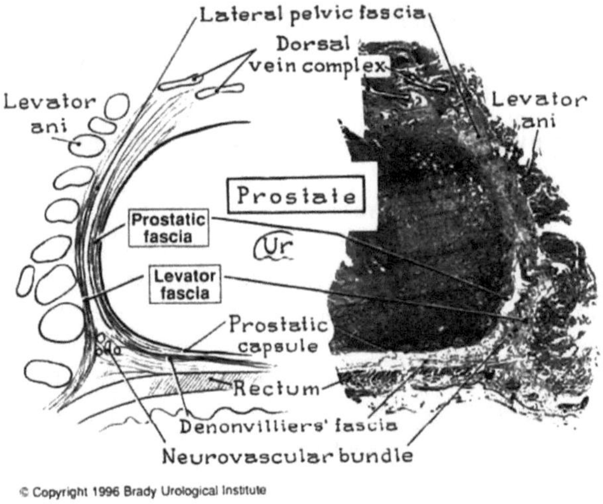

Fig. 7 Cross section of adult prostate demonstrating the posterolaterally situated neurovascular bundle running between the layers of the lateral pelvic fascia – the levator fascia lies lateral, and the prostatic fascia lies medial to the bundle. © Brady Urological Institute (Permission obtained from Professor Patrick C. Walsh of the Brady Urological Institute, Johns Hopkins Hospital.)

Takenaka's anatomic studies highlighted the lattice-like distribution of the NVB on the lateral surface of the prostate, demonstrating that the NVB is more a network of multiple fine dispersed nerves than a distinct structure [85]. Kiyoshima et al. also described that the dispersed nerve fibers are located between the prostate capsule and the lateral pelvic fascia [86]. Similarly, Eichelberg et al. demonstrated that only 46–66% of all nerves were found in the classical posterolateral location, while 21–29% were found on the anterolateral surface of the prostate [87].

The Tri-zonal Concept

Tewari and colleagues [88, 89] proposed that the periprostatic nerves consistently fell into three broad surgically identifiable zones: the proximal neurovascular plate (PNP), the predominant neurovascular bundle (PNB), and the accessory neural pathways (ANP) (Fig. 9). The predominant neurovascular bundles are usually located in a posterolateral groove on the side of the prostate. Significant variations in the location, shape, course, and composition of this bundle occur. They can be widespread on the rectum, Denonvilliers' fascia, and lateral prostatic fascia, or they can be circumscribed on the posterolateral groove enclosed in the triangular space. The PNB is closely related to the prostatic pedicle and prostatic fascia, and its branches can sometimes be intermingled with the lateral pedicles of the prostate (Fig. 10). Tissue planes also may be obliterated due to periprostatic inflammation,

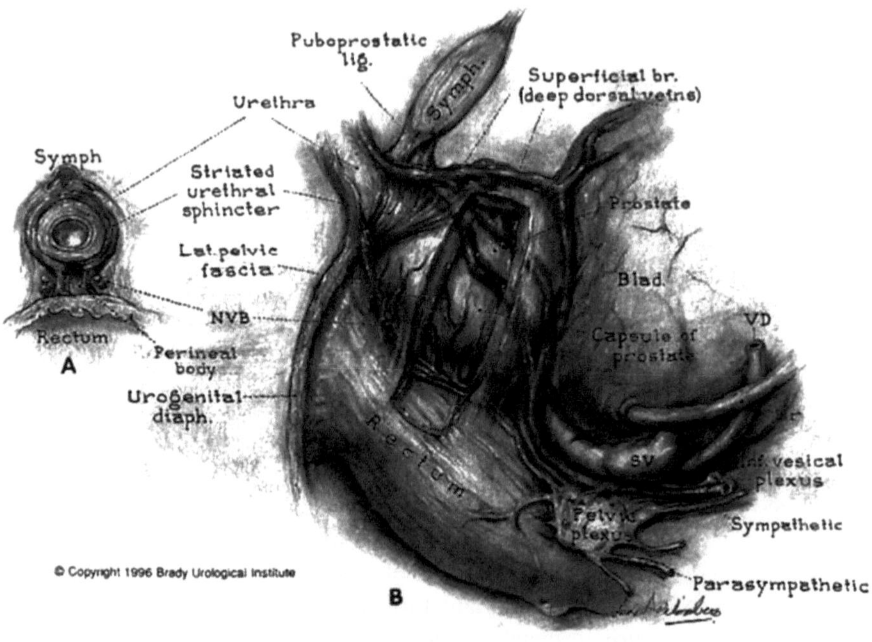

Fig. 8 (**a**) Cross section of membranous urethra just distal to the prostatic apex, demonstrating the relationship of the neurovascular bundle to the striated urethral sphincter and the perineal body. (**b**) Lateral view of the neurovascular bundle, tracing its course from the pelvic plexus through the layers of the lateral pelvic fascia distally to lie lateral to the membranous urethra. © Brady Urological Institute (Permission obtained from Professor Patrick C. Walsh of the Brady Urological Institute, Johns Hopkins Hospital.)

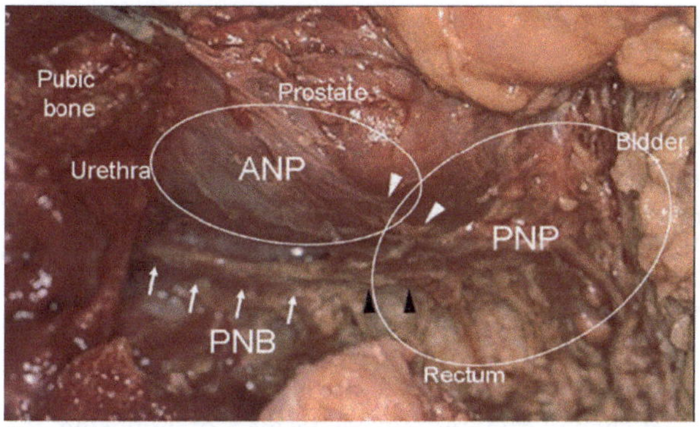

Fig. 9 Gross anatomy photograph (*right*) showing the proximal neurovascular plate (PNP) and predominant neurovascular bundle (PNB). © Tewari et al. [89] (Reprinted with permission from Urology Times Clinical Edition 2008;3:s4–12.)

tumor-induced desmoplasia, or extraprostatic extension, and resolving hemorrhage can make a dissection difficult.

Correlating their anatomic findings from cadaveric dissections with intraoperative video footage and final histology slides, Tewari's group observed accessory neural pathways in several locations around the prostate: specifically, between the prostatic and lateral prostatic fascia, posterior to the prostate and in the layers of Denonvilliers' fascia, in several planes between the layers of periprostatic fascia, and even in the outer layers of the prostatic capsule. The superficial layer of Denonvilliers' fascia has cross-communicating fibers between the left and right neurovascular bundles. Distally, these bundles coalesce to form a retroapical plexus. In up to 35% of cases, this distal plexus penetrates the rectourethralis muscle (Fig. 11). As this area is the final exit pathway for the cavernous and retroapical nerves, these delicate structures may easily be damaged during urethral transection and anastomosis.

Fascial Planes Surrounding the Prostate Capsule

The lateral pelvic fascia (LPF) – a multilayered fascial covering – surrounds the prostatic capsule. The medial, well-defined component of the LPF is known as the prostatic fascia and directly wraps around the prostate capsule. The laterally defined part of LPF is the levator fascia, which lies on the levator muscles. Interposed between the prostatic fascia and the levator fascia are the periprostatic venous plexus and the neurovascular tissue that travel distally to supply the sphincter, urethra, and cavernous tissue. These neural fibers can travel close to the vessels, or occasionally, independently, on the surface of prostate or laterally on

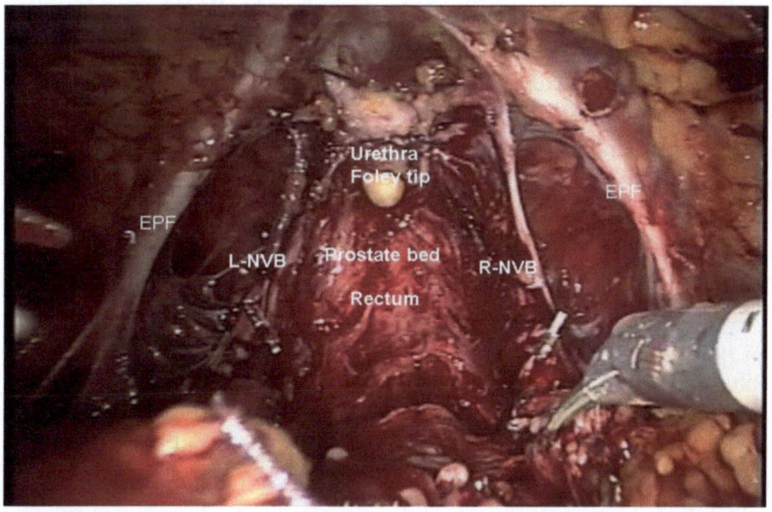

Fig. 10 View of the neurovascular bundles (NVBs) in the prostatic fossa after removal of the prostate gland. Note that the NVBs are closely related to the prostatic pedicle and prostatic fascia, and its branches can sometimes be intermingled with the lateral pedicles of the prostate. © Tewari et al. [89] (Reprinted with permission from Urology Times Clinical Edition 2008;3: s4–12.)

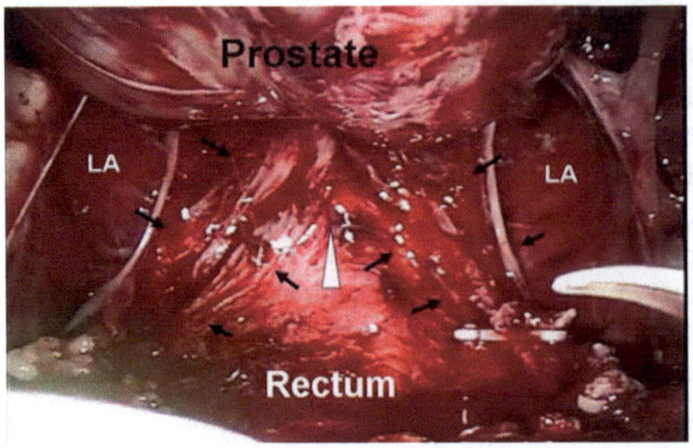

Fig. 11 Retroapical region of prostate has a rich plexus of nerves formed by cross-communicating fibers between the left and right neurovascular bundles and fibers. (LA, Levator ani; *black arrows*, neural tissue). © Tewari et al. [89] (Reprinted with permission from Urology Times Clinical Edition 2008;3:s4–12.)

the rectum. Some of these vessels remain subcapsular for a short distance before dipping into the prostatic tissue. Excessive blunt dissection of these vessels can create an artificial transcapsular plane resulting in a capsular incision.

Operative Strategies for Preservation of Sexual Function

Postprostatectomy erectile dysfunction arises chiefly from injury to the erectogenic nerves, as evidenced by studies reporting a correlation between the number of preserved neurovascular bundles and recovery of potency [37, 76, 79]. Diminished innervation of the corpora cavernosa tissue prevents the release of nitrous oxide (NO) from NANC nerves, decreases the production of cyclic nucleotides within the vascular smooth muscle, and causes impairment of vascular engorgement. Vascular injuries, namely arterial insufficiency and veno-occlusive leakage, have also been proposed as possible etiologies for PPED, although the evidence for this is still early [90–92]. In their systematic review of the literature, Montorsi and colleagues concluded that properly selected patients undergoing nerve-sparing radical prostatectomy by experienced surgeons should be able to achieve unassisted or medically assisted erections following surgery [93].

Maneuvers in Radical Retropubic Prostatectomy

Based on their anatomic elucidations of the neurovascular bundles, Walsh [95] proposed the following maneuvers to avoid inadvertent NVB injury during open retropubic radical prostatectomy:

- Securing venous backbleeding on the anterior prostate after ligation and division of the dorsal venous complex – this should be achieved with a V-shaped running suture instead of apposing the edges toward the midline, as the latter causes medial displacement of the NVB at the apex, making accurate dissection difficult;
- Transecting the membranous urethra at the lateral edges only and refraining from blind dissection of the prostatic apex;
- Releasing the superficial layer of the lateral pelvic fascia, which facilitates dissection of the posterolateral groove between the prostate and the rectum posteriorly, and aids in appreciation of the NVBs;
- Avoiding excessive traction on the NVBs during the posterolateral dissection by gently rolling the prostate side to side;
- Careful dissection of the seminal vesicles to avoid injury to distal branches of the inferior hypogastric plexus.

Alternative approaches to preservation of the NVBs described by Ruckle and Zincke [96], Scardino [97], and Klein [98] involve incising the lateral pelvic fascia medial to the NVBs on the anterolateral prostate prior to apical dissection and division of the deep venous complex. Use of surgical loupes for optical magnification of the operative field has also been reported to improve earlier return of potency and lower rate of positive surgical margins following open RP [99, 100].

Alternatives to Electrocautery

Collateral thermal injury to the neurovascular bundles during radical prostatectomy is a well-recognized phenomenon. Tissue coagulation is achieved with temperatures above 45°C; tissue denaturation ensues at 57–60°C and protein coagulation at temperatures above 65°C [101]. Ong and colleagues elegantly demonstrated a decrease in erectile function following application of thermal energy to the neurovascular bundles in a canine model [102]. In their series of robotic-assisted radical prostatectomies, Ahlering et al. reported that avoidance of thermal energy results in nearly a fivefold improvement in early return of sexual function and that thermal injury induces a pronounced but mostly recoverable injury after 2 years from time of surgery [103]. Recently, Tewari's group [104] also reported that bipolar cautery during robotic-assisted radical prostatectomy (RARP) causes significantly higher and more persistent rise in temperature to tissues within 1 cm of its use, compared to monoploar cautery applied at the same distance, challenging the widely held belief that bipolar cautery causes less collateral tissue damage. Using a porcine model, Khan et al. [105] also demonstrated that the lateral prostatic pedicles serve as a heat sink during bladder neck transection using cautery, protecting the NVBs from thermal injury.

Various alternatives to thermal energy have been proposed during RARP. Ahlering and colleagues [106] reported their experience placing laparoscopic bulldog clamps on the lateral pedicles 1 cm from the prostate, followed by division of the lateral pedicles with cold scissors. After mobilization of the neurovascular bundle off the prostatic capsule, FloSeal^{TM} was applied along its entire length and the NVB covered with a dry 1-cm × 4-cm sheet of Gelfoam^{TM}. The bulldog clamps were sequentially withdrawn following completion of prostatectomy, and 3-0 figure-of-eight sutures used for hemostasis of bleeding from the lateral pedicles. In the same year, Shalhav's group [107] reported 47% of patients returning to baseline potency at 1 month after RARP using an antegrade dissection of the neurovascular bundle that avoided the use of clips or monopolar cautery.

Gill and colleagues [108, 109] from the Cleveland Clinic reported a different approach to lateral pedicle ligation during laparoscopic radical prostatectomy. In their antegrade technique, the lateral prostatic pedicles were first controlled with atraumatic bulldog clamps, then divided using cold scissors, and the NVBs preserved with blunt and sharp dissection. Hemostasis was then secured with superficial suturing of the transected pedicle (Fig. 12). Using real-time Doppler transrectal ultrasound guidance, they demonstrated that application of bulldog clamps on the lateral pedicles did not impair blood flow through the NVBs throughout this maneuver. More recently, these investigators reported their preliminary experience comparing the KTP laser against ultrasonic shears and athermal cold Endoshear^{TM} scissors dissection of the lateral pelvic fascia during laparoscopic unilateral NVB mobilization in a canine radical prostatectomy model [110]. Measuring peak intracavernous pressure upon cavernous nerve stimulation both acutely and at 1 month follow-up in 36 dogs, they found that the KTP laser was comparable to the athermal technique (Fig. 13), and superior to the ultrasonic shears, for preserving cavernous nerve function. In addition, intraoperative thermography revealed less collateral thermal spread from the KTP laser than from the ultrasonic shears. These animal studies suggest laser energy as a less traumatic alternative for periprostatic fascial dissection, and their feasibility in human trials is awaited.

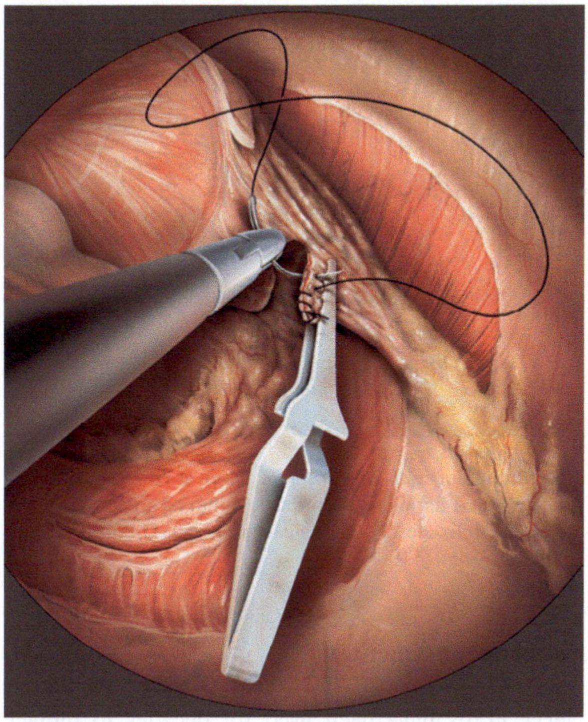

Fig. 12 Control of lateral prostatic pedicles using atraumatic bulldog clamps. The clamps are placed close to the prostate and the pedicles divided with cold Endoshear scissors. Bleeding vessels are then secured with superficial 4-0 sutures. © BJU International – Haber et al. [109] (Reprinted with permission from Urology Times Clinical Edition 2008;3:s4–12.)

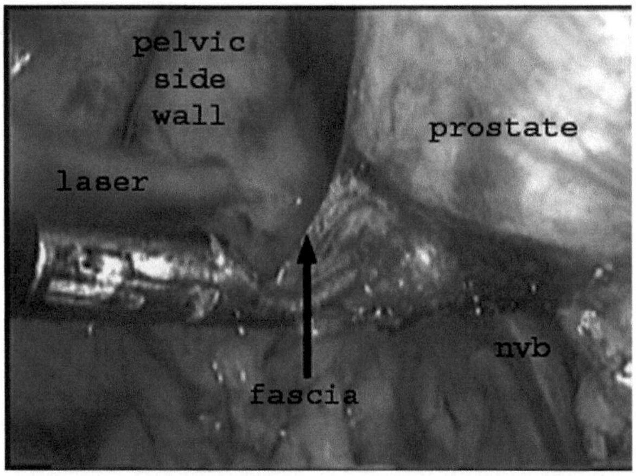

Fig. 13 Intraoperative use of KTP laser at 6 W via 200 μm fiber delivered through custom-made 5 mm laparoscopic instrument to mobilize left NVB in a canine model. © Elsevier Inc. – Gianduzzo et al. [110]

Nerve Reconstruction

Nerve grafts have been used for decades to replace damaged or divided sensorimotor nerves. In 1991, Quinlan and Walsh first reported successful return of erectile function in rats using interposition cavernous nerve grafts after iatrogenic denervation [111]. Kim and Scardino [112, 113] subsequently reported excellent results using bilateral sural interposition nerve grafts (SNG) in 23 erstwhile potent patients with aggressive cancer undergoing nonnerve-sparing retropubic radical prostatectomy with deliberate wide NVB resection, compared to a control group of 12 men undergoing similar surgery who did not have SNG. Of the patients receiving bilateral SNG, 26% had spontaneous medically unassisted erections sufficient for penetrative intercourse, 26% reported spontaneous erections insufficient for intercourse, and 43% had intercourse with sildenafil. The greatest return of potency occurred at 18 months follow-up, although none of the patients reported erections before 5 months. This technique was subsequently adopted for both laparoscopic [114] and robotic-assisted [115] radical prostatectomy, with similar encouraging results. However, results of a randomized phase II trial by investigators at MD Anderson Cancer Center, Houston, in a cohort of 107 men undergoing unilateral nerve-sparing radical prostatectomy, failed to demonstrate any additional improvement of potency with unilateral sural nerve grafting at 2 years following surgery [116].

Tewari and colleagues [117] reported an alternative approach of nerve advancement using end-to-end reconstruction of the neurovasucular bundle after partial resection in clinically high-risk patients with MRI evidence of extracapsular extension of disease, most of whom had T3 disease at final histology. In these patients who demonstrated fibrotic tissue around the NVBs, athermal partial resection of the NVBs was performed outside the lateral pelvic fascia. The proximal and distal ends of the NVB were then mobilized off and approximated without tension using 6-0 polypropylene interrupted sutures (Fig. 14). At a median of 20 months follow-up, five of these seven patients reported recovery erections with or without phosphodiesterase inhibitors and a median SHIM score of 18.

Atala's group [118] reported significant recovery of erectile function in adult male Sprague–Dawley rats with bilateral cavernous nerve excision, using acellular nerve matrices processed from donor rat corporal nerves for interposition nerve grafting. Subsequent electromyography of the acellular nerve grafts at 3 months after surgery demonstrated adequate intracavernosal pressures, confirming their feasibility as an alternative to autologous nerve grafts in aiding recovery of cavernosal nerve function. Other innovative approaches being developed in animal models include use of embryonic stem cells [119] and growth factors [120] to augment cavernous nerve regeneration. While exciting, final applicability of these new strategies in humans remains to be seen.

Periprostatic Planes of Fascial Dissection

Recent anatomic studies by Costello [84], Takenaka [85], and Kiyoshima [86] demonstrated significant variation of the periprostatic nerves from the classical description of the distinct neurovascular bundles found in the posterolateral grooves of the prostate (see above). Correlating their intraoperative observations during robotic-assisted radical prostatectomy with histological specimens, Menon and colleagues from the Vattikuti Urology Institute, Detroit, recognized that numerous nerve bundles are present in the different layers of fascia enveloping the prostate. Deviating from Walsh's accepted technique [83] of leaving prostatic fascia on the prostatectomy specimen, Menon et al. [121, 122] adopted an aggressive approach to nerve sparing called the "Veil of Aphrodite" technique,

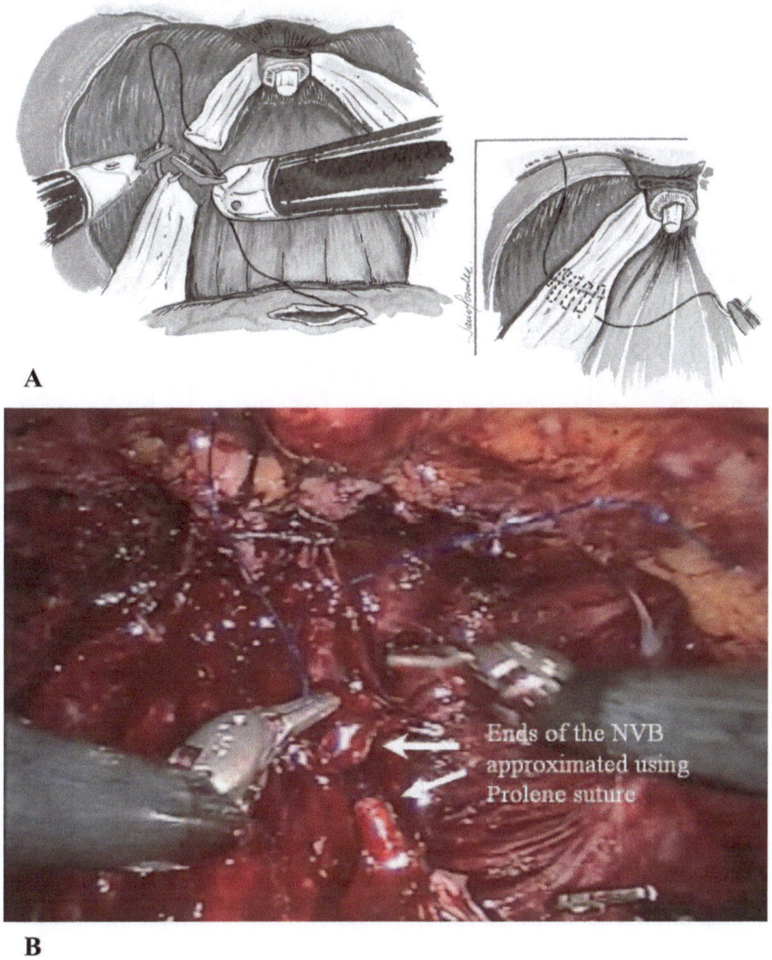

Fig. 14 (**a**) Pictorial representation of nerve advancement technique following partial neurovascular bundle resection. (**b**) Intraoperative view of approximation of cut ends of NVB using 6-0 polypropeline suture with da Vinci® robotic assistance. © Mary Ann Liebert Inc. – Martinez-Salamanca et al. [117]

wherein the lateral pelvic fascia is dissected down to the glistening prostatic capsule surface and the veil of periprostatic tissue teased away in a relatively avascular plane (Fig. 15). In their cohort of 154 men, 96% reported return of potency (either with or without medical assistance) at 12 months follow-up, with a positive margin rate of 5% [123]. Adopting this aggressive intrafascial approach of dissection down to the shiny prostatic capsule for laparoscopic radical prostatectomy, Stolzenburg [124] also reported return of potency in 89.7% of their patients aged less than 55 years at 12 months following surgery, with margin positivity rates of 4.5% in pT2 and 29.4% in pT3 disease. Interestingly, Walsh's group [125] also adopted this approach in performing high anterior release of the levator fascia during bilateral nerve-sparing retropubic RP and reported improved sexual function without compromise of surgical margins.

Balancing Nerve Preservation with Cancer Control: Cornell Risk-Stratified Approach

Striving to balance the competing goals of cancer clearance with preservation of potencty, we adopt a risk-stratified approach toward nerve sparing according to the patient's likelihood of ipsilateral EPE at our institution (Fig. 16). The patient's PSA, Gleason score, percentage of cancer in the biopsy, number of positive cores, presence of unilateral vs. bilateral positive cores

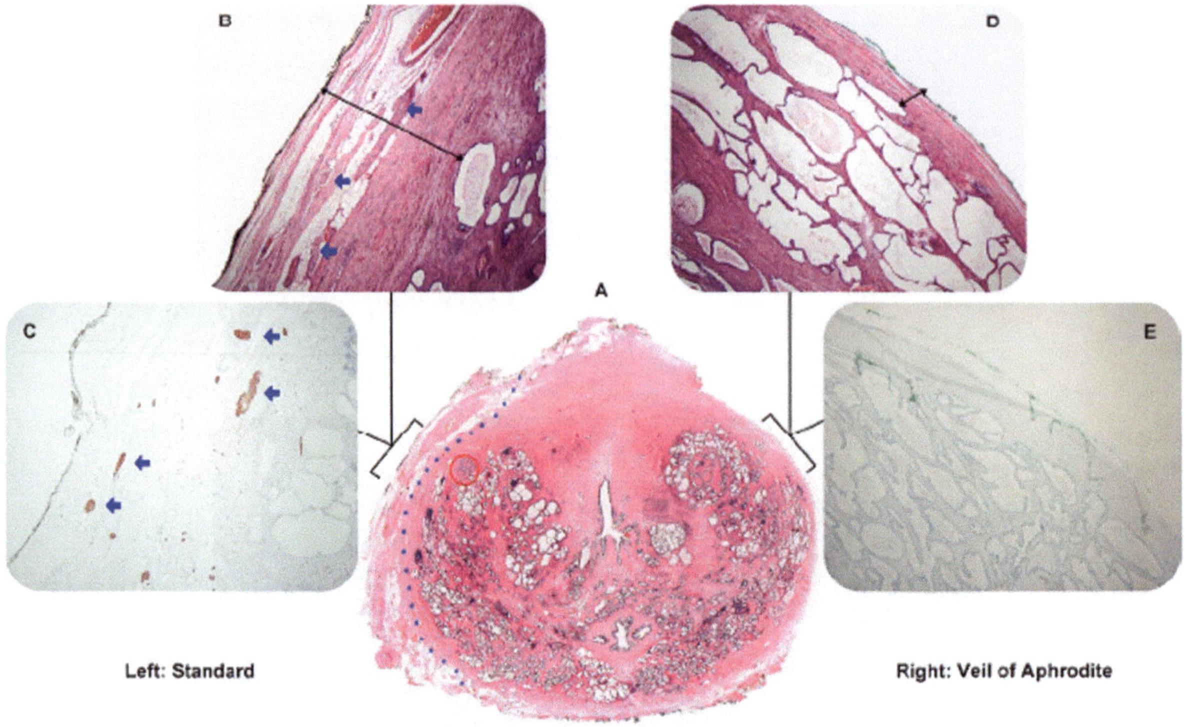

Fig. 15 (**a**) H&E of whole mount radical prostatectomy specimen demonstrating Walsh's conventional nerve-sparing technique on *left* and "Veil of Aphrodite" technique on the *right*. Note the presence of tumor (*red circle*) and the lateral pelvic fascia on the *left*, and absence of LPF external to the prostatic capsule on the *right*. (**b, c**) H&E of the lateral pelvic fascia, demonstrating nerve bundles and extended margin to the capsule. (**d, e**) Absence of LPF and close proximity of margin to the capsule. © Elsevier – Savera et al. [122]

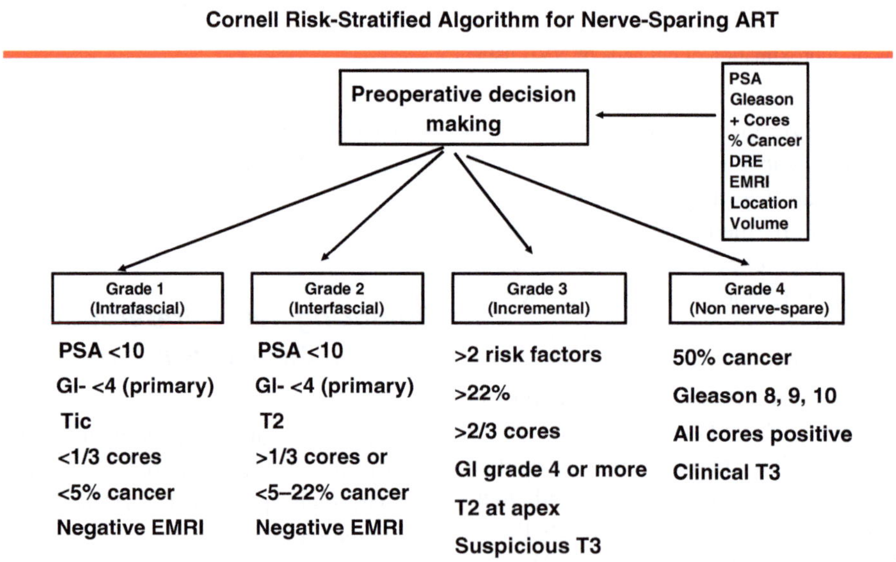

Fig. 16 Risk-stratified algorithm for nerve-sparing athermal nerve-sparing robotic radical prostatectomy

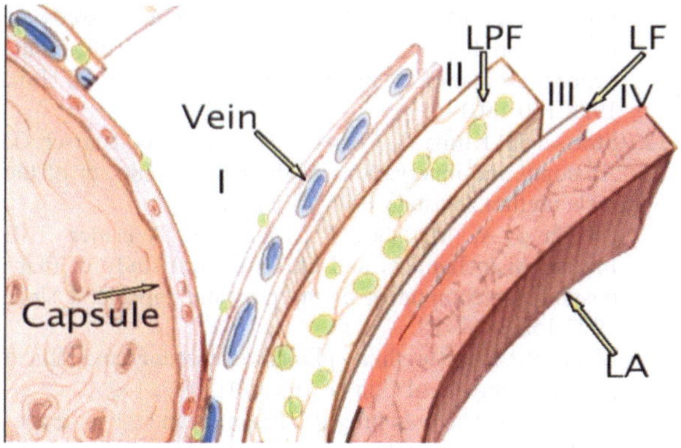

Fig. 17 Layers of fascia enveloping prostatic capsule demonstrating the planes of dissection for differing grades (I–IV) of nerve sparing

(used as a surrogate for high-volume cancer or multifocality), clinical stage, and findings of the endorectal magnetic resonance imaging in terms of cancer localization, volume, status of capsule, and periprostatic tissue are some parameters that we regularly use to select patients for a nerve-sparing prostatectomy. Our approach to nerve sparing during robotic prostatectomy involves varying degrees of preservation of the nerve fibers in the various fascial planes (Fig. 17). We refer to them as follows:

Grade 1 approach – Incision of the Denonvilliers' fascia and LPF is taken just outside the prostatic capsule. We perform this only for patients with no-to-minimal risk of EPE.

Grade 2 approach – Incision through the Denonvilliers' fascia (leaving deeper layers on the rectum) and LPF is taken just outside the layer of veins of the prostate capsule – this preserves most large neural trunks and ganglions, and is used for patients at low risk of EPE.

Grade 3 (partial/incremental nerve-sparing) approach – Incision is taken through the outer compartment of LPF, excising all layers of Denonvilliers' fascia. This is performed for patients with moderate risk of EPE because some of the medial trunks are killed while lateral trunks are preserved.

Grade 4 (non-nerve-sparing approach) – These patients have high risk for EPE, and essentially, in traditional terms, they are not candidates for nerve sparing. Here we perform wide excision of the LPF and Denonvilliers' fascia containing the majority of the periprostatic neurovascular tissues. In some of these patients, we may attempt nerve advancement of the identifiable ends of the neurovascular bundle: a donor site and using the same neural tissue, instead of interposing a dissimilar, devascularized nerve graft.

In addition, we have adopted the following modifications to our athermal robotic nerve-sparing technique: (a) minimizing periprostatic dissection to avoid traction/transaction of the delicate nerves; (b) limiting dissection to the midline during bladder neck transection, as this will protect the predominant neurovascular plate (PNP) from thermal/mechanical injury; (c) adopting athermal dissection of the seminal vesicles, as this should cause the least damage to the PNP and hypogastric nerve; and (d) avoiding use of cautery during the posterolateral prostate dissection.

We have found that in our cohort of potent men who meet selection criteria for aggressive bilateral grade 1 nerve sparing (PSA <10 ng/dl, clinical stage $\leq$ T2, primary Gleason grade <4, cancer volume <5% in all cores, and absence of cues suggestive of extraprostatic extension on endorectal MRI and during surgery), 95% of these hitherto potent men had partial erections with and without the use of PDE5 inhibitors and 86% had erection sufficient for penetrative intercourse at a mean follow-up of 26 weeks [126].

Acknowledgments Dr. Tan discloses that he receives financial support from the *Ferdinand C. Valentine Fellowship In Urologic Research, New York Academy of Medicine;* the *John Steyn Travelling Fellowship in Urology, Royal College of Surgeons of Edinburgh;* and the *Medical Research Fellowship, National Medical Research Council, Singapore.*

Dr. Tewari discloses that he receives a research grant from *Intuitive Surgical Inc, Sunnyvale, CA.*

References

1. Jemal A, Siegel R, Ward E, et al. Cancer statistics, 2009. CA Cancer J Clin. 2009;59:225–49.
2. Penson DF, Rossignol M, Sartor AO, Scardino PT, Abenhaim LL. Prostate cancer: epidemiology and health-related quality of life. Urology. 2008;72Suppl 6A: 3–11.
3. Quinn M, Babb P. Patterns and trends in prostate cancer incidence, survival, prevalence and mortality. Part 1: International comparisons. BJU Int. 2002;90: 162–73.

4. Lu-Yao GL, Yao S. Population based study of long-term survival in patients with clinically localized prostate cancer. Lancet. 1997;349:906–910.
5. D'Amico DV, Whittington R, Malkowicz SB, et al. Biochemical outcome after radical prostatectomy, external beam radiation therapy, or interstitial radiation therapy for clinically localized prostate cancer. JAMA. 1998;280(11):969–74.
6. Bill-Axelson A, Holmberg L, Ruutu M, et al. Radical prostatectomy versus watchful waiting in early prostate cancer. N Engl J Med. 2005;352(19):1977–84.
7. Bill-Axelson A, Holmberg L, Filen F, et al. Radical prostatectomy versus watchful waiting in localized prostate cancer: the Scandinavian prostate cancer group-4 randomized trial. J Natl Cancer Inst. 2008;100(16):1144–54.
8. Klein EA, Ceizki J, Kupelian PA, Mahadevan A. Outcomes for intermediate risk prostate cancer: are there advantages for surgery, external radiation or brachytherapy? Urol Oncol. 2009;27(1):67–71.
9. Tewari A, Johnsson CC, Devine G, Crawford ED, Gamito EJ, Demers R, Menon M. Long-term survival probability in men with clinically localized prostate cancer: a case-control, propensity modeling study stratified by race, age, treatment and co-morbidities. J Urol. 2004;171: 1513–19.
10. Wilt TJ, MacDonald R, Rutks I, Shamliyan TA, Taylor BC, Kane RL. Systematic review: comparative effectiveness and harms of treatments for clinically localized prostate cancer. Ann Int Med. 2008;148:435–48.
11. Su L. Role of robotics in modern urologic practice. Curr Opin Urol. 2009;19:63–4.
12. Tan GY, Goel RK, Kaouk JH, Tewari AK. Technological advances in robotic-assisted laparoscopic surgery. Urol Clin N Am. 2009;36:237–49.
13. Berryhill R Jr, Jhaveri J, Yadav R, et al. Robotic prostatectomy: a review of outcomes compared with laparoscopic and open approaches. Urology. 2008;72:15–23.
14. Ficarra V, Novara G, Artibani W, et al. Retropubic, laparoscopic and robot-assisted radical prostatectomy: a systematic review and cumulative analysis of comparative studies. Eur Urol. 2009. doi:10.1016/j.eururo. 2009.01.036.
15. Marsh DM, Lepor H. Predicting continence following radical prostatectomy. Curr Urol Rep. 2001;2:248–52.
16. MacDiarmid SA. Incontinence after radical prostatectomy: pathophysiology and management. Curr Urol Rep. 2001;2:209–13.
17. Fowler FJ, Barry MJ, Lu-Yao G, et al. Effect of radical prostatectomy on patient quality of life: results from a Medicare survey. Urology. 1995;45:1007–13.
18. Brown JA, Elliott DS, Barrett DM. Postprostatectomy urinary incontinence: a comparison of the cost of conservative versus surgical management. Urology. 1998;51(5):715–20.
19. Stolzenburg JU, Schwalenberg T, Horn L-C, Neuhaus J, Constantinides C, Liatsikos EN. Anatomical landmarks of radical prostatectomy. Eur Urol. 2007;51:629–39.
20. Tan GY, El Douaihy Y, Te AE, Tewari AK. Scientific and technical advances in continence recovery following radical prostatectomy. Exp Rev Med Dev. 2009;6(4): 431–53.
21. Burnett AL, Mostwin JL. In situ anatomical study of the male urethral sphincteric complex: relevance to continence preservation following major pelvic surgery. J Urol. 1998;160:1301–6.
22. Strasser H, Klima G, Poisel S, Horninger W, Bartsch G. Anatomy and innervations of the rhabdosphincter of the male urethra. Prostate 1996;28:24–31.
23. Elbadawi A, Mathews R, Light JK, Wheeler TM. Immunohistochemical and ultrastructural study of rhabdosphincter component of the prostatic capsule. J Urol. 1997;158:1819–28.
24. Myers RP. Male urethral sphincteric anatomy and radical prostatectomy. Urol Clin N Am. 1991;18:211–27.
25. Steiner MS. The puboprostatic ligament and the male urethral suspensory mechanism: an anatomic study. Urology. 1994;44:530–4.
26. Juenemann KP, Lue TF, Schmidt RA, Melchior H, Tanagho EA. Neuroanatomy and clinical significance of sacral and pudendal nerve anatomy. J Urol. 1988;139: 74–80.
27. Hollabaugh RS Jr, Dmochowski RR, Steiner MS. Neuroanatomy of the male rhabdosphincter. Urology. 1997;49:426–34.
28. Eastham JA, Kattan MW, Rogers E, et al. Risk factors for urinary incontinence after radical prostatectomy. J Urol. 1996;156:1707–13.
29. Sacco E, Prayer-Galetti T, Pinto F. Urinary incontinence after radical prostatectomy: incidence by definition, risk factors and temporal trend in a large series with a long-term follow-up. BJU Int. 2006;97(6):1234–41.
30. Coakley FV, Eberhardt S, Kattan MW, et al. Urinary continence after radical retropubic prostatectomy: relationship with membranous urethral length on preoperative endorectal magnetic resonance imaging. J Urol. 2002;168:1032–5.
31. Nyugen L, Jhaveri J, Tewari A. Surgical technique to overcome anatomical shortcoming: balancing post-prostatectomy continence outcomes of urethral sphincter lengths on preoperative magnetic resonance imaging. J Urol. 2008;179:1907–11.
32. Paperal P, Akin O, Sandhu JS, et al. Recovery of urinary continence after radical prostatectomy: association with urethral length and urethral fibrosis measured by preoperative and postoperative endorectal magnetic resonance imaging. Eur Urol. 2008. doi: 10.1016/j.eururo.2008.08.057.
33. Park R, Martin S, Goldberg JD, Lepor H. Anastomotic strictures following radical prostatectomy: insights into incidence, effectiveness of intervention, effect on continence, and factors predisposing to occurrence. Urology. 2001;57:742–6.
34. Begg CB, Riedel ER, Bach PB, Kattan MW, Schrag D, Warren JL, Scardino PT. Variations in morbidity after radical prostatectomy. N Engl J Med. 2002;346(15): 1138–44.
35. Bianco FJ Jr, Reidel ER, Begg CB, Kattan MW, Scardino PT. Variations among high volume surgeons in the rate of complications after radical prostatectomy: further evidence that technique matters. J Urol. 2005;173:2099–13.
36. Wilt TJ, Shamliyan TA, Taylor BC, MacDonald R, Kane RL. Association between hospital and surgeon radical

prostatectomy volume and patient outcomes: a systematic review. J Urol. 2008;180:820–29.
37. Kundu SD, Roehl KA, Eggener SE, et al. Potency, continence and complications in 3,477 consecutive radical retropubic prostatectomies. J Urol. 2004;172:2227–31.
38. Burkhard FC, Kessler TM, Fleischmann A, Thalmann GN, Schumacher M, Studer UE. Nerve sparing open radical retropubic prostatectomy – does it have an impact on urinary continence? J Urol. 2006;176(1):189–95.
39. Konety BR, Sadetsky N, Carroll PR, CaPSURE Investigators. Recovery of urinary continence following radical prostatectomy: the impact of prostate volume – analysis of data from the CaPSURE database. J Urol. 2007;177(4):1423–25.
40. Boczko J, Erturk E, Golijanin D, et al. Impact of prostate size in robot-assisted radical prostatectomy. J Endourol. 2007;21(2):184–8.
41. Oefelein MG. Prospective predictors of urinary continence after anatomical radical retropubic prostatectomy: a multivariate analysis. World J Urol. 2004;22:267–71.
42. Eden CG, Richards AJ, Ooi J, Moon DA, Laczko I. Previous bladder outlet surgery does not affect medium-term outcomes after laparoscopic radical prostatectomy. BJU Int. 2007;99(2):399–402.
43. Walsh PC, Partin AW, Epstein JI. Cancer control and quality of life following anatomical radical retropubic prostatectomy: results at 10 years. J Urol. 1994;152(5):1831–6.
44. Lepor H, Kaci L, Xue X. Continence following radical retropubic prostatectomy using self-reporting instruments. J Urol. 2004;171:1212–5.
45. Seckiner I, Yesili C, Mungan NA, Aykanat A, Akduman B. Correlations between the ICIQ-SF score and urodynamic findings. Neurourol Urodyn. 2007;26:492–4.
46. Thüroff J, Abrams P, Andersson KE, et al. Guidelines on urinary incontinence. In: Aus G, editors. European Association of urology (EAU) guidelines. Arnhem, the Netherlands: European Association of Urology; 2008. pp. 3–7.
47. van Randenborgh H, Paul R, Kubler H, Breul J, Hartung R. Improved urinary continence after radical retropubic prostatectomy with preparation of a long, partially intraprostatic portion of the membranous urethra: an analysis of 1013 consecutive cases. Prostate Cancer Prostat Dis. 2004;7:253–7.
48. Nyugen L, Jhaveri J, Tewari A. Surgical technique to overcome anatomical shortcoming: balancing post-prostatectomy continence outcomes of urethral sphincter lengths on preoperative magnetic resonance imaging. J Urol. 2008;179:1907–11.
49. Rocco F, Carmignani L, Aquati P, et al. Restoration of posterior aspect of rhabdosphincter shortens continence time after radical retropubic prostatectomy. J Urol. 2006;175:2201–6.
50. Rocco F, Luca Carmignani L, Acquati P, et al. Early continence recovery after open radical prostatectomy with restoration of the posterior aspect of the rhabdosphincter. Eur Urol. 2007;52:376–83.
51. Rocco B, Gregori A, Stener S, et al. Posterior reconstruction of the rhabdosphincter allows a rapid recovery of continence after transperitoneal videolaparoscopic radical prostatectomy. Eur Urol. 2007;51:996–1003.
52. Nguyen MM, Kamoi K, Stein RJ, et al. Early continence outcomes of posterior musculofascial plate reconstruction during robotic and laparoscopic prostatectomy. BJU Int. 2008;101:1135–9.
53. Licht MR, Klein EA, Tuason L, Levin H. Impact of bladder neck preservation during radical prostatectomy on continence and cancer control. Urology. 1994;44:883–7.
54. Lepor H, Chan S, Melamed J. The role of bladder neck biopsy in men undergoing radical retropubic prostatectomy with preservation of the bladder neck. J Urol. 1998;160(6):2435–9.
55. Shelfo SW, Obek C, Soloway MS. Update on bladder neck preservation during radical retropubic prostatectomy: impact on pathological outcome, anastomotic strictures and continence. Urology. 1998;51(1):73–8.
56. Srougi M, Nesrallah LJ, Kauffman JR, Nesrallah A, Leite KR. Urinary continence and pathological outcome after bladder neck preservation during radical retropubic prostatectomy: a randomized prospective trial. J Urol. 2001;165(3):815–8.
57. Deliveliotis C, Protogerou V, Alargorf E, Varkarakis J. Radical prostatectomy: bladder neck preservation and puboprostatic ligament sparing – effect on continence and positive margins. Urology. 2002;60(5):855–58.
58. Bianco FJ, Grignon DJ, Sakr WA, et al. Radical prostatectomy with bladder neck preservation: impact of a positive margin. Eur Urol. 2003;43(5):461–6.
59. Cambio AJ, Evans CP. Minimising postoperative incontinence following radical prostatectomy: considerations and evidence. Eur Urol. 2006;50:903–13.
60. Walsh PC, Marschke PL. Intussusception of the bladder neck leads to earlier continence after radical prostatectomy. Urology. 2002;59(6):934–8.
61. Wille S, Varga Z, von Knobloch R, Hofmann R. Intussusception of bladder neck improves early continence after radical prostatectomy: results of a prospective trial. Urology. 2005;65(3):524–7.
62. Thiel DD, Igel TC, Brisson TE, Heckman MG. Outcomes with an alternative anastomotic technique after radical retropubic prostatectomy: 10-year experience. Urology. 2006;68:132–6.
63. Srougi M, Paranhos M, Leite KM, Dall'Oglio M, Nesrallah L. The influence of bladder neck mucosal eversion and early urinary extravasation on patient outcome after radical retropubic prosatatectomy: a prospective controlled trial. BJU Int. 2005;95(6):757–60.
64. Steiner MS. Continence-preserving anatomic radical retropubic prostatectomy: the "no-touch" technique. Curr Urol Rep. 2000;1:20–7.
65. Stolzenburg JU, Liatsikos EN, Rabenalt R, et al. Nerve sparing endoscopic extraperitoneal radical prostatectomy – effect of puboprostatic ligament preservation on early continence and positive margins. Eur Urol. 2006;49(1):103–11.
66. Tewari AK, Bigelow K, Rao S, et al. Anatomic restoration technique of continence mechanism and preservation of puboprostatic collar: a novel modification to achieve early urinary continence in men undergoing robotic prostatectomy. Urology. 2007;69:726–31.
67. Takenaka A. Tewari AK, Leung RA, et al. Preservation of the puboperineoplasty for early recovery of urinary incon-

tinence after robotic prostatectomy: anatomic basis and preliminary outcomes. Eur Urol. 2007;51:433–40.
68. Tewari A, Jhaveri J, Rao S, et al. Total reconstruction of the vesico-urethral junction. BJU Int. 2008;101:871–7.
69. Hollabaugh RS, Dmochowski RR, Kneib TG, Steiner MS. Preservation of putative continence nerves during radical retropubic prostatectomy leads to more rapid return of urinary continence. Urology. 1998;51:960–7.
70. John H, Hauri D, Leuener M, Reinecke M, Maake C. Evidence of trigonal denervation and reinnervation after radical retropubic prostatectomy. J Urol. 2001;165:111–3.
71. Catarin MV, Manzano GM, Nobrega JA, Almeida FG, Srougi M, Bruschini H. The role of membranous urethral afferent autonomic innervation in the continence mechanism after nerve sparing radical prostatectomy: a clinical and prospective study. J Urol. 2008;180:2527–31.
72. Tan GY, Jhaveri JK, Tewari AK. Anatomic restoration technique (ART): a biomechanics based approach for early continence recovery following minimally invasive radical prostatectomy. Urology. 2009;74(3):492–6.
73. Raina R, Agarwal A, Zippe CD. Management of erectile dysfunction after radical prostatectomy. Urology. 2005;66:923–9.
74. Penson DF, Feng Z, Kuniyuki A, McClerran D, Albertsen PC, Deapen D, et al. General Quality of life 2 years following treatment for prostate cancer: what influences outcomes? Results from the Prostate Cancer Outcomes Study. J Clin Oncol. 2003;21:1147–54.
75. Kirschner-Hermanns R, Jakse G. Quality of life following radical prostatectomy. Crit Rev Oncol Hematol. 2002;43:141–51.
76. McCullough AR. Rehabilitation of erectile function following radical prostatectomy. Asian J Androl. 2008;10(1):61–74.
77. Quinlan DM, Epstein JI, Carter BS, Walsh PC. Sexual function following radical prostatectomy: influence of preservation of neurovascular bundles. J Urol. 1991;145:998–1002.
78. Rabbani F, Stapleton AM, Kattan MW, Wheeler TM, Scardino PT. Factors predicting recovery of erections after radical prostatectomy. J Urol. 2000;164(6):1929–34.
79. Dubbelman YD, Dohle GR, FH Schroder. Sexual function before and after radical retropubic prostatectomy: a systematic review of prognostic indicators for a successful outcome. Eur Urol. 2006;50:711–20.
80. Walz J, Graefen M, Huland H. Basic principles of anatomy for optimal surgical management of prostate cancer. World J Urol. 2007;25:31–38.
81. Walsh PC, Donker PJ. Impotence following radical prostatectomy: insight into etiology and prevention. J Urol. 1982;128:492–7.
82. Lepor H, Gregerman M, Crosby R, mostofi FK, Walsh PC. Precise localization of the autonomic nerves from the pelvic plexus to the corpora cavernosa: a detailed anatomical study of the adult male pelvis. J Urol. 1985;133:207–12.
83. Walsh PC. Anatomic radical prostatectomy: evolution of surgical technique. J Urol. 1998;160:2418–24.
84. Costello AJ, Brooks M, Cole OJ. Anatomical studies of the neurovascular bundle and cavernosal nerves. BJU Int. 2004;94:1071–6.
85. Takenaka A, Murakami G, Matsubara A, et al. Variation in course of cavernous nerve with special reference to details of topographic relationships near prostatic apex: histologic study using male cadavers. Urology. 2005;65:136–42.
86. Kiyoshima K, Yokomizo A, Yoshida T, et al. Anatomic features of periprostatic tissue and its surroundings: a histological analysis of 79 radical retropubic prostatectomy specimens. Jpn J Clin Oncol. 2004;34:463–68.
87. Eichelberg C, Erbersdobler A, Michl U, Schlomm T, Salomon G, Graefen M, et al. Nerve Distribution along the Prostatic Capsule. Eur Urol. 2007;51(1):105–11.
88. Tewari A, Takenaka A, Mtui E, Horninger W, Peschel R, Bartsch G, Vaughan ED. The proximal neurovascular plate and the tri-zonal neural architecture around the prostate gland: importance in the athermal robotic technique of nerve-sparing prostatectomy. BJU Int. 2006;98:318–23.
89. Tewari A, Tan GY, Dorsey PJ Jr, Yadav R, Ramanathan R, Patel N, Takenaka A. Optimizing erectogenic outcomes during athermal robotic prostatectomy: a risk-stratified tri-zonal approach. Urol Times Clinical Edition. 2008;3:s4–s12.
90. Kim ED, Blackburn D, McVary KT. Post-radical prostatectomy penile blood flow: assessment with color Doppler ultrasound. J Urol. 1994;152:2276–9.
91. Mulhall JP, Slovick R, Hotaling J, et al. Erectile dysfunction after radical prostatectomy: haemodynamic profiles and their correlation with the recovery of erectile function. J Urol. 2002;167:1371–5.
92. Kawanishi Y, Lee KS, Kimura K, Kojima K, Yamamoto A, Numata A. Effect of radical retropubic prostatectomy on erectile function, evaluated before and after surgery using color Doppler ultrasonography and nocturnal penile tumescence monitoring. BJU Int. 2001;88:244–7.
93. Montorsi F, Briganti A, Salonia A, Rigatti P, Burnett AL. Current and future strategies for preventing and managing erectile dysfunction following radical prostatectomy. Eur Urol. 2004;45:123–33.
94. Bianco F, kattan M, Eastham J, Scardino P, Mulhall JP. Surgeon and surgical volume as predictors of erectile function outcomes following radical prostatectomy. J Sex Med. 2004;1:33.
95. Walsh PC. Anatomic radical retropubic prostatectomy. In: Walsh PC, Retik AB, Vaughan ED Jr, Wein AJ, editors. Campbell's urology, volume 4 chapter 90. 8th ed. Philadelphia, PA: WB Saunders Co; 2002. pp. 3107–29.
96. Ruckle HC, Zincke H. Potency sparing radical retropubic prostatectomy: a simplified anatomical approach. J Urol. 1995;153:1875–7.
97. Goad JR, Scardino PT. Modifications in the technique of radical prostatectomy to minimize blood loss. Atlas Urol Clin North Am. 1994;3:65–80.
98. Klein EA, Kupelian PA, Tuason L, Levin HS. Initial dissection of the lateral fascia reduces the positive margin rate in radical prostatectomy. Urology. 1998;51:766–73.
99. Chuang MS, O-Connor RC, Laven BA, Orvieto MA, Brendler CB. Early release of the neurovascular bundles and optical loupe magnification lead to improved and earlier return of potency following radical retropubic prostatectomy. J Urol. 2005;173:537–9.

100. Magera JS, Inman BA, Slezak JM, Bagniewski SM, Sebo TJ, Myers RP. Increased optical magnification from 2.5x to 4.3x with technical modification lowers the positive margin rate in open radical retropubic prostatectomy. J Urol. 2008;179:130–5.
101. Lantis JC, Durville FM, Connolly R, Schwaitzberg SD. Comparison of coagulation modalities in surgery. J Laparosc Adv Surg Tech. 1998;8:381–94.
102. Ong AM, Su LM, Varkarakis I, et al. Nerve sparing radical prostatectomy: effects of hemostatic energy sources on the recovery of cavernous nerve function in a canine model. J Urol. 2004;172:1318–22.
103. Ahlering TE, Rodriquez E, Skarecky DW. Overcoming obstacles: nerve-sparing issues in radical prostatectomy. J Endourol. 2008;22:745–9.
104. Mandhani A, Dorsey PJ Jr, Ramanathan R, et al. Real time monitoring of temperature changes in neurovascular bundles during robotic radical prostatectomy: thermal map for nerve-sparing radical prostatectomy. J Endourol. 2008;22:2313–7.
105. Khan F, Rodriguez E, Finley DS, Skarecky DW, Ahlering TE. Spread of thermal energy and heat sinks: implications for nerve-sparing robotic prostatectomy. J Endourol. 2007;21:1195–8.
106. Ahlering TE, Eichel L, Chou D, Skarecky DW. Feasibility study for robotic radical prostatectomy cautery-free neurovascular bundle preservation. Urology. 2005;65:994–7.
107. Chien GW, Mikhail AA, Orvieto MA, et al. Modified clipless antegrade nerve preservation in robotic-assisted laparoscopic radical prostatectomy with validated sexual function evaluation. Urology. 2005;66:419–23.
108. Gill IS, Ukimura O, Rubinstein M, et al. Lateral pedicle control during laparoscopic radical prostatectomy: refined technique. Urology. 2005;65:23–7.
109. Haber G, Aron M, Ukimura O, Gill IS. Energy-free nerve-sparing laparoscopic radical prostatectomy: the bulldog technique. BJU Int. 2008;102:1766–9.
110. Gianduzzo TRJ, Colombo JR, Haber GP, et al. KTP laser nerve sparing radical prostatectomy: comparison of ultrasonic and cold scissor dissection on cavernous nerve function. J Urol. 2009;181:2760–6.
111. Quinlan DM, Nelson RJ, Walsh PC. Cavernous nerve grafts restore erectile function in denervated rats. J Urol. 1991;145:380–3.
112. Kim ED, Scardino PT, Hampel O, et al. Interposition of sural nerve restores function of cavernous nerves resected during radical prostatectomy. J Urol. 1999;161:188–92.
113. Kim ED, Nath R, Slawin K, Kadmon D, Miles BJ, Scardino PT. Bilateral nerve grafting during radical retropubic prostatectomy: extended follow-up. Urology. 2001;58:983–7.
114. Turk IA, Deger S, Morgan WR, Davis JW, Schelhammer PF, Loening SA. Sural nerve graft during laparoscopic radical prostatectomy: initial experience. Urol Oncol. 2002;7:191–4.
115. Kaouk JH, Desai MM, Abreu SC, Papay F, Gill IS. Robotic assisted laparoscopic sural nerve grafting during radical prostatectomy: initial experience. J Urol. 2003;170:909–12.
116. Davis JW, Chang DW, Chevray P, et al. Randomized phase II trial evaluation of erectile function after attempted unilateral cavernous nerve-sparing retropubic radical prostatectomy with versus without unilateral sural nerve grafting for clinically localized prostate cancer. Eur Urol. 2009;55:1135–44.
117. Martinez-Salamanca JI, Rao S, Ramanathan R, et al. Nerve advancement with end-to-end reconstruction after partial neurovascular bundle resection: a feasibility study. J Endourol. 2007;21:830–5.
118. Conolly SS, Yoo JJ, Abouheba M, Soker S, McDougal WS, Atala A. Cavernous nerve regeneration using acellular nerve grafts. World J Urol. 2008;26:333–9.
119. Bochinski D, Lin GT, Nunes L, et al. The effect of neural embryonic stem cell therapy is a rat model of cavernosal nerve injury. BJU Int. 2004;94:904–9.
120. Hsieh PS, Bochinski DJ, Lin GT, et al. The effect of vascular endothelial growth factor and brain-derived neurotrophic factor on cavernosal nerve regeneration in a nerve-crush rat model. BJU Int. 2003;92:470–5.
121. Kaul S, Bhandari A, Hemal A, Savera A, Shrivastava A, Menon M. Robotic radical prostatectomy with preservation of prostatic fascia: a feasibility study. Urology. 2005;66:1261–5.
122. Savera AT, Kaul S, Badani K, Stark AT, Shah NL, Menon M. Robotic radical prostatectomy with the "veil of Aphrodite" technique: histologic evidence of enhanced nerve sparing. Eur Urol. 2006;49:1065–74.
123. Kaul S, Savera A, Badni K, Fumor M, Bhandari A, Menon M. Efficacy of Vattikuti Institute prostatectomy with veil of Aphrodite nerve sparing: an analysis of 154 consecutive patients. BJU Int. 2006;97:467–72.
124. Stolzenburg JU, Rabenalt R, Do M, et al. Intrafascial nerve-sparing endoscopic extraperitoneal radical prostatectomy. Eur Urol. 2008;53:931–40.
125. Nielsen ME, Schaeffer EM, Marschke P, Walsh PC. High anterior release of the levator fascia improves sexual function following open radical retropubic prostatectomy. J Urol. 2008;180:2557–64.
126. Dorsey P Jr, Tan G, Jhaveri J, Patel N, El Douaihy Y, Vaughan E Jr, Tewari A. Early return of potency and orgasmic function during aggressive bilateral intrafascial nerve-sparing during trizonal athermal robotic prostatectomy: a prospective cohort study. (Abstract) CUAJ. 2009; 3(3 Suppl 1):S11 (POD-3.03).

Complications of Laparoscopic and Robotic-Assisted Radical Cystectomy

Ahmed M. Mansour, James O. Peabody, and Khurshid A. Guru

Keywords Cystectomy · Bladder · Cancer Laparoscopy · Robotics

Introduction

Bladder cancer is the fourth most common cancer in men and the eighth most common cancer in women in the United States [1]. Radical cystectomy is considered the standard therapeutic modality for muscle-invasive bladder cancer [2–4]. Most recently, minimally invasive approaches have been shown to offer considerable benefit in reduction of both major and minor morbidities as well as overall reduction in hospital stay [5].

Despite the feasibility and safe employment of laparoscopic radical cystectomy (LRC) for the management of muscle-invasive cancer of the bladder [6], it has not been established universally over the last 15 years. At present, LRC remains difficult to learn and master and thus it has not gained widespread popularity owing to its technical difficulty. The technique for robot-assisted radical cystectomy (RARC) was developed based on the principles of open and laparoscopic surgery with modification using the da Vinci surgical system. The technical advantages that robotic assistance offers, such as magnified 3D vision, endowrist, and ability to perform fine complex surgical repair, have been employed [6, 7]. After the initial reports of robot-assisted radical cystectomy by Menon and colleagues [7, 8], the surgical techniques and outcomes have been reproduced at other institutions.

At Roswell Park Cancer Institute, an effort has been made to improve upon the original technique of RARC, without oncologic compromise. With over 180 robotic radical cystectomies performed since the initiation of the robotic-assisted radical cystectomy program in 2005, cumulative experience has been gained and the technique has been well established.

Technique of Robot-Assisted Radical Cystectomy

The technique modified at Roswell Park Cancer Institute is described.

Operative Steps for Male Cystoprostatectomy

Surgical Development of Avascular Spaces

Once the ports are placed the key landmarks in the pelvis are examined. Examining and freeing of the lateral paracolic space especially sigmoid adhesions is helpful. The goal is to define three avascular spaces (periureteral, lateral pelvic space, and anterior rectal

K.A. Guru (✉)
Department of Urology, Roswell Park Cancer Institute, Buffalo, NY, USA
e-mail: khurshid.guru@roswellpark.org

R. Ghavamian (ed.), *Complications of Laparoscopic and Robotic Urologic Surgery*,
DOI 10.1007/978-1-60761-676-4_19, © Springer Science+Business Media, LLC 2010

spaces) and to complete a full anatomic dissection of all critical portions of RARC.

Development of Periureteral Space

Peristalsis of the ureter with aid of magnification and 3D vision helps in defining the landmarks for identification and delineation of the spaces (Fig. 1). The incision of the posterior peritoneum is carried out with separation of the visceral fascia and identification of the ureter in the loose areolar tissue. The periureteral space is opened with mobilization and dissection of the ureter distally up to the uretero-vesical junction. Preservation of the periureteral adventitial tissue is critical to ensure viability. Proximal mobilization of the ureter is carried out up to the aortic bifurcation which will later aid in completion of an extended lymph node dissection. One of the caveats in this technique is to avoid early clipping of the ureter during the initial dissection. The intact distal ureters act as a landmark in identifying the lateral pedicles and ensure negative surgical margins.

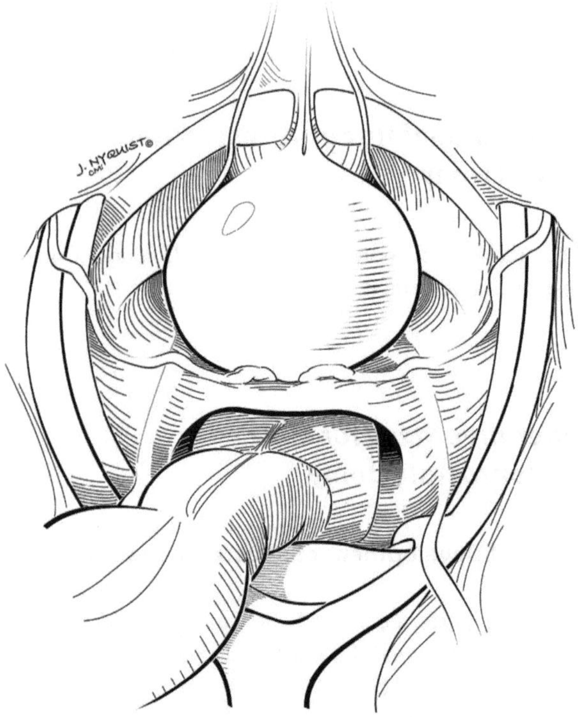

Fig. 1 Anatomical landmarks for the technique of spaces

Development of Lateral Pelvic Space

After completion of the dissection of the periureteral space, incision of the posterior peritoneum is carried parallel and lateral to the umbilical ligaments onto the anterior abdominal wall above the superior pubis ramus. This helps one in developing the second space, namely the lateral pelvic space. The avascular areolar space is opened following the medial curve of the pubic bone rami. The vas deferens is seen traversing across and underneath the posterior peritoneum and is divided to access the lateral pelvic space. The bladder is still left attached to the anterior abdominal wall and provides natural anterior retraction. Once the avascular lateral pelvic space is developed, one is able to identify the levator ani muscle on the lateral pelvic side wall and medially the lateral and posterior aspect of the bladder. Once dissection of periureteral and lateral pelvic spaces is complete, one should be able to identify the distal ureter up to the uretero-vesical junction at the medial edge of the dissection and the vascular pedicle arising from the anterior division of the internal iliac (hypogastric) artery. The external iliac vessels as well as the obturator nerve and vessels are recognized on the lateral aspect of the pelvic space.

Both the periureteral and lateral pelvic spaces are separated by the ureter and the postero-lateral pedicle arising from the internal iliac vessels. The external iliac vessels, obturator nerve, and vessels constitute the lateral boundary of both the spaces (Fig. 2).

Development of Anterior Rectal Space

Once the periureteric and lateral avascular spaces are defined bilaterally the anterior rectal space is developed. The two lateral incisions of the posterior peritoneum are joined together at the peritoneal reflection of the pouch of Douglas (Fig. 3). The dissection of this space is carried distally as far as the apex of the prostate. The plane between the anterior sheath of Denonvillier's fascia and the rectum is easily accessible. Blunt dissection following the anterior rectal wall is continued caudally. Using a zero degree lens, the anterior rectal fibers which are adherent to the apex of the prostate can be clearly seen. Careful blunt and sharp dissection using a cold round tip scissors is preferred to separate the rectum from the prostatic apex.

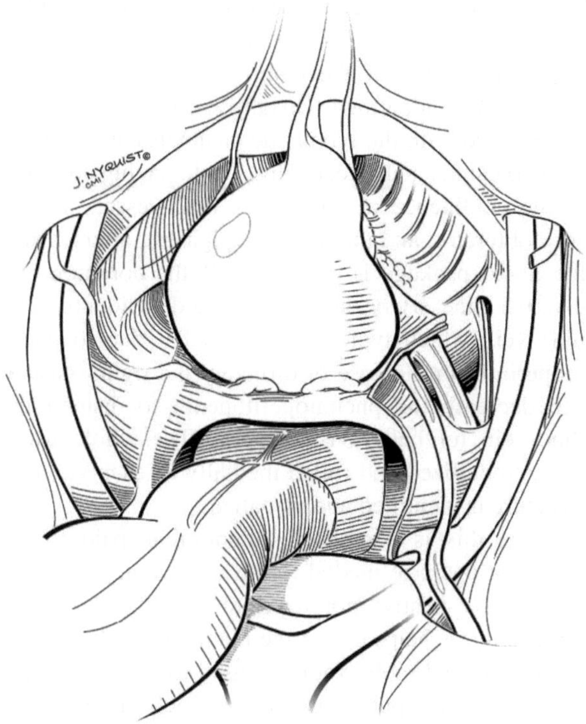

Fig. 2 Periureteric and lateral pelvic spaces

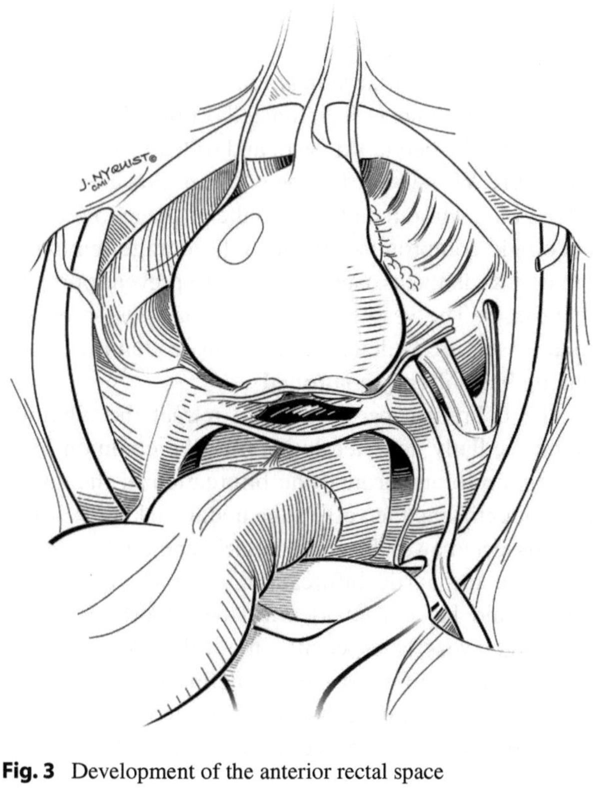

Fig. 3 Development of the anterior rectal space

Use of electrocautery hook or a hot shear scissors in this area may result in rectal injury.

Control of Vascular Pedicles and Mobilization of Neurovascular Bundles

The bladder is left suspended from the anterior abdominal wall while posterior dissection is completed. Anterior and lateral traction on the bladder using the fourth arm with a cobra grasper helps in exposing the lateral vascular pedicles of the bladder. The distal UV junction is identified and the ureters are ligated with two Weck Hem-o-lok clips. The distal ureteral margins are sent for frozen section. Based on the tumor stage and need for nerve preservation, the dissection is carried either near the base of the bladder at the tip of the seminal vesicles or behind the plane of the Denonvillier's fascia. An endovascular stapling device or Hem-o-lok clips can be used to secure the lateral pedicles in an expeditious fashion. In a patient with locally advanced disease where a non-nerve-sparing radical excision is contemplated, we advocate wider excision of pedicle with the endovascular stapler. The landmark for identifying the inferior vesical pedicle is the appearance of the "fat pad." After controlling the inferior vesical vessels, the endopelvic fascia is opened bilaterally.

Anterior Exposure and Apical Dissection

Incision of the median and medial umbilical ligaments to release the bladder from the anterior abdominal wall is carried out once the posterior dissection is complete. The bladder will drop posteriorly. Dissection of the retropubic fat is performed and the superficial dorsal vein is cauterized. Suture ligation of the deep venous complex is performed; further release of the prostate is accomplished once the deep dorsal complex is incised. Once the proximal membranous urethra is skeletonized, the urethral catheter is removed. A Hem-o-lok clip is applied just distal to the apex of the prostate to prevent urine spillage. After incision of the urethra the specimen is placed in a retrieval bag and removed from the pelvic cavity. The pelvic cavity is irrigated and the area is examined for any bleeding. Control of any bleeding and irrigation of the pelvis with sterile water is thoroughly performed with approximately 1 l of irrigation.

Crossing of the Ureter

Once the extended lymph node dissection is completed, the ureters are evaluated for length and further mobilization. The ureters are mobilized as proximal as possible with the ureter held retracted with the fourth robotic arm or the right assistant. Occasionally one may need to sacrifice the branch of the common iliac vessels feeding the ureter for further mobilization. The lateral edge of the right side of the posterior peritoneum is lifted and dissection carried with the mobilization of the sigmoid. The sigmoid is left suspended by the fourth robotic arm while performing the posterior dissection. After the dissection the right assistant passes a laparoscopic grasper underneath the dissected space and the console surgeon is able to see the protruding tips of the grasper on the left side. The left ureter is passed into the jaws of the laparoscopic grasper and transferred underneath the sigmoid colon across to the right side.

Lymph Node Dissection in Robot-Assisted Radical Cystectomy

Release and Roll technique

Once the cystectomy specimen is moved away from the pelvic cavity, adequate space is available for the node dissection. The ureter has already been mobilized proximally allowing one to view the vessels below the aortic bifurcation.

Our initial approach starts with retraction of the posterior peritoneum by the right-sided assistant with a Micro-France grasper. The gonadal vessels and the genitofemoral nerve are identified. The nodal tissue is mobilized off the psoas muscle by dividing the fibroareolar attachments while paying attention and avoiding any injury to the genitofemoral nerve. The nodal tissue is lifted off the muscle and swept medially by point cauterizing the small fibro-vascular attachments, which are controlled and incised by the round tip scissors.

This tissue package is dissected medially en bloc in what we describe as the "release and roll" technique. The edge of the common and external iliac artery can be identified. Distally the node of Cloquet is dissected with the lymphatic channels cauterized or clipped using small Weck clips, while paying attention to the confluence of circumflex iliac vessels, accessory obturator, and the inferior epigastric artery. Once the nodal package is dissected off the common and external iliac artery, attention is paid to identify the iliac vein which typically appears flat due to pneumoperitoneum. In case of difficulty the right assistant can decrease the pneumoperitoneum to distend the iliac vein for better visualization. The whole package is mobilized and rolled medially as each vascular structure is identified and visualized.

Once this is completed, attention is paid to the obturator package medial to the iliac vein. The nodal package is gently mobilized to identify the pubic bone and this helps define the plane of the dissection. Further medial mobilization is used to clear the nodal package off the pubic bone after which the obturator nerve is identified and skeletonized. Occasionally, the obturator vessels may need to be sacrificed to completely clean the obturator fossa for complete retrieval of the nodal package. Once this package is mobilized, the obturator package is removed from underneath the proximal external iliac vein around the obturator nerve. The nodal package is skeletonized off the iliac vessels, nerve, and the pelvic side wall and rolled medially into the pelvis. We believe that the whole package has to be left en bloc without cutting into the package to prevent oncologic compromise. We also discourage removing the nodes via the assistant port site to prevent port site metastasis. The vessels of the anterior division of the iliac vessels are skeletonized and can be identified after having been already controlled.

The cobra grasper is used to retract the sigmoid colon medially and clearly identify the common iliac vessels up to and around the bifurcation of the aorta. After identifying the vessels the nodal package is lifted and dissected away from the vessels and clipped proximally at the aortic bifurcation. After the dissection one should be able to identify the underlying common iliac vessels especially the vein. Once this is completed, attention is paid to define the triangle of Marcille. The investing fascia is dissected off the psoas fascia in order to mobilize the iliac vessels medially.

The fascia is dissected distally for easy mobilization. Arterial branch of the common iliac artery needs to be controlled as it enters the psoas muscle. Once this vessel is controlled attention is paid to the collapsed hidden iliac vein from which the nodal package has been removed without injuring the obturator nerve. At completion of the development of the "space of Marcille," the obturator nerve can be seen exiting the psoas muscle. The nodal package from each side is placed in endo-catch bags and removed when the incision for the diversion is made. After completion of the node dissection aggressive sterile water irrigation is carried out again and thorough hemostasis is achieved before proceeding to the lymph node dissection on the other side.

Complications of Robotic-Assisted Radical Cystectomy

Radical cystectomy is a technically challenging procedure that carries the potential for serious complications [2–4, 9, 10]. Moreover, the incidence of muscle-invasive disease peaks in the seventh decade of life, when comorbid conditions are frequently coexistent (e.g., coronary artery disease, atherosclerosis, cerebrovascular accidents) [11, 10, 12]. The mortality and morbidity inherent to the procedure are expectedly high, and although advances in perioperative medical care, anesthetic management, and surgical techniques have lowered mortality to less than 3%, early postoperative morbidity (i.e., within 30 days) still exceeds 30% following open surgery [13, 9, 14, ,11, 10, 12, 15].

Most complications of RARC are identical to the comparable open approach, and management would likewise be identical. These complications can be divided into medical and surgical complications and further into two subgroups, namely major and minor or more recently according to the Dindo–Clavien classification system (Table 1). Published series are limited with respect to patient number and long-term follow-up, therefore complication rates have not been well established for comparison (Table 2). This chapter will focus on the early and delayed complications associated with RARC and intestinal urinary diversion.

Cystectomy-Related Complications

Hemorrhage

Hemorrhage is a common complication of open radical cystectomy that can occur intraoperatively or in the delayed setting. The bladder, prostate, and vagina are highly vascular organs and are drained by a rich venous supply that necessitates meticulous dissection and careful and secure vascular control [26]. Pneumoperitoneum and 3D visualization create an excellent working environment and gently compress tissues. This results in remarkable hemostasis and contributes to the reduction of intraoperative blood loss. The 3D vision and the 10× magnification provided by the da Vinci system enable precise dissection and allow prevention of vascular injuries. However, a sound understanding of the pelvic anatomy and adherence to the proper surgical technique remain the cornerstone of preventing significant bleeding.

The blood supply to the anterior pelvic organs is derived primarily from the anterior division of the internal iliac artery (superior vesical, inferior vesical, uterine, internal pudendal, obturator, and the inferior gluteal arteries). Developing the periureteric space and the anterior rectal space as described previously helps define the bladder pedicle, thus making identification, ligation, and division of the individual branches of the internal iliac artery easy and bloodless.

The dorsal venous complex (DVC) is a major vascular structure that must be controlled prior to the removal of the cystectomy specimen. In open surgery the DVC can be the cause of troublesome bleeding if not adequately controlled. However, the pneumoperitoneum in robotic cystectomy causes marked reduction in bleeding from the DVC to the extent that some surgeons prefer raising the pneumoperitoneum to 20 mmHg and dividing the DVC prior to securing it. We prefer controlling the DVC using an absorbable 2-0 suture prior to its division close to the apex of the prostate.

Attention must be paid during lymph node dissection in robotic-assisted radical cystectomy to avoid major vascular injury. Several caveats in performing the dissection have proved helpful. Cold scissor dissection and bipolar point cauterization are used for small blood vessels and lymphatic channels to prevent bleeding. Avoiding the monopolar hook in the surgeon's

Table 1 Complications of robotic-assisted radical cystectomy according to the Dindo–Clavien classification system

Grades	Organ system	Description	Menon et al. [7]	Rhee et al. [16]	Galich et al. [17]	Abraham et al. [18]	Lowentritt et al. [19]	Murphy et al. [20]	Ng et al. [21]	Pruthi et al. [22]	Guru et al. [unpublished data]
Grade 1	Other	Wound infection (opened at bedside)							4		2
		FUO							2		
Grade II	Cardiac	Afib							4		
		Arrhythmia							1		6
		MI				1			1		1
	Pulmonary	PE							2		3
		Pneumonia							1		
	Gastrointestinal	*C. difficile* colitis							3		2
		Ileus		1		2		1	13		9
		SBO			1					8	
	Renal	UTI							14		5
	Other	Sepsis							2		6
		DVT							5		3
		Depression							0		
		Transfusion		4		6		1	1		
		Postoperative Bleed	1	1					2		2
		Abscess			1				5		
		Fungal infection							1		
		Pyelonephritis							1		
		Bilharziasis	13								
		Port site metastasis									
Grade IIIa	Renal	Ureteral obstruction							3	1	1
		Urinary leak				1		1	2		
		Renal failure							4		1
		Anastomotic stricture							0		
	Other								0		
Grade IIIb	Gastrointestinal	Rectal injury						1	0		
		EC fistula			1				1		
	Renal	Urinary fistula							1		
	Other	Dehiscence							1		
		Open conversion					1		0		
		Return to OR	1						?		
		Nerve injury				1					
		Hernia							2		
Grade IV	ICU management								1		3
Grade V	Death								0	5	

Table 2 Concurrent series of robotic-assisted radical cystectomy

Authors	N	Urinary diversion	Age	Mean OR Time	EBL	Hospital stay	Complications
Menon et al. [7]	17	Ileal conduit (3)	–	260	150	–	Re-exploration for postoperative bleed (1)
		Neobladder (14)		308			Bilharziasis (13)
Beecken et al. [23]	1	Intracorporeal W neobladder	–	510	200	5	Nil
Balajii et al. [24]	2	Ileal conduit	60	690	1118	6	Nil
Hemal et al. [25]	24	Ileal conduit (4)	–	290	200	–	Minimal blood loss and morbidity
		W pouch (16)					
		T pouch (2)					
		Double chimney (2)					
Rhee et al. [16]	7	Ileal conduit	60	638	479	11	57% Transfusion rate (4)
							Port site hematoma (1) Ileus (1)
Galich et al. [17]	13	Ileal conduit (6)	70	697	500	8	Enterovesical fistula + SBO (1) abscess (1)
		Neobladder (5)					
		Indiana pouch (2)					
Abraham et al. [18]	14	Ileal conduit (14)	76.5	419	212	5.8	42.8% Transfusion rate
							28% Complication rate: Ileus (2) Urine leak (1) MI (1), Incomplete transaction of L t obturator nerve
Lowentritt et al. [19]	5	Ileal conduit (4)	69.5	350	300	5	Initial open conversion for hypercapnia (1) not reported
Murphy et al. [20]	23	Ileal conduit	–	397	278	11	Ileus, postoperative bleed, rectal injury
		Studer pouch					
Ng et al. [21]	83	Ileal conduit (47)	70.9	375	460	5.5	Cellulitis, dehiscence, renal failure, ureteral obstruction, urinary fistula/leak, FUO, PNA, UTI, abscess, pyelonephritis, ileus, fungal infection, SBO, *C. difficile* colitis, GI bleed, hematemesis, EC fistula, arrhythmia, MI, transfusion (1), rash, dehydration, DVT, PE
		Indiana pouch (10)					
		Neobladder (26)					
Pruthi et al. [22]	50	Ileal conduit (30)	63.9	302.4	268.2	4.5	FUO, anastomotic leak, others previously reported in Pruthi et al. 2008 [14]
		Neobladder (20)					
Guru et al. 2009 (unpublished data)	150	Neobladder (7) Ileal conduit (137) Intracorporeal ileal conduit (6)	70.5	343	577.8	7.55	Open conv (2), vasc injection (1), postoperative heme (2), ileus (9), bowel obstruction (8), pancreatitis (1), UTI (5), ureteral stricture (1), ARF (1), MI (1), dysrhythmia (6) cardiac arrest (1), pulmonary failure (1), sepsis/infection (6), *C. difficile* infection (2), wound dehiscence (3), wound infection (3), DVT/PE (3), transfusion reaction (1)

FUO fever of unknown origin, *PNA* pneumonia, *UTI* urinary tract infection, *infn* infection, *SBO* small bowel obstruction, *EC fistula* enterocutaneous fistula, *MI* myocardial infarction, *DVT* deep vein thrombosis, *PE* pulmonary embolism early experience helps in avoiding thermal injury to the vessels. We believe that LND performed after cystectomy has several advantages as cystectomy leaves adequate space to perform LND and allows the ability to stay away from the tissue planes of the bladder. Exposure and development of the triangle of Marcille facilitates appropriate application of the 3D vision, magnification, and maneuverability of the Endowrist® arms to perform LND within the narrow space behind the iliac vessels [13].

Even with meticulous inspection at the completion of a procedure, a vascular injury may go unrecognized and may not become manifest until the postoperative period. Therefore, the surgeon must always be vigilant in recognizing these injuries promptly. Physical signs of tachycardia, hypotension, oliguria or anuria, ecchymosis, abdominal or pelvic distention or pain, a new bruit, or loss of previously palpable pulses in the immediate postoperative period could indicate internal hemorrhage. Laboratory studies may demonstrate anemia, acidosis, electrolyte disturbances, elevated lactate dehydrogenase, or renal insufficiency or failure. Radiographic tests may reveal hematoma formation, ongoing hemorrhage, loss of arterial blood flow, or an arteriovenous fistula. If a major arterial injury is suspected in the immediate postoperative period, surgical exploration may be warranted for confirmation.

In contemporary robotic cystectomy series, four patients have experienced surgically related postoperative bleeding, three of whom required a return to the operating room, and open exploration [27, 7, 28, 20].

Rectal Injury

Rectal injury as a complication of radical cystectomy remains an entity with potentially grave consequences if not recognized intraoperatively. Prospective identification of the patients at risk and sound adherence to the anatomical planes during dissection can help in avoiding this complication. Factors predisposing to rectal injury include bulky posterior bladder masses, extensive repeated prior transurethral resection of bladder tumors, prior pelvic surgery, and preoperative radiotherapy.

Understanding the fascial layers between the bladder and the rectum is crucial for minimizing the risk of rectal injury. During development of the posterior space, it is important to incise the Denonvillier's fascia sharply and under vision. This is facilitated by utilizing the 0° lens of the da Vinci system. Subsequently, the plane between the posterior sheath of Denonvillier's fascia and the rectum is developed. This is achieved by sweeping down the rectum by blunt and sharp dissection until the urethra is reached. This plane may be obliterated in patients with posterior bulky tumors, thus sharp dissection should be used to enter this space.

It is mandatory to test the rectum for any injuries after removal of the bladder, especially in cases with difficult posterior dissection. This is achieved by filling the pelvis with saline and insufflating air via a rectal tube. This maneuver is also used to identify the rectum in cases of bulky posterior tumors or previous pelvic procedures.

Once identified, a rectal injury should be repaired in two layers. After debridement of the edges, the mucosa is closed with special care to invert the mucosa into the bowel lumen, this is further reinforced by a second layer of interrupted non-absorbable sutures. If possible the interpositioning of an omental flap over the site of the injury is advised [29]. However, if the defect is considerable, the contamination is significant or impaired healing is expected as a result of previous pelvic irradiation and diversion of the fecal stream by means of a colostomy is recommended.

The incidence of rectal injury in open cystectomy series ranges from 0.3 to 9.7% [2–4]. Two cases of rectal injuries have been reported until now in RARC series. In these cases, the rectum was repaired in two layers in one patient without the need for fecal diversion [27] while a colostomy was required for the other patient [20].

Prolonged Postoperative Ileus

Postoperative ileus is the delay in the coordinated movements of the gastrointestinal tract. It is a common postoperative complication after radical cystectomy and urinary diversion which leads to longer hospital stay, significant perioperative morbidity, and increased health-care costs. Several factors responsible for the pathogenesis of postoperative ileus have been elucidated. These include an imbalance between the sympathetic, parasympathetic, and intrinsic nervous system of the small intestine and the colon and the possible role of inflammatory mediators [30]. Following open radical cystectomy, the incidence of prolonged ileus ranges from 7 to 23% [2–5, 9, 12]. In the reported robotic cystectomy series the incidence ranges from 5 to 12% [20, 31, 27].

Several measures have been proposed for reduction of postoperative ileus. In minimally invasive surgery, gentle manipulation of the intestines and decreased exposure of intestines result in more rapid postoperative recovery of the intestinal motility. Limiting the use of intravenous opioids and supplementing narcotics with nonsteroidal anti-inflammatory drugs may be helpful. Following RARC, patients are found to require less opiate analgesics than those who underwent open surgery [32]. There are no prospective, randomized trials that validate the use of prokinetic agents (e.g., metoclopramide) in the resolution of postoperative ileus. Early ambulation, contrary to the popular belief, has no demonstrable effect on expediting the resolution of postoperative ileus. However, ambulation should be encouraged for the prevention of atelectasis, pneumonia, and DVT [30]. Kouba et al. were the first to demonstrate an improved recovery of postoperative ileus after bowel surgery with chewing gum. Chewing has been shown to increase secretion from the salivary glands and liver, as well as an increase in plasma concentrations of certain hormones (gastrin, neurotensin, pancreatic polypeptide, and cholecystokinin) which are involved in vagal afferent stimulation of smooth muscle fibers important in gastrointestinal motility [33].

In the absence of clinical and radiological signs of an intra-abdominal complication, paralytic ileus is likely to resolve with conservative management. Correction of the electrolyte imbalances, particularly hypokalemia, hyponatremia, and hypomagnesemia, is important to restore bowel function. A search for additional causes such as an abscess from intestinal anastomotic or urine leaks should also be considered. Adequate bowel decompression is crucial to hasten the recoverability of intestinal motility and prevent nausea, vomiting, abdominal distension, and pain. Poorly decompressed bowel in the setting of unresolved ileus may result in significant fluid shifts and potentially stresses the enteric anastomosis predisposing to anastomotic leaks.

Bowel Obstruction

Mechanical bowel obstruction that occurs early in the postoperative period following radical cystectomy is commonly caused by fibrinous adhesions before they become organized to form permanent fibrous bands; a loop of small bowel may get stuck to the raw surface from the cystectomy or pelvic lymph node dissection. It may also result from internal herniation, volvulus, anastomotic edema, intraperitoneal hematoma, or abscess [34].

Several tricks proved useful in preventing postradical cystectomy bowel obstruction. In cases of extracorporeal diversion care should be given at the end of the operation before abdominal wall closure to restore the anatomical arrangement of the intestine in the abdominal cavity. The mesentery of the small intestine should be adequately closed to avoid internal herniation. After ileal conduit diversion, the posterior peritoneum should be utilized to cover the ileal conduit (retroperitonalization of the conduit), thus preventing the entrapment of the bowel loops between the conduit and the abdominal wall. Finally the omentum should be spread to the pelvis to cover the abdominal contents preventing adhesions between raw surfaces and the abdominal wall.

Mechanical bowel obstruction gives rise to central and colicky pain that may be associated with borborygmus in contrast to postoperative ileus which is painless. The pain is eased by vomiting, which with prolonged obstruction is excessive and becomes feculent. The abdomen can feel tense and is tympanitic, but tenderness and guarding may not be evident unless the bowel is ischemic from gross distension or strangulation or if there is an abscess or inflammatory mass. This may not be easily palpable in a grossly distended abdomen. The bowel sounds are usually hyperactive and high pitched in mechanical obstruction coinciding with attacks of colic. However, with prolonged mechanical obstruction bowel sounds may become infrequent as the bowel becomes paralytic and dilated [35].

An erect plain abdominal film confirms the diagnosis by demonstrating a dilated small intestine with air-fluid levels. A CT scan is essential in mechanical obstruction and in non-resolving paralytic ileus particularly if associated with signs of sepsis or when it develops after return of bowel activity as this may herald the onset of an intra-abdominal complication.

The initial management is conservative and includes bowel rest, intestinal decompression with nasogastric tube aspiration, resuscitation (intravenous fluid and electrolyte replacement), and hemodynamic monitoring. The passage of flatus or liquid stool, diminishing abdominal distension and nasogastric aspirates, and the return of bowel sounds are reliable clinical indicators of resolving obstruction which can be confirmed by abdominal X-ray films.

Laparotomy should be considered if there is no improvement or earlier if obstruction is progressing. The presence of abdominal signs such as fever, a markedly elevated white cell count, a base deficit, and absent bowel sounds are suggestive of strangulation. Laparotomy is carried out under prophylactic broad-spectrum antibiotics to prevent the translocation of bacteria through the bowel wall and to minimize the consequences of contamination from inadvertent or planned enterotomy. The surgical procedure involves the division of adhesions and bands, release of internal herniation, reduction of a volvulus, resection, or proximal diversion of a narrowed anastomosis or an inflammatory mass. In order to facilitate abdominal closure the bowel contents are milked retrogradely into the stomach and drained via a nasogastric tube or by suction via an enterotomy [36].

Bowel Leak/Enterocutaneous Fistula

The development of bowel leak after RARC is a devastating complication with significant morbidity and mortality. The findings of fever, wound infection, and elevation of white blood cells and delayed return of bowel function should raise the suspicion of a potential bowel leak from the bowel anastomosis or unrecognized enterotomy. The diagnosis is confirmed when enteric contents are found leaking through the wound or surgically placed drains. If there is no prudent external evidence of a fistula, a CT scan with water-soluble oral contrast typically reveals extravasation from the bowel lumen into an intra-abdominal or pelvic collection [37].

Once the diagnosis is confirmed, the decision to begin a trial of conservative management is dependent on the presence or absence of peritonitis or sepsis [37]. If the patient is well drained, the fistula drainage is controlled and in the absence of clinical peritonitis or intra-abdominal abscess formation, a trial of conservative management is warranted [38]. The patient should be followed with proximal decompression by means of a nasogastric tube, and total parenteral nutrition (TPN) should be initiated. TPN has proved to increase the rate of spontaneous closure by inducing bowel hypoactivity. Furthermore, it prepares the patient from a nutritional standpoint for reoperation if the fistula fails to close spontaneously.

The use of somatostatin in the conservative management of enterocutaneous fistula is controversial. While it has been shown to decrease the fistula output thus making it possible to manage fluid, electrolyte, and protein imbalance, the therapeutic advantage of reducing the time to fistula closure has not been proven in clinical trials [38, 39]. Only 50% of postoperative bowel fistulas close spontaneously within 4–6 weeks in the absence of distal obstruction or loss of intestinal continuity. The remainder of the patients should be explored electively to repair the fistula and restore intestinal continuity. Reoperation should be delayed for at least 3–4 months after surgery [38].

Emergency laparotomy is indicated in patients displaying peritonitis or signs of sepsis with suspected or proven intraperitoneal abscesses, who have failed or not amenable to percutaneous drainage. The goal of laparotomy is to drain any abdominal or pelvic loculated abscesses and to cleanse the abdominal cavity utilizing copious amounts of irrigation. Under optimal conditions, fistulas are excised with the involved segment of intestine with primary anastomosis with or without proximal diversion. Alternatively, the excised bowel ends are exteriorized as a stoma and mucous fistula and occasionally a diverting stoma proximal to the fistula can be sufficient as in anastomotic leaks [26]. In the reported RARC series, two cases developed enterocutaneous fistulas which were managed successfully by conservative measures [31].

Venous Thromboembolism

Several risk factors predispose radical cystectomy patients to a higher incidence of venous thromboembolism. Most of bladder cancer patients are elderly, with usually long history of smoking and concurrent pulmonary morbidities. They undergo a lengthy procedure with significant fluid shifts and postoperatively are at risk of morbidities and prolonged immobility [40, 41]. Evidence has accumulated in the form of randomized clinical trials that prove the effect of primary thromboprophylaxis in the reduction of deep venous thrombosis (DVT), pulmonary embolism, and fatal pulmonary complications [40, 41]. In Roswell Park Cancer Institute, we utilize weight-adjusted prophylactic dose of low molecular weight heparin (LMWH) together with intermittent pneumatic compression devices (IPC) and graduated compression stockings (GCS) as routine thromboprophylaxis regimen for all patients undergoing RARC.

Wound Infection/Fascial Dehiscence

Wound infection and fascial dehiscence are well-known postoperative complications following open radical cystectomy. The incidence of wound infection and dehiscence after open radical cystectomy ranges from 3 to 6% and 1 to 3%, respectively. However, in the RARC series owing to smaller wounds required for extracorporeal diversion, wound infection and dehiscence are expected to be less. Acutely, there can be a dehiscence of the entire wound with the dramatic results of exposure of the viscera. In the acute setting what is required is an urgent return to the operating room. Poor tissue handling along with too tight a closure and poor patient nutrition are the usual important contributing factors. When faced with an acute abdominal dehiscence, the wound edges can be freshened and the wound re-sutured only if the surgeon is confident of obtaining a tension-free repair of healthy, well-vascularized tissue. Occasionally, in case of minor fascial separation, it may be possible to delay immediate repair for several months in the absence of frank evisceration or incarceration of bowel [26].

Diversion-Related Complications

Extracorporeal urinary diversion is still the standard of care. However, in the future with the development of technology, instrumentations, tissue engineering, absorbable bowel stapling devices, and with further refinement of surgical technique, the entire procedure may be done completely intracorporeally with equal efficiency and less morbidity.

Urine Leak

Persistent leakage of urine from the pouch or the conduit may occur in the postoperative period [42]. Routine stentograms or pouchograms before catheter removal have proven not to be necessary [43, 44]. The diagnosis can be confirmed by estimation of creatinine from the output of the tube drain, or by a pouchogram. Urine leaks can be managed conservatively in the majority of cases with proximal diverting drainage. Antegrade stenting of the leaking ureteroileal anastomosis may be an option following proximal drainage until the leak stops. Finally open exploration is the last resort in rare cases of persistent leakage despite proximal diversion [42]. Anastomotic rates can be decreased with employment of single J stents at the time of the diversion procedure.

Ureteroenteric Anastomotic Stricture

The incidence of ureteroenteric anastomotic stricture ranges from 4 to 20% in recent series [2–5, 9, 12]. Eighty percent are diagnosed within the first year. Most anastomotic strictures are non-malignant and are due to technical causes such as anastomosis under tension, angulation, twisting, or inadequate mucosa to mucosa anastomosis [42]. Left side is more prone to develop stricture (60% in most of the series) [2, 3, 9] due to longer dissection needed to cross the ureter to the other side. Endoscopic treatment should be tried as the primary form of treatment. Dilatation can be attempted either by balloon or by semirigid fascial dilators. Other techniques include endo-incision using cold knife or electro-incision [45, 46]. Revision surgery is the ideal treatment. However, it is usually not an easy operation and inadvertent injuries are frequently unavoidable. Careful atraumatic dissection of the ureter should always be carried out. Viable ureter is usually shorter than expected and mobilization of the pouch may be needed and sometimes a pouch flap or a new bowel segment may be required to bridge the defect [47].

Conclusion

Robot-assisted radical cystectomy (RARC) has evolved to provide a minimally invasive alternative to the standard open approach. It can be accomplished with low morbidity and with the advantages of less transfusion rates, earlier recoverability of bowel function, and shorter hospital stay. Complications following RARC are comparable to those of open surgery and are managed similarly.

References

1. Jemal A, Tiwari R, Murray T, et al. Cancer statistics, 2004. CA Cancer J Clin. 2004;54:8–29.
2. Ghoneim MA, el-Mekresh MM, el-Baz MA, el-Attar IA, Ashmallah A. Radical cystectomy for carcinoma of the bladder: critical evaluation of the results in 1026 cases. J Urol. 1997;158:393–9.
3. Ghoneim MA, Abdel-Latif M, El-Mekresh M, Abol-Enein H, Mosbah A, Ashamallah A, Elbaz MA. Radical cystectomy for carcinoma of the bladder: 2,720 consecutive cases 5 years later. J Urol. 2008;180: 121–7.
4. Hautmann RE, Gschwend JE, de Petriconi RC, Kron M, Volkmer BG. Cystectomy for transitional cell carcinoma of the bladder: results of a surgery only series in the neobladder era. J Urol. 2006;176:486.
5. Guillotreau J, Gamé X, Mouzin M, Doumerc N, Mallet R, Sallusto F, Malavaud B, Rischmann P. Radical cystectomy for bladder cancer: morbidity of laparoscopic versus open surgery. J Urol. 2009;181:554–9.
6. Haber GP, Crouzet S, Gill IS. Laparoscopic and robotic assisted radical cystectomy for bladder cancer: a critical analysis. Eur Urol. 2008;54:54–62.
7. Menon M, Hemal AK, Tewari A, et al. Nerve sparing robot-assisted radical cystoprostatectomy and urinary diversion. BJU Int. 2003;92:232–6.
8. Menon M, Hemal AK, Tewari A, et al. Robot assisted radical cystectomy and urinary diversion in female patients: technique with preservation of the uterus and vagina. J Am Coll Surg 2004;198:386–93.
9. Chang SS, Cookson MS, Baumgartner RG, Wells N, Smith JA Jr. Analysis of early complications after radical cystectomy: results of a collaborative care pathway. J Urol. 2002;167:2012–6.
10. Hollenbeck BK, Miller DC, Taub D, Dunn RL, Khuri SF, Henderson WG, et al. Identifying risk factors for potentially avoidable complications following radical cystectomy. J Urol. 2005;174:1231–7.
11. Clark PE, Stein JP, Groshen SG, Cai J, Miranda G, Lieskovsky G, et al. Radical cystectomy in the elderly. Comparison of survival between younger and older patients. Cancer 2005;103:546–52.
12. Novotny V, Hakenberg OW, Wiessner D, Heberling U, Litz RJ, Oehlschlaeger S, et al. Perioperative complications of radical cystectomy in a contemporary series. Eur Urol. 2007;51:397–402.
13. Guru KA, Sternberg K, Wilding GE, Tan W, Butt ZM, Mohler JL, Kim HL. The lymph node yield during robot-assisted radical cystectomy. BJU Int. 2008;102:231–4.
14. Chang SS, Baumgartner RG, Wells N, Cookson MS, Smith JA Jr. Causes of increased hospital stay after radical cystectomy in a clinical pathway setting. J Urol. 2002;167: 208–11.
15. Soulie M, Straub M, Game X, Seguin P, De Petriconi R, Plante P, et al. A multicenter study of the morbidity of radical cystectomy in select elderly patients with bladder cancer. J Urol. 2002;167:1325–8.
16. Rhee JJ, Lebeau S, Smolkin M, Theodorescu D. Radical cystectomy with ileal conduit diversion: early prospective evaluation of the impact of robotic assistance. BJU Int. 2006;98:1059–63.
17. Galich A, Sterrett S, Nazemi T, Pohlman G, Smith L, Balaji KC. Comparative analysis of early perioperative outcomes following radical cystectomy by either the robotic or open method. JSLS. 2006;10:145–50.
18. Abraham JB, Young JL, Box GO. Comparative analysis of laparoscopic and robotic-assisted radical cystectomy with ileal conduit urinary diversion. J Endourol. 2007;21: 1473–80.
19. Lowentritt BH, Castle EP, Woods M, Davis R, Thomas R. Robot-assisted radical cystectomy in women: technique and initial experience. J Endourol. 2008;22:709–12.
20. Murphy DG, Challacombe BJ, Elhage O, O'Brien TS, Rimington P, Shamim KM, Dasgupta P. Robotic-assisted laparoscopic radical cystectomy with extracorporeal urinary diversion: initial experience. Eur Urol. 2008;54: 570–80.
21. Ng CK, Kauffman EC, Lee MM, Otto BJ, Portnoff A, Ehrlich JR, Schwartz MJ, Wang GJ, Scherr DS. A comparison of postoperative complications in open versus robotic cystectomy. Eur Urol. 2010;57(2):274–81.
22. Pruthi RS, Stefaniak H, Hubbard JS, Wallen EM Robotic anterior pelvic exenteration for bladder cancer in the female: outcomes and comparisons to their male counterparts. J Laparoendosc Adv Surg Tech A. 2009;19: 23–7.
23. Beecken WD, Wolfram M, Engl T, Bentas W, Probst M, Blaheta R, Oertl A, Jonas D, Binder J. Robotic-assisted laparoscopic radical cystectomy and intra-abdominal formation of an orthotopic ileal neobladder. Eur Urol. 2003;44:337–9.
24. Balaji KC, Yohannes P, McBride CL, Oleynikov D, Hemstreet GP 3rd. Feasibility of robot-assisted totally intracorporeal laparoscopic ileal conduit urinary diversion: initial results of a single institutional pilot study. Urology. 2004;63(1):51–5.
25. Hemal AK, Abol-Enein H, Tewari A, et al. Robotic radical cystectomy and urinary diversion in the management of bladder cancer. Urol Clin North Am. 2004;31: 719–29.
26. Taneja S, Smith R, Ehrlich R, editors. Complications of urologic surgery. Prevention and management. 3rd ed. Philadelphia, PA: W. B. Saunders; 2001.

27. Guru KA, Kim HL, Piacente M, Mohler JL. Robot-assisted radical cystectomy and pelvic lymph node dissection: initial experience at Roswell Park Cancer institute. Urology. 2007;69:469–74.
28. Pruthi RS, Wallen EM. Is robotic radical cystectomy an appropriate treatment for bladder cancer? Short-term oncologic and clinical follow-up in 50 consecutive patients. Urology. 2008;72:617–22.
29. Kozminski M, Konnak KW, Grossman HB. Management of rectal injuries during radical cystectomy. J Urol. 1989;142:1204–5.
30. Maffezzini M, Campodonico F, Canepa G, Gerbi G, Parodi D. Current perioperative management of radical cystectomy with intestinal urinary reconstruction for muscle-invasive bladder cancer and reduction of the incidence of postoperative ileus. Surg Oncol. 2008;17:41–8.
31. Wang GJ, Barocas DA, Raman JD, Scherr DS. Robotic vs. open radical cystectomy: prospective comparison of perioperative outcomes and pathological measures of early oncological efficacy. BJU Int. 2007;101:89–93.
32. Guru KA, Wilding GE, Piacente P, Thompson J, Deng W, Kim HL, Mohler J, O'Leary K. Robot-assisted radical cystectomy versus open radical cystectomy: assessment of postoperative pain. Can J Urol. 2007;14:3753–6.
33. Kouba G, Wallen P, Pruthi MM. Gum chewing stimulates bowel motility in patients undergoing radical cystectomy with urinary diversion. J Urol. 2007;70:1053–6.
34. Varkarakis IM, Chrisofos M, Antoniou N, Papatsoris A, Deliveliotis C. Evaluation of findings during re-exploration for obstructive ileus after radical cystectomy and ileal-loop urinary diversion: insight into potential technical improvements. BJU Int. 2007;99:893–7.
35. Cappell MS, Batke M. Mechanical obstruction of the small bowel and colon. Med Clin North Am. 2008;92:575–97.
36. Torer N, Nursal TZ, Tufan H, Can F, Bal N, Tarim A, Moray G, Haberal M. Effect of manual bowel decompression (milking) in the obstructed small bowel. Am J Surg. 2008;195:807–13.
37. Foster CE, Lefor AT. General management of gastrointestinal fistulas. Recognition, stabilization, and correction of fluid and electrolyte imbalances. Surg Clin North Am. 1996;76:1019–33.
38. Lloyd DA, Gabe SM, Windsor AC. Nutrition and management of enterocutaneous fistula. Br J Surg. 2006;93:1045–55.
39. Mulvihill S, Pappas TN, Passaro E Jr, Debas HT. The use of somatostatin and its analogs in the treatment of surgical disorders. Surgery. 1986;100:467–76.
40. Amin A, Stemkowski S, Lin J, Yang G. Appropriate thromboprophylaxis in hospitalized cancer patients. Clin Adv Hematol Oncol. 2008;6:910–20.
41. McGarry LJ, Thompson D. Retrospective database analysis of the prevention of venous thromboembolism with low-molecular-weight heparin in acutely III medical inpatients in community practice. Clin Ther. 2004;26:419–30.
42. Farnham SB, Cookson MS. Surgical complications of urinary diversion. World J Urol. 2004;22:157–67.
43. Pantuck AJ, Weiss RE, Cummings KB. Routine stentograms are not necessary before stent removal following radical cystectomy. J Urol. 1997;158:772–5.
44. Ankem MK, Han KR, Hartanto V, Perrotti M, Decarvalho VS, Cummings KB, Weiss RE. Routine pouchograms are not necessary after continent urinary diversion. Urology. 2004;63:435–7.
45. Pappas P, Stravodimos KG, Kapetanakis T, Leonardou P, Koutallelis G, Adamakis I, Constantinides C. Ureterointestinal strictures following Bricker ileal conduit: management via a percutaneous approach. Int Urol Nephrol. 2008;40:621–7.
46. Kurzer E, Leveillee RJ. Endoscopic management of ureterointestinal strictures after radical cystectomy. J Endourol. 2005;19:677–82.
47. Tal R, Sivan B, Kedar D, Baniel J. Management of benign ureteral strictures following radical cystectomy and urinary diversion for bladder cancer. J Urol. 2007;178:538–42.

Complications of Laparoscopic and Robotic Reconstructive Procedures for Urinary Incontinence and Pelvic Organ Prolapse

Alvaro Lucioni and Kathleen C. Kobashi

Keywords Incontinence · Pelvic prolapsed · Complications · Laparoscopy

Introduction

Recognition of the impact of pelvic floor disorders in women has increased significantly in recent years. A contemporary study evaluating the prevalence of pelvic floor disorders including urinary incontinence and pelvic organ prolapse in US women demonstrated that 23.7% of women complain of at least one pelvic floor disorder [1]. Approximately 10% of women undergo surgery for either urinary incontinence or pelvic organ prolapse in their lifetime [2]. With increase acknowledgement of the high prevalence of pelvic floor disorders in women the surgical management of these disorders becomes more important. Together with this increase in surgical management of pelvic floor disorders we have also seen an increase in the utilization of minimally invasive surgical treatments. As urologists and gynecologists become more familiar with the use of laparoscopy and robotic-assisted procedures, these skills are being applied to treat pelvic floor disorders. Advantages of the laparoscopic approach include improved visualization of the pelvis due to laparoscopic magnification and insufflation effects, shorter hospital stays, and decreased post-operative pain and recovery time. Given this increase in the use of the laparoscopic approach, the understanding of surgical techniques and complications of these procedures becomes more important. The purpose of this chapter is to briefly review the different laparoscopic techniques used to treat pelvic floor disorders and provide a thorough analysis of the complications reported with each technique.

Laparoscopic Treatment for Stress Urinary Incontinence

The surgical management of stress urinary incontinence (SUI) in women has significantly changed in the last decade. During the second half of the 20th century the open Burch colposuspension became the standard of care for treatment of SUI [3]. Given the success of the open Burch colposuspension, Lui and Paek attempted the first laparoscopic Burch colposuspension in 1991 [3]. However, the procedure was not optimal and with the introduction of the midurethral sling by Ulmsten, the use of the laparoscopic Burch colposuspension quickly fell out of favor. Nevertheless as some surgeons are still utilizing this minimally invasive approach review of the procedure and its complications is warranted.

Laparoscopic Burch Coloposuspension

The open Burch colposuspension was introduced by Burch in 1961 and since then it has undergone a few modifications [4]. The procedure restores the bladder

A. Lucioni (✉)
The Continence Center at Virginia Mason Medical Center, 1100 Ninth Ave, Mailstop C7-URO, P.O. Box 900, Seattle, WA 98101, USA
e-mail: alvaro.lucioni@vmmc.org

R. Ghavamian (ed.), *Complications of Laparoscopic and Robotic Urologic Surgery*,
DOI 10.1007/978-1-60761-676-4_20, © Springer Science+Business Media, LLC 2010

neck to its normal retropubic position by approximating the paravaginal fascia to Cooper's ligament. The laparoscopic Burch colposuspension utilizes the same surgical principles as the open approach.

Prior to surgery some surgeons advocate the use of bowel preparation. After general anesthesia is induced, the patient is placed in a low lithotomy position with Trendelenburg as necessary. A Foley catheter is placed to drain the bladder. The procedure can be performed either extraperitoneally or intraperitoneally. The former has been associated with shorter operative times and fewer bladder injuries, while the latter provides a larger operating space and the ability to perform concomitant intraperitoneal surgery [5, 6]. The extraperitoneal approach also avoids the development of intraperitoneal pelvic adhesions and provides a shorter learning curve, but does have a higher risk of CO_2 absorption leading to pneumomediastinum and pneumothorax [7, 8]. Three ports are placed, one periumbilical, one in the right, and one in the left lower quadrant just lateral to their respective epigastric vessels, approximately 3 cm medial and superior to the anterior superior iliac spine. In the extraperitoneal approach the space of Retzius is dissected using a balloon or finger with the aid of pneumodissection. The paravaginal fascia and Copper's ligaments are then identified. The use of absorbable or nonabsorbable suture has been described to approximate these two structures. A study by Persson and Wolner-Hanssen advocated the use of two sutures on each side given a higher success rate compared to only one suture [9]. Studies comparing suture placement versus mesh placement demonstrated higher success rates with suture [10]. Tensioning of the sutures is more difficult in the laparoscopic approach given lack of tactile sensation. Cystoscopy after suture placement is recommended to rule out bladder injury.

Success rates for the laparoscopic approach range between 80 and 92%. Unfortunately most of these studies are short term and thus durable long-term results comparing open versus laparoscopic approach are needed. Though previous studies demonstrated decreased use of pain medication and shorter hospital stay with the laparoscopic approach, a recent randomized study by Carey et al. did not demonstrate any difference in either variable [11]. However, Carey et al. did show a faster return to normal activities in patients undergoing the laparoscopic compared to open approach.

Other Laparoscopic Procedure for Stress Urinary Incontinence

With the introduction of the robotic-assisted laparoscopic procedure in urology and gynecology and given the success of the laparoscopic colposuspension, surgeons have started to use the robotic system to perform colposuspension. The shorter learning curve while using the robotic system has allowed surgeons to overcome the suturing difficulties in the laparoscopic procedure. Khan et al. reported the successful use of the robotic system to perform colposuspension [12]. However, further study is needed to evaluate the efficacy of the robotic system for this operation.

Other laparoscopic surgeries reported for the management of SUI include laparoscopic-assisted suburethral sling placement. The space of Retzius is dissected laparoscopically and a midurethral dissection is performed transvaginally. The sling material is then passed from the vaginal incision to the retropubic space and secured laparoscopically to the Cooper's ligament. Phelps et al. reported on their experience with this technique [13]. They successfully performed a laparoscopic-assisted suburethral sling placement in 63 patients with overall satisfaction of 89%.

Complications of Laparoscopic Colposuspension

The overall complication rate for laparoscopic Burch colposuspension is higher compared to the open approach with complication rates of 8–22% for the former and 5–8% for the latter. Most studies report that surgical skill is critical in preventing complications.

Lower Urinary Tract Injury

Bladder injury is the most common major intraoperative complication during laparoscopic colposuspension with rates ranging between 2.2 and 18% and occurs more commonly in women who have undergone previous pelvic surgery [3, 7, 14–18]. Table 1 summarizes the intraoperative complications in selected studies reporting their results after of laparoscopic colposuspension.

Table 1 Complications after laparoscopic Burch colposuspension

			Intraoperative/perioperative, n (%)						Long-term complication, n (%)		
Study	n	Follow-up (months)	Bladder injury	Ureteral injury	Bowel injury	Bleeding	UTI	Wound	Urinary retention	Urinary urgency/OAB	POP
Radomski et al. [23]	46	17.3	0	0	0	2	0	NA	1	0	2
Liu et al. [25]	433	NA	8 (1.8)	2 (0.5)	NA	NA		NA	15 (3.5)	14 (3.2)	2 (0.5)
Kitchener et al. [21]	144	24	4 (2.8)	0	1 (0.7)	1 (0.7)	8 (5.7)	1 (0.7)	NA	NA	NA
Carey et al. [11]	96	44.4	5 (5.2)	0	0	1 (1.0)	NA	NA	NA	47 (62.7)	NA
Moore et al. [22]	33	18.6	2 (6.1%)	0	1 (3.0)	0	NA	NA	NA	NA	NA
Cooper et al. [7]	113	8.4	11 (9.7)	0	1 (0.9)	1 (0.9)	NA	NA	NA	9 (8.0)	1 (0.9)

Laparoscopic bladder injury could be detected intraoperatively by direct observation of urine or fluid in the operative field or by gaseous distention of the urinary bag. Once injury is detected, the opening in the bladder should be closed with absorbable suture. The bladder should be drained for at least 5 days post-operative with longer catheterization times depending on the size of the injury and quality of the repair. A cystogram can be obtained prior to removal of the catheter.

Post-operative presentation of inadvertent bladder injury includes a constellation of symptoms including abdominal pain and distention, nausea and vomiting, hematuria, urine drainage from wounds with or without infection, and sepsis. Laboratory findings may include elevated white blood cell count and elevated creatinine level secondary to urine reabsorption. Radiographic studies may demonstrate free fluid in the abdomen with possible bowel findings suggestive of ileus. Diagnostic studies include either fluoroscopic cystogram (with post-drainage films) or computed tomography (CT) cystogram. Either study may demonstrate contrast extravasation. Depending on the site (extraperitoneal if that approach was used) and size of the injury, abdominal exploration may be needed. Small injuries may heal via a conservative approach maximizing bladder drainage with a large bore Foley catheter and/or suprapubic tube and the use of broad spectrum antibiotics. If an urinoma is present percutaneous drainage may be warranted, particularly if evidence of infection is apparent. In case of larger injuries or failure of conservative management, particularly if the injury is intraperitoneal, abdominal exploration and closure of the injury are warranted.

Placement of sutures into the bladder or urethra can be detected by direct laparoscopic visualization of the sutures placed into the bladder or by cystoscopy after placement of the sutures. If such injury is noted, the sutures should be removed and replaced. Post-operative presentation of sutures into the bladder may include hematuria, urinary urgency, and/or recurrent urinary tract infection (UTI), any of which may present as an immediate or delayed symptom in relation to surgery. Cystoscopy is warranted to evaluate foreign material in the bladder or urethra. Imaging studies may demonstrate calcifications over the suture. Management of these injuries may require abdominal exploration to remove the foreign material from the urinary tract.

There have also been studies reporting injury to the distal ureter, but most of these are rare and the reported cases only include partial ureteral obstruction secondary to angling of the distal ureter by the colposuspension [3, 19]. Ureteral obstruction should be suspected in any patient presenting with worsening renal function or flank pain. Imaging studies may demonstrate hydronephrosis with hydroureter. Management includes ureteral stenting or abdominal exploration with ureterolysis. In rare occasions ureteral reimplantation may be necessary.

Surgeons utilizing mesh for their suspension during laparoscopic colposuspension should also be aware of the risk of mesh or track erosion. There are two cases reported in the literature describing tack erosion into the bladder in which patients presented with lower abdominal pain, dyspareunia, urinary urgency, and recurrent UTI [20]. These cases were managed by abdominal exploration and removal of the tacks and mesh material.

Other Intraoperative and Perioperative Complications

Though bladder injury is the most common intraoperative complication, other possible morbidities include bowel injury, vaginal injury, and bleeding. With regard to bowel injury, most studies report less than 1% risk. A review by Cooper et al. reported one possible enterotomy in a group of 113 patients that was oversewn laparoscopically [7]. Kitchener et al. reported one (0.7%) bowel injury in the laparoscopic group compared to none in the open colposuspension group [21]. Moore et al. reported one serosal tear in an early series of 33 patients that was oversewn laparoscopically [22]. When bowel injury occurs the recommendation is to attempt to repair the enterotomy laparoscopically. If this is not possible then conversion to an open procedure may be necessary. Unrecognized bowel injury may present postoperatively with abdominal pain at one of the port sites or frank peritoneal signs, or sepsis.

Vaginal injury has also been reported but occurs very infrequently with only one study reporting a vaginal tear in a series of 113 patients [7]. Once recognized, vaginal tears can be repaired laparoscopically with absorbable suture.

Though most studies comparing the open and laparoscopic approaches for colposuspension demonstrate decrease estimated blood loss in the latter, intraoperative blood vessel injury and excessive blood loss during laparoscopic colposuspension have been reported. Studies describe epigastric vessel injury during port placement as well as obturator vessel injury during pelvic dissection [7, 11]. When injury to a vessel occurs the pneumoperitoneum can be used to the surgeon's advantage. Abdominal pressure may be temporarily increased to up to 20 cm H_2O to decrease blood loss and better identify the bleeding vessel. A laparoscopic bipolar instrument or clips may be used for hemostasis. Post-operative hemorrhage is similarly uncommon. Kitchener et al. reported on one patient who had blood loss greater than 500 ml (Kitchener). An earlier study by Radomski and Herschorn described two patients (4%) with post-operative bleeding, only one of whom required blood transfusion [23].

Reported perioperative morbidities after laparoscopic colposuspension include urinary tract infection, pneumonia, transient urinary retention, and wound infection. UTI has been reported to occur similarly in both open and laparoscopic procedures at rates of 5–6% [21]. UTI should be suspected when patients present with symptoms suggestive of a lower urinary tract infection, including dysuria, frequency, urgency, and/or hematuria. A urinalysis and urine cultures should be sent and depending on clinical suspicion, the patient could be started empirically on antibiotic medication. Patients who present with recurrent UTI's should be evaluated for a foreign object in the lower urinary tract and proper voiding function. Transient urinary retention after laparoscopic colposuspension is rare with rates ranging between 1 and 3% [3, 23–25]. Management of transient urinary retention includes clean intermittent catheterization versus indwelling catheter or suprapubic tube placement.

Wound infection occurs more commonly in the open colposuspension, with reported rates ranging between 5 and 8% in the open and less than 1% in the laparoscopic approaches. Small bowel obstruction has also been reported in a patient undergoing laparoscopic colposuspension [26].

Long-Term Complications After Laparoscopic Burch Colposuspension

Urinary Urgency

Patients with stress urinary incontinence often have associated overactive bladder (OAB) symptoms. Some early studies suggested that treatment of OAB was not necessary prior to proceeding with a retropubic anti-incontinence procedure given that in many instances OAB symptoms would subside after the procedure [27]. Although most practitioners would now advocate controlling OAB prior to proceeding with a sling, this is beginning to change with increasing experience with midurethral slings. Studies evaluating the risk of urgency after open colposuspension show that risk almost doubles if OAB symptoms were present prior to surgery [28]. Laparoscopic colposuspension series suggest a risk of developing OAB after surgery of 2.8–9% [3, 7, 15, 23, 29–32]. The decrease in OAB symptoms in the laparoscopic series compared to the open series has been attributed to the decrease in periurethral and pericolpium dissection and the fact that the sutures are tied with less tension [33]. Despite some studies suggesting a decreased incidence of OAB in the laparoscopic series, a randomized study comparing the open and laparoscopic approaches by Carey et al. did not demonstrate any difference between the groups [11]. The rate of urinary urgency and detrusor overactivity were 22 and 13% versus 28 and 11% for the open and laparoscopic groups, respectively.

Patients who developed OAB usually experience resolution of their symptoms within 3 months of surgery. While symptomatic, patients may be treated temporarily with anticholinergic medication. Persistent OAB symptoms after surgery warrant cystoscopy to rule out the presence of intravesical or intraurethral foreign objects and urodynamic study to evaluate for an obstructive voiding pattern. Symptoms of OAB could be treated with anticholinergic medication and behavioral modification. Patients with refractory symptoms may require neuromodulation, off-label use of intradetrusor botulinum toxin injection, or augmentation cystoplasty.

Urinary Retention

The rates of urinary retention after laparoscopic colposuspension range between 1 and 3% with far fewer patients developing long-term retention [3, 23–25]. This represents a rate lower than the 5% reported following open colposuspension [28]. Causes of urinary retention include overcorrection of the urethral axis due to incorrect placement or excessive tension of the sutures, denervation resulting from extensive dissection of the perivesical tissues, and pre-operative voiding dysfunction. Patients with a history of voiding dysfunction, urinary retention, or urodynamic findings of high capacity, high compliance, and poor bladder sensation are at increase risk of developing post-operative urinary retention and should be counseled appropriately.

Transient urinary retention should be managed with clean intermittent catheterization if possible. Patients who cannot perform self-catheterization may need chronic catheterization or suprapubic tube placement. If return to normal voiding after surgery is delayed, cystoscopy and urodynamic evaluation is warranted. However, it must be noted that many women with post-operative obstruction may not demonstrate the classic finding of high voiding pressure and low flow. One must ultimately use the urodynamic findings in conjunction with the clinical findings to determine the need for urethral release or urethrolysis. Video urodynamic evaluation or voiding cystourethrogram demonstrating a retropubically angulated or fixed urethra may also be helpful in determining the need for urethral release.

Pelvic Organ Prolapse

Development of pelvic organ prolapse is a well-known complication of open Burch colposuspension. Since the laparoscopic approach follows the principles of the open approach, a similar rate of pelvic organ prolapse occurs after laparoscopic colposuspension. By altering the vaginal and bladder base anatomy, colposuspension allows for the development of organ prolapse, specifically, via worsening of the posterior vaginal wall support. Wiskind et al. reported that 27% of patients undergoing Burch colposuspension developed prolapse requiring surgical repair [34, 35]. In the laparoscopic literature the rate of prolapse ranges between 11 and 30%, with rectocele (11–30%) and enterocele (1–6%) being the most common. Because of this high incidence of posterior prolapse some authors propose obliterating the cul-de-sac and performing an enterocele or rectocele repair at the same time.

In order to better determine the risk of organ prolapse development, a thorough pelvic exam prior to surgery is necessary. Cystoceles, enteroceles, apical prolapse, and symptomatic rectoceles should be repaired concomitantly with the colposuspension. Patients without posterior prolapse should be counseled on the risk of prolapse development. The authors recommend only treating rectoceles that are symptomatic (e.g., stool trapping requiring vaginal splinting to facilitate evacuation). However, rectocele repairs have approximately a 10% chance of developing pain and dyspareunia and thus patient should be well advised of this possibility.

Laparoscopic Treatment of Pelvic Organ Prolapse

Pelvic organ prolapse (POP) encompasses defects in any of the three pelvic compartments: anterior, apical, and posterior. Apical defects have traditionally been addressed via a transabdominal approach. Although all three compartments can be repaired transvaginally. Transvaginal approaches provide faster recovery times and preferred cosmetic results when compared to transabdominal procedures, but transabdominal procedures provided excellent and likely superior long-term results [36, 37]. With the advancement in minimally invasive transabdominal surgery, namely laparoscopic and robotic-assisted procedures, surgeons are using these approaches for repair of apical defects and, occasionally, anterior and posterior defects. Recent evidence suggests that these procedures may provide the long-term efficacy of open transabdominal surgery with the benefits of recovery times comparable to that of vaginal surgery [38, 39]. The goal of this section is to provide a brief review of the multiple laparoscopic and robotic-assisted procedures available for POP repair and then review in detail the incidence, diagnosis, and management of complications of these procedures. Given the larger experience with the use of laparoscopic sacrocolpopexy for repair of apical defects the focus of the complication analysis will be on this procedure.

Available Laparoscopic Procedures for Management of Pelvic Organ Prolapse

Laparoscopic Cystocele Repair

Transvaginal colporrhaphy, with or without synthetic or biograft, is the most common procedure used for cystocele repair. Despite its common use, failure rates of 10–70% have been reported [40–42]. Following the successful use of laparoscopic Burch colposuspension for SUI, pelvic surgeons began to apply laparoscopic skills and the surgical principles of the transvaginal approach to the repair of cystoceles. Laparoscopic port placement is similar to that use during laparoscopic colposuspension. The bladder is mobilized; the space of Retzius developed; and the bladder neck, Cooper's ligament, and the lateral detachment of the endopelvic fascia from the arcus tendinous fasciae pelvis (ATFP) are identified. With insertion of a vaginal manipulator the edges of the pubocervical fascia are identified and approximated to the ATFP with non-absorbable sutures. These sutures should also incorporate vaginal tissue and the obturator internus and iliopectineal ligaments.

Behnia-Willison reported on their experience with laparoscopic cystocele repair in 212 patients (42 underwent concomitant hysteropexy or colpopexy and 47 underwent concomitant posterior repair) [43]. With a mean follow-up of 14.2 months, the objective cure rate, defined as POP-Q stage 0 or 1, was 76%. Eighteen of the 23 women with residual central defects underwent graft-reinforced anterior colporrhaphy.

Laparoscopic Rectocele Repair

The transvaginal approach remains the most common approach for repair of posterior compartment defects [44]. However, there are a few limited reports on the laparoscopic transabdominal approach for rectocele repair. The key steps of the procedure involve careful dissection of the rectovaginal space, securing of the perineal body to the rectovaginal septum, closure of rectovaginal defects with absorbable sutures, and, if needed, levator ani plication. Lyons et al. reported their results of laparoscopic rectocele repair with polyglactin mesh in 20 patients. They found that with 12 month follow-up, 16 of the patients had resolution of the symptoms [45]. Another report by Thornton et al. compared the laparoscopic versus the transanal approach for rectocele repair. After 44 month follow-up, they noted a higher success rate with the transanal repair. Only 28% of the patients who underwent laparoscopic repair reported more than 50% symptom improvement.

Laparoscopic Apical Prolapse Repair

Multiple laparoscopic procedures for apical prolapse repair have been described, including laparoscopic vaginal vault or uterine uterosacral ligament fixation, laparoscopic sacrocolpopexy, laparoscopic culdoplasty using the Moschowitz and Halban procedures, and laparoscopic enterocele excision and closure. The laparoscopic uterosacral fixation and sacrocolpopexy are the most commonly reported and thus will comprise the focus of the apical discussion. During laparoscopic uterosacral ligament fixation the vaginal apex is approximated to the distal aspect of the uterosacral ligaments using non-absorbable sutures (care must be taken to identify the ureter, usually located 1–1.5 cm lateral to the uterosacral ligament). The rectovaginal fascia is then approximated to a more proximal aspect of the uterosacral ligaments. For the uterine suspension, a non-absorbable suture is placed through the full thickness of the uterosacral ligament at the level of the ischial spine and then again at its insertion point into the lower uterine segment. Most studies reporting outcomes using uterosacral ligament fixation have short follow-up and thus results must be interpreted with caution. The longest follow-up was reported by Medina and Tacaks who demonstrated a significant improvement in the prolapse stage from an average POP-Q stage 2 to stage 0 at a follow-up of almost 16 months. No patients had symptomatic prolapse and no intraoperative complications were reported.

The most commonly reported laparoscopic apical repair is the sacrocolpopexy. For the laparoscopic approach an intraumbilical or periumbilical port and two lower quadrant 10–12 mm ports are utilized. One or two ancillary ports may be placed at the level of the umbilicus lateral to the rectus muscle. If the robotic-assisted technique is used, then a 12 mm camera port is placed (supraumbilical), two 8 mm robotic arm ports are placed 8 cm from the midline and 17 cm from the symphysis pubis, and two assistant ports are placed (a 10 mm port 3 cm above the right anterior superior iliac spine and a right-sided 5 mm port 8 cm lateral to the camera port) (Fig. 1).

As is typical of minimally invasive techniques, the laparoscopic or robotic-assisted laparoscopic sacrocolpopexy applies the surgical principles of the open abdominal sacrocolpopexy. Using an EEA sizer or other vaginal obturators to facilitate the dissection, a

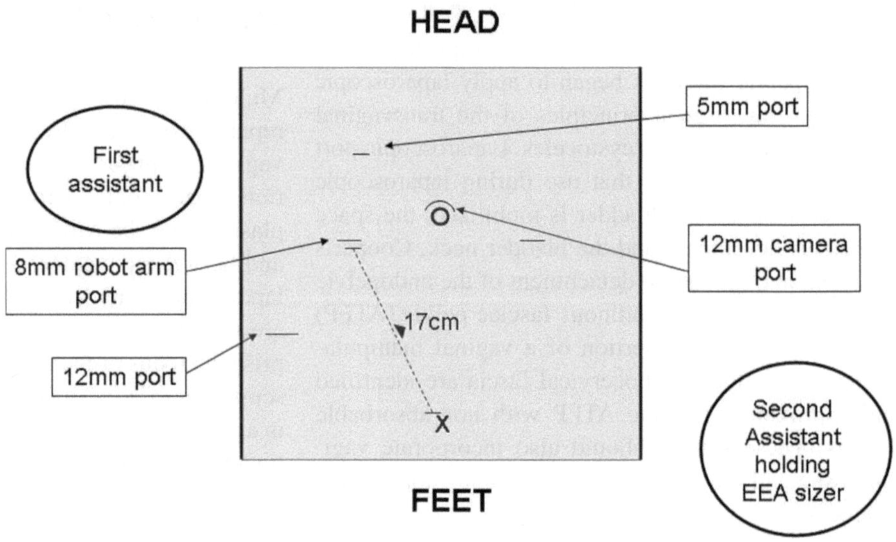

Fig. 1 Port placement for robotic-assisted laparoscopic sacrocolpopexy

peritoneal flap is dissected off the vaginal cuff. Care is taken to avoid injury to the bladder (catheter in place). The sacral promontory is then identified and the pre-sacral space is exposed. The sigmoid is retracted to the left with the use of an anchoring suture to the abdominal wall to provide excellent exposure of the posterior peritoneum and the vaginal apex. The sacral periosteum is carefully exposed with care taken to avoid any pre-sacral veins. The posterior peritoneum is then opened, connecting the vaginal peritoneal flap to the pre-sacral space. Next, a Y-shape synthetic mesh or biologic graft is secured to the anterior and posterior aspects of the vaginal apex with full thickness passes of non-absorbable sutures. The base of the mesh or graft is then secured to the pre-sacral ligaments and the periosteum with either two non-absorbable sutures or two bone anchors. The graft is secured with no tension. Most surgeons advocate retroperitonealization of the mesh to minimize the risk of adhesions and bowel obstruction. However, some surgeons have suggested that this step is unnecessary [46].

Hysterectomy can be performed concomitantly with the sacrocolpopexy. Given the higher incidence of mesh erosion in this patient population, however, surgeons have reported on the use of a supracervical hysterectomy in select patients [46].

A recent comprehensive review of laparoscopic sacrocolpopexy in a metaanalysis of greater than 1000 patients revealed an overall satisfaction rate of 94.4% with a mean follow-up of 25 months [47]. The mean operative time was 158 min with a 2.7% conversion to open rate and a 1.6% early reoperation rate. The authors conclude that the laparoscopic sacrocolpopexy outcomes uphold the outcomes of the gold standard abdominal sacrocolpopexy but that longer prospective and randomized trials are needed to further evaluate the laparoscopic approach. So far most preliminary reports of the robotic-assisted laparoscopic sacrocolpopexy have shown this procedure to be equally as successful as the laparoscopic approach [48–50].

Complications of Laparoscopic Pelvic Organ Prolapse Repair

Of all the laparoscopic procedures described for the treatment of POP, the laparoscopic sacrocolpopexy is the most commonly performed and the procedure with the most extensive follow-up. Given this, the following discussion will focus on complications described specifically in relation to the laparoscopic sacrocolpopexy.

Intraoperative and Perioperative Complications (Table 1)

Lower Urinary Tract Injury

Injuries to the bladder can occur during dissection of the peritoneal flap from the vaginal cuff. Often after hysterectomy the bladder can be adhered to the anterior vaginal wall as well as the vaginal cuff. Distending the bladder with saline solution through a catheter may help identify the boundaries of the bladder and aid in the dissection. Bladder injury can also occur during closure of the peritoneal flap via inadvertent placement of suture into the bladder. To avoid this injury the needle should be passed just 2–3 mm from the edge of the peritoneal flap. Sarlos et al. reported four bladder injuries in a series of 101 patients undergoing laparoscopic sacrocolpopexy [51]. All of the injuries were repaired laparoscopically and patients required Foley catheterization for 7 days. One of the patients presented 6 months postoperatively with dysuria and hematuria and was noted to have mesh erosion into the bladder. The patient underwent a laparoscopic cystotomy with partial resection of the anterior mesh and bladder repair. Another cohort study comparing open to laparoscopic sacrocolpopexy by Paraiso et al. described six (10.7%) and two (3.3%) cystotomies or bladder sutures in the laparoscopic and open group, respectively [39]. A recent review of 11 series of laparoscopic sacrocolpopexies by Ganatra et al. showed that there were 24 bladder injuries reported in a total of 1197 patients (2%) (Table 2) [47].

Table 2 Complications of laparoscopic sacrocolpopexy

Complication	n	%
Intraoperative	69	5.8
Bladder injury	24	2.0
Bowel Injury	20	1.7
Vessel injury	14	1.2
Vaginal injury	5	0.4
Ureteral injury	1	0.1
Return to OR		
Repair of prolapse recurrence	42	3.5
Treat de novo SUI	45	3.8
Mesh removal	21	1.8
Urethrolysis	4	0.3
Long term		
Mesh erosion	29	2.7
Recurrent prolapse	119	9.9
Anterior	50	4.2
Apical	18	1.5
Posterior	51	4.3
Urinary dysfunction	183	18.2
SUI	107	10.6
Mixed incontinence	39	3.9
Urinary retention	20	2.0
Bowel dysfunction	90	9.8
Sexual dysfunction	68	7.8

Source: Adapted from Ganatra et al. [47] (Reprinted with permission from Elsevier Limited, UK)

Ureteral injury could occur during exposure of the sacral periosteum or development of the retroperitoneal flap. One ureteral injury requiring reoperation has been reported in the literature during laparoscopic sacrocolpopexy (0.01%) [52]. Evaluation and management of bladder and ureteral injuries is similar to that described in the complication of laparoscopic colposuspension. It must be noted that there may be a higher risk of mesh erosion into the bladder in these patients.

Bowel Injury

Both small and large bowel injuries have been described in the laparoscopic sacrocolpopexy literature. A prospective study evaluating the efficacy and safety of laparoscopic sacrocolpopexy in 101 patients reported three rectal injuries [51]. One was repaired laparoscopically and the other required conversion to an open procedure. One patient had an unrecognized thermal rectal injury that caused sepsis and required reoperation with bowel diversion. No small bowel injuries were reported in this series. In their comprehensive literature review, Ganatra et al. reported a total of 15 (1.2%) small bowel injuries and 5 (0.04%) rectal injuries [47]. Bowel injury, when unrecognized, can lead to significant morbidity and mortality. Patients may require reoperation with temporary bowel diversion and are at high risk for wound infection. Injuries recognized intraoperatively can be repaired laparoscopically or in an open fashion with usually minimal morbidity. Although pre-operative bowel preparation would minimize the risk of infection broadening the spectrum of perioperative antibiotics in the case of bowel injury is recommended.

Vaginal Injury

Dissection of the peritoneal flap off the vaginal cuff is occasionally challenging due to scarring and adhesions. Use of a vaginal obturator is helpful in facilitating the dissection, but vaginal injury is still possible. Cheret et al. in 2001 reported on 44 patients undergoing laparoscopic sacrocolpopexy. In their series, they had one vaginal injury [53]. Revoir et al. reported three vaginal injuries in their series of 131 patients undergoing laparoscopic sacrocolpopexy [52]. A more recent review of the status of laparoscopic sacrocolopexy,

Ganatra et al. reported a total of five vaginal injuries (0.4% of patients) [47]. Vaginal injuries can be closed with absorbable suture. Depending on the size and location of the injury, these patients may be at higher risk of developing vaginal mesh extrusion. In cases of vaginal injury or thin vaginal wall the authors advocate consideration of an interpositional biologic graft between the vaginal injury and the mesh.

Infection

Although earlier studies reported on a decreased risk of wound infection in laparoscopic compared to open procedures, Paraiso et al. reported a significantly higher number of wound infections in their laparoscopic (10.7%) compared to the open sacrocolpopexy group (3.3%) [39]. There is one case report on the literature describing osteomyelitis following sacrocervicopexy [54]. The patient presented with lower back pain and vaginal discharge. Magnetic resonance imaging revealed discitis, an epidural abscess at the L5 to S1 level, and a fistulous tract extending from the rectovaginal space to the vertebrae. The patient required surgical exploration with hysterectomy and removal of the infected Mersilene mesh. This may be certainly be related more to the graft or anchoring technique than to the surgical approach.

Long-Term Complications

Mesh Erosion or Extrusion

Several types of mesh materials have been used during laparoscopic sacrocolpopexy, including polyethylene tetraphthalate (Mersilene), polyester single-side silicone-covered mesh (Cousin Biotech), polypropylene (Prolene by Ethicon and Marlex by Coloplast) [46, 55, 56]. The ideal mesh material should be strong, pliable, durable, and allow for appropriate tissue in-growth to minimize the risk of infection and extrusion. There are no prospective studies evaluating the use of different mesh types.

The rate of mesh erosion or extrusion after POP repair varies significantly depending on the length of follow-up, the mesh material, and the amount of mesh used. Evaluation of mesh erosion rates must be performed cautiously with care taken to identify each of these factors that may affect the occurrence of erosion. In the open abdominal sacrocolpopexy literature, the rate of mesh erosion varies between 3 and 12% [37, 57]. Review of laparoscopic sacrocolpopexy series by Ganatra et al. reported an overall erosion rate of 2.7%, with rates ranging from 0 to 9% [47]. Interestingly, the reports describing the highest erosion rates where those in studies with the longest follow-up [58, 59]. The mean time to erosion varied between 6 and 36 months.

When comparing open to laparoscopic sacrocolpopexy, Paraiso et al. found a higher erosion rate in the laparoscopic group (3.6%) versus the open group (1.6%) [39]. It should be noted that this cohort study only has a mean follow-up of 13 months. Stephanian et al. reported their extrusion rate after laparoscopic sacrocolpopexy with or without concomitant hysterectomy [60]. With a mean follow-up of 12 months, the overall extrusion rate was 5 in 446 patients (1.1%). Three of the extrusion occurred in patients undergoing concurrent hysterectomy and two in patients with history of hysterectomy. There was no statistical significant difference between both groups.

Patients with vaginal mesh extrusion may present with complaints of vaginal discharge, usually bloody, and abdominal or pelvic pain. Pelvic examination reveals extrusion of the mesh. Given that extrusion commonly presents at the vaginal apex, careful examination must be performed. Occasionally anesthesia may be necessary for patient comfort and adequate retraction and exposure to facilitate identification of a point of extrusion. Cystoscopy should also be performed to rule out mesh erosion into the bladder and/or a vesicovaginal fistula. Reports on mesh excision in the office have shown successful results. However, since most mesh erosions occur at the vaginal apex, the authors recommend mesh excision in the operating room. During mesh excision it is critical to mobilize the edges of vaginal epithelium surrounding the extrusion area and close the defect without tension. A sufficient area of mesh should be excised such that adequate tissue mobilization can be achieved. In cases of significant mesh extrusion a transabdominal approach may with complete excision of the mesh material be warranted. Despite complete removal of the mesh patients typically continue to experience appropriate vaginal support [39].

Partial removal of the extruded mesh with closure of the vaginal defect may be difficult. If enough vaginal epithelium cannot be mobilized for closure, an interpositional biologic graft may be helpful. Patel et al. presented his results using porcine small intestine submucosa for closure of large vaginal mesh extrusion defects in 10 patients [61]. With a follow-up of 10 months he reports no recurrent mesh extrusion. In patients who are at higher risk of developing mesh extrusion due to vaginal or bladder injury, one may consider the use of a biological material for reconstruction. The biograft can be used either as an interposition graft or as the Y-shaped suspension material. Ross et al. reported on the use of porcine dermis as an interpositional graft in the arms of the Y-shaped mesh in 31 patients. With a follow-up of 2 years there were no vaginal extrusions encountered [62].

Most authors describe retroperitonealization of the mesh after sacrocolpopexy to prevent bowel adhesion and mesh erosion. However, closure of the retroperitoneum does risk ureteral, bowel, or vessel injury. Elneil et al. presented their experience on 128 patients with mean follow-up of 19 months undergoing open sacrocolpopexy without burial of the mesh and found no cases of bowel injury by the mesh [63]. No randomized control trial has been performed evaluating the need for retroperitonealization of the mesh and thus no definite recommendations can be put forth at this time.

Patients who undergo concomitant hysterectomy at the time of sacrocolpopexy may have an increased risk of mesh extrusion at the vaginal apex. Subtotal hysterectomy with cervical preservation has been suggested to reduce the risk of erosion [46]. However, caution must be taken given the risk of cancer in the retained cervix. Descargues reported on 3 women in a series of 154 who were found to have cancer in their hysterectomy specimens after sacrocolpopexy [64].

Voiding Dysfunction

Evaluation of urinary symptoms prior to surgical correction of POP is critical. Patients should be evaluated for adequate voiding function as well as for the presence of urinary incontinence. Urodynamic evaluation may be required for complete evaluation of voiding function and to evaluate for the need of a concomitant anti-incontinent procedure. The need for a concomitant sling or Burch at the time of sacrocolpopexy has been extensively evaluated and is beyond the focus of this chapter [2, 42, 65]. At this point, it is unclear if all women undergoing sacrocolpopexies require concomitant anti-incontinence procedures. Clearly there are risks associated with additional procedures and the risks are not negligible (urinary retention, urethral or bladder injury, mesh extrusion, urinary dysfunction). The authors recommend that all women with symptoms of SUI or who demonstrate SUI in urodynamic evaluation (with or without reduction of their prolapse) should undergo a concomitant anti-incontinence procedure. Patients without SUI prior to surgery should be counseled on the potential for of development of de novo SUI after POP repair.

Dyspareunia and Bowel Dysfunction

With the increase is vaginal length after sacrocolpopexy one would expect that patients would experience less dyspareunia. However, 7.8% of patients complain of sexual dysfunction after laparoscopic sacrocolpopexy. The incidence of dyspareunia may be even higher in patients who undergo a concomitant rectocele repair. Management of these patients can be challenging. Use of trigger point injections may be considered in those patients in whom specific points of tenderness can be identified.

Some patients undergoing laparoscopic sacrocolpopexy may have temporary bowel dysfunction. Ganatra et al. reported a 9.8% incidence of bowel dysfunction after laparoscopic sacrocolpopexy, including constipation, anal pain, and fecal incontinence [47]. Most of these symptoms resolved within 6 months of surgery. There was only one case of fecal incontinence reported and this occurred in a patient who was also undergoing concomitant sphincteroplasties [59].

Recurrence of Pelvic Organ Prolapse

Unfortunately there is no clear definition of success after POP repair and thus no standard definition of failure after POP repair. Most authors would agree that resolution of POP symptoms as well as pelvic exam showing no evidence of POP would define success. Most studies evaluating the efficacy of sacrocolpopexy define recurrence of POP as prolapse extending beyond the hymen or onset of new prolapse symptoms [66]. However, symptoms do not correlate with physical exam findings of severity of POP, thus making the evaluation of POP recurrence more difficult [1]. POP recurrence rates are also complicated by the fact that long-term data are lacking. Most studies report their results with follow-up times less than 2 years and thus long-term failures are not assessed. More long-term studies evaluating repair failures are needed.

With a mean follow-up of 24.6 months, Ganatra reported a recurrence rate of 9.9% in 11 series of laparoscopic sacrocolpopexy [47]; 6.2% of these patients required reoperation for POP recurrence. It is unclear if these patients were symptomatic. However, it must be noted that only 1.5% of all patients have apical prolapse repair with the remainder developing anterior or posterior defects that may or may not have been addressed at the time of initial sacrocolpopexy.

Conclusions

With the increased use of laparoscopy and robotic-assisted procedures in pelvic floor reconstruction surgeons must be versed in the potential risks of the procedures. Most laparoscopic procedures follow their respective surgical principles of the open procedure and thus, not surprisingly, studies to date have shown similar results. However, more long-term studies are needed to evaluate the long-term success and complications of these procedures.

References

1. Nygaard I, Barber MD, Burgio KL, et al. Prevalence of symptomatic pelvic floor disorders in US women. JAMA. 2008;300:1311.
2. Olsen AL, Smith VJ, Bergstrom JO, et al. Epidemiology of surgically managed pelvic organ prolapse and urinary incontinence. Obstet Gynecol. 1997;89:501.
3. Liu CY. Laparoscopic retropubic colposuspension (Burch procedure). A review of 58 cases. J Reprod Med. 1993;38:526.
4. Burch JC. Cooper's ligament urethrovesical suspension for stress incontinence. Nine years' experience – results, complications, techniques. 1968. Am J Obstet Gynecol. 2002;187:512.
5. Frankel G, Kantipong M. Sixteen-month experience with video-assisted extraperitoneal laparoscopic bladder neck suspension. J Endourol. 1995;9:259.
6. Raboy A, Hakim LS, Ferzli G, et al. Extraperitoneal endoscopic vesicourethral suspension. J Laparoendosc Surg. 1993;3:505.
7. Cooper MJ, Cario G, Lam A, et al. A review of results in a series of 113 laparoscopic colposuspensions. Aust N Z J Obstet Gynaecol. 1996;36:44.
8. Wolf JS Jr, Monk TG, McDougall EM, et al. The extraperitoneal approach and subcutaneous emphysema are associated with greater absorption of carbon dioxide during laparoscopic renal surgery. J Urol. 1995;154:959.
9. Persson J, Wolner-Hanssen P. Laparoscopic Burch colposuspension for stress urinary incontinence: a randomized comparison of one or two sutures on each side of the urethra. Obstet Gynecol. 2000;95:151.
10. Zullo F, Palomba S, Russo T, et al. Laparoscopic colposuspension using sutures or prolene meshes: a 3-year follow-up. Eur J Obstet Gynecol Reprod Biol. 2004;117:201.
11. Carey MP, Goh JT, Rosamilia A, et al. Laparoscopic versus open Burch colposuspension: a randomised controlled trial. BJOG. 2006;113:999.
12. Khan MS, Challacombe B, Rose K, et al. Robotic colposuspension: two case reports. J Endourol. 2007;21:1077.
13. Phelps JY, Lin L, Liu CY. Laparoscopic suburethral sling procedure. J Am Assoc Gynecol Laparosc. 2003;10:496.
14. Brenner B. Comparing the laparoscopic Burch colposuspension and the suburethral sling. N Z Med J. 2001;114:146.
15. Meltomaa S, Haarala M, Makinen J, et al. Endoscopic colposuspension with simplified extraperitoneal approach. Tech Urol. 1997;3:216.
16. Saidi MH, Gallagher MS, Skop IP, et al. Extraperitoneal laparoscopic colposuspension: short-term cure rate, complications, and duration of hospital stay in comparison with Burch colposuspension. Obstet Gynecol. 1998;92:619.
17. Myers DL, Peipert JF, Rosenblatt PL, et al. Patient satisfaction with laparoscopic Burch retropubic urethropexy. J Reprod Med. 2000;45:939.
18. Speights SE, Moore RD, Miklos JR. Frequency of lower urinary tract injury at laparoscopic Burch and paravaginal repair. J Am Assoc Gynecol Laparosc. 2000;7:515.
19. Ferland RD, Rosenblatt P. Ureteral compromise after laparoscopic Burch colpopexy. J Am Assoc Gynecol Laparosc. 1999;6:217.
20. Albright TS, Garlich CL, Iglesia CB. Complications after laparoscopic Burch with hernia mesh and surgical tacks. Obstet Gynecol. 2006;108:718.
21. Kitchener HC, Dunn G, Lawton V, et al. Laparoscopic versus open colposuspension—results of a prospective randomised controlled trial. BJOG. 2006;113:1007.
22. Moore RD, Speights SE, Miklos JR. Laparoscopic Burch colposuspension for recurrent stress urinary incontinence. J Am Assoc Gynecol Laparosc. 2001;8:389.
23. Radomski SB, Herschorn S. Laparoscopic Burch bladder neck suspension: early results. J Urol. 1996;155:515.
24. Liu CY. Laparoscopic treatment for genuine urinary stress incontinence. Baillieres Clin Obstet Gynaecol. 1994;8:789.

25. Liu CY. Laparoscopic treatment of stress urinary incontinence. Obstet Gynecol Clin North Am. 1999;26:149.
26. Margossian H, Pollard RR, Walters MD. Small bowel obstruction in a peritoneal defect after laparoscopic Burch procedure. J Am Assoc Gynecol Laparosc. 1999;6:343.
27. McGuire EJ, Lytton B, Kohorn EI, et al. The value of urodynamic testing in stress urinary incontinence. J Urol. 1980;124:256.
28. Leach GE, Dmochowski RR, Appell RA, et al. Female Stress Urinary Incontinence Clinical Guidelines Panel summary report on surgical management of female stress urinary incontinence. The American Urological Association. J Urol. 1997;158:875.
29. Nezhat CH, Nezhat F, Nezhat CR, et al. Laparoscopic retropubic cystourethropexy. J Am Assoc Gynecol Laparosc. 1994;1:339.
30. Miannay E, Cosson M, Lanvin D, et al. Comparison of open retropubic and laparoscopic colposuspension for treatment of stress urinary incontinence. Eur J Obstet Gynecol Reprod Biol. 1998;79:159.
31. Fatthy H, El Hao M, Samaha I, et al. Modified Burch colposuspension: laparoscopy versus laparotomy. J Am Assoc Gynecol Laparosc. 2001;8:99.
32. Ou CS, Rowbotham R. Five-year follow-up of laparoscopic bladder neck suspension using synthetic mesh and surgical staples. J Laparoendosc Adv Surg Tech A. 1999;9:249.
33. Paraiso MF, Walters MD. Laparoscopic surgery for stress urinary incontinence and pelvic organ prolapse. Clin Obstet Gynecol. 2005;48:724.
34. Kwon CH, Culligan PJ, Koduri S, et al. The development of pelvic organ prolapse following isolated Burch retropubic urethropexy. Int Urogynecol J Pelvic Floor Dysfunct. 2003;14:321.
35. Wiskind AK, Creighton SM, Stanton SL. The incidence of genital prolapse after the Burch colposuspension. Am J Obstet Gynecol. 1992;167:399.
36. Benson JT, Lucente V, McClellan E. Vaginal versus abdominal reconstructive surgery for the treatment of pelvic support defects: a prospective randomized study with long-term outcome evaluation. Am J Obstet Gynecol. 1996;175:1418.
37. Nygaard IE, McCreery R, Brubaker L, et al. Abdominal sacrocolpopexy: a comprehensive review. Obstet Gynecol. 2004;104:805.
38. Hsiao KC, Latchamsetty K, Govier FE, et al. Comparison of laparoscopic and abdominal sacrocolpopexy for the treatment of vaginal vault prolapse. J Endourol. 2007;21:926.
39. Paraiso MF, Walters MD, Rackley RR, et al. Laparoscopic and abdominal sacral colpopexies: a comparative cohort study. Am J Obstet Gynecol. 2005;192:1752.
40. Sand PK, Koduri S, Lobel RW, et al. Prospective randomized trial of polyglactin 910 mesh to prevent recurrence of cystoceles and rectoceles. Am J Obstet Gynecol. 2001;184:1357.
41. Weber AM, Walters MD, Piedmonte MR, et al. Anterior colporrhaphy: a randomized trial of three surgical techniques. Am J Obstet Gynecol. 2001;185:1299.
42. Maher C, Baessler K, Glazener CM, et al. Surgical management of pelvic organ prolapse in women: a short version Cochrane review. Neurourol Urodyn. 2008;27:3.
43. Behnia-Willison F, Seman EI, Cook JR, et al. Laparoscopic paravaginal repair of anterior compartment prolapse. J Minim Invasive Gynecol. 2007;14:475.
44. Daneshgari F, Paraiso MF, Kaouk J, et al. Robotic and laparoscopic female pelvic floor reconstruction. BJU Int. 2006;98 Suppl 1:62.
45. Cundiff GW, Fenner D. Evaluation and treatment of women with rectocele: focus on associated defecatory and sexual dysfunction. Obstet Gynecol. 2004;104:1403.
46. Gadonneix P, Ercoli A, Salet-Lizee D, et al. Laparoscopic sacrocolpopexy with two separate meshes along the anterior and posterior vaginal walls for multicompartment pelvic organ prolapse. J Am Assoc Gynecol Laparosc. 2004;11:29.
47. Ganatra AM, Rozet F, Sanchez-Salas R, et al. The current status of laparoscopic sacrocolpopexy: a review. Eur Urol. 2009;55(5):1089.
48. Ayav A, Bresler L, Hubert J, et al. Robotic-assisted pelvic organ prolapse surgery. Surg Endosc. 2005;19:1200.
49. Daneshgari F, Kefer JC, Moore C, et al. Robotic abdominal sacrocolpopexy/sacrouteropexy repair of advanced female pelvic organ prolaspe (POP): utilizing POP-quantification-based staging and outcomes. BJU Int. 2007;100:875.
50. Elliott DS, Krambeck AE, Chow GK. Long-term results of robotic assisted laparoscopic sacrocolpopexy for the treatment of high grade vaginal vault prolapse. J Urol. 2006;176:655.
51. Sarlos D, Brandner S, Kots L, et al. Laparoscopic sacrocolpopexy for uterine and post-hysterectomy prolapse: anatomical results, quality of life and perioperative outcome-a prospective study with 101 cases. Int Urogynecol J Pelvic Floor Dysfunct. 2008;19:1415.
52. Rivoire C, Botchorishvili R, Canis M, et al. Complete laparoscopic treatment of genital prolapse with meshes including vaginal promontofixation and anterior repair: a series of 138 patients. J Minim Invasive Gynecol. 2007;14:712.
53. Cheret A, Von Theobald P, Lucas J, et al. Laparoscopic promontofixation feasibility study in 44 patients. J Gynecol Obstet Biol Reprod (Paris). 2001;30:139.
54. Downing KT. Vertebral osteomyelitis and epidural abscess after laparoscopic uterus-preserving cervicosacropexy. J Minim Invasive Gynecol. 2008;15:370.
55. Rozet F, Mandron E, Arroyo C, et al. Laparoscopic sacral colpopexy approach for genito-urinary prolapse: experience with 363 cases. Eur Urol. 2005;47:230.
56. Wattiez A, Mashiach R, Donoso M. Laparoscopic repair of vaginal vault prolapse. Curr Opin Obstet Gynecol. 2003;15:315.
57. Kohli N, Walsh PM, Roat TW, et al. Mesh erosion after abdominal sacrocolpopexy. Obstet Gynecol. 1998;92:999.
58. Higgs PJ, Chua HL, Smith AR. Long term review of laparoscopic sacrocolpopexy. BJOG. 2005;112:1134.
59. Ross JW, Preston M. Laparoscopic sacrocolpopexy for severe vaginal vault prolapse: five-year outcome. J Minim Invasive Gynecol. 2005;12:221.
60. Stepanian AA, Miklos JR, Moore RD, et al. Risk of mesh extrusion and other mesh-related complications after laparoscopic sacral colpopexy with or without concurrent laparoscopic-assisted vaginal hysterectomy: experience of 402 patients. J Minim Invasive Gynecol. 2008;15:188.

61. Patel M. A reconstructive option for large vaginal mesh exposures using a porcine small intestinal submucosa graft. SUFU 2009 Annual Meeting, Las Vegas, Nevada, 2009.
62. Ross JW. The use of a xenogenic barrier to prevent mesh erosion with laparoscopic sacrocolpopexy. J Minim Invasive Gynecol. 2007;14:470.
63. Elneil S, Cutner AS, Remy M, et al. Abdominal sacrocolpopexy for vault prolapse without burial of mesh: a case series. BJOG. 2005;112:486.
64. Descargues G, Collard P, Grise P. Surgical management of pelvic organ prolapse in women: laparoscopic or vaginal sacrocolpopexy? Gynecol Obstet Fertil. 2008;36:978.
65. Brubaker L, Cundiff GW, Fine P, et al. Abdominal sacrocolpopexy with Burch colposuspension to reduce urinary stress incontinence. N Engl J Med. 2006;354:1557.
66. Beer M, Kuhn A. Surgical techniques for vault prolapse: a review of the literature. Eur J Obstet Gynecol Reprod Biol. 2005;119:144.

Complications of Single Port Laparoscopic and Robotic Surgery

Wesley M. White, Raj K. Goel, and Jihad H. Kaouk

Keywords Single port · Laparoscopy · Robotics · Single incision · Complications

Introduction

Any new surgical approach or technique requires a stringent inquisition of its relative merits and risks. When laparoscopic cholecystectomy was introduced nearly two decades ago, a small rise in complications during the learning curve of the procedure was accepted by both physicians and patients given the tangibly lessened morbidity and shortened convalescence that were associated with the approach [1]. Single port laparoscopy was conceptualized and refined over the last 18 months in an attempt to further reduce patient discomfort and to improve cosmesis. Collectively, over 200 single port urologic procedures have been successfully completed and include both extirpative and reconstructive indications [2–4]. Thus far, results have been generally favorable with a modicum of complications commensurate with any new technique. However, the superiority of the single port approach as compared to standard laparoscopy has yet to be firmly established [4]. Given that the single port approach is, at least in the short term, demonstrating only marginal differential benefit, complications with single port surgery must be critically evaluated. This chapter will offer a brief review of the single port laparoscopic literature with an emphasis on reported complications and finally outline our algorithm for addressing single port adverse events.

Review of Single Port Surgery

Since its inception, success during laparoscopic surgery has been predicated on instrument triangulation that obviates internal and external clashing, the judicious placement of ancillary ports for optimized exposure, and the use of primarily rigid operative instruments for secure tissue grasping and dissection [5]. Single port surgery runs contrary to these axioms and invokes questions regarding the practicality and technical ease of the approach. Indeed, when the initial reports of single port laparoscopic surgery appeared in the general surgical and gynecologic literature several decades ago, its broad application was severely hindered by instrument clashing secondary to in-line placement [6–8]. The most significant barrier at that time included ill-adapted instruments and platforms that precluded safe tissue handling and/or yielded cumbersome instrument clashing. Single port surgery has reemerged within the last year as flexible tip laparoscopes and coaxial flexible operating instruments have become commercially available [2, 9]. These newer instruments afford the operating surgeon improved range of motion, the ability to 'triangulate' instruments despite in-line placement, better control and exposure of the operative field, improved ergonomics, and decreased surgeon fatigue (Fig. 1).

J.H. Kaouk (✉)
Section of Laparoscopic and Robotic Urology, Glickman Urological and Kidney Institute, Cleveland Clinic, Cleveland, OH, USA
e-mail: kaoukj@ccf.org

R. Ghavamian (ed.), *Complications of Laparoscopic and Robotic Urologic Surgery*,
DOI 10.1007/978-1-60761-676-4_21, © Springer Science+Business Media, LLC 2010

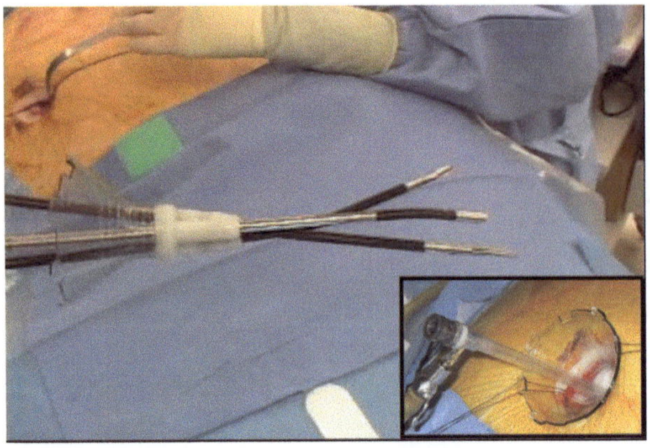

Fig. 1 Intraoperative image of a multichannel port used during single port surgery. Inserted in parallel through the port is a 5 mm laparoscope with a flexible tip. Also inserted are two curved laparoscopic instruments to minimize clashing of instruments during surgery

The culmination of these aforementioned technical innovations was the first published series of single port laparoscopic surgery in urology in 2008. At the Cleveland Clinic, we detailed our initial experience with 10 patients who underwent single port extirpative and reconstructive renal and pelvic procedures [2]. All procedures were successfully completed without conversion or the use of ancillary ports. In general, outcomes were favorable with no significant complications. Although the authors enthusiastically trumpeted the arrival of single port surgery in earnest, they did concede that myriad logistical difficulties would hinder the broad application of the approach.

Following this initial report, numerous centers have published their experience with single port urologic surgery with a variable focus on site-specific or procedure-specific outcomes [10–13] (Table 1). Many of these centers employed alternative ports, platforms, and instruments in an attempt to overcome many of the limitations previously discussed. The vast majority of procedures were successfully completed without the need for conversion to standard laparoscopy. Judicious use of assistant ports was necessary, in some situations, to improve exposure of the operative field and to offer increased patient safety. A detailed analysis of reported adverse events will be discussed later in this chapter.

In late 2008, an expert panel was convened during the Cleveland Clinic Medical Innovation Summit regarding the state of the art and future of minimally invasive urologic surgery [14]. The focus of discussion centered primarily on single port or Laparoendoscopic single-site (LESS) surgery and natural orifice translumenal endoscopic surgery (NOTES). While the purpose of the panel was neither to generate a consensus statement on the future of these aforementioned approaches nor debate the superiority of LESS and NOTES as compared to standard laparoscopy, a transparent accord was reached and an equally pressing need defined. The take-home message was that existing instrumentation is less than optimal and continued technical innovation is warranted to nourish LESS and NOTES. Specific mention was made of the need for a purpose-built robotic operating platform that could potentially overcome many of the logistical issues inherent to NOTES and LESS and shorten the considerable learning curve associated with these techniques. The panel concurred that the pragmatic and innovative application of existing robotic technology would not only improve laparoscopy in its current form but also foster and delineate the genuine feasibility of NOTES and the practicable reproducibility of LESS.

Having now completed over 150 single port urologic procedures, we feel comfortable with the approach and have seen benefit with respect to pain control and cosmesis. In our hands, we believe single port surgery to be non-inferior to standard laparoscopy for select patients. However, no randomized controlled trials have been performed which demonstrates statistically significant improved outcomes with the single port approach. We are therefore hesitant to proclaim its superiority. Ultimately, if single port surgery is to be more than a fad, the learning curve must be curtailed and instrumentation streamlined and improved. We anticipate that a purpose-built robotic platform may allow single port surgery to become generalizable much as its introduction made laparoscopic prostatectomy accessible to the general urologist.

Single Port Surgical Complications – Review of the Literature

In general, the complications encountered with single port laparoscopic surgery are analogous to those experienced with standard laparoscopic surgery. Indeed, with the exception of obtaining access to the peritoneal cavity or retroperitoneal space and closure of

Table 1 Summary of selected single port urologic surgery series

	N	Procedure(s)	Complications	Type of complication(s)
Kaouk et al. [2]	10	Renal and pelvic extirpative and reconstructive	1	Blood transfusion
Desai et al. [3]	2	Nephrectomy and pyeloplasty	0	N/A
Raman et al. [4]	11	Nephrectomy		
Gill et al. [12]	4	Donor nephrectomy	0	N/A
Kaouk et al. [20]	7	Partial nephrectomy	0	N/A
Kaouk et al. [21]	4	Radical prostatectomy	1	Recto-urethral fistula
Desai et al. [22]	4	Renal and pelvic reconstructive	0	N/A
White et al. [10]	8	Retroperitoneal	0	N/A
White et al. [11]	10	Sacral colpopexy	0	N/A
White et al. [17]	100	Cumulative renal and pelvic extirpative and reconstructive	10	Transfusion (6); ICU admission (1); recto-urethral fistula (1); UTI (1); DVT (1)
Stein et al. [13]	4	Pyeloplasty, nephrectomy, and partial nephrectomy	1	Transfusion
Aron et al. [23]	5	Partial nephrectomy	1	Bleeding/pulmonary embolism
Ponsky et al. [24]	1	Radical nephrectomy	0	N/A
Desai et al. [19]	30	Enucleation of the prostate	5	Bleeding (3); bowel Injury (1); mortality (1)
Rane et al. [25]	5	Nephrectomy	2	Not reported

the port site, the operative steps are identical with the two approaches. The literature cites an expected complication rate of approximately 5% during laparoscopic urologic surgery. In a review published in 1999, of over 2,000 laparoscopic procedures performed at multiple centers in Germany, 107 complications (4.4%) were reported [15]. The majority of complications were vascular in nature (1.7%), with hollow viscous injury (1.1%) and infectious complications (0.8%) less common. Injuries secondary to trocar placement occurred in 0.2% of cases. Of note, the complication rate was 13.3% for the first 100 procedures and averaged 3.6% thereafter.

In 2002, Vallancien and colleagues in France examined their complications during over 1,300 laparoscopic procedures [16]. In this series, bowel injury (1.2%), vascular injury (0.5%), and ureteral injuries (0.8%) were reported. The overall transfusion rate was 2.4%. Operative conversion was required in 1.2% of cases and reoperation was required in 2.4% of cases. The authors concluded that laparoscopic surgery was associated with essentially the same risks as any open surgery.

One would expect a distinct but not profound rise in the incidence of surgical complications with the single port approach. Although the aforementioned German study cited a considerably higher complication rate (13.3 vs. 3.6%) during their first 100 laparoscopic cases, these adverse events occurred during the surgeons' learning curve and would be expected with any profoundly new surgical approach [15]. While single port surgery does present ergonomic challenges and a radically different philosophical approach to laparoscopic surgery, the operative steps are essentially identical to those of standard laparoscopy. As such, adverse events should be expected but at a lower rate than during the initial learning curve with laparoscopy.

In 2008, Kaouk and colleagues at the Cleveland Clinic published their initial experience with single port laparoscopic surgery in urology [2]. A total of 10 patients underwent renal cryotherapy ($n = 4$), wedge kidney biopsy ($n = 1$), radical nephrectomy ($n = 1$), and abdominal sacral colpopexy ($n = 4$). Access was obtained under direct vision, and the Uni-X Single Port Access Laparoscopic System (Pnavel Systems, Morganville, NJ) was used as the operating platform of choice. One patient undergoing renal cryoablation required a transfusion of 3 U of packed RBCs (Clavien Class II surgical complication). Of note, the patient had baseline chronic anemia, and a post-operative computed tomography scan revealed only a small perinephric hematoma.

Rane and colleagues subsequently reported their experience with single port urologic surgery in 2008 [9]. Five patients underwent simple nephrectomy (2), orchiectomy (1), orchiopexy (1), and ureterolithotomy (1). No complications were reported with respect to access, intraoperative complications, or post-operative adverse events. Specific to the single port technique, the authors felt that obtaining access with the R-Port (Olympus Surgical, Orangeburg, NJ) was controlled and safe. In general, the R-Port is placed once direct visual access to the abdominal cavity is achieved. The port is then inserted with an introducer that has a blunt but still pointed tip (Fig. 2). The authors speculated that intra-abdominal vascular and visceral injury and abdominal wall bleeding may be minimized with use of such a port and introducer.

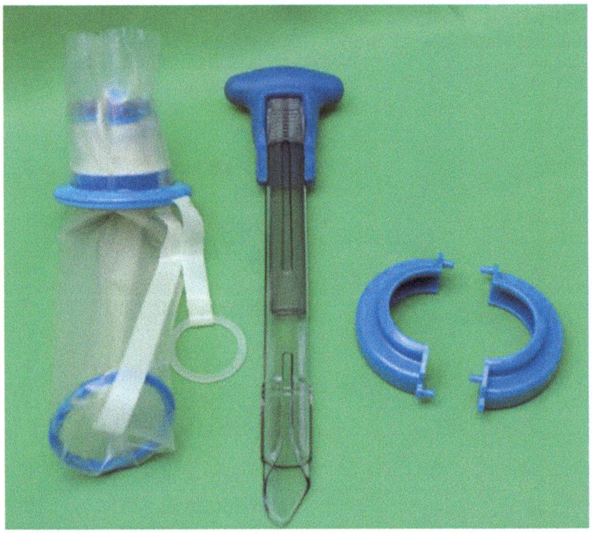

Fig. 2 Photo of a R-Port device used during single port laparoscopy. Note that this multichannel port includes a trocar for insertion. While the trocar allows for easier port insertion, risk of intra-abdominal injury using this trocar should be considered to avoid complications

In 2009, White and colleagues reported their single-center experience with over 100 single port laparoscopic procedures [17]. Using the Clavien Classification system, the authors detailed their short-term and long-term complications [18]. During the immediate post-operative period, surgical complications occurred in six patients. Six patients required a blood transfusion for symptomatic anemia (Clavien Class II) and one patient required a blood transfusion and developed an upper extremity deep venous thrombosis (Clavien Class II). Three patients experienced delayed adverse events. One patient developed an iatrogenic culture-documented urinary tract infection (Clavien Class II) that required oral antibiotics. One patient following radical prostatectomy developed a recto-urethral fistula that required operative intervention to correct (Clavien Grade IIIb). An additional patient had post-operative bleeding following partial nephrectomy and required readmission to the intensive care unit, transfusion, and angioembolization (Clavien Grade IVa). The overall rate of adverse events was 10%. Significant surgical complications occurred in 2%.

Irwin and colleagues recently reported their multicenter outcomes with a focus on conversions from single port laparoscopic to standard laparoscopic procedures and independent complications with single port surgery [18]. The study was procedure specific and was limited only to nephrectomy, adrenalectomy, and pyeloplasty. One hundred forty-five procedures were attempted with the single port approach. Ten procedures (6.8%) required conversion to conventional laparoscopy. The cited reasons for conversion included failure to progress in five patients, inability to safely perform reconstruction in three patients, and control of bleeding in the remaining two patients. Complications occurred in 10.3% of single port procedures. No additional details or insight regarding the nature or severity of complications was reported.

Recently, Desai and colleagues reported their multi-center experience with single port laparoscopy. In this series, the majority of patients underwent benign reconstructive procedures including single port transvesical enucleation of the prostate and dismembered pyeloplasty. Complications were reported. In a separate study of the same population, Desai and colleagues focused on outcomes following single port transvesical enucleation of the prostate. A total of 30 patients underwent adenoma enucleation for symptomatic BPH through a multichannel port positioned transvesically. Reported complications included bleeding requiring transfusion in three patients, bowel injury in one patient, and one immediate post-operative death due to bleeding in a Jehovah's Witness patient [19].

In our personal experience, complications with single port laparoscopy are largely analogous to those we encounter during standard laparoscopic cases. However, the ability to satisfactorily address intraoperative complications, especially bleeding, can be extremely challenging with the single port approach. For example, in our series of over 100 patients, conversion to standard laparoscopy was required during two renal procedures secondary to bleeding from venous tributaries. When additional ports were placed, the operative field was quickly evacuated and the bleeding easily controlled. The ability to evacuate the field rapidly, expose the offending vessel, and securely obtain hemostasis can be extremely challenging. The operating surgeon is compromised not only by the inherent difficulties with in-line instrument placement but also by the lack of flexibility with some of the commercially available ports. That is, several of the single ports offer limited access with 10 mm ports, thereby restricting what instruments can be employed to control the bleeding. This issue can be even more challenging during single port robotic surgery in which the assistant port is often difficult to access and/or the suction/irrigator has limited range of motion with the robot docked. Without question, there is a smaller margin of error afforded with LESS, and conversion to standard laparoscopy, especially during one's learning curve, should not be construed as a complication but rather surgical 'common sense' that serves the best interests of the patient (Clayman RV, April 28, 2009, personal communication).

Lack of progress is occasionally encountered during our single port operations. With savvy and experience, we have learned to persevere through difficult anatomy and ergonomic challenges to realize satisfactory outcomes. Troubleshooting is to be expected and an experienced team is critical. In general, operative times in our single port procedures are only marginally longer than with standard laparoscopy [10, 11, 17]. Indeed, longer operative times should be expected initially with the single port approach as one develops the requisite skill set to obtain reproducible outcomes.

Patient selection cannot be over-emphasized as it pertains to the avoidance of complications during surgery. In our experience, ergonomic challenges occur more commonly with taller patients and among those with a higher BMI. This is particularly true during single port renal procedures owing to the comparatively long distance between the umbilicus and the upper pole of the kidney. Despite these challenges, an elevated BMI has not been proven to be associated with a higher rate of conversion to conventional laparoscopy or with adverse events during single port surgery [18]. The aforementioned narrow margin for surgical error similarly applies to patient selection. The only reported mortality in the single port literature occurred following a single port enucleation of the prostate on a Jehovah's Witness patient. Although speculative, patients with no margin for error may be better served with better-established surgical approaches.

Conclusions

Single port laparoscopy represents a very new and exciting frontier in minimally invasive surgery. This approach has the potential to offer patients improved cosmesis, decreased post-operative pain, and shortened convalescence as compared to conventional laparoscopy (Fig. 3). Thus far, outcomes have been favorable in the majority of published series with little to no comparative trials that validate the inferiority or superiority of the single port approach. Based on the existing literature, complications with single port laparoscopy are of a similar nature and occur with a similar frequency to those experienced during standard laparoscopy.

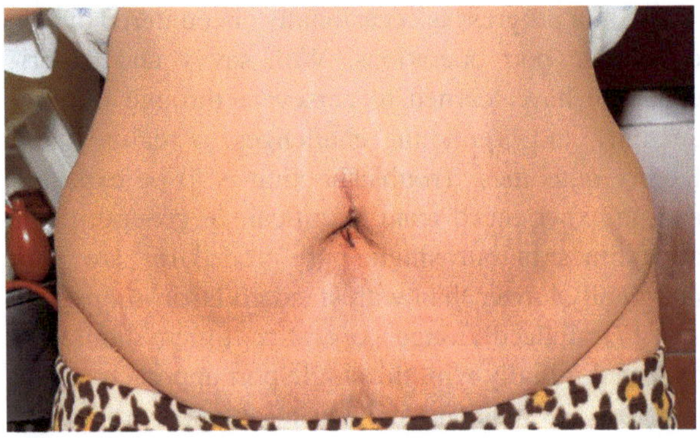

Fig. 3 Surgical scar image at 1 month follow-up after a single port laparoscopic donor nephrectomy

References

1. Gilchrist BF, Vlessis AA, Kay GA, et al. Open versus laparoscopic cholecystectomy: an initial analysis. J Laparoendosc Surg. 1991;1:193–6.
2. Kaouk JH, Haber GP, Goel RK, et al. Single-port laparoscopic surgery in urology: initial experience. Urology. 2008;71:3–6.
3. Desai MM, Rao PP, Aron M, et al. Scarless single port transumbilical nephrectomy and pyeloplasty: first clinical report. BJU Int. 2008;101:83–8.
4. Raman JD, Cadeddu JA, Rao P, et al. Single-incision laparoscopic surgery: initial urological experience and comparison with natural-orifice transluminal endoscopic surgery. BJU Int. 2008;101:493–6.
5. Bishoff JT, Kavoussi LR. Laparoscopic surgery of the kidney. In: Kavoussi LR, Novick AC, Partin AW, Peters CA, Wein AJ, editors. Campbell-Walsh urology. 9th ed. Philadelphia, PA: Saunders; 2007. pp. 1759–809.
6. Wheeless CR. A rapid, inexpensive and effective method of surgical sterilization by laparoscopy. J Reprod Med. 1969;3:65–9.
7. Pelosi MA, Pelosi MA 3rd. Laparoscopic hysterectomy with bilateral salpingo-oophorectomy using a single umbilical puncture. N J Med. 1991;88:721–6.
8. D'Alessio A, Piro E, Tadini B, et al. One-trocar transumbilical laparoscopic-assisted appendectomy in children: our experience. Eur J Pediatr Surg. 2002;12:24–7.
9. Rane A, Kommu S, Eddy B, et al. Clinical evaluation of a novel laparoscopic port (R-port) and evolution of the single laparoscopic port procedure (SLiPP). J Endourol. 2007;21 Suppl 1:A22–3.
10. White WM, Goel RK, Kaouk JH. Single port laparoscopic retroperitoneal surgery: initial operative experience and comparative outcomes. Urology. 2009;73(6):1279.
11. White WM, Goel RK, Swartz MA, et al. Single port laparoscopic abdominal sacral colpopexy: initial experience and comparative outcomes. Urology. 2009;74(5):1008–12.
12. Gill IS, Canes D, Aron M, et al. Single port transumbilical (E-NOTES) donor nephrectomy. J Urol. 2008;180: 637–41.
13. Stein RJ, White WM, Goel RK, et al. Robotic laparoendoscopic single-site surgery using GelPort as the access platform. Eur Urol. 2010;57(1):132–6.
14. 2008 Medical Innovation Summit Cleveland Clinic, Cleveland, OH. November 10–12, 2008.
15. Fahlenkamp D, Rassweiler J, Fornara P, et al. Complications of laparoscopic procedures in urology: experience with 2,407 procedures at 4 German centers. J Urol. 1999;162:765–70.
16. Vallancien G, Cathelineau X, Baumert H, et al. Complications of transperitoneal laparoscopic surgery in urology: review of 1,311 procedures at a single center. J Urol. 2002;168:23–6.
17. White WM, Haber GP, Goel RK, et al. Single port urologic surgery: single center experience with the first 100 cases. Urology. 2009;74(4):801–4.
18. Irwin BH, Berger A, Tracy CR, et al. Factors leading to conversion from single port to conventional laparoscopy: a multi-institutional study. J Urol. 2009;181:531.
19. Desai MM, Berger A, Aron M, et al. Single-Port Transvesical Enucleation of the Prostate (STEP): clinical experience. J Urol. 2009;181:699.
20. Kaouk JH, Goel RK. Single-port laparoscopic and robotic partial nephrectomy. Eur Urol. 2009;55(5):1163–9.
21. Kaouk JH, Goel RK, Haber GP, et al. Single-port laparoscopic radical prostatectomy. Urology. 2008;72: 10.1190–3.
22. Desai MM, Stein R, Rao P, et al. Embryonic natural orifice transumbilical endoscopic surgery (E-NOTES) for advanced reconstruction: initial experience. Urology. 2009;73:182–7.
23. Aron M, Canes D, Desai MM, et al. Transumbilical single-port laparoscopic partial nephrectomy. BJU Int. 2008;103:516–21.
24. Ponsky LE, Cherullo EE, Sawyer M, et al. Single access site laparoscopic radical nephrectomy: initial clinical experience. J Endourol. 2008;22:663–6.
25. Rane A, Ahmed S, Kommu SS, et al. Single-port 'scarless' laparoscopic nephrectomies: the United Kingdom experience. BJU Int. 2009;104(2):230–3.

Complications of Ablative Renal Procedures

Chad R. Tracy and Jeffrey A. Cadeddu

Keywords Ablation · Laparoscopy · Cryotherapy · Radiofrequency · Complication

Introduction

Increasing use of sonography, computed tomography (CT), and magnetic resonance imaging (MRI) has led to a rapid rise in the discovery of small renal tumors and an increase in detection of renal cell cancer (RCC). Although these incidentally discovered masses tend to be smaller and of lower grade than symptomatic lesions [1, 2], the majority (65–80%) of these tumors are renal cell carcinomas (RCC) when pathologically analyzed [3]. In addition, nearly 60% of these lesions will exhibit growth during active surveillance (mean 0.26 cm/year), such that given a long life expectancy, lesions in younger patients may grow sufficiently to become symptomatic or to metastasize [4].

While radical nephrectomy has traditionally been considered the "gold standard" for treatment of renal masses, nephron-sparing surgery has developed into a widely accepted alternative given intermediate-term and long-term cancer control rates similar to radical nephrectomy [5, 6]. Laparoscopic partial nephrectomy improves postoperative pain and shortens convalescence when compared to open surgery, but the surgery is technically demanding and associated with complication rates similar to open partial nephrectomy [7, 8]. Due to these limitations and the increased detection of tumors in younger patients, there is an ongoing interest toward development of minimally invasive therapies for renal tumors, including tissue ablative techniques.

In situ ablation methods such as radiofrequency ablation (RFA) and cryotherapy offer potential benefits compared to the extirpative approach, including a decreased complication rate, shorter convalescence, absence of an ischemic period, and the possibility of using intravenous sedation over general anesthesia [2, 9]. All of these potential benefits are clearly desirable in the increasingly older, sicker patients who represent an increasing proportion of patients with incidental renal masses. While these potential benefits make renal tumor ablation attractive for both patient and surgeon, successful cancer control and an ability to recognize potential complications of therapy are required prior to broad adoption of these technologies.

Indications and Anatomic Considerations

Prospective clinical trials validating the clinical indications for renal mass ablation are lacking in the literature. Early studies of ablation included primarily patients with compromised renal function, multiple or bilateral tumors, or those patients who were determined to be poor surgical candidates due to significant co-morbidities. As experience has increased and results have continued to appear promising, more

J.A. Cadeddu (✉)
Clinical Center for Minimally Invasive Surgery, University of Texas Southwestern Medical Center, Dallas, TX, USA
e-mail: jeffrey.cadeddu@utsouthwestern.edu

R. Ghavamian (ed.), *Complications of Laparoscopic and Robotic Urologic Surgery*,
DOI 10.1007/978-1-60761-676-4_22, © Springer Science+Business Media, LLC 2010

treatments are being carried out on healthier patients with solitary small renal masses. Candidates for ablation generally include patients with small solid renal masses (<4 cm) with contrast enhancement (≥10–12 Hounsfield Units) on computed tomography (CT) or magnetic resonance imaging (MRI). In addition, tumors must be located > 0.5 cm from the ureteropelvic junction or renal pelvis and >1 cm from segmental renal vessels. Ablation is offered as an alternative to open partial nephrectomy, laparoscopic partial nephrectomy, or laparoscopic radical nephrectomy in these patients.

Ablative technologies may be performed through either a percutaneous approach or a laparoscopic approach based on tumor location. Injury to adjacent organs, including bowel, liver, spleen, and the renal collecting system, may lead to significant morbidity. In order to avoid these injuries, anterior tumors within 1 cm of colon or small bowel and those in close proximity to the ureter or renal pelvis should be managed with a laparoscopic approach. Posterior or laterally based tumors that are far removed from adjacent structures may be ablated percutaneously under CT or MR guidance [10].

Technique for Percutaneous Ablation

Prior to percutaneous ablation, CT imaging is performed in order to confirm tumor accessibility and intravenous contrast is administered in order to further delineate the lesion. A 20-Gauge Chiba needle is directed to the rim of the tumor and the CT scan is repeated. If positioning is correct, the ablative probe is advanced to the rim of the tumor. With RFA, the tines are deployed in order to create an ablation zone approximately 5–10 mm beyond the tumor margin. In CA, one or more cryoneedles are placed in order to completely ablate the mass based on the size of the tumor and the size of the probes being used. After the probe has been placed, an 18-Gauge true-cut biopsy needle is used to obtain 2–3 biopsy specimens. Biopsy should not be performed prior to probe placement, as bleeding from the tumor may obscure the radiographic appearance of the mass. After confirmation of probe placement based on CT, we routinely carry out RFA ablation using the RITA Medical Systems (Angiodynamics, Queensbury, NY) model 1500 RF generator coupled to the 14-Gauge Starburst XL probe. Ablation is based on manufacturer's recommendations (less than 2 cm ablated for 5 min, 2–3 cm for 7 min, and over 3 cm for 8 min), with a 30 s cool-down period followed by a second ablation cycle of identical duration. CA is performed by monitoring the size of the ice ball based on intraoperative imaging (CT or Ultrasound) or by placement of temperature-sensing probes at the periphery of the lesion. The primary ablation is complete once the ice ball reaches approximately 5–10 mm beyond the tumor margin and then a second ablation is typically performed following a period of active thawing. With RFA, tract ablation is performed by withdrawing the tines into the probe and then gradually removing the probe through Gerota's fascia, keeping probe temperature above 70°C.

Technique for Laparoscopic Ablation

After induction of general anesthesia, the patient is positioned in the modified flank position at 30–45° and three trocars are placed with a 12 mm trocar in the umbilicus, a 5 mm trocar one-third of the way down between the xiphoid and umbilicus, and a 12 mm trocar in the mid-clavicular line 2–4 cm below the umbilicus. After the lesion is exposed by reflecting the bowel and dissecting the perinephric fat, a laparoscopic ultrasound probe is brought through the inferior laparoscopic port in order to confirm the lesion characteristics including size and depth of penetration. The ablation probe(s) is introduced through a separate stab incision along a perpendicular orientation to the tumor surface and probe placement is confirmed by intraoperative ultrasound. Once probe placement is confirmed, ablation is carried out as detailed above. Biopsies during laparoscopic CA can be performed prior to probe placement using a biopsy needle, but must be performed prior to ablation. Conversely, we routinely perform RFA biopsies using a 5 mm toothed biopsy forceps *after* the ablation is complete in order obtain larger tissue samples and prevent intraoperative hemorrhage. We have previously shown that post-ablation biopsies are fully interpretable by pathologists and equivalent to pre-treatment biopsy specimens [11]. Whereas real-time monitoring of ablation during laparoscopic RFA is not possible due to radiofrequency interference and formation of microbubbles, ultrasound is routinely employed to monitor the size of the growing ice ball during laparoscopic CA.

Safety and Complications

Complications following ablative treatment of renal masses are relatively uncommon, with one multi-institutional study reporting an overall complication rate of 11% [12]. Of these complications the majority are minor with major complications occurring in less than 2% of cases [12]. However, up to 20% of complications may require hospital readmission, procedural intervention, or transfusion [12]. Laparoscopic ablation tends to have a higher rate of complications when compared to the percutaneous ablation, with an estimated one-third of laparoscopic ablation complications occurring as a result of laparoscopic technique [12]. Complications decrease significantly, regardless of surgical approach, with increasing operative experience.

While laparoscopic access appears to be associated with a higher complication rate, comparing cryosurgical ablation to radiofrequency ablation is more difficult based on a lack of randomized trials. Cryoablation and radiofrequency ablation studies vary in how they report results as well as in how the procedure is performed (equipment, ablation time, generator used, etc.). Overall, the majority of complications do not appear to be significantly different between the two modalities. One theorized advantage to cryotherapy may be that, in the absence of puncture to the collecting system, direct freezing of the urothelium rarely leads to the development of urinary fistula [13, 14]. However, there have been several reports of urinary fistula or collecting system injury following radiofrequency ablation [15, 16] and recently cryoablation [17]. On the other hand, significant bleeding (requiring a blood transfusion) has been seen in up to 27.8% of patients undergoing laparoscopic cryoablation and 11.1% of patients undergoing percutaneous cryoablation [18], compared to a rate less than 1% in most of the larger series on radiofrequency ablation [19, 20].

In order to prevent or at least minimize the risk of complications with percutaneous and laparoscopic ablation, it is important to recognize potential pitfalls

Table 1 Avoidance maneuvers and management of complications from ablative renal procedures

Complication	Avoidance maneuvers	Management
General Surgical Considerations Underlying medical conditions Coagulopathy	Thorough history, physical, and pre-operative work-up	Complication specific Anticoagulation stopped pre-operatively based on specific medication
Damage to surrounding structures Intra-renal collecting system Extra-renal collecting system Pleural cavity/Lung Colon Liver Spleen Posterior body-wall nerves	Appropriate position-specific pre-operative imaging Use of "finder needle" Hydro-dissection of surrounding tissues Strong consideration to laparoscopic approach	Conservative management generally effective Failure of conservative management may require operative intervention, including: ureteral stent placement, fecal diversion, or splenectomy based on specific injury Repair of any injury found during initial laparoscopic ablation
Intraoperative and postoperative hemorrhage Renal bleeding Body wall (intercostal arteries)	RFA – tract ablation during probe removal CA – avoidance of multiple probes if possible; avoid removing probes prior to thawing of ice ball Avoid placing probes directly subcostal	Conservative management generally effective Use of hemostatic agents and direct pressure during laparoscopic ablation Serial imaging for persistent hematomas Angioembolization if bleeding is persistent
Body wall/Skin complications Pain/Paresthesia Electrical skin burns (RFA) Freezer damage (CA)	RFA – do not ablate tract outside of Gerota's fascia RFA – place grounding pads appropriately	Oral pain medications Most injuries heal over time
Infectious complications Urinary tract infection Perinephric abscess	Pre-operative urine cultures in at risk patients	Perioperative prophylaxis Treat urinary tract infections pre-operatively when possible Pathogen-specific antibiotics
Complications unrelated to ablation technique Anesthetic risks Surgical risks	Appropriate pre-operative screening and medical work-up	Complication-specific

in technique and to plan appropriately in order to prevent unnecessary morbidity. Indeed, it has been demonstrated that as surgeons become more familiar with these techniques, complication rates diminish with experience [12]. Complications can be broadly separated into general surgical considerations, damage to surrounding structures (including the urinary tract), intraoperative and postoperative hemorrhage, abdominal wall injury, infection, and complications unrelated to the surgical technique, such as respiratory difficulty following anesthesia (Table 1).

General Surgical Considerations

There are few strict contraindications to renal mass ablation including an uncorrected coagulopathy and the patient's overall medical condition. Patients should have pre-operative coagulation studies (PT/PTT) and should be held from all medications that may alter platelet activity, including aspirin and clopidogrel. Patients with known bleeding disorders should be optimized with the help of a hematologist in order to prevent significant bleeding during the procedure. If concern remains for risk of bleeding or if anticoagulation must be restored immediately after ablation, RFA as a coagulative technology may be preferred over cryoablation. In regard to the patient's overall health, all patients should undergo a detailed medical and surgical history, with more focused studies (e.g., EKG, chest radiograph) if required due to patient age or risk factors for medical disease.

When performing percutaneous ablation, the choice of anesthesia should be a joint decision between surgeon and patient. While local anesthesia may be favored in many institutions, some authors have indicated that ablation success may be lower under sedation when compared to general anesthesia [21]. Patients treated under sedation may become uncomfortable during long or complex ablation procedures, such that use of general anesthesia may be more favorable under these circumstances. In addition to patient comfort, general anesthesia may allow for more precise probe placement by allowing control of ventilation, such that probe placement and renal position is reproducible throughout the procedure.

General contraindications to laparoscopic surgery apply to laparoscopic ablation, including multiple intra-abdominal adhesions, history of peritonitis, bowel distention, and severe chronic obstructive pulmonary disease (COPD). As previously mentioned laparoscopy should be considered the primary approach for all patients with anterior lesions and for those with lesions located within close proximity to other intra-abdominal organs, as intraoperative dissection allows for an increased margin for safely avoiding adjacent structures.

Damage to Surrounding Structures

Complications from damage to surrounding intra-abdominal organs can be minimized through appropriate patient selection, pre-operative planning, and good surgical technique. In this regard, pre-operative imaging is essential in order to determine if a tumor should be managed with a laparoscopic or percutaneous approach. All patients scheduled for ablative renal procedures should, at a minimum, undergo a supine spiral CT scan in order to delineate tumor margins with respect to renal anatomy and surrounding organs. In those patients with lateral tumors or tumors near surrounding organs, patients should undergo further imaging in order to determine whether there will be a suitable access tract to their tumor. For instance, a patient who has difficult access to the tumor due to the spleen lying within close proximity may be placed in the right lateral decubitus position over a small kidney cushion in order to role the spleen anteriorly and allow for direct percutaneous access. Patients with anterior tumors, tumors close to the collecting system, or without a suitable access tract on pre-operative imaging, should be scheduled for laparoscopic ablation. Ideal patients for percutaneous treatment are those with posterior tumors, those with tumors located > 0.5 cm from the ureteropelvic junction or renal pelvis, and those with tumors at least 1 cm from surrounding bowel.

During percutaneous access, damage to surrounding organs can be limited with the employment of a "finder needle" prior to placement of the ablation probe(s). Once the lesion location and a clear access path have been confirmed by planning CT, a 20-Gauge Chiba needle is directed such that the tip of the needle is located adjacent to the rim of the central portion of the tumor. By using a small caliber needle, it is possible to have a trial of probe placement without introducing the risk of organ damage associated with the larger probe. Once the needle is placed, its distance and approximate angle can be judged in order to appropriately place the treatment needle(s).

Involvement of the urinary tract in the ablation zone may present as minor hematuria, hematuria with significant clots, or obstruction of urinary drainage due to urothelial damage. Patients with hematuria should be managed conservatively. Retrograde renal cooling during radiofrequency ablation may protect the urothelium, though this technique is rarely used in clinical practice [22]. If hematuria is significant, continuous bladder irrigation may be instituted, though this is rarely helpful due to clots forming in the renal pelvis rather than the bladder. If hematuria results in significant bleeding, some patients may require selective angioembolization. Permanent urothelial damage may present as either calyceal obstruction (Fig. 1) or ureteral obstruction if damage occurs at the UPJ or distally. In extreme cases, damage to the urinary tract may result in perirenal urinoma formation or cutaneous urinary fistula. While calyceal obstruction may be observed conservatively, patients with ureteral obstruction or urine leakage from the collecting system should be managed with insertion of an indwelling ureteral stent. Patients with significant urinoma accumulation should have a percutaneous drain placed.

Injury to the pleural cavity resulting in pneumothorax or hemothorax can occur if probes are placed above the 12th rib in order to treat upper pole lesions. These complications are typically recognized during the procedure as either breathing difficulties or, with percutaneous access, on routine imaging during tumor treatment. If a simple pneumothorax is identified, it may be treated by aspiration using a small needle inserted into the pleural space at the conclusion of the case. As lung parenchymal injury is rare, placement of a chest tube should be performed sparingly. Nevertheless, large or persistent pneumothorax or hemothorax should be managed with chest tube insertion and overnight observation. Postoperatively, chest pain or shortness of breath should trigger suspicion of pneumothorax and prompt performance of an upright chest radiograph.

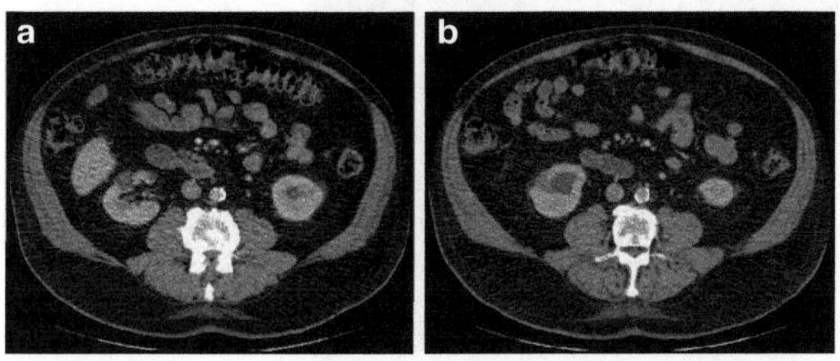

Fig. 1 Follow-up imaging 18 months after undergoing right RFA demonstrates (**a**) adequate ablation of a right renal mass with (**b**) subsequent development of a lower pole hydrocalyx secondary to a stenotic infundibulum. The hydrocalyx continues to be followed and remains unchanged after 4 years

Colon injury following renal mass ablation is exceedingly rare and should be largely preventable with appropriate surgical technique. During percutaneous access, tumors within close proximity to bowel may be dissected free from the treatment area by injecting saline in order to hydro-dissect tissues and develop a safe working space around the tumor [23–25]. However, reproducibility and surgeon familiarity with the patient's anatomy may make these lesions more suitable for the laparoscopic approach where the bowel can be safely removed from the operative field. Patients with colon damage should be managed along with a general surgical consultation. Patients with a controlled colon-nephric fistula should be initially managed with placement of a ureteral stent, while those with a persistent fistula or with colon-cutaneous fistulas may require surgical diversion or a trial of total peripheral nutrition (TPN) [26, 27]. Patients with frank colon perforation and signs of peritonitis should be managed with prompt surgical exploration.

When treating posterior tumors percutaneously, it is important to be cognizant of the nerves running along the posterior body wall. Damage to these nerves or to the surrounding musculature can lead to severe postoperative pain [28]. In addition, damage to the genitofemoral nerve, resulting in severe paresthesias, has been reported [25]. This complication can be avoided by positioning the patient so that the tumor falls away from the body wall or by hydro-dissecting the plane between kidney and body wall [25]. For patients with multiple posterior tumors or with limited perinephric fat between the kidney and the body wall, strong consideration should be given to the laparoscopic approach where the kidney can be physically moved away from the body wall.

Intraoperative and Postoperative Hemorrhage

Intraoperative or postoperative hemorrhage may occur in up to 11–27% of patients undergoing ablative renal procedures [18]. The primary risk factor for hemorrhage is the use of multiple probes for treatment of larger renal masses. In addition, cryosurgery may have an increased rate of hemorrhage due to ice ball "fracture" where parenchymal lacerations may develop between adjacently placed cryoprobes. In order to decrease this complication during CA, probes should be given adequate time to thaw, as premature removal increases the risk of tumor fracture. Although perirenal hematoma formation is relatively common (Fig. 2), significant bleeding requiring blood transfusion is rare. If bleeding is noticed during the procedure, the ablation should proceed as planned, as the ablation may slow or stop the bleeding focus, particularly with the cauterizing effect of RFA. Bleeding during laparoscopic ablation can be managed with the use of hemostatic agents including FloSeal (Baxter Healthcare Co., Deerfield, IL) and Surgicel (Ethicon Inc., Somerville, NJ) combined with direct pressure using laparoscopic graspers or the face of the ultrasound probe. If bleeding continues post-ablation, the hematoma may be monitored with serial imaging with consideration given to selective angioembolization.

Abdominal Wall/Skin Complications

The most common complication following renal tumor ablation is pain or paresthesia at the percutaneous probe insertion site, occurring in up to 8% of patients [29]. Early generations of cryotherapy probes did not contain thermal insulation around the proximal portion of the probe, such that the entire probe was cooled, often leading to pain and freezer burn injuries to the skin surface. With newer versions of the cryoprobes, however, an insulating sheath has dramatically reduced

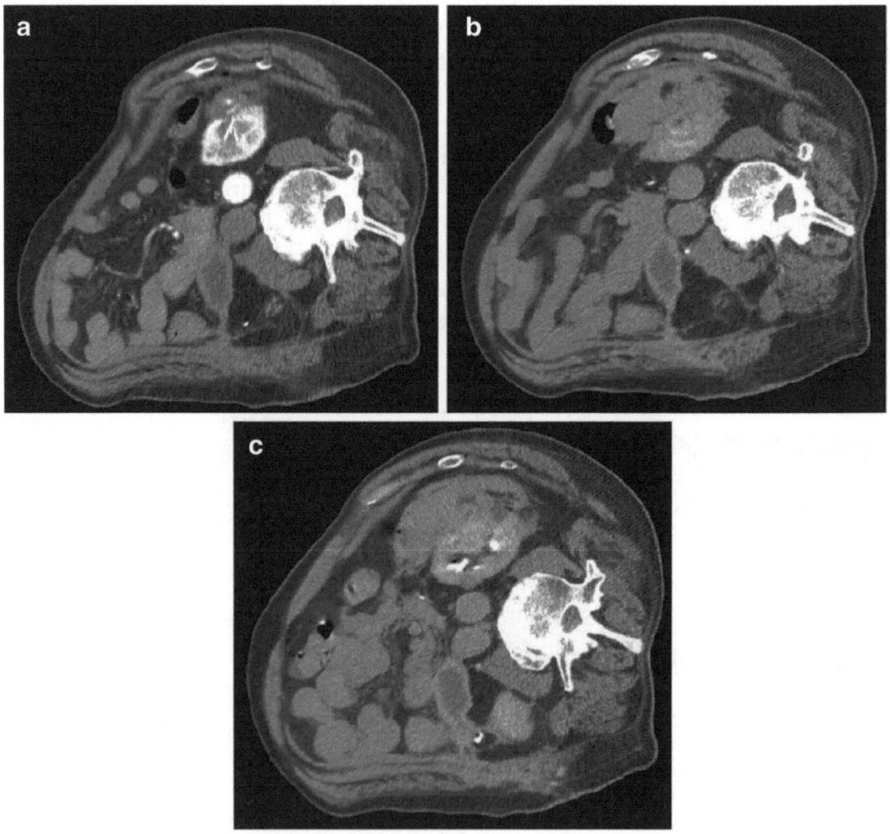

Fig. 2 RFA of left endophytic renal mass complicated by perinephric hematoma. (**a**) Initial tine placement within the left renal mass leads to the immediate development of a small perinephric hematoma that (**b, c**) expands around the lateral aspect of the kidney before stabilizing. This patient was managed conservatively with overnight observation without further sequelae

these complications. With RFA the active portion of the probe is located on at the distal most portion, so that heat is only generated within the targeted tissue. While heat may be conducted to adjacent tissues, the probe itself does not generate heat at the skin surface. Neural injury from RFA, therefore, does not typically occur during the ablation procedure, but rather occurs during tract ablation. In order to prevent inadvertent nerve damage, the tract ablation should be carried out only long enough to remove the probe from the kidney and surrounding Gerota's fascia. Pain and/or paresthesia following ablation is generally self-limited and may be adequately treated with oral pain medications, though persistent pain has been reported [29]. Patients with posteriorly located tumors should be counseled that they may have increased periprocedural narcotic requirements and may elect to undergo a laparoscopic approach [28].

As with any percutaneous needle placement, ablative renal procedures risk damage to the abdominal wall vasculature. While the majority of these injuries are difficult to avoid, care should be taken to minimize damage to intercostal arteries by avoiding needle placement directly below the ribs. When injury to a vessel occurs during percutaneous ablation, it is typically visualized during the procedure with routine imaging (Fig. 3). Bleeding from a vessel may not be immediately identified during laparoscopic ablation, though there should be significant concern if blood is seen tracking down or around the ablation probe. As with renal bleeding, the expanding hematoma may be observed with serial imaging (if rapidly expanding) or serial hematocrits (if stable), with only the rare case requiring angiographic embolization.

Electrical skin burns following radiofrequency ablation should be incredibly rare. Radiofrequency ablation requires placement of grounding pads on in order to complete the electrical circuit and allow return of the monopolar alternating current to the generator. Because of the high amounts of energy used with radiofrequency ablation, improper placement of the pads may result in severe burns to the skin where the pads are located [30]. In order to prevent injury, two grounding pads are used (one the posterior of each thigh) and should be placed at exactly the same level on each leg. As energy returning to the generator travels in the shortest arc, the pads should be placed perpendicular to the long axis of the thigh to increase surface area for energy dissipation.

Infectious Complications

Postoperative infection following tumor ablation, in the absence of a large hematoma or urinoma, is exceedingly rare. Patients at risk for infection are those with

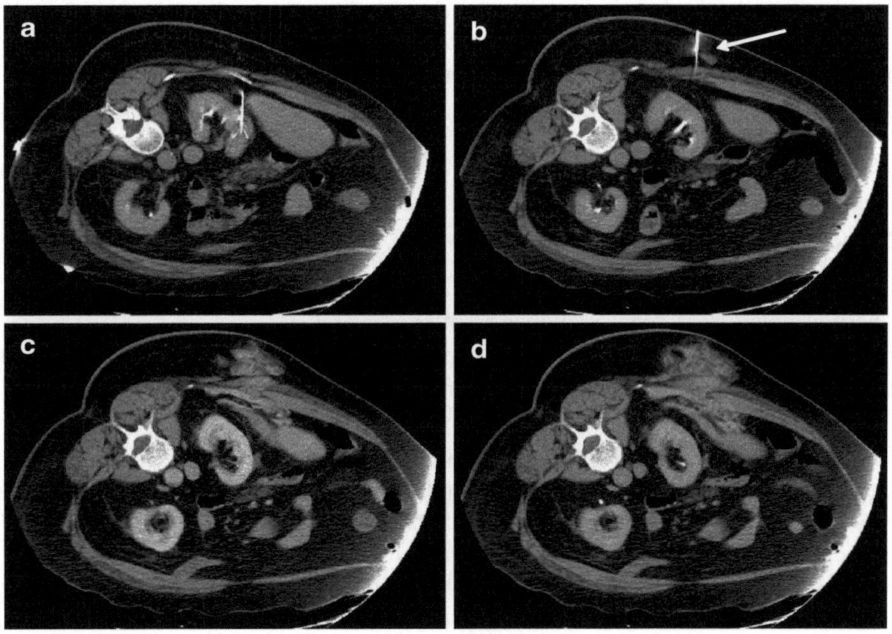

Fig. 3 Radiofrequency ablation of a 2.5 cm mesophytic right renal mass complicated by intercostal vessel injury. (**a**) Initial tine placement in the mass. (**b**) A small hematoma (*arrow*) developed in the subcutaneous tissue, followed by significant expansion over the next 20 min (**c, d**). Hematoma formation was self-limited and the patient was managed conservatively

chronic colonization of the urinary tract (e.g., Ileal conduit) or active infection at the time of procedure [17, 31]. When infectious complications do occur, they typically present anywhere from one week to 6 months as a chronic drainage or retroperitoneal abscess. Patients at risk for urinary tract infection should be screened by urine culture and treated appropriately prior to their ablation procedure. While we routinely administer perioperative prophylactic antibiotics at the time of the surgery, some authors suggest broad-spectrum coverage 2 days prior and two weeks after surgery for patients at high risk of infection [31].

Complications Unrelated to Ablative Technique

Patients undergoing renal mass ablation are typically older and sicker than those who undergo partial nephrectomy [32]. Because this tends to be a more at risk population, all patients undergoing percutaneous ablation should undergo thorough medical screening in order to decrease the likelihood of surgical complications. Even with appropriate screening, however, ablative renal procedures continue to carry the risks of any surgical procedure ranging from atrial fibrillation to respiratory failure [33, 34]. In addition to the risks of percutaneous ablation, laparoscopic ablation carries risks specific to the laparoscopic approach including the possibility of open conversion, damage to intra-abdominal organs during access or dissection, and the development of postoperative ileus [12].

Conclusion

Thermal ablation of renal malignancy offers several benefits over extirpative surgery including improved convalescence, minimal postoperative pain, and, in the case of percutaneous ablation, the ability to be performed on an outpatient basis. However, current limitations of ablative surgery, including potential damage to surrounding organs and the intra- and extra-renal collecting system, limits its applicability to a subset of patients with renal malignancy. A thorough knowledge of the procedure and of the potential complications and pitfalls is essential in order to perform ablative renal procedures in a safe and effective manner.

References

1. Pantuck AJ, Zisman A, Rauch MK, Belldegrun A. Incidental renal tumors. Urology. Aug 1 2000;56(2):190–6.
2. Luciani LG, Cestari R, Tallarigo C. Incidental renal cell carcinoma-age and stage characterization and clinical implications: study of 1092 patients (1982–1997). Urology. Jul 2000;56(1):58–62.
3. Remzi M, Memarsadeghi M. Small incidental renal tumors. Evaluation and biological parameters. Urologe A. May 2007;46(5):478, 480–74.
4. Abouassaly R, Lane BR, Novick AC. Active surveillance of renal masses in elderly patients. J Urol. Aug 2008;180(2):505–8; discussion 508–9.
5. Lane BR, Novick AC, Babineau D, Fergany AF, Kaouk JH, Gill IS. Comparison of laparoscopic and open partial nephrectomy for tumor in a solitary kidney. J Urol. Mar 2008;179(3):847–51; discussion 852.
6. Gill IS, Kavoussi LR, Lane BR, et al. Comparison of 1,800 laparoscopic and open partial nephrectomies for single renal tumors. J Urol. Jul 2007;178(1):41–6.
7. Matin SF, Gill IS, Worley S, Novick AC. Outcome of laparoscopic radical and open partial nephrectomy for the sporadic 4 cm or less renal tumor with a normal contralateral kidney. J Urol. Oct 2002;168(4 Pt 1):1356–9; discussion 1359–60.
8. Ramani AP, Desai MM, Steinberg AP, et al. Complications of laparoscopic partial nephrectomy in 200 cases. J Urol. Jan 2005;173(1):42–7.
9. Allaf ME, Varkarakis IM, Bhayani SB, Inagaki T, Kavoussi LR, Solomon SB. Pain control requirements for percutaneous ablation of renal tumors: cryoablation versus radiofrequency ablation – initial observations. Radiology. Oct 2005;237(1):366–70.
10. Ogan K, Jacomides L, Dolmatch BL, et al. Percutaneous radiofrequency ablation of renal tumors: technique, limitations, and morbidity. Urology. Dec 2002;60(6):954–8.
11. Margulis V, Matsumoto ED, Lindberg G, et al. Acute histologic effects of temperature-based radiofrequency ablation on renal tumor pathologic interpretation. Urology. Oct 2004;64(4):660–3.
12. Johnson DB, Solomon SB, Su LM, et al. Defining the complications of cryoablation and radio frequency ablation of small renal tumors: a multi-institutional review. J Urol. Sep 2004;172(3):874–7.
13. Sung GT, Gill IS, Hsu TH, et al. Effect of intentional cryo-injury to the renal collecting system. J Urol. Aug 2003;170(2 Pt 1):619–22.
14. Warlick CA, Lima GC, Allaf ME, et al. Clinical sequelae of radiographic iceball involvement of collecting system during computed tomography-guided percutaneous renal tumor cryoablation. Urology. May 2006;67(5):918–22.
15. Janzen NK, Perry KT, Han KR, et al. The effects of intentional cryoablation and radio frequency ablation of renal

tissue involving the collecting system in a porcine model. J Urol. Apr 2005;173(4):1368–74.
16. Gervais DA, Arellano RS, McGovern FJ, McDougal WS, Mueller PR. Radiofrequency ablation of renal cell carcinoma: part 2. Lessons learned with ablation of 100 tumors. AJR Am J Roentgenol. Jul 2005;185(1):72–80.
17. Brown DB, Bhayani SB. Persistent urine leak after cryoablation of a renal tumor in a patient with an ileal conduit. J Vasc Interv Radiol. Oct 2007;18(10):1324–7.
18. Finley DS, Beck S, Box G, et al. Percutaneous and laparoscopic cryoablation of small renal masses. J Urol. Aug 2008;180(2):492–8; discussion 498.
19. Hegarty NJ, Gill IS, Desai MM, Remer EM, O'Malley CM, Kaouk JH. Probe-ablative nephron-sparing surgery: cryoablation versus radiofrequency ablation. Urology. Jul 2006;68 Suppl 1:7–13.
20. Park S, Cadeddu JA. Outcomes of radiofrequency ablation for kidney cancer. Cancer Control. Jul 2007;14(3): 205–10.
21. Hui GC, Tuncali K, Tatli S, Morrison PR, Silverman SG. Comparison of percutaneous and surgical approaches to renal tumor ablation: metaanalysis of effectiveness and complication rates. J Vasc Interv Radiol. Sep 2008;19(9):1311–20.
22. Margulis V, Matsumoto ED, Taylor G, Shaffer S, Kabbani W, Cadeddu JA. Retrograde renal cooling during radio frequency ablation to protect from renal collecting system injury. J Urol. Jul 2005;174(1):350–2.
23. Clark TW, Malkowicz B, Stavropoulos SW, et al. Radiofrequency ablation of small renal cell carcinomas using multitined expandable electrodes: preliminary experience. J Vasc Interv Radiol. Mar 2006;17(3): 513–9.
24. Farrell MA, Charboneau JW, Callstrom MR, Reading CC, Engen DE, Blute ML. Paranephric water instillation: a technique to prevent bowel injury during percutaneous renal radiofrequency ablation. AJR Am J Roentgenol. Nov 2003;181(5):1315–7.
25. Lee SJ, Choyke LT, Locklin JK, Wood BJ. Use of hydrodissection to prevent nerve and muscular damage during radiofrequency ablation of kidney tumors. J Vasc Interv Radiol. Dec 2006;17(12):1967–9.
26. Weizer AZ, Raj GV, O'Connell M, Robertson CN, Nelson RC, Polascik TJ. Complications after percutaneous radiofrequency ablation of renal tumors. Urology. Dec 2005;66(6):1176–80.
27. Vanderbrink BA, Rastinehad A, Caplin D, Ost MC, Lobko I, Lee BR. Successful conservative management of colorenal fistula after percutaneous cryoablation of renal-cell carcinoma. J Endourol. Jul 2007;21(7):726–9.
28. Baker M, Anderson JK, Jaffer O, Trimmer C, Cadeddu JA. Pain after percutaneous radiofrequency ablation of renal tumors. J Endourol. Jun 2007;21(6):606–9.
29. Farrell MA, Charboneau WJ, DiMarco DS, et al. Imaging-guided radiofrequency ablation of solid renal tumors. AJR Am J Roentgenol. Jun 2003;180(6):1509–13.
30. McDougal WS, Gervais DA, McGovern FJ, Mueller PR. Long-term followup of patients with renal cell carcinoma treated with radio frequency ablation with curative intent. J Urol. Jul 2005;174(1):61–3.
31. Wah TM, Irving HC. Infectious complications after percutaneous radiofrequency ablation of renal cell carcinoma in patients with ileal conduit. J Vasc Interv Radiol. Sep 2008;19(9):1382–5.
32. Hruby G, Reisiger K, Venkatesh R, Yan Y, Landman J. Comparison of laparoscopic partial nephrectomy and laparoscopic cryoablation for renal hilar tumors. Urology. Jan 2006;67(1):50–4.
33. Bandi G, Wen CC, Hedican SP, Moon TD, Lee FT Jr, Nakada SY. Cryoablation of small renal masses: assessment of the outcome at one institution. BJU Int. Oct 2007;100(4):798–801.
34. Hinshaw JL, Shadid AM, Nakada SY, Hedican SP, Winter TC 3rd, Lee FT Jr. Comparison of percutaneous and laparoscopic cryoablation for the treatment of solid renal masses. AJR Am J Roentgenol. Oct 2008;191(4):1159–68.

Complications of Laparoscopic and Robotic Pediatric Urologic Surgery

Sean T. Corbett

Keywords Pediatric urology · Laparoscopy · Robotics · Complications

Overview

Laparoscopy was a relatively new adjunct in the treatment armamentarium for adult urologic diseases 15 years ago, but it has now become the standard of care in many cases and its applications continue to expand. In pediatric urology the search for appropriate indications for laparoscopic interventions has only recently graduated from its infancy. There is still significant debate among pediatric urologists regarding the benefits of laparoscopic and robotic surgery in infants and children where one could argue that the goal has always been minimally invasive surgery or invasive surgery through small incisions. As pioneers in laparoscopic and robotic techniques in the world of pediatric urology continue to expand the horizons for these techniques they must use caution and balance the drive to expand the field with good patient care. It is also crucial that they play a vital role in the development of the new technology rather than await its arrival. Perhaps much has been learned from the previous lessons of our adult counterparts and the learning curve will be less steep and the technology more broadly applicable. Only time will tell.

Laparoscopic surgery in the practice of pediatric urology up until recently has remained within the larger academic centers of excellence primarily due to the difficulty of learning the techniques and the limitations of the equipment available. However, as the technology continues to improve and now with the benefit of the da Vinci® robotic system, the boundaries of minimally invasive surgery within the pediatric population are expanding at an exponential rate and in a greater number of surgeons' hands. In addition, as the newer generation urologists finish their training programs, a greater number of them are receiving laparoscopic and robotic training in residency and fellowship, which has improved their comfort level [1]. This in turn has resulted in a significant increase in those with endoscopic skills willing to tackle endoscopy in children and infants. Even surgeons with minimal or no formal laparoscopic training have begun to incorporate endoscopic surgery into daily practice with the help of mentorship programs [2]. Another reason we are seeing an increase in the number of endoscopic procedures being performed in the pediatric population is for the same reason we have realized its expansion in the adult population: the robot. Where few laparoscopic surgeons have mastered the fine suturing techniques required for laparoscopic procedures within pediatric urology, the surgical precision of the robot has provided a level of enhancement over laparoscopy that allows a greater number of surgeons to tackle these procedures and continue to push its applicability.

There are certainly challenges unique to the pediatric population that continue to challenge those pursuing minimally invasive surgery and which warrant special consideration. The wide range in size of the patients, both inside and out, makes it difficult to standardize equipment and set up, and so surgeons must

S.T. Corbett (✉)
Department of Urology, University of Virginia,
P.O. Box 800422, Charlottesville, VA 22908-0422, USA
e-mail: stc2u@virginia.edu

R. Ghavamian (ed.), *Complications of Laparoscopic and Robotic Urologic Surgery*,
DOI 10.1007/978-1-60761-676-4_23, © Springer Science+Business Media, LLC 2010

maintain a great degree of flexibility in their approach to these patients and make appropriate adjustments with each case. These limitations can, if not appropriately considered, increase the complications experienced in these operations.

Recognizing the limitations of himself as well as his equipment should be the responsibility of the surgeon to minimize the potential complications that may arise and manage them appropriately when they do.

Although the utility of laparoscopy and robotic surgery remains to be defined, the continued evolution of technology and experience will allow us to push the boundaries of minimally invasive surgery in pediatric urology. However, we must remember that excessive expectations can impede successful development and, in fact, have deleterious effects.

Complications are an undeniable event for all those that operate; they are a statistical fact of life and if a surgeon is not encountering complications then he is probably not operating. As surgeons we are better to expect complications in order that we may be better prepared when they are encountered. This is not to say that surgeons are helpless in their ability to anticipate, avoid, and effectively deal with complications, but rather, by being prepared a surgeon can improve the likelihood of a favorable outcome. In the words of Finagle: "Whatever can go wrong will go wrong, and at the worst possible time, in the worst possible way," so be ready.

As new technologies are incorporated into practice, so too will new complications be observed. Hopefully, with more time and experience the accumulated results will demonstrate that laparoscopy and robotic surgery are not just exciting new technologies useful to a few, but rather innovative approaches to be embraced by the majority and ultimately accepted as the standard of care. We must always heed the experience of the pioneers that have gone before us if we are to be successful and continue to do no harm.

Procedures

The limits of laparoscopy and robotic surgery are constantly being tested. In 1976 Cortesi et al. introduced laparoscopy into urological practice, when they performed laparoscopy to diagnose non-palpable testes [3]. The application did not advance past this for the next 15 years, however, as non-palpable testes remained the only indication for laparoscopy. The last 20 years, however, have been witness to an exponential increase in the indications for laparoscopy in pediatric urology (Fig. 1) [4]. The use of the robot to assist with surgery may push those indications further yet, although the technology needs to catch up to the creativity of the pioneers of laparoscopic and robotic surgery in infants and children.

Procedures:

1. Diagnostic
   i. Cryptorchidism
   ii. Intersex conditions
   iii. Hernia
2. Extirpative surgery
   i. Nephrectomy
   ii. Partial nephrectomy
   iii. Adrenalectomy
   iv. Urachal cysts
   v. Gonadectomy and Müllerian remnants
3. Reconstructive surgery
   i. Orchiopexy
   ii. Hernia
   iii. Varicocele
   iv. Pyeloplasty
   v. Antireflux surgery
   vi. Continent diversion and augmentation

Fig. 1 List of the more common procedures performed endoscopically in the pediatric urologic population

As noted above, laparoscopy for diagnosis has been in use for over 30 years in the case of the non-palpable testis. Laparoscopic orchiopexy was not performed until the mid 1990s, but has become common practice in many centers [5, 6]. The utility of diagnostic laparoscopy for intersex conditions and for the evaluation of hernias is also invaluable. Clearly the adult urologists have proven the benefits of laparoscopy in extirpative surgery with nephrectomy, which has now become the standard of care and only to a slightly lesser degree partial nephrectomy. In children the partial nephrectomy is almost always performed for duplication anomalies versus the adult world where partial nephrectomy is nearly always performed for malignancy [7, 8]. Extirpative techniques have also been applied to urachal anomalies and intersex conditions for gonadectomy and Müllerian remnants [9]. As far as reconstructive surgery in pediatric urology, laparoscopy remains in its infancy although its potential is great [10, 11]. Many procedures have been attempted, but few have been used with any frequency except in the hands of a few obstinate surgeons. Robotic surgery will likely permit more surgeons to use laparoscopic methods for pediatric urology. In most tertiary centers orchiopexy and hernia repairs are performed routinely and certainly pyeloplasty has also become more common [6, 10, 12–15]. Less commonly surgeons have been performing antireflux surgery and complex upper tract reconstruction in children with duplex collecting systems [16, 17], as well as a host of procedures for neurogenic patients, including, continent diversion and augmentation. The technical aspects of the major procedures have not yet been refined to the extent that allows for broad applicability, but that time will likely come.

Patient Selection

Although initial experiences in laparoscopy in pediatric urology were tackled in the young adult and adolescent populations, rightfully so, we have also started to see the age and size boundaries tackled in ways that were difficult to conceptualize previously. As technology continues to advance the size of the patient has become less of a limitation or contraindication, although there remain those surgeons that question the utility of laparoscopy and robotic-assisted laparoscopy (RAL) in place of a single small incision. Can minimally invasive surgery be more minimally invasive? While we ponder this, we must remember that children and infants are more than just little adults. The wide range in size and anatomic variability that exists between the infant and the adolescent requires flexibility and the ability to adjust appropriately. Although landmarks and abnormalities in children are typically palpable this is not always the case as we have seen due to rising rates of obesity in the younger populations. Obesity in particular will continue to plague pediatric urologists, as there is no sign that the current upward trend in obesity will change anytime soon. In the most capable hands, laparoscopy in obese children has for the most part proven easier than open surgery although access can sometimes be a challenge and remains a limitation for the less dogged surgeon.

The robot continues to expand the applicability of laparoscopic surgery to a greater number of pediatric urologic surgeons but it also poses a unique set of challenges based on its size relative to this patient population. It can be a challenge to see, let alone access the patient once the robot is engaged and these limitations must be borne in mind by the surgical and anesthetic teams in case emergency access becomes necessary.

In general, most laparoscopic and robotic surgeons in pediatric urology still try to avoid procedures in the very young and very small patient, but again, the boundaries continue to expand as attempts at fetal laparoscopic and robotic procedures have been undertaken by some centers in animal models to help determine their feasibility. Pediatric urologists are continuing to push the envelope irrespective of patient age or size, refusing to be limited in these regards.

Contraindications

As surgeon's experience with evolved technologies continues to improve we find ourselves less encumbered or limited by what may have been considered a contraindication in the recent past. There will always be some relatively constant absolute contraindications such as uncorrectable coagulopathy, pregnancy, bowel obstruction, and generalized peritonitis. However, the list of relative contraindications decreases regularly especially in very capable hands. Even in pediatric urology, where the size of the patient was thought to limit the applicability of laparoscopy and more recently robotic-assisted laparoscopy to the larger child or adolescent we continue to push the limits. Diagnostic laparoscopy has been in the armamentarium of most pediatric urologists now for over 20 years but technological advances have amplified our ability to manage these patients. The role of endoscopic surgery in pediatric urology is evolving rapidly; its limits are yet to be determined.

Laparoscopy Versus Robotic Surgery

Laparoscopy in pediatric urology offers significant benefits to patients as it has in the adult population. We have seen its applicability expanded from its initial use as an adjunct to diagnosis in the case of the undescended, non-palpable testicle to extirpative surgery in the case of partial nephrectomy and more recently to reconstructive surgery in the case of pyeloplasty. The laparoscopic interface improves visualization with the use of magnification. In addition, the surgeon maintains his ability to utilize tactile feedback for tissue dissection and knot tying.

The emerging role of the robot in laparoscopy highlights the impact this technology is having on minimally invasive surgery as a whole. Its utility has been realized in several fields to date and pediatric urology is quickly recognizing its potential as well. The technology is novel and expensive, but the initial results are promising and warrant further development and utilization. Where few surgeons have been able to master the skills required for advanced laparoscopy, especially fine suturing, the robotic systems have more than leveled the playing field, however, it is at a significant cost as the robotic systems (da Vinci® – Intuitive Surgical Inc., Sunnyvale, CA; Zeus® – Computer Motion, Santa Barbara, CA) remain costly and outside the budget of smaller hospitals/institutions. The robotic interface provides the surgeon with several advantages: magnified, three-dimensional (3D) vision, tremor reduction by digitization of hand movements, and superior maneuverability of robotic instruments [18]. The improved visualization likely supplants a surgeon's normal dependence on tactile cues and drives the surgeon to adopt visual cues. A potential disadvantage to the robot in pediatric urology is the immensity of the equipment in relation to the patient size. If the surgeon or anesthesiologist requires immediate access to the patient, this may present a huge problem. The entire robotic team (surgeon, anesthesiologist, and nursing staff) must be prepared for emergency situations at any time and clearly establish paths of access to the patient before the procedure commences [19]. With either modality, laparoscopy, or robotic-assisted laparoscopy, and early in the learning curve, surgeons are less likely to encounter complications if they are assisted or receive adequate proctoring by someone with more experience [2].

Complications

Laparoscopic urological procedures represent about 10–15% of all laparoscopic procedures performed in children [20], but reports of complication rates are few in number in pediatric urologic literature although we are beginning to see reports surface (Tables 1 and 2) [13, 21–24]. Complications can occur at any time in any procedure, for the purposes of this text they will be divided based on the time they occur during the case: with anesthesia or positioning, during port placement, in the midst of the procedure, during port closure, or postoperatively (Fig. 2).

Anesthesia

Any potential benefits of laparoscopic surgery involve exposing the patient to physiological derangements which are not part of conventional open surgery [25]. In children the differences in anatomy and physiology compared to adults are relatively minor, but there are significant differences in neonates and infants compared to adults. Laparoscopy requires the formation of a working area in the peritoneal cavity or, in some cases, extraperitoneally. In either case there is an increase in intra-abdominal pressure (IAP), which is determined by the compliance of the abdominal cavity and the volume of gas insufflated. Carbon dioxide (CO_2) is the insufflatant of choice given its solubility and non-combustion properties, however, it can have physiologic consequences when absorbed that warrant careful monitoring. CO_2 is rapidly absorbed across

Table 1 Comparison of complication rates among published series for laparoscopic surgery in the pediatric population

Author	Date	Length of review (years)	Total no. cases	% Complications (no. complications)	Dominant procedure	% Postoperative complications (no. complications)
C. Esposito [21]	1997	10	430	1.8 (8)	Mixture	n/a
D. Fahlenkamp [13]	1999	*6 (4 centers)	2407	4.4 (107)	Mixture	n/a
C. Esposito [45]	2001	*3 (8 centers)	211	3.8 (8)	Varicocele	9 (19)
L. Baker [14]	2001	*10 (10 centers)	299	5 (15)	Orchiopexy	n/a
C. Esposito [23]	2003	*3 (8 centers)	701	2.7 (19)	Mixture	n/a
C. Passerotti [24]	2008	10	806	2 (16)	Mixture	n/a

*Multiple centers utilized for data collection

Table 2 Comparison of complication rates among published series for laparoscopic renal procedures in the pediatric population

Author	Year	Number of cases	Type of renal surgery	% Complications (no. Complications)	% Open conversion (no. conversions)	% Postoperative complications (no. complications)
P. Caione [46]	2000	20	Retroperitoneal renal biopsy	5 (1)	5 (1)	n/a
S. Micali [33]	2001	31	Retroperitoneal renal surgery	6 (2)	0 (0)	n/a
J. Valla [38]	2003	24	Retroperitoneal partial nephrectomy	37.5 (9)	12.5 (3)	20 (5)
P. Borzi [36]	2004	185	Nephrectomy and partial nephrectomy	0 (0)	3 (6)	n/a
F. Atug [10]	2005	7	RAL pyeloplasty	0 (0)	0 (0)	n/a
R. Lee [12]	2006	33	RAL pyeloplasty	3 (1)	0 (0)	n/a
L. Piaggio [47]	2006	14	Partial nephrectomy	14 (2)	0 (0)	n/a
D. Yee [48]	2006	8	RAL pyeloplasty	12 (1)	0 (0)	n/a
H. Singh [49]	2007	19	Laparoscopic pyeloplasty	0 (0)	0 (0)	5 (1)
I. Ravish [50]	2007	15	Laparoscopic pyeloplasty	13 (2)	0 (0)	6.7 (1)

Complications:

1. Anesthetic
   a. Respiratory
   b. Cardiovascular
2. Positioning
   a. Orthopedic
   b. Neurologic
3. Access
   a. Vascular Injury
   b. Viscous Injury
      i. Bowel Perforation
      ii. Bladder perforation
      iii. Liver or splenic injury
   c. Thoracic
      i. Subcutaneous Emphysema
      ii. Pneumomediastinum
      iii. Pneumopericardium
      iv. Pneumothorax
4. Intraoperative
   a. Vascular injury
   b. Viscous injury
5. Postoperative
   a. Hemorrhage
   b. Infection
   c. Incisional hernia

Fig. 2 Complications encountered during endoscopic surgery

the peritoneum and leads to a resultant increase in total body CO_2 content. Ventilation must be altered in response to this increase to avoid hypercarbia and respiratory acidosis. As it is, oxygenation is impaired in most patients during general anesthesia but these effects are exacerbated in laparoscopic procedures with increases in IAP and further reduction of the functional residual capacity (FRC) of the lungs and total thoracic compliance while airway resistance is increased. A reverse Trendelenburg position is often used in laparoscopic cases and this can further impair lung function.

The cardiovascular system can also be affected for many of the same reasons that the pulmonary system is affected. The IAP causes compression of both the venous and arterial vessels. The preload volume delivered to the right atrium decreases with compression of the vena cava, while the increased pressure on the aorta along with the increased sympathetic tone results in an increased cardiac afterload and a reduction of cardiac output [26]. These effects can be minimized by preoperative volume expansion. Cardiac arrhythmias can also result from increased vagal tone and hypercarbia. These effects can be limited by hyperventilating the patient, decreasing the CO_2 insufflation pressures, and using antiarrhythmic medications where appropriate [18].

Overall, these complications are rare as anesthesiologists and surgeons are well versed in these types of procedures now, nonetheless, special consideration must be given, especially to infants and neonates where the surface area available for absorption is greater. Insufflation pressures must also be altered accordingly for the size of the patient. Pulmonary function is less impaired following laparoscopic abdominal procedures and recovers more quickly compared to equivalent open surgical procedures, even in the very obese [25]. Finally, everyone involved in a robotic case must be aware of the potential difficulty accessing a small patient in the case where emergency access is required. Both the surgical and anesthesia teams must prepare clear paths of access to the patient prior to commencing the procedure. The surgeons must be prepared to rapidly undock the robot when necessary.

Positioning

Perhaps in no other urologic operation are the positioning, padding, and start of the procedure so important and so potentially fraught with complications as they are in laparoscopic and robotic-assisted laparoscopic procedures [27]. To ensure optimal exposure of the operative field the patient must be properly positioned on the operating room table. This is also vital to minimize the risk of neuromuscular injuries, which, for the most part, are easily preventable injuries. For infants and small children given their small size this is less problematic, however, in the older child and adolescents they are at greater risk, especially as the body mass index rises and the duration of the case is extended. Adequate padding of pressure points with the judicious use of gel pads and/or egg crate foam on the operating room tables will decrease the risk of injury. Equally important is to avoid extremes of flexion, extension, or torque in order to further limit the risk of injury. Wrapping the patients' arms at their sides and using split leg tables or placing the patients' legs in padded stirrups may also prevent injury. Once the patient's position is set, securing the patient to the bed with tape, straps, or a beanbag will prevent unwanted movement of the patient when the bed positioned is altered, for example, during a pyeloplasty where the bed can be rotated laterally or during a ureteral reimplant with the bed in steep Trendelenburg. This is especially true in the case of robotic-assisted laparoscopic procedures once the robot is docked as any degree of movement can result in significant injury to the small patient or dramatically affect the small working space. A secure position may be problematic for the anesthesiologist if he has not been involved with the process, as access will be limited once the case is initiated; undoubtedly this is the case during a robotic-assisted laparoscopic procedure. Failure to progress during a procedure must also be an indication for conversion to an open surgical procedure; the surgeon must be cognizant of this and keep track of time. The exact rate of neuromuscular injuries in pediatric laparoscopic and robotic surgery is unknown but surveys of adult populations have demonstrated a rate of 2.7% [28].

Certainly, another important concern in the pediatric population is the shear size of the da Vinci® robot in relation to the patient (Fig. 3). Positioning of the robot to facilitate its use on these small patients can be a challenge for even the most experienced pediatric urologist. In a small child or infant, the robot may completely obscure them from view during the case let alone provide ready access should an emergency situation arise. The entire robotic team should have a plan established prior to beginning the case for emergency access, including rapid undocking of the robot. At the very least being prepared for an emergency situation may help ward off untoward events.

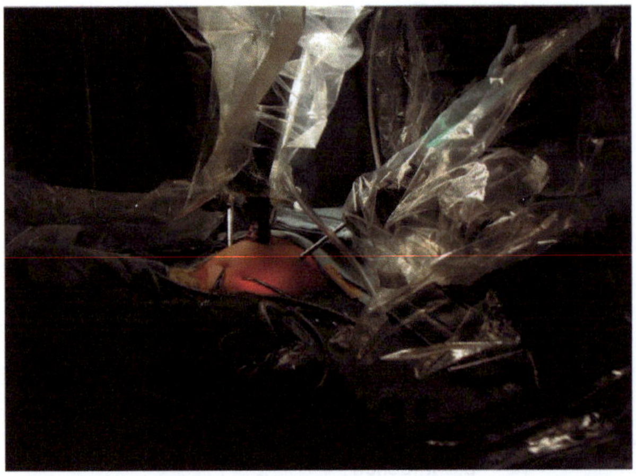

Fig. 3 "Night light": da Vinci® robot docked over infant during robotic-assisted laparoscopic pyeloplasty

Access (Fig. 3)

Port placement is of paramount importance to assure the success of the operation; without a doubt this is the case in infants and small children (Fig. 3). The small working space in children requires careful consideration in port placement and operative strategy (Fig. 4). In robotic surgery, special consideration must be given to the robot itself, its size, and relative immobility. Additionally, in robotic surgery a certain amount of the cannula must be within the abdominal cavity to permit the point of no movement (the virtual center) to be at the abdominal wall [19]. Even with small cannulae the working area can be rapidly encroached upon. To combat this, the surgeon must adjust the port of entry further away from the actual operating area: in the case of renal procedures this may be closer to the midline whereas for pelvic procedures this will be higher in the abdomen. In actuality this is an issue in very small children and infants, but not such a problem in older children and adolescents.

It is the surgeon's preference on how he wishes to obtain access, but most surgeons will adopt a technique that consistently works for them; one that is comfortable and reproducible. Although being knowledgeable in multiple access techniques will improve a surgeon's versatility should one technique not work. If a peritoneal approach is desired then a Veress needle or an open or Hasson technique can be used. The Veress needle technique is a blind procedure that depends on a surgeon's sense of touch as the needle "pops" into the peritoneal cavity. Virtually any blood vessel, hollow viscera, or solid organ can be injured with the placement of the Veress needle and first trocar (Fig. 5). The surgeon should always bear in mind that in very thin patients and in children the aorta may lie only a few centimeters below the skin. However, Veress needle punctures are generally safe and require no further intervention, whereas lesions caused by a trocar can have devastating consequences [21]. The Veress technique may be associated with slightly higher complication rate compared to open techniques, but the complication rates are low overall [14, 21–24, 29, 30], and most series demonstrate that as experience grows complication rates decline [24]. Passerotti et al. demonstrated a complication rate of 2.0 and 0.8% for the Veress technique and the open or Hasson technique, respectively, in 785 laparoscopic procedures performed by 10 different surgeons, however, this difference did not achieve statistical significance [24].

The risk of entry-related complications can be limited by decompression of the stomach and bladder at the outset of the case, as well as a firm grasp of the underlying anatomy especially where the patient has been previously operated on. The port of entry can be adjusted to avoid underlying deep and superficial epigastric vessels in or where there is scar tissue from a previous procedure that may indicate the presence of adhesions below or in the case of the obese

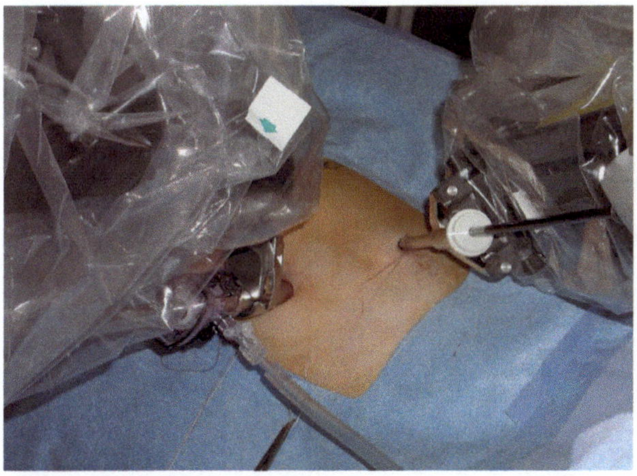

Fig. 4 Port placement in infants during robotic-assisted laparoscopic surgery is of paramount importance: notice proximity of cannulae in this case

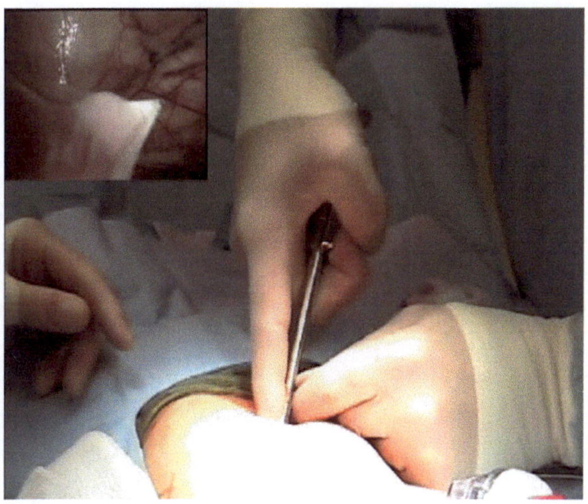

Fig. 5 Veress technique to avoid past pointing

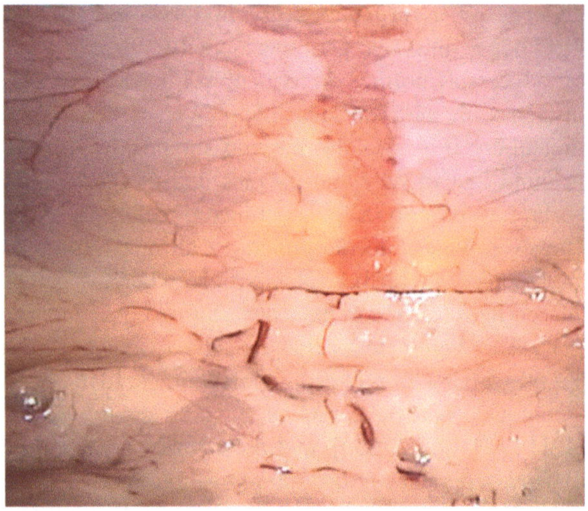

Fig. 6 Blood tracking from access port

child. The use of multiple trocar sites makes injury to superficial and deep epigastric vessels more likely. These injuries can be recognized by blood dripping down the trocar into the abdomen or from a hematoma formation around the site of trocar insertion (Fig. 6). If such injuries occur, several techniques are available for management [31]. Minimal bleeding can often be controlled by coagulation of the parietal peritoneum above and below the trocar sheath or with tamponade using a Foley catheter balloon inflated through the trocar site. For more severe bleeding a full-thickness abdominal wall suture can be placed under laparoscopic control. If all else fails, then direct exploration of the wound may be required.

Consideration must also be given to the pressure required to insert the needle (Fig. 5); aggressive needle placement can easily result in vascular or visceral injury (Figs. 6 and 7). After placement of the needle, position in the peritoneal cavity should be confirmed by aspiration to assure no return of visceral fluid, followed by injection of saline for the "drop test" which should allow the saline to "drop" into the peritoneal cavity. Where there is doubt the sequence can be repeated or the needle replaced. A low intraperitoneal pressure after commencement of the insufflation reaffirms correct placement.

On the other hand, an open technique may theoretically reduce the amount of injuries by allowing direct visual placement of cannulae into the peritoneum. However, this can be cumbersome and visceral and vascular injuries can still occur (Fig. 8) [22, 24, 32]. Once access is obtained, the remaining trocars should be placed under direct vision to limit the risk of injury. Again, overzealous trocar placement can result in visceral or vascular injury. Skin incisions should be adequate to accommodate the size of the trocar being used, thus reducing the amount of downward force necessary for insertion. In most children and especially in infants, using the light from the camera can identify subcutaneous abdominal wall vessels (Fig. 3) such as the epigastrics and subsequently allow the surgeon to avoid them by adjusting trocar placement accordingly. Non-bladed trocars can also reduce the complication rates by decreasing the risk of vascular injuries and creating smaller defects. The use of landmarks such as the xiphoid process, umbilicus, and pubic symphysis will

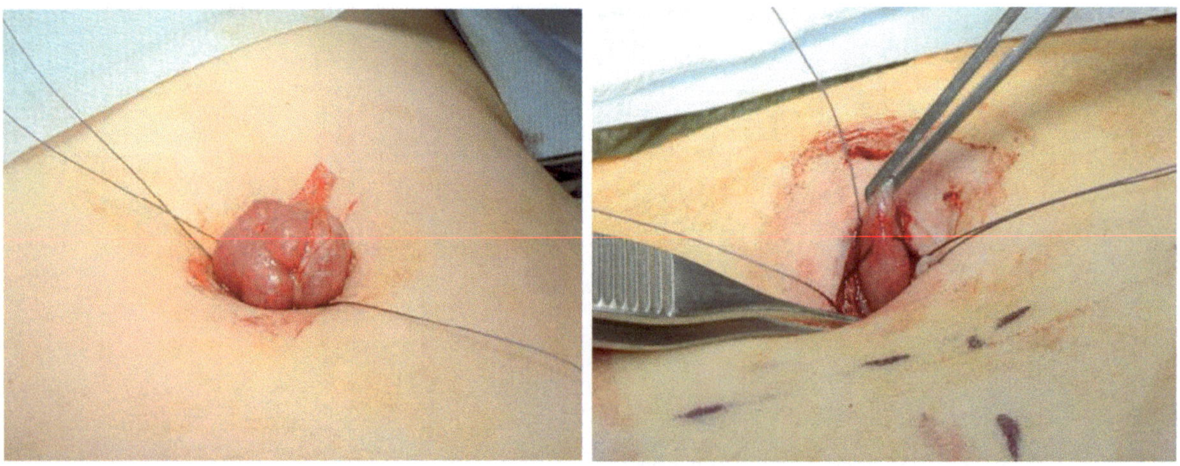

Fig. 7 Bowel perforation with initial access recognized and repaired primarily

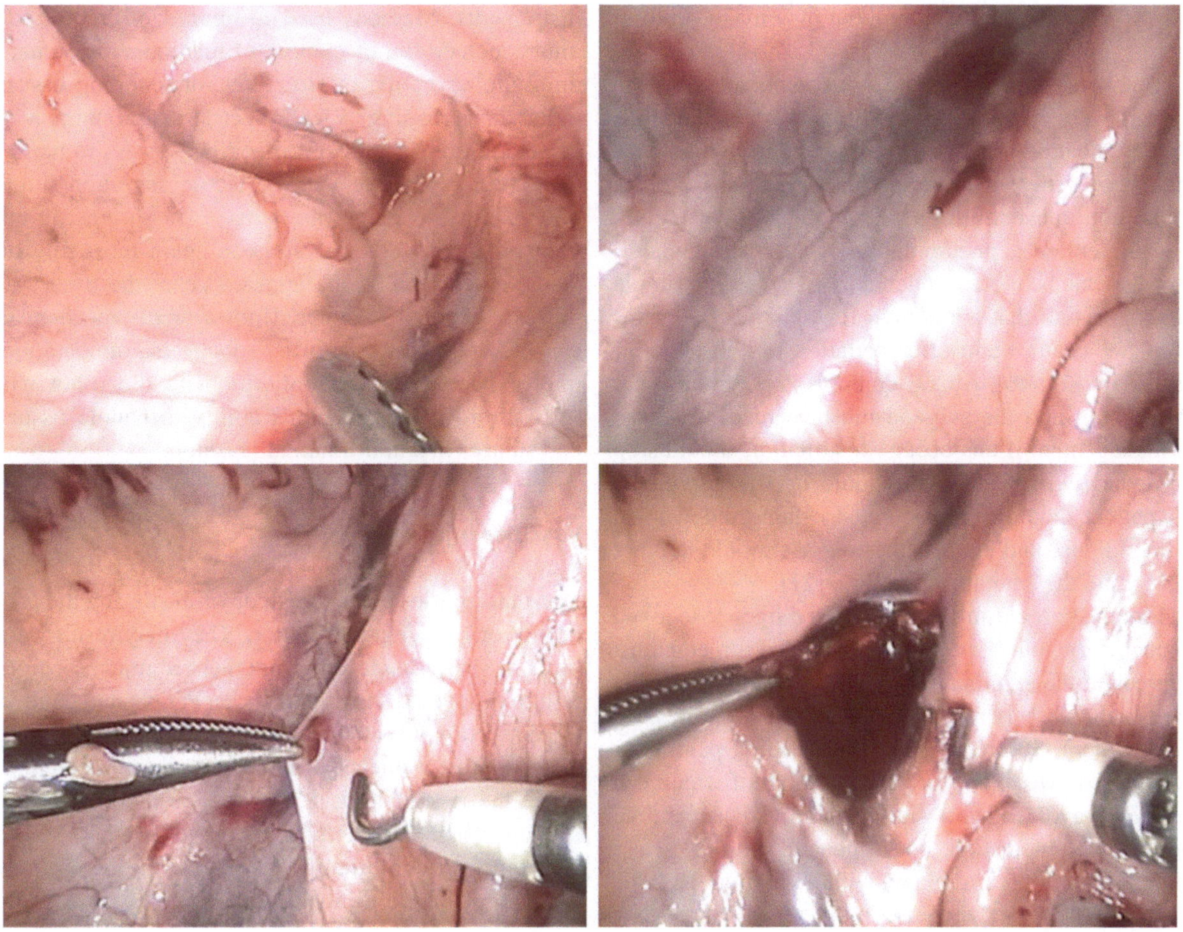

Fig. 8 Iatrogenic iliac vessel injury noted by appearance of ecchymosis over iliac vessels and presence of bloody fluid in cul-de-sac

minimize misadventure, although, with either the open or the closed techniques, port placement may have to be adjusted for previous scars, underlying adhesions, and extremes of body habitus. If additional trocars are needed these should be placed under direct vision to reduce the risk of complications.

Finally, the location of port placement will vary with the type of surgery being performed and the surgeon preference. In the case of a retroperitoneal approach for renal, adrenal, or retroperitoneal lymph node access, for example, additional challenges may arise [33–36]. Anatomically, the surgeon will have to adjust his perspective compared to a transperitoneal approach. The use of landmarks like the psoas muscle is vital for orientation. Blind entry techniques can be utilized but an optical access trocar allows visualization of tissue planes and facilitates safe entry [33]. Working space is limited even in adults and the pediatric surgeon must take this into consideration in his population. The working space itself can either be developed bluntly by the surgeon's finger, the use of a dilating balloon, or bluntly with the laparoscope. In this situation the surgeon wants to avoid entry into the peritoneal cavity as it will further limit the working space [37, 38]. After insufflation is attained, additional trocars can be placed under direct vision. With experience a laparoscopic retroperitoneal approach is safe [39] and affords great visualization of the retroperitoneal structures, including the ureter down to the level of the bladder which can be more difficult to access via a transperitoneal approach. The principle of triangulation of instruments is difficult to observe at times with this approach which has little bearing on dissection but may make suturing more challenging [38].

The insufflatant can also cause complications, aside from the cardiovascular and pulmonary complications already mentioned above, if it migrates from the working space. The subcutaneous or scrotal diffusion is trivial and uneventful, whereas thoracic involvement, causing either a pneumothorax or a pneumomediastinum, can be more problematic. In general, a simple puncture is all that is required for treatment, and this does not occur again after deflation of the abdominal cavity [21, 40]. A CO_2 embolus is potentially life threatening and the surgeon must be ready to assist in management if this occurs. Insufflation should stop immediately, the abdomen should be decompressed, the patient should be repositioned with head down and right side up, and the anesthesiologist should attempt to aspirate the embolus if possible [27].

Finally, port closure deserves due diligence to avoid unnecessary injury or complications. The surgeon must appreciate the significance of this final portion of the case – the case is not over until the last sutures are placed. Poor closure can result in bleeding pain, poor cosmesis, bowel injury or herniation, all of which can easily be avoided. Port sites vary in size depending on the instrumentation, but in general, port sites less than 5 mm are not associated with herniation. Robotic surgery unfortunately requires more generous incisions to accommodate the instruments. However, da Vinci® has recently developed an 8 mm camera and continues to work on developing smaller instruments as its applications are expanded in the pediatric populations. Until then, larger incisions will still be required which means a greater risk for herniation and poor cosmesis unless judicious port closure is performed.

Intraoperative

In laparoscopy, the tactile cues that an open surgeon relies on are different and this requires an adjustment that only improves with increased laparoscopic experience. Robot-assisted laparoscopic surgery lacks tactile feedback altogether and further adjustment is required with this modality. In this case the surgeon must rely on visual cues provided for by the enhanced visualization in place of the tactile cues. Caution must be exercised in handling tissues to avoid crush effects from robotic instruments. Methods used to minimize direct tissue injury include the placement of traction sutures, handling the adventitia of structures, or scooping tissues rather than grasping. A well-placed traction suture may serve additional purpose to facilitate access to particular areas [19]. The lack of tactile sensation limits one's ability to gauge the tension on sutures during knot tying as well. The surgeon again must rely on visual clues such as the appearance of the tissues as they are brought together. Until a tactile mechanism can be incorporated into the robotic instrumentation, only experience and familiarity with the robot will truly improve the surgeon's ability to handle tissues and sutures in a non-traumatic fashion.

Vascular Injury

Vascular injuries can occur at any time during the procedure or in a delayed fashion. They may result from blunt or sharp dissection, from thermal injury, or from failure of vascular ligation devices. Patient and deliberate dissection, knowing the anatomy, and maintaining visualization of one's instruments at all times can minimize the risk of injury, however, no blood vessel is immune (Fig. 9). Vascular anomalies of the kidneys are common and although preoperative imaging may assist in detection of aberrant anatomy preoperatively

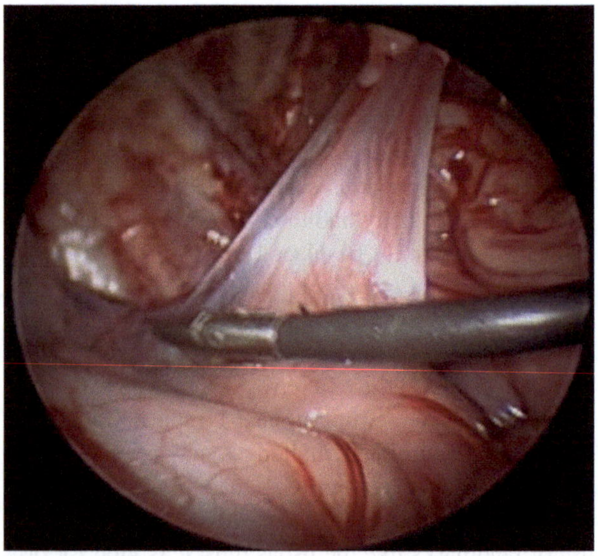

Fig. 9 Orchiopexy procedure with iliac vessels clearly visible: Know your anatomy and keep your instruments in view

this is not always the case. In order to avoid surgical misadventure, maintaining orientation with respect to the patient's internal anatomy, cautious dissection, and visualization of one's instruments at all times is crucial. In laparoscopic cases the assistant driving the camera can play a huge role in this respect. If the camera is rotated or the image is not centered it can lead to surgeon disorientation, resulting in untoward events. Vessels have been confused on occasion, resulting in devastating, sometimes fatal, consequences. The surgeon must recognize landmarks and readily identifiable anatomic structures and proceed from known to unknown. If bleeding does occur, the key, irrespective of the size of the vessel, is not to panic. Often the insufflation pressure can be used to one's advantage and increased to assist with control until appropriate instruments can be obtained. In addition, direct pressure can be applied while a suction irrigator is placed to enhance visibility. This will allot the surgeon time to determine how he will approach the injured vessel: whether to observe and control bleeding, convert to open surgery, or consult vascular surgery if needed. Small vessels will often stop on their own or with the application of thermal energy or a vascular ligation device.

In the case of medium and larger vessels, the surgeon must thoroughly and rapidly assess the situation to develop a strategy to fix the injury at hand. Even larger vessels can be repaired in a controlled manner; again the key is not to panic but to use the resources available. Consideration of potential bleeding complications before the procedure starts will ensure that the appropriate instruments are available when a complication does arise. However, one must be able to recognize his own ability to rapidly gain control of the situation, either laparoscopically or by converting to an open procedure, and, most importantly, when necessary get help.

Viscous Injury

Visceral injuries can also occur during a laparoscopic or robotic-assisted laparoscopic procedures [21, 32].

Hollow Viscous Injury

Bowel or bladder injury may occur with initial trocar placement or during the case itself. When detected it should receive prudent attention. Even small injuries may have devastating sequelae if unrecognized and thus not addressed [41]. However, often these injuries can be repaired easily and with minimal effort. Patients having undergone previous abdominal procedures are at risk of underlying adhesions; the surgeon must be prepared from this and the patient appropriately counseled during discussion of the surgical procedure, as these patients are more likely to be converted to an open procedure. The abdomen should always be carefully inspected following port placement irrespective of the technique used. If a small bowel injury is noted (a serosal abrasion or small perforation) the bowel may be pulled up through the port site incision and repaired primarily or this may be done laparoscopically depending on the surgeon's comfort level (Fig. 7) [24]. Large bowel injuries may also be repaired in this manner. In any case, a general surgery consult is probably warranted if the surgeon remains uncomfortable or the injury is large. The surgeon must maintain awareness of the patient's anatomy, keep the instruments in the visual field at all times, take care to avoid cautery injury, and exercise good control of the tissues throughout the case to decrease the risk of injury. Due diligence may not be enough, and a bowel injury may go unnoticed. The surgeon must be able to identify the signs and symptoms of an unrecognized bowel injury (severe, single trocar site pain, diarrhea, leucopenia, and abdominal distention) in the postoperative period to avoid dire consequences (acute cardiopulmonary collapse secondary to sepsis) often within 96 h postoperatively. Fortunately the rate of bowel injury associated with endoscopic surgery is rare, but the consequences may be terrible [41].

Bladder injuries can occur in laparoscopic surgery in a similar fashion to any other hollow viscous. Decompression of the bladder with a Foley catheter and syringe-assisted drainage at the outset of the case will minimize this risk, but not eliminate it especially if there has been previous surgery such as a vesicostomy or inguinal surgery. As always, the surgeon should exercise careful dissection and maintain a high index of suspicion, especially when hematuria is observed. Filling and emptying the bladder during the procedure and the utilization of dyes may demonstrate the presence of injury intraoperatively. Although rare, bladder injury can occur and present a spectrum of complications and thus require a range of care [6, 42, 43]. Intraoperatively the surgeon may note hematuria, often a finding associated with a bladder perforation; however, small perforations and occasionally large perforations may not be associated with hematuria at all. The surgeon must maintain a high index of suspicion, especially in the case of difficult dissection or when something "doesn't look or feel quite right." Another clue during the case that may indicate the presence of a bladder injury is pneumovesicum; recognized by distention of the urinary drainage bag by the insufflatant. If suspected intraoperative cystoscopy or instillation of methylene blue or indigo carmine can help identify injuries, however, a bladder injury may still go unrecognized [6]. These patients can then present in the postoperative period with abdominal distention, decreased urine output, nausea, vomiting and laboratory irregularities (elevated serum Creatinine or blood urea nitrogen secondary to absorption of urine from the peritoneum). Evaluation with a bladder ultrasound or plain film of the abdomen can demonstrate ascites. A cystogram can demonstrate a perforation. Depending on when and what type of injury is detected will dictate the repair necessary; which may range from Foley catheter placement to open or endoscopic repair. The operative approach for repair will depend on the surgeon, but he should choose the approach that he is most comfortable with and that will provide optimal repair of the injury. Endoscopic repair of bladder injuries has been reported in numerous settings [44].

Solid Organ Injury

The liver, spleen, pancreas, kidneys, and testicles can all be injured during endoscopic surgery. Cavalier port placement can cause significant insult. The same principles of careful port placement should be applied as discussed above. In most cases, small injuries, with the Veress needle for example, may have little consequence. Whereas larger insults, as can occur with trocar placement, may necessitate repair either by the primary surgeon or from a consult service. The surgeon must maintain his cool and handle the situation at hand in a controlled manner utilizing the equipment he has at his discretion until either more appropriate instrumentation is available, the case is converted to an open procedure, or expert consultation arrives. Often times a suction device and a laparoscopic sponge may be all that is necessary to gain control of the situation or at least buy the surgeon time to determine the appropriate course of action. In case of large trocar injuries, it is often prudent to leave the trocar intact while converting the endoscopic procedure to an open one. After initial access has been obtained, all remaining ports should be placed under direct vision. It will be much more difficult to defend oneself in court for injuries incurred during port placement that was performed blindly when there was already a camera port in position. Thermal energy devices can cause significant injury if not properly used. The surgeon should carefully inspect these instruments prior to utilization to assure that they are functioning properly. In addition, he must have an understanding of the distance the energy can travel when applied.

Testicular injury can occur directly either to the cryptorchid testicle, to the vas deferens, or to the vasculature supplying the testicle. Injury may be immediately apparent; damage to the spermatic vessels, which may necessitate a first stage Fowler–Stephens orchiopexy. The insult may also not be realized until much later with testicular atrophy. The surgeon needs to exercise great care in performing orchiopexy and avoid vigorous dissection as the vasculature or vas deferens can be easily injured and repair can be difficult potentially requiring autotransplant.

Postoperative

Complications during this period can be divided into those that occur early and those occurring late. In the immediate perioperative period the patient can develop hypercarbia, shoulder pain, or vomiting if the surgeon fails to evacuate CO_2 at the end of surgery; this can impair spontaneous ventilation by splinting the diaphragm. Most surgeons are aware of this and will evacuate the insufflatant as the ports are removed. Bleeding can also occur from major vessels internally to small superficial vessels. Large vessel bleeds can be devastating in this population as pediatric patients can crash hard and fast without much warning. The surgeon must have a high index of suspicion, especially if the hemostatic device used during the case did not function well. In these cases the patient can be rushed to back to the operating theater for immediate evaluation either laparoscopically or more likely open. Additional complications that can occur later in the postoperative period include infection and herniation. The increasing obesity rates among the pediatric population may contribute to an increase in infections of the incisions. Judicious closure of the tissue layers will minimize potential dead space and decrease the risk of seroma formation and the likelihood of infection. Depending on the procedure most urologists will give the patient a dose of prophylactic antibiotics within 1 h of commencing the procedure, which will further limit the infection risk. Incisional hernias may also occur, but in general for port sites 5 mm or less the risk is negligible. In most infants and children it is often easy to find the fascia and perform a simple closure quickly. The obesity rates may impede our ability to do this easily.

Pediatric urologists utilizing either laparoscopic or robotic-assisted laparoscopic techniques should anticipate complications. This is best accomplished with a three-tiered strategy of prevention, recognition, and management.

Prevention should center on the surgeon's knowledge of the inherent risks associated with any procedure, but especially those specific to individual procedures. Anticipation of these risks and recognizing that there are certain situations that are more complication-prone, such as difficult access, limited vision, scarring, and unusual anatomy will minimize the likelihood of misadventure or at least keep the surgeon prepared should problems arise. The surgeon's adherence to safe technique will further limit complications. Access, whether open or Veress, can be performed easily and safely (Fig. 6). The method of entry is dependent on surgeon preference, which lends itself to the development of a certain comfort level thus reinforcing the preference. The open technique allows the surgeon to maintain visualization at all times whereas the Veress needle technique is a blind technique that requires caution as one can easily past point and cause iatrogenic injury. To confirm placement the saline test aspirate or drop test may be performed. Once inside the peritoneal cavity the surgeon must maintain awareness of the anatomy, visualize the instruments at all times, practice good cautery care, and exercise tissue control.

Recognition of complications should develop with experience but newer endoscopic surgeons should anticipate complications especially early in their development. Complications can and will occur at all stages of development, even in the most experienced hands. Higher levels of experience are likely necessary to create a significant difference in complication rates; the learning curve may not plateau until a new generation of surgeons is born who have learned from current practitioners and with further evolution of the technology. Additionally, ongoing laparoscopic surgical volume appears to relate to complication rates [24]. Knowing what can go wrong at any time during the case, during access or in the midst of the procedure or even in the postoperative period, will enhance the surgeon's ability to recognize and therefore manage complications earlier and possibly minimize the consequences. A growing level of experience will improve the surgeon's ability to manage complications as they occur.

Conclusions

Complications in surgery will happen and the surgeon needs to anticipate this. The surgeon's goal should be to minimize the number of complications that occur and he should take the appropriate steps to assure that this happens, including, patient selection, choosing the best operation based on the indications, and using meticulous technique. In short, the surgeon should anticipate complications in order to prevent, recognize, and manage complications effectively, and thus minimize the untoward consequences. Fortunately, laparoscopic and robotic complications in pediatric urology are rare; nonetheless, they can be significant. Patients, families, and surgeons need to understand that minimally invasive surgery is not synonymous with minimal risk of complications. New technologies, although providing novel means to treat patients, must continue to be assessed critically to prevent inappropriate utilization and potential complications. This is especially true in the pediatric population where the assessment of laparoscopy is difficult and few standards exist. We must not be lulled into a false sense of security given the low rates of complications in laparoscopic and RAL procedures in the pediatric populations. A good surgeon will always be ready to deal with complications; they will, unfortunately, occur.

Parting Comments

The roles of laparoscopy and more recently robotic-assisted laparoscopic surgery in pediatric urology are constantly evolving and will continue to do so as the technology evolves and the experience of the surgeons increases. Complications will continue to occur for all skill levels from the beginner to the expert laparoscopic or robotic surgeon; this should not restrict us in our abilities and desires to expand the boundaries of care utilizing these modalities. However, we must proceed with caution and always with the patient's interests in the forefront.

Acknowledgments I would like to give a special thanks to Dr. Lars J. Cisek and Dr. Craig A. Peters for contributing images.

References

1. Shay BF, Thomas R, Monga M. Urology practice patterns after residency training in laparoscopy. J Endourol. 2002; 16 (4): 251–6.
2. Farhat W, Khoury A, Bagli D, McLorie G, El-Ghoneimi A. Mentored retroperitoneal laparoscopic renal surgery in children: a safe approach to learning. Br J Urol Int. 2003;92:4.
3. Cortesi N, Ferrari P, Zambada E. Diagnosis of bilateral abdominal cryptorchidism by laparoscopy. Endoscopy. 1976;8:33–4.
4. Peters CA. Laparoscopic and robotic approach to genitourinary anomalies in children. Urol Clin N Am. 2004;31:11.
5. Jordan GH, Winslow BH. Laparoscopic single stage and staged orchiopexy. J Urol. 1994;152.
6. Hsieh MH, Bayne A, Cisek LJ, Jones EA, Roth DR. Bladder injuries during laparoscopic orchiopexy: incidence and lessons learned. J Urol. 2009;182(1):280–4; discussion 284–5.
7. Janetschek G, Seibold J, Radmayr C, Bartsch G. Laparoscopic heminephroureterectomy in pediatric patients. J Urol. 1997;158:1928–30.
8. Winfield HN, Donovan JF, Lund GO, Kreder KJ, Stanley KE, Brown BP, et al. Laparoscopic partial nephrectomy: initial experience and comparison to the open surgical approach. J Urol. 1995;153:1409–14.
9. Khurana S, Borzi PA. Laparoscopic management of complicated urachal disease in children. J Urol. 2002;168: 1526–8.
10. Atug F, Woods M, Burgess S, Castle E, Thomas R. Robotic assisted laparoscopic pyeloplasty in children. J Urol. 2005;174:1440–2.
11. Savage JGV, Yohannes P. Laparoscopic antegrade continence enema in situ appendix procedure for refractory constipation and overflow fecal incontinence in children with spina bifida. J Urol. 2000;164:1084–7.
12. Lee RS, Retik AB, Borer JG, Peters CA. Pediatric robot assisted laparoscopic dismembered pyeloplasty: comparison with a cohort of open surgery. J Urol. 2006;175: 683–7.
13. Fahlenkamp D, Rassweiler J, Fornara P, Frede T, Loening SA. Complications of laparoscopic procedures in urology: experience with 2,407 procedures at 4 German centers. J Urol. 1999;162:765–71.
14. Baker L, Docimo S, Surer I, Peters C, Cisek L, Diamond D, et al. A multi-institutional analysis of laparoscopic orchidopexy. Br J Urol Int. 2001;87:484–9.
15. Schwab CW, Casalae P. Bilateral dismembered laparoscopic pediatric pyeloplasty via a transperitoneal 4-port approach. J Urol. 2005;174:1091–3.
16. Lowe GJ, Canon SJ, Jayanthi VR. Laparoscopic reconstructive options for obstruction in children with duplex renal anomalies. Br J Urol Int. 2007;101:227–30.
17. Kutikov A, Nguyen M, Guzzo T, Canter D, Casale P. Laparoscopic and robotic complex upper-tract reconstruction in children with a duplex collecting system. J Endourol. 2007;21(6):621–4.
18. Appledorn SV, Costello AJ. Complications of robotic surgery and how to prevent them. In: Patel VR, editor. Robotic urologic surgery. 1st ed. London: Springer; 2007. pp. 169–78.
19. Peters CA. Applications of robotics in pediatric urologic surgery. In: Patel VR, editor. Robotic urologic surgery. 1st ed. London: Springer; 2007. pp. 179–87.
20. Tam P. Laparoscopic surgery in children. Arch Dis Children. 2000;82:240.
21. Esposito C, Ascione G, Garipoli V, De Bernardo G, Esposito G. Complications of pediatric laparoscopic surgery. Surg Endosc. 1997;11:655–7.
22. Peters CA. Complications in pediatric urological laparoscopy: results of a survey. J Urol. 1996;155: 1070–3.
23. Esposito C, Lima M, Mattioli G, Mastoianni L, Centonze A, Monguzzi GL, et al. Complications of pediatric urological laparoscopy: mistakes and risks. J Urol. 2003;169:1490–2.
24. Passerotti CC, Nguyen HT, Retik AB, Peters CA. Patterns and predictors of laparoscopic complications in pediatric urology: the role of ongoing surgical volume and access techniques. J Urol. 2008;180:681–5.
25. Wedgewood J, Doyle E. Anesthesia and laparoscopic surgery in children. Paediatric Anaesthesia. 2001;11: 391–9.
26. Halachmi S, El Ghoneimi A, Bissonnette B, Zaarour C, Bagli DJ, McLorie GA, et al. Hemodynamic and respiratory effect of pediatric urological laparoscopic surgery: a retrospective study. J Urol. 2003;170:1651–4.
27. Waxman S. How to avoid the medicolegal pitfalls of laparoscopy. Urol Times. 2009;37(5):24–7.
28. Wolf JS Jr, Marcovich R, Gill I. Survey of neuromuscular injuries to the patient and surgeon during urologic laparoscopic surgery. Urology. 2000;55:831–6.
29. Peters CA. Laparoscopy in pediatric urology. Curr Opin Urol. 2004;14:67–73.
30. El-Ghoneimi A. Paediatric laparoscopic surgery. Curr Opin Urol. 2003;13:329–35.
31. LE Saville, Woods M. Laparoscopy and major retroperitoneal vascular injury. Surg Endosc. 1995;9:1096–100.

32. Sadeghi-Nejad H, Kavoussi LR, Peters CA. Bowel injury in open technique laparoscopic cannula placement. Urology. 1994;43(4):559–60.
33. Micali S, Caione P, Virgili G, Capozza N, Scarfini M, Micali F. Retroperitoneal laparoscopic access in children using a direct vision technique. J Urol. 2001;165:4.
34. El-Ghoneimi A, Valla JS, Steyaert H, Aigrain Y. Laparoscopic renal surgery via a retroperitoneal approach in children. J Urol. 1998;160:1138–41.
35. Kobashi KC, Chamberlin DA, Rajpoot D, Shanberg AM. Retroperitoneal laparoscopic nephrectomy in children. J Urol. 1998;160:1142–4.
36. Borzi PA, Yeung CK. Selective approach for transperitoneal and extraperitoneal endoscopic nephrectomy in children. J Urol. 2004;171:814–6.
37. Olsen LH, Jorgensen TM. Computer assisted pyeloplasty in children: the retroperitoneal approach. J Urol. 2004;171:2629–31.
38. Valla J-S, Breaud J, Carfagna L, Tursini S, Steyaert H. Treatment of ureterocele on duplex ureter: upper pole nephrectomy by retroperitoneoscopy in children based on a series of 24 cases. Eur Urol. 2003;43:426–9.
39. Meraney AM, Samee AA-E, Gill IS. Vascular and bowel complications during retroperitoneal laparoscopic surgery. J Urol. 2002;168:4.
40. Berci G. Complications of laparoscopic surgery. Surg Endosc. 1994;8:165–8.
41. Bishoff JT, Allaf ME, Kirkels W, Moore RG, Kavoussi LR, Schroder F. Laparoscopic bowel injury: incidence and clinical presentation. J Urol. 1999;161(3):887–90.
42. Ostrzenski A, Ostrzenska KM. Bladder injury during laparoscopic surgery. Obstet Gynecol Surv. 1998;53.
43. Taskin O, Wheeler JM. Laparoscopic repair of bladder injury and laceration. J Am Assoc Gynecol Laparosc. 1995;2.
44. Colegate-Stone TJ, Raymond T, Khot U, Dickinson IK, Parker MC. Laparoscopic management of iatrogenic bladder injury and bladder stone formation following laparoscopic inguinal herniorrhaphy. Hernia. 2008;12.
45. Esposito C, Monguzzi G, Gonzalez-Sabin MA, Rubino R, Montinaro L, Papparella A, et al. Results and complications of laparoscopic surgery for pediatric varicocele. J Pediatr Surg. 2001;36(5):767–9.
46. Caione P, Micali S, Rinaldi S, Capozza N, Lais A, Matarazzo E, et al. Retroperitoneal laparoscopy for renal biopsy in children. J Urol. 2000;164:1080–3.
47. Piaggio L, Franc-Guimond J, Figueroa TE, Barthold JS, Gonzalez R. Comparison of laparoscopic and open partial nephrectomy for duplication anomalies in children. J Urol. 2006;175:2269–73.
48. Yee DS, Shanberg AM, Duel BP, Rodriguez E, Eichel L, Rajpoot D. Initial comparison of robotic-assisted laparoscopic versus open pyeloplasty in children. Urology. 2006;67:599–602.
49. Singh H, Ganpule A, Malhotra V, Manohar T, Muthu V, Desai M. Transperitoneal laparoscopic pyeloplasty in children. J Endourol. 2007;21(12):1461–6.
50. Ravish IR, Nerli RB, Reddy MN, Amarkhed SS. Laparoscopic Pyeloplasty compared with open pyeloplasty in children. J Endourol. 2007;21(8):897–902.

Medicolegal Aspects of Minimally Invasive Urologic Surgery

Maxwell V. Meng and Michael H. Hsieh

Keywords Laparoscopy · Medicolegal · Legal · Complications

Introduction

Among the myriad concerns and complexities for the practicing urologist, the potential for medical malpractice claims is one of the most troubling and frustrating situations. The physician is often unknowledgeable and poorly prepared for these events, with little emphasis on this aspect of medicine in either medical school or residency training. Only when these unfortunate cases arise does one obtain on-the-job training regarding our legal system, tort law, risk management, and how to avoid malpractice litigation. Herein we discuss relevant medicolegal issues for urologists performing laparoscopic and robotic-assisted procedures.

Overview of the Problem

The common perception is that there is a medical malpractice crisis in the United States. From the physicians' perspective, patients are increasingly litiginous with an explosion of baseless claims and large, jury-decided damage awards. In addition, medical malpractice premium costs are steadily rising with a concomitant reduction in the number of liability carriers. From the patients' perspective, there is an epidemic of medical mistakes from uncaring doctors within an impersonal medical system. These have only been reinforced by recent publications. A report compiled by the Committee on Quality of Health Care in America, published by the Institute of Medicine, stated that between 45,000 and 98,000 people die each year as the result of medical errors, making it the eighth leading cause of death in the United States [1]. Other popular books – with alarmist titles such as *Internal Bleeding: The Truth Behind America's Terrifying Epidemic of Medical Mistakes* and *Wall of Silence: The Untold Story of the Medical Mistakes that Kill and Injure Millions of Americans* – highlight the frequency of medical errors and suggest ways to improve the system of medical care delivery [2, 3].

These issues are particularly relevant and important for laparoscopy and robotics in urology. Indeed, while improvements in information technology may aid in the reduction of errors such as adverse drug events and improve medical record keeping, the introduction of new techniques in minimally invasive surgery and the rapid application to complex operations may initially lead to an increase in complications and must be carefully considered.

Definitions

Tort law addresses civil, rather than criminal, wrongs not arising out of contractual obligations. In a medical malpractice suit, the key of tort liability is negligence.

M.V. Meng (✉)
Department of Urology, University of California, San Francisco, 1600 Divisadero St., San Francisco, CA 94138, USA
e-mail: mmeng@urology.ucsf.edu

R. Ghavamian (ed.), *Complications of Laparoscopic and Robotic Urologic Surgery*,
DOI 10.1007/978-1-60761-676-4_24,

Four elements must be proven for negligence: (1) a duty was owed; (2) a duty was breached; (3) the breach caused an injury; and (4) damages occurred [4]. Clearly, a legal duty exists in the patient-doctor relationship and is established when the surgeon undertakes an operation on a patient. Determining whether a duty of care was breached assesses whether the healthcare provider adhered to a standard of reasonable care, as determined by members of the profession, and thus relies predominantly on expert opinion. In many states, the only test for duty of care is whether the harm to the plantiff from the defendant's actions was foreseeable; however, in California a complex test including multiple factors is applied to determine whether a duty of care exists in a negligence action (Table 1). Then, it must be established that the breach of duty was a proximate cause of the injury. Without damages, whether pecuniary or emotional, there is no basis for a claim even if the physician was negligent. The resulting damages can be divided into direct (lost earnings), indirect (pain and suffering), and punitive.

Do medical malpractice cases actually reflect medical errors and poor patient care, or does the American medicolegal system encourage frivolous suits? Studdert et al. reviewed a random sample of 1,452 closed malpractice claims [5]. Few cases (3%) had no verifiable medical injuries and 37% did not involve errors. Moreover, the absence of errors did not result in compensation in most cases (73%); conversely most cases that involved injuries due to error resulted in compensation (73%). The authors concluded that while frivolous claims are not uncommon, they do not typically result in compensation. Among the total expenditures in these claims, overhead costs of the system, including defense attorneys and contingency fees for the plantiffs' attorneys, accounted for 54% of the compensation paid to the plantiffs.

These data have raised criticism of the existing medical malpractice system and supported efforts at tort reform, such as establishing special medical malpractice courts and limiting non-economic damages. Whether these measures will ultimately benefit both patients and physicians remains unclear and is included in the current efforts of changing the way medical care is delivered nationally. An analysis of malpractice cases involving urologists between 1984 and 2005 did not suggest instituting caps on non-economic awards in specific states had an impact on the number of suits or size of the verdict or settlement [6]. The most common clinical areas involved in the suits included oncology and endourology, although the frequency of seemingly minor complications in routine procedures (e.g., retrograde ejaculation and urinary retention with transurethral resection of the prostate) underscores the importance of thorough discussion and pre-operative patient preparation. In the review of 469 malpractice claims in urology from Perrotti et al., 96 of these alleged negligent surgery (20%) [7]. Laparoscopic pelvic lymph node dissection accounted for four claims without other laparoscopic or robotic operations noted during the study period (1985–2004). However, this may merely reflect a period before the widespread proliferation of laparoscopic and robotic-assisted surgery, as well as the typical delay (2–5 years) in resolution of malpractice claims. Most reports note a high incidence of claims involving urologic oncology [8]. Interestingly, a prior review of claims during

Table 1 Factors determining whether a duty of care exists (California tort)

Foreseeability of harm to the injured party
Degree of certainty s/he suffered injury
Closeness of connection between the defendant's conduct and the injury suffered
Moral blame attached to the defendant's conduct
Policy of preventing future harm
Extent of burden to the defendant and consequences to the community of imposing duty of care with resulting liability for breach
Availability, cost, and prevalence of insurance for the risk involved
Social utility of the defendant's conduct from which the injury arose

Ballard v. Aribe, 41 Cal. 3d 564, 572 n.6 (1986)
Rowland v. Christian, 69 Cal. 2d 108 (1968)
Parsons v. Crown Disposal Co., 15 Cal. 4th 456 (1997)

the popularization of endoscopic procedures (1995–1999) found that endourologic procedures resulted in the greatest incidence of surgical claims, while claims related to prostatectomy proved to be most expensive with mean cost of $185,345 [9].

Malpractice and Minimally Invasive Surgery

The adoption of new technology and surgical techniques will be inevitably associated with a learning curve and a potential for increase in complications. Urologists are fortunate to have the experiences of the general surgeons and gynecologists with their introduction of laparoscopic procedures into clinical practice to serve as a model. In a report from the Physician Insurers Association of America, claims related to laparoscopic cholecystectomy were the most common, followed by exploratory laparoscopy, tubal ligation, and laparoscopically assisted vaginal hysterectomy [10]. McLean found that despite increased formal training during residency, the nature of injuries leading to malpractice litigation after laparoscopic cholecystectomy changed very little over time with persistence of bile duct (≈70%), bowel (≈10%), and vascular (≈10%) injuries [11, 12]. It is important to note that over 80% of injures were missed and few cases (15%) were converted to open procedures. Other international reviews of malpractice cases in laparoscopic cholecystectomy also stress the importance of (1) early identification of injury and (2) conversion when appropriate [13, 14]. What is also clear is the fact that the introduction of laparoscopic cholecystectomy resulted in an increase of a previously uncommon complication, bile duct injury, but that nearly 25 years of experience has not further reduced this rate much below 1 in 200 cases (0.1–0.5%) [15].

A nation-wide review of all hysterectomies performed in Finland between 2000 and 2005 demonstrated a reduction in major complications from laparoscopic hysterectomy (1.8–1.0%), as well as for injuries to the urinary tract (1.4–0.7%) [16]. Despite a reduction in complications with experience, other studies have demonstrated that the laparoscopic approach may still have higher rates of urinary tract injury (bladder and ureter) compared with traditional abdominal hysterectomy [17]. While laparoscopic cholecystectomy accounted for 51% of Physician Insurers Association of America claims in the United States, nearly half of claims outside of the United States involved gynecologic laparoscopy. An analysis of data from 1990 to 1997 revealed that tubal occlusion is associated with the highest litigation rate for gynecologic laparoscopists compared with all other surgical procedures [18].

The accumulated experience and evidence from the application of minimally invasive techniques in other specialties point to several fundamental principles. First, the primary duty is to the patient, and the considerations of liability or malpractice are secondary to patient safety and best-practice guidelines. Second, minimally invasive procedures are likely to result in increased complications early in the surgeon's experience and that explicit disclosure is mandatory. Third, communication with the patient and family before the operation, during the hospitalization, and after discharge is essential in routine cases but even more important after an adverse event has occurred. Most cases of medical errors do not result in malpractice claims, and an important element is communication and honesty, both of which reinforce trust with the patient. Fourth, complications arising from laparoscopy are often missed and that heightened awareness is essential. This is particularly true given the limited field of view, dark operative environment, reduction in tactile feedback, and dissociation from the patient in robotic surgery. Moreover, delays in diagnosis often lead to more serious complications. Despite the smaller incisions visible to the patients, it should be emphasized that minimally invasive surgery still has major risks and that the underlying risks associated with the operation itself remain essentially unchanged when compared with the corresponding open procedure. The minimally invasive approach does not necessarily equate with minimal risk or complications. Fifth, the potential need for conversion to open exists for any surgeon in all patients, and that this should not be viewed as a complication nor as a failure; rather, the decision to do so should reflect the objective assessment of the situation and recognition of the best method to manage a complication or failure to progress, and thus is the result of good intra-operative judgment.

Informed Consent

Although the ethical obligation of providing the relevant information to patients is not new, the legal concept of informed consent is a development over the past century. In Schloendorff v. Society of New York Hospitals (1914), the judge opined: "Every human being of adult years and sound mind has a right to determine what shall be done with his own body; and a surgeon who performs an operation without his patient's consent commits an insult for which he is liable in damages" [19]. This was furthered by the case of Natanson v. Kline (1960), where the court held that the physician was "obligated to make a reasonable disclosure to the appellant of the nature and probably consequences of the suggested or recommended cobalt irradiation treatment, and he was also obligated to make a reasonable disclosure of the dangers within his knowledge which was incidence to, or possible in, the treatment he proposed to administer" [20]. This was expanded in the case of Canterbury v. Spence (1972), where "the inherent and potential hazards of the proposed treatment, the alternatives to that treatment, if any, and the results likely if the patient remains untreated" needed to be disclosed to the patient [21]. Thus, informed consent represents the *process* where the patient is informed about the treatment options, alternatives to these options, the potential risks and complications of the treatments, the intended benefits of treatment, and reasonable expectations [22]. It is important to note that informed consent is not simply a form or statement, which is necessary, but is the process of communication and dialogue between the physician and patient; thus, a signed alone consent form does not guarantee consent.

Table 2 summaries critical elements of informed consent. Several additional recent reviews in the urologic literature discuss these issues in more detail [22, 23]. In obtaining consent, the patient must be competent, informed, and consent voluntarily. The informed consent process should be adequately documented in the medical records to provide evidence that the physician disclosed and explained the relevant information. In the Australian Law Reform Commission document, it was recommended that the physician discuss the magnitude of possible harm by addressing specific severe adverse events and that there is a greater obligation to disclose risks that are more likely to occur [24]. For laparoscopic and robotic operations, explicit mention should be made of injury to blood vessels, bowel, bladder, and other organs, as well as the potential need to convert to an open procedure in some cases. The degree of disclosure is often confusing and a matter of debate and uncertainty. The process of informed consent has been governed primarily by case law, rather than statute, although many states now have incorporated this into written law. In the English tort law, the Bolam test has been applied to the level of disclosure necessary, where the standard of care and reasonableness are determined by peers or similarly qualified specialist (rather than the court or patients) [25]. Subsequently, the Bolitho case questioned the sole reliance on professionals in setting the standard of care (professional community standard) and shifted toward a patient-based standard (reasonable patient standard) [26]. Indeed, in the United Kingdom the approach has evolved to what exists in the United States where disclosure is not necessarily based on what a "reasonable doctor" would disclose under similar circumstances but rather on what a "reasonable patient" would wish to know. The New York Department of Health issued a memorandum that outlines the importance of making the patient aware of the learning curve and the surgeon's experience [27].

The Australian Law Reform Commission provides further factors to consider during the informed consent process, taking into consideration patient variability and individuality (Table 3). In the United States, broad guidelines and standards regarding informed consent have been provided by organizations such as the American Medical Association as well

Table 2 Essential elements of informed consent requiring discussion and disclosure

Diagnosis
Purpose of treatment or procedure
Risks and benefits of treatment or procedure
Alternatives, including risks and benefits
Risks and benefits of not receiving treatment

Table 3 Factors to be considered during the informed consent process

Personality of patient
Intelligence of patient
Temperament of patient
Whether patient wants information, and to what detail
Whether patient asks questions
Patient's level of reasonable understanding
Nature of treatment
Magnitude of possible harm
Likelihood of risk

Source: Adapted from Australian Law Reform Commission

as American College of Surgeons, as well as the Centers for Medicare and Medicaid Services and Joint Commission on Accreditation of Healthcare Organizations. In contrast, the United Kingdom's regulatory General Medical Council details clearly and specifically the responsibilities of the surgeon in the informed consent process, and the Department of Health has mandated use of model consent documentation [28].

The actual consent form should be obtained and documented in the medical records. Although this is often done in the pre-operative holding area, most urologic (and minimally invasive) procedures are elective and the consent can be signed in advance of the operation. In addition, providing printed materials regarding the procedure may be helpful to better inform the patient and family and further document disclosure of relevant information. A study of patients undergoing laparoscopic operations suggested that patients were uniformly pleased to receive standardized information sheets at the pre-operative consultation summarizing the techniques and the risks [29]. Although some (41%) were worried by the explanations of the risks, no patients cancelled their surgery nor reported less confidence in the surgeon. Most patients (95%) found this system of informed consent necessary. A retrospective review of consent forms for transurethral resection of the prostate and radical prostatectomy at the Atlanta Veterans Affairs Medical Center revealed that information on the purpose and benefits of treatment was missing in 4.4% and deficient in 22.6% [30]. All consents were either missing or deficient in mention of alternative treatment options. General and procedure specific risks were inconsistently documented. For example, while urinary incontinence and erectile dysfunction were mentioned in 92 and 97%, respectively, rectal injury was documented in only 44% and bladder neck contracture in 29%. These findings led to the implementation of an electronic, procedure-specific consent form system with high patient preference (96%) compared with traditional paper consents.

Specific Considerations in Urology

Other portions of this book cover the nature and incidence of procedure-specific complications and their management. However, examination of general complications reveals aspects of laparoscopy the surgeon should be aware of and that have litiginous risk.

The mortality rate of laparoscopic operations is low and comparable to corresponding open procedures. In large series of patients in the general surgery and gynecologic literature, the complication rate is less than 5% and mortality occurs in 1 per 1,000 to 20,000 patients [31]. However, it must be kept in mind that many of these are retrospective reviews and that the true incidence of morbidity and mortality may be underestimated. In addition, the nature of operations performed in the earlier era of laparoscopy is less complex than many contemporary urologic procedures and that gynecologic laparoscopy consists of many diagnostic procedures performed in the relatively young, healthy female population.

Risks factors for increased complications with laparoscopy include patient-related variables such as prior abdominal surgery, number and severity of medical comorbidities, obesity, male gender, older age, and diabetes mellitus. Thus, specific patient characteristics affect the decision of whether a laparoscopic/robotic approach is appropriate and should guide in the counseling of the patient and decision making during surgery and in the peri-operative period [32].

Patient Positioning

Urologists are familiar with the importance of meticulous patient positioning and padding in cases involving high lithotomy and full flank configurations. Similar care must be used in laparoscopic and robotic operations, especially given the inability to easily examine or reposition the patient intra-operatively and often extreme configurations (i.e., steep Trendelenburg). A recent review of over 600 laparoscopic renal operations identified rhabdomyolysis in four patients (0.67%), similar to other reports [33]. Factors associated with rhabdomyolysis included greater body mass index, longer operative time, lateral decubitus position, use of the kidney rest, and male gender. The sequelae of rhabdomyolysis may include a prolonged period of recovery and long-term disability, such as long-term pain and numbness and need for an ambulation assistance device [34, 35]. This has also been reported after both open and robotic prostatectomy and may be compounded by the lithotomy and Trendelenburg positions as well as the use of a firm beanbag. In combination with the intraperitoneal insufflation pressure, rhabdomyolysis may play a role in the increased incidence of acute renal failure in patients undergoing robot-assisted prostatectomy [36]. Ulnar neuropathy, while generally transient, has been reported and suggests the need for greater attention to padding of the upper extremities and keeping the operative time to less than 5 h [37]. In 1651 laparoscopic cases, neuromuscular injuries occurred in 2.7% and included, in descending frequency, abdominal wall neuralgia, extremity sensory deficit, extremity motor deficit, clinical rhabdomyolysis, shoulder contusion, and back spasm [38]. It is important to note that this was prior to the proliferation of robotic prostatectomy.

Anesthetic Considerations

Laparoscopy and the associated use of intra-abdominal insufflation result in unique considerations for the anesthesia team, and the pathophysiology of CO_2 at 15 mmHg pressure is covered elsewhere. From a legal perspective, the urologic surgeon must not only understand the effects of the increased intra-abdominal pressure but recognize and be aware of problems arising from this, and know how to manage complications [39]. In general the physiologic changes such as reduced venous return to the heart, increased peak airway pressure, and hypercarbia are of no consequence to the patient, or surgeon, and can be managed by the anesthesiologist. Patients with severe chronic obstructive pulmonary disease (COPD) may be able to undergo minimally invasive surgery successfully, but require heightened awareness of complications. In COPD, CO_2 is less efficiently eliminated and hypercarbia may develop even with hyperventilation. Frequent testing for hypercarbia via arterial blood gases should be performed and insufflation pressure may need to be lowered below 15 mmHg. In some patients with COPD, laparoscopic procedures cannot be successfully performed due to intolerance of pneumoperitoneum and require conversion to open surgery.

Deep Vein Thrombosis

The American Urological Association has published a best-practice statement for the prevention of deep vein thrombosis (DVT) in patients undergoing urologic surgery [40]. The Panel recommended the use of intermittent pneumatic compression devices at the time of surgery. Patients at "high-risk" for DVT may require the use of heparin. Overall, the risk of venous thromboembolism in laparoscopic and robotic-assisted operations appears low, with rates between 0.2 and 1.2% [41, 42]. A non-randomized study did not find a reduction in thrombotic complications (1.2%) in patients undergoing upper retroperitoneal laparoscopic surgery receiving either subcutaneous-fractionated heparin or sequential compression devices [42]. However, heparin was associated with an increase in major (7 vs. 2.9%) and minor hemorrhagic complications. An international review of 5,951 patients undergoing laparoscopic or robotic prostatectomy found a 0.5% incidence of symptomatic DVT [43]. Risks of DVT included prior DVT (OR 13.5), current smoking (OR 2.8), larger prostate (OR 1.18), re-exploration (OR

20.6), longer operative time (OR 1.05), and longer hospitalization (OR 1.05).

Laparoscopic Access

Procedure-based surveys of laparoscopic access injuries show a relatively low incidence ranging from 3 per 1,000 to 5 per 10,000. However, this critical and necessary aspect of the operation is associated with significant potential morbidity and the object of malpractice claims. A review of all malpractice claims from the largest liability carrier in the Netherlands found that entry-related complications accounted for 18% of all laparoscopy-related claims [44]. Nearly all cases (95%) utilized a closed (needle) technique and the majority (54%) were not identified during the surgery. Although there were no deaths, claims were filed for longer hospital stay and related costs, and payments were made in 57% of the settled claims. Chandler et al. identified 594 injuries arising from access injuries within two databases – claims reported to the Physicians Insurers Association of America (1980–1999) and events related to medical devices reported to the U.S. FDA (1995–1997) [45]. The majority of injuries occurred during general surgical procedures (67%) and 76% of injuries involved either bowel or retroperitoneal vascular injuries. More importantly, almost half of bowel injuries went unrecognized for at least 24 h. Overall morality in this cohort was 13% and was associated with delayed diagnosis, age greater than 59 year, and major visceral vascular injury. A subsequent study of trocar injuries demonstrated that no method or device is completely safe and confirmed the importance of early diagnosis and management [46]. Disposable trocars with safety shields and direct-viewing trocars were still associated with major vascular and bowel injuries. In 629 trocar injuries, the mortality rate was 5%; of these deaths, 81% were related to vascular injury and 19% were related to bowel injury. In the fatal vascular events, the aorta (23%) and inferior vena cava (15%) were most commonly involved. In only a single case was device malfunction confirmed to be have occurred, suggesting surgeon variables, rather than mechanical, play the primary role in access-related injury. Contrary to common clinical practice, there is no advantage of (1) the radially expanding access system nor to (2) lifting the abdominal wall during Veress needle insertion [47]. The only potential advantages of a direct trocar entry technique, compared with Veress needle, are avoiding extraperitoneal insufflation (OR 0.06) and failed entry (OR 0.22).

A systematic review of avalable literature and survey of clinical practice has led to a proposed 10-step guideline for safe closed laparoscopic entry (Table 4) [48]. Although not validated, these types of information regarding approach and technique should be reviewed and familiar to the urologist [45, 48, 49]. Most experts would agree that (1) the bladder and stomach should be decompressed prior to initial entry, (2) the surgeon should be facile with both closed and

Table 4 Proposed 10-step guidelines for closed laparoscopic access

1. Suitability criteria: Consider site and type of entry based on prior abdominal surgery, obesity, extremely thin habitus, know adhesions
2. Safety criteria: patient should be flat with empty bladder; abdomen should be palpated for aorta and masses; check Veress needle
3. Incision: 10 mm incision
4. Insertion of Veress needle: at 90° to the skin in a controlled fashion, < 2 cm of needle tip
5. No movement of Veress needle after insertion to avoid converting a possible focal injury to a large complex tear
6. Safety of abdominal pressure check of Veress placement: should be < 10 mmHg
7. Safety abdominal pressure check for primary trocar: should be 25 mmHg to maximize safe distance between anterior abdominal wall and abdominal contents
8. Vertical primary trocar insertion: inserted in a controlled two-handed screwing fashion vertically at 90° to the skin, only the tip of the trocar inserted through the abdominal wall
9. Injury check: 360° laparoscopic examination for intraperitoneal organ injury
10. Avoiding the epigastric vessels for secondary trocas: insert under direct vision in a controlled two-handed manner at 90° to the skin

Source: Adapted from Varma [48]

open (Hasson) entry techniques, and (3) secondary trocars should be placed under direct vision.

Vascular Injury

Injury to both major and minor vessels may occur during minimally invasive surgery [50–53], likely in the range of 0.05% for major injuries. Most of these occur during establishment of initial access and pneumoperitoneum, as discussed above, but can be overlooked or missed completely. The key is awareness of the potential for these injuries and early identification and management; delayed presentation is more likely to be associated with greater morbidity and mortality.

Injury to the epigastric vessels is a complication unique to minimally invasive surgery resulting from trocar placement through the rectus muscle. These can be avoided by direct visualization of trocar placement and knowledge of where the vessels are located; if recognized, management is relatively straightforward with suture occlusion of the vessels.

Rates of major vascular injury during the urologic operation itself do not appear to be higher than the corresponding open procedure. In addition, the presence of pneumoperitoneum may aid in tamponade of small vessels and minor oozing. However, meticulous hemostasis is more important during minimally invasive procedures where adequate visualization is essential and the ability to manage bleeding is limited. Thus avoiding and preventing significant bleeding during dissection are mandatory to successful laparoscopic and robotic surgery. Although many tools are available to aid in vascular control and achieving hemostasis, all have the potential to fail and are not fail-proof. This has been well documented in examination of the FDA MAUDE database, with malfunction of both endovascular staplers (0.38–1.7%) and clips [54–57]. It should be noted that the manufacturer of the Hem-o-lok clip (Weck Closure Systems) has issued a warning against the use of the polymer self-locking clip in controlling the renal artery during laparoscopic donor nephrectomy.

The intra-operative management of a major vascular injury relies on surgeon experience, specific situation, and good judgment. Older studies of laparoscopic complications revealed that over 80% of patients with major vascular injuries managed without laparotomy died and overall mortality is around 10% [58, 59]. As skill and experience have increased as well as the availability of the da Vinci robot, complex vascular reconstruction and repair are possible; nevertheless, one should consider conversion to open in the presence of a recognized major vascular injury or bleeding from an unknown source [60–62]. From a legal perspective, the occurrence of a major vascular injury is not evidence of error nor negligence, but it is the subsequent management, whether appropriate or successful, that becomes the point of litigation.

Bowel Injury

In addition to vascular injury, damage to the bowel results in major complications and potential for medicolegal risk. These occur primarily during insertion of the first trocar or establishment of pneumoperitoneum, or during dissection of adhesions. As mentioned, prior abdominal surgery should raise awareness of the potential for increased risk of bowel injury. In over 1,283 cases using the optical access trocar, bowel injury occurred in 0.08% [63]. In an earlier review of 915 patients undergoing laparoscopic urological procedures, bowel perforation occurred in 0.2% of cases and bowel "abrasion" occurred in 0.6%, which was comparable to a review of the literature (0.13–0.9%) [64]. The majority (69%) of injuries were not recognized at the time of surgery and 80% required laparotomy to repair the injury. In addition to delayed diagnosis, the post-operative presentation was atypical with signs of severe pain at a single trocar site, abdominal distention, diarrhea, and leukopenia. Half of the injuries were caused by electrocautery.

As with vascular injuries, careful access via either needle or Hasson technique and bowel dissection should minimize the incidence of bowel injury. Prevention includes keeping instruments in the visual field at all times, careful lysis of adhesions, judicious application of thermal energy, and maintaining a high index of suspicion. Any injury noted during surgery should be promptly addressed, whether with a suture or resection and formal repair. The threshold for consultation with a general surgeon should be low both for appropriate management and for minimizing liability.

Much discussion revolves around the "best" laparoscopic energy source and which has the least risk of thermal damage to surrounding tissue and the bowel. Despite various studies and data, none are completely safe and thus the surgeon must be vigilant. Monopolar electrocautery may cause injury due to inadvertent activation on unintended tissue, lateral spread during intended use, direct coupling, and capacitive coupling. The surgeon must be knowledgeable about these mechanisms and carefully inspect all instruments prior to use for breaks in insulation. Active electrode monitoring has been incorporated into newer generators and detects current leak associated with insulation failure or capacitive coupling, automatically shutting down the generator in these circumstances. Cold sharp dissection with scissors may be the best method around bowel and adhesions.

Given the frequent delay in the diagnosis of bowel injuries, careful monitoring and examination of the patient after surgery is essential. Only subtle signs and symptoms may be present, and the surgeon should not hesitate to evaluate for unsuspected bowel injury. Computed tomography with oral contrast is the best imaging modality and delayed images or surgical exploration may be necessary if the concern for bowel injury persists.

Laparoscopic and robotic prostatectomy are associated with a risk of rectal injury (<1%), comparable to that from open retropubic prostatectomy [65–67]. If recognized intra-operatively, these can be repaired at the time without need to convert to open surgery.

Conversion to Open

The inability to complete an operation in a minimally invasive fashion should not be viewed as failure or a complication, and the pre-operative consultation with the patient and consent need to include this possibility. It is difficult to predict which patients or cases may require conversion, although rates of conversion decrease with surgeon experience. Siqueira et al. reported a conversion rate of 6.1% in 292 consecutive patients undergoing laparoscopic renal surgery [68]. "Simple" nephrectomy had the highest rate of elective conversion, while live donor nephrectomy required emergent conversion in 60%. As mentioned, conversion may be necessary in situations when there is failure to progress or a complication cannot be managed laparosopically or using the robot.

Wound Closure

A seemingly minor and often overlooked aspect of minimally invasive surgery is port site and incision closure. Traditional practice has been to close the fascia of trocar sites 10 mm and greater to reduce the incidence of hernias (1%). However, non-bladed trocars and radially dilating systems are thought to be less traumatic and associated with less risk of incisional hernias due to separation, rather than cutting, of the fascia. Case reports still document hernias with these types of trocars and should still be closed if $\geq$10 mm.

Bird et al. compared various sites of specimen extraction after laparoscopic radical nephrectomy [69]. Incisional hernias occurred in 2.3% and were more frequently associated with the paramedian site compared with lower quadrant and umbilical locations. Others have suggested that a transverse, lower flank incision cutting of the muscle resulted in a high rate of incisional hernias (17%) and that a low midline, muscle splitting or Pfannenstiel incision may be preferable [70].

Unique Aspects of the Pediatric Population

Urologic laparoscopy in children features a unique set of issues which can contribute to risks of complications and resulting malpractice torts. The technical difficulty of pediatric urologic laparoscopy can vary widely from case to case, depending on patient body habitus, surgeon skill, patient anatomy, and the specific procedure. Many children requiring urologic surgery are small infants or have chronic contractures that make optimal positioning difficult. Younger children exhibit less peritoneal excursion during insufflation, which results in a shorter distance between the access trocar or needle and the intra-abdominal viscera. This can be exacerbated by the need to use reduced insufflation pressures (12 mmHg) in children. A single institution series reported an overall 2% complication rate for urologic laparoscopic procedures performed on children, with the vast majority related to access [71]. Veress needle versus open access was not significantly different with regard to complication rates. Complications not related to access included vessel injury, small bowel injury, bleeding requiring conversion, bladder perforation, and vas deferens injury. Finally, children undergoing major urologic reconstruction are often reoperative with extensive scarring in the surgical field (e.g., failed pyeloplasty, exstrophy, spina bifida), which may further predispose these patients to complications.

Generally speaking, adoption of minimally invasive techniques has been slower in pediatric urology relative to other disciplines of urology. Hence, many pediatric urologists have less experience with laparoscopic approaches. For example, a higher rate of obstruction has been reported to occur early in the learning curve for pediatric laparoscopic pyeloplasty [72]. Chertin et al. reported that ureteral injury during pediatric laparoscopic partial nephrectomy led to open conversion early in their learning curve [73]. Based on the Boston Children's experience, pediatric urologists who perform more than 12 laparoscopic procedures annually have lower complication rates [71].

Although patient-specific factors and the learning curve are unavoidable, there are a number of measures that can be taken in order to minimize risks of complications. Perhaps even more so than in adult urology, clear and thorough communication with parents, including informed consent, is a key component to pre-operative preparation. There are a burgeoning number of pediatric-specific minimally invasive surgery workshops for urologists. These courses may help reduce the duration of the learning curve. Finally, the identification of the root causes of complications in pediatric urologic laparoscopy may decrease complication rates. For instance, a recent case series reported that bladder injuries during laparoscopic orchiopexy may be more likely to occur when either no urethral catheter is placed pre-operatively or a catheter is placed but merely placed to passive drainage. The authors recommended that urethral catheters be placed for all laparoscopic orchiopexies, to aspirate all urine from the bladder at the beginning of surgery and to fill and empty the bladder to clearly delineate it during the procedure [74]. Finally, unlike adult laparoscopy, it may be advisable to close small umbilical port sites in children. Yee and Duel reported an omental hernia through a 3 mm umbilical port site made with a bladeless trocar during diagnostic laparoscopy [75].

Future Considerations

The field of minimally invasive surgery in urology is rapidly evolving, with the introduction of new techniques (e.g., laparoendoscopic single site surgery) as well as continued popularization of the robot to increasingly complex procedures [76]. These changes have medicolegal implications and as urologic surgeons we should consider the role we should play in addressing issues of training and tort reform.

Innovations in Minimally Invasive Surgery

We are blessed in the field of urology to have continuous improvements in equipment and technique as well as entirely new procedures. These advances have been provided by pioneering surgeons and technological developments. Indeed, much of current operative urology was unheard of (and unimaginable) just 20 years ago. How are these innovations balanced against the ethical and legal obligations to the patient and society? All surgeons should review the excellent discussion contained in a recent dialogue among experts across a variety of disciplines [77]. Despite the rapid growth of laparoscopic and robotic surgery without clinical trials, we should be more cautious in the adoption of new operations with unproven safety and benefits. Whether it is feasible to prove the efficiency, effectiveness, equanimity, and economy of new procedure remains to be determined, but without such evidence exposure to medicolegal risks will exist.

Training and Credentialing

Even if a new technique or operation is proven safe and effective, questions arise regarding the dissemination to practicing urologists. There is clearly a learning curve for new procedures, as evidenced by the experience with laparoscopic renal surgery and robotic prostatectomy. This issue was encountered with the introduction of laparoscopic cholecystectomy and resulted in guidelines offered by the State of New York Department of Health [78]. The document recommended specific credentialing guidelines for surgeons learning the operation outside of a traditional surgical residency program including (1) specifically outlining the characteristics of a short course for those interested in learning the operation, (2) mandating participation as an assistant surgeon in a sufficient number of cases (5–10), and (3) subsequently requiring supervision by a credentialed surgeon during the first 10–15 cases as responsible surgeon. The Society of American Gastrointestinal and Endoscopic Surgeons has also presented privileging guidelines for laparoscopic and thoracosopic techniques (http://www.sages.org/sagespublication.php?doc=14). Within urology, recommendations have been made regarding robotic urological surgery [79]. In the future, brief weekend courses are likely to be insufficient from both regulatory and ethical points of view, and there will be greater reliance on structured programs of didactics, surgical simulators, mentored and proctored surgical experience, and demonstration of proficiency [80–82].

Expert Testimony

The medical expert witness plays an important role in medical liability cases given the reliance on peers in establishing the standard of medical care. The American Urological Association has a developed a policy as well as an affirmation statement (http://www.auanet.org/content/guidelines-and-quality-care/policy-statements/e/expert-witness-testimony-in-medical-liability-cases.cfm). Other professional societies have instituted standards to regulate conduct and enforce these through formal disciplinary procedures (American Medical Association Guidelines H-265) [83]. The goals of addressing the expert witness issue are not to limit plantiff claims or physician liability, but to ensure responsible and expert testimony for both sides.

Tort Reform

The topic of tort reform is controversial and currently closely linked with the efforts at radically altering the healthcare system in the United States. The objectives of such changes should include minimizing incentives for frivolous suits, reducing costs of malpractice litigation, increasing the number and affordability of liability carriers while preserving the ability of patients to bring legitimate suits and collect for damages. Ultimately these goals may best be achieved by improving patient care and safety through continued education, adherence to guidelines and clinical pathways, individual physician responsibility, and oversight and enforcement by specialty organizations.

Costs have come to the forefront as an issue in the medical system (http://www.ama-assn.org/ama1/pub/upload/mm/-1/mlrnow.pdf). The median jury award in medical liability cases have tripled from 1997 to 2006, increasing from $157,000 to $487,5000 and the mean award is $637,134 in 2006. This has occurred despite many states having instituted caps on non-economic damages. Settlements have also increased from medians of $100,000 to $204,500 over the same period. Recent data suggest that medical liability represents a growing component of U.S. tort costs (12.2%), outpacing the yearly growth compared with other torts (11.1 vs. 8.4% per year). Whether the threat of malpractice claims leads to "defensive" medicine, and further costs to the system, is unclear, but likely does not improve physician cost-effectiveness. Thus, reforming the system may address costs, improve physician practice, and increase efficiency. Interestingly, the Kaiser Permanente medical group has utilized an arbitration system for several decades. At the time of enrollment, patients sign an agreement that prohibits a malpractice claim from going to traditional court (in most cases) and uses an arbitration system. This eliminates the need for either a jury or specialized medical court system, improves the resolution of cases within a mandated 18 months, and has been upheld as both reasonable and constitutional.

Summary

Minimally invasive surgery is here to stay in urology and is only likely to increase its role in all areas. So too is the necessity for tort law which dates back to antiquity [84]. The Code of Hammurabi contains 282 laws, including ones dealing with fee schedules for surgical services and penalties, with "eye for an eye" justice – "If a physician make a large incision with the operating knife, and kill him, or open a tumor with the operating knife, and cut out the eye, his hands shall be cut off."

Individual physicians can make an impact on the medicolegal situation by improving knowledge and avoidance of potential complications, conveying appropriate information to patients in both verbal and written forms, obtaining and documenting truly informed consent, communicating with patients and family after adverse events occur, and continually improving and acquiring technical skills. The role of medical organizations and specialized societies is to provide guidance and tools for surgeon training and establishing credentialing mechanisms, as well as advocating for tort reform. However, it must be kept in mind that the ultimate objectives of addressing medicolegal issues are to provide the best and most up-to-date care for patients while ensuring their safety and to guarantee a fair and efficient system to recover damages in cases of negligence.

References

1. Committee on Quality of Health Care in America, Institute of Medicine. To err is human: building a safer health system. Washington, DC: National Academy Press; 2000.
2. Wachter RM, Shojania K. Internal bleeding: the truth behind America's terrifying epidemic of medical mistakes. New York: Rugged Land; 2004.
3. Gibson T, Singh JP. Wall of silence: the untold story of the medical mistakes that kill and injure millions of Americans. Washington, DC: LifeLine Press; 2003.
4. The Four Elements of Medical Malpractice. Yale New Haven medical center: issues in risk management; 1997.
5. Studdert DM, Mello MM, Gawande AA, et al. Claims, errors, and compensation payments in medical malpractice litigation. N Engl J Med. 2006;354:2024–33.
6. Hsieh MH, Tan AG, Meng MV. Medical malpractice in American urology: 22-year national review of the impact of caps and implication for contemporary practice. J Urol. 2008;179:1944–9.
7. Perrotti M, Badger W, Prader S, Moran ME. Medical malpractice in urology, 1985-2004: 469 consecutive cases closed with indemnity payment. J Urol. 2006;178:2537–9.
8. Sherman C. Urologists hit by malpractice crisis. Renal Urol News. 2005; vol. 42–43, July/August.
9. Kahan SE, Goldman HB, Marengo S, Resnick MI. Urological medical malpractice. J Urol. 2001; 165:1538.
10. Physicians Insurers Association of America. What is PIAA? http://www.thepiaa.org/about_piaa/what_is_piaa.htm
11. McLean TR. Risk management observations from litigation involving laparoscopic cholecystectomy. Arch Surg. 2006;141:643–8.
12. Kern KA. Malpractice litigation involving laparoscopic cholecystectomy. Arch Surg. 1997;132:392–8.
13. Kienzle HF. Malpractice in laparoscopic cholecystectomy. Results of cases recently considered by the Expert Commission. Zentralbl Chir. 1999;124:535–41.
14. de Reuver PR, Wind J, Cremers JE, et al. Litigation after laparoscopic cholecystectomy: an evaluation of the Dutch arbitration system for medical malpractice. J Am Coll Surg. 2008;206:328–34.
15. A prospective analysis of 1518 laparoscopic cholecystectomies. The Southern Surgeons Club. N Engl J Med. 1991;324:1073–8.
16. Brummer THI, Sepålå, Hårkki PSM. National learning curve for laparoscopic hysterectomy and trends in hysterectomy in Finland 2000–2005. Hum Reprod. 2008;23:840–5.
17. Johnson N, Barlow D, Lethaby A, et al. Surgical approach to hysterectomy for benign gynaecological disease. Cochrane Database Sys Rev. 2006;2:CD003677.
18. Owolabi T. Minimizing risks of laparoscopy. J Soc Obstet Gynaecol Can. 2000;22:974–6.
19. Schloendorff v. Society of New York Hospitals, 1914;211 NY 125.
20. Natanson v. Kline, 186 Kan 393, 350 P.2d 1093; 1960.
21. Canterbury c. Spence, 464 F.2d 772, 789 U.S. Court of Appeals, District of Columbia; 1972.
22. Jones B. Legal aspects of consent. BJU Int. 2000;86: 275–9.
23. Reynard J, Marsh H. The development of consent from Bolam to Chester: what you need to know and what your patients are entitled to know. BJU Int. 2009;103:1458–61.
24. Australian Government National Health and Medical Research Council. General Guidelines for Medical Practitioners on Providing Information to Patients. Commonwealth of Australia; 2004.
25. Bolam v. Fiern Hospital Management Committee; 1957.
26. Bolitho v. City and Hackney Health Authority; 1997.
27. New York State Department of Health Memorandum H-18, June 12, 1992.
28. Department of Health. Good practice in consent implementation guide: consent to examination or treatment. HSC 2001/023. London: Department of Health; 2001.
29. Wijtenburg E, Navez B, Cambier E, Guiot P. Patient's opinion about written information before laparoscopy: a consecutive series of 100 cases. Acta Chir Belg. 2002;102:17–9.
30. Issa MM, Setzer E, Charaf C, et al. Informed versus uninformed consent for prostate surgery: the value of electronic consents. J Urol. 2006;176:694–9.
31. Bonjer HJ, Hazebroek EJ, Kazemier G, et al. Open versus closed establishment of pneumoperitoneum in laparoscopic surgery. Br J Surg. 1997;84:599–602.
32. Proceedings of the Association of Trial Lawyers of America Annual Convention. 2002;1:1–4.
33. Glassman DT, Merriam WG, Trabulsi EJ, et al. Rhabdomyolysis after laparoscopic nephrectomy. JSLS. 2007;11:432–7.

34. Reisiger KE, Landman J, Kibel A, Clayman RV. Laparoscopic renal surgery and the risk of rhabdomyolysis: diagnosis and treatment. Urology. 2005;66:29–35.
35. Shaikh S, Nabi G, McClinton S. Risk factors and prevention of rhabdomyolysis after laparoscopic nephrectomy. BJU Int. 2006;98:960–2.
36. Li, J-R, Cheng C-L, Weng W, et al. Acute renal failure after prolonged pneumoperitoneum in robot-assisted prostatectomy: a rare complication report. J Robotic Surg. 2008;1:1863.
37. Cadeddu JA, Wolfe JS Jr, Nakada S, et al. Complication of laparoscopic procedures after concentrated training in urological laparoscopy. J Urol. 2001;166:2109–11.
38. Wolf JS Jr, Marcovich R, Gill IS, et al. Surgery of neuromuscular injuries to the patient and surgeon during urologic laparoscopic surgery. Urology. 2000;55:831–6.
39. Wolf JS Jr, Stoller ML. The physiology of laparoscopy: basic principles, complications and other considerations. J Urol. 1994;152:294–302.
40. Forrest JB, et al. Best practice statement for the prevention of deep vein thrombosis in patient undergoing urologic surgery. Baltimore: American Urological Association; 2008.
41. Rassweiler J, Fornara P, Weber M. Laparoscopic nephrectomy: the experience of the laparoscopic working group of the German Urologic Association. J Urol. 1998;160: 18–21.
42. Montgomery JS, Wolf JS Jr. Venous thrombosis prophylaxis for urologic laparoscopy: fractionated heparin versus sequential compression devices. J Urol. 2005;173:1623–6.
43. Secin FP, Jiborn T, Bjartell AS, et al. Multi-institutional study of symptomatic deep venous thrombosis and pulmonary embolism in prostate cancer patients undergoing laparoscopic or robot-assisted laparoscopic radical prostatectomy. Eur Urol. 2008;53:134–45.
44. Wind J, Cremers JE, van Berge Henegouwen MI, et al. Medical liability insurance claims on entry-related complications in laparoscopy. Surg Endosc. 2007;21:2094–9.
45. Chandler JG, Corson SL, Way LW. Three spectra of laparoscopic entry access injuries. J Am Coll Surg. 2001;192:478–90.
46. Bhoyrul S, Vierra MA, Hezhat CR, et al. Trocar injuries in laparoscopic surgery. J Am Coll Surg. 2001;192:677–83.
47. Ahmad G, Duffy JM, Phillips K, Watson A. Laparoscopic entry techniques. Cochrane Database Syst Rev. 2008;16(2):CD006583.
48. Varma R, Gupta JK. Laparoscopic entry techniques: clinical guideline, national survey, and medicolegal ramifications. Surg Endosc. 2008;22:2686–97.
49. Collins S, Lehman DS, McDougall EM, et al. AUA handbook of laparoscopic and robotic fundamentals. Baltimore: American Urological Association. 2008.
50. Nordestgaard AG, Bodily KC, Osborne RW Jr, Buttorff JD. Major vascular injuries during laparoscopic procedures. Am J Surg. 1995;169:543–5.
51. Gill IS, Kavoussi LR, Clayman RV, et al. Complications of laparoscopic nephrectomy in 185 patients: a multi-institutional review. J Urol. 1995;154:479–83.
52. Roviaro GC, Varoli F, Saguatti L, et al. Major vascular injuries in laparoscopic surgery. Surg Endosc. 2002;16:1192–6.
53. Guloglu R, Dilege S, Aksoy M, et al. Major retroperitoneal vascular injuries during laparoscopic cholecystectomy and appendectomy. L Laparoendosc Adv Surg Tech A. 2001;14:73–6.
54. Chan D, Bishoff JT, Ratner L, et al. Endovascular gastrointestinal stapler device malfunction during laparoscopic nephrectomy: early recognition and management. J Urol. 2000;164:319–21.
55. Deng DY, Meng MV, Nguyen HT, et al. Laparoscopic linear cutting stapler failure. Urology. 2002;60:415–9.
56. Hsi RS, Saint-Elie DT, Zimmerman GJ, Baldwin DD. Mechanisms of hemostatic failure during laparoscopic nephrectomy: review of Food and Drug Administration database. Urology. 2007;70:888–92.
57. Andonian S, Okeke Z, Okeke DA, et al. Device failures associated with patient injuries during robot-assisted laparoscopic surgeries: a comprehensive review of FDA MAUDE database. Can J Urol. 2008;15:3912–6.
58. Thiel R, Adam JB. Venous dissection injuries during laparoscopic urological surgery. J Urol. 1996;155:1874–6.
59. Soderstrom RM. Injuries to major blood vessels during endoscopy. J Am Assoc Gyn Lap. 1997;4:395–8.
60. Safi KC, Teber D. Laparoscopic repair of external iliac transection during laparoscopic radical prostatectomy. J Endourol. 2006;20:237–9.
61. Castillo OA, Peacock L, Vitagliano G, et al. Laparoscopic repair of an iliac artery injury during radical cystoprostatectomy. Surg Laparosc Endosc Percutan Tech. 2008;18:31508.
62. Hemal AK, Goel A. External iliac vein injury and its repair during laparoscopic radical cystectomy. JSLS. 2004;8: 81–3.
63. Thomas MA, Rha KH, Ong AM, et al. Optical access trocar injuries in urological laparoscopic surgery. J Urol. 2003;170:61–3.
64. Bishoff JT, Allaf ME, Kirkels W, et al. Laparoscopic bowel injury: incidence and clinical presentation. J Urol. 1999;161:887–90.
65. Yee DS, Ornstein DK. Repair of rectal injury during robotic-assisted laparoscopic prostatectomy. Urology. 2008;72:428–31.
66. Blumberg JM, Lesser T, Tran VQ, et al. Management of rectal injuries sustained during laparoscopic radical prostatectomy. Urology. 2009;73:163–6.
67. Brown JA, Garlitz C, Gomella LG, et al. Perioperative morbidity of laparoscopic radical prostatectomy compared with open radical retropubic prostatectomy. Urol Oncol. 2004;22:102–6.
68. Siqueira TM Jr, Kuo RL, Gardner TA, et al. Major complications in 213 laparoscopic nephrectomy cases: the Indianapolis experience. J Urol. 2002;168:1361–5.
69. Bird VG, Au JK, Sandman Y, et al. Comparison of different extraction sites used during laparoscopic radical nephrectomy. J Urol. 2009;18:1565–70.
70. Elashry OM, Guisti G, Nadler RB, et al. Incisional hernia after laparoscopic nephrectomy with intact specimen removal: cavast emptor. J Urol. 1997;158:363–9.
71. Passerotti CC, Nguyen HT, Retik AB, Peters CA. Patterns and predictors of laparoscopic complications in pediatric urology: the role of ongoing surgical volume and access techniques. J Urol. 2008;180:681–5.

72. Braga LH, Pippi-Salle J, Lorenzo AJ, et al. Pediatric laparoscopic pyeloplasty in a referral center: lessons learned. J Endourol. 2007;21:738–42.
73. Chertin B, Ben-Chaim J, Landau EH, et al. Pediatric transperitoneal laparoscopic partial nephrectomy: comparison with an age-matched group undergoing open surgery. Pediatr Surg Int. 2007; 23:1233–6.
74. Hsieh MH, Bayne A, Cisek LJ, et al. Bladder injuries during laparoscopic orchiopexy: incidence and lessons learned. J Urol. 2009;182:280–4.
75. Yee DS, Duel BP. Omental herniation through a 3-mm umbilical trocar site. J Endourol. 2006;20:133–4.
76. Irwin BH, Rao PP, Stein RJ, Desai MM. Laparoendoscopic single site surgery in urology. Urol Clin North Am. 2009;36:223–35.
77. Cooper JD, Clayman RV, Krummel TM, et al. Inside the operating room – balancing the risks and benefits of new surgical procedures. Cleve Clin J Med. 2008;75:S37–54.
78. State of New York Laparoscopic Surgery Memorandum, 1992, Series 92–20.
79. Zorn KC, Gautam G, Shalhav AL, et al. Training, credentialing, proctoring, and medicolegal risks of robotic urological surgery: recommendation of the society of urologic robotic surgeons. J Urol. 2009;182(3):1126–32.
80. Hammond L, Ketchum J, Schwartz BF. Accreditation council on graduate medical education technical skills competency compliance: urologic surgical skills. J Am Coll Surg. 2005;201:454–7.
81. Marguet CG, Young MD, L'Esperance JO, et al. Hand assisted laparoscopic training for postgraduate urologists: the role of mentoring. J Urol. 2004;172:286–9.
82. Schwartz BF. Training requirement and credentialing for laparoscopic and robotic surgery – what are our responsibilities? J Urol. 2009;182(3):828–9.
83. Kesselheim AS, Studdert DM. Professional oversight of physician expert witnesses: an analysis of complaints to the Professional Conduct Committee of the American Association of Neurological Surgeons, 1992–2006. Ann Surg. 2009;249(1):168–72.
84. Halwani TM, Takrouri MSM. Medical laws and ethics of Babylon as read in Hammurabi's code. 2009. http://www.ispub.com/journal/the_internet_journal_of_law_healthcare_and_ethics/volume_4_number_2_24/article/medical_laws_and_ethics_of_babylon_as_read_in_hammurabi_s_code_history.html.

Subject Index

Note: The letters 'f' and 't' following locators refer to figures and tables respectively.

R. Ghavamian (ed.), *Complications of Laparoscopic and Robotic Urologic Surgery*,
DOI 10.1007/978-1-60761-676-4, © Springer Science+Business Media, LLC 2010

M

N

R